Diagnosis and Management of Cholangiocarcinoma

James H. Tabibian
Editor

Diagnosis and Management of Cholangiocarcinoma

A Multidisciplinary Approach

Springer

Editor
James H. Tabibian
Division of Gastroenterology
Department of Medicine
Olive View-UCLA Medical Center
Sylmar, CA
USA

David Geffen School of Medicine at UCLA
Los Angeles, CA
USA

ISBN 978-3-030-70935-8 ISBN 978-3-030-70936-5 (eBook)
https://doi.org/10.1007/978-3-030-70936-5

This Springer imprint is published by the registered company Springer Nature Switzerland AG
The registered company address is: Gewerbestrasse 11, 6330 Cham, Switzerland

Preface

Cholangiocarcinoma is a generally rare yet impactful, heterogeneous, and, in many ways, enigmatic malignancy of the biliary tract that can occur anywhere along its course, from the intrahepatic radicles that line the canals of Hering on down to the common bile duct and hepatopancreatic ampulla. Despite all cholangiocarcinoma, irrespective of anatomical location, being of biliary epithelial origin (by definition), the disease embodies a wide epidemiological, biological, and clinical spectrum of subtypes. Although cholangiocarcinoma is often aggressive, screening modalities are lacking, and most patients are asymptomatic until advanced stages of disease. Insofar as it is becoming more common worldwide, cholangiocarcinoma, considering its relatively high morbidity and mortality and limited therapeutic options, poses a critical biomedical and public health problem.

Advances in delineating the molecular events that lead to the development and progression of cholangiocarcinoma have lagged in relation to other, more common and anatomically accessible malignancies that are typically easier to model and study. As such, it may come as no surprise that significant advances in treatment approaches, as seen for instance in breast or colorectal cancer, have correspondingly not been realized. However, on the heels of progress in other areas of cancer research, recent studies have shed light on the pathogenesis of cholangiocarcinoma, which not only help explain the apparent heterogeneity of this disease, but also lend great promise in the clinical arena. Indeed, in parallel with the enhanced understanding of the molecular biology of cholangiocarcinoma have come developments in other areas, including but not limited to clinical epidemiology, noninvasive imaging, histopathology, endoscopic management, targeted chemotherapy, surgical oncology, disease biomarkers, surveillance, and modeling. While these developments have improved our ability to care for patients with cholangiocarcinoma, there is still much to be learned and accomplished, as evidenced by the ongoing diagnostic challenges, limited treatment options, and relatively high morbidity and mortality which continue to be associated with this disease.

In this context, I was very pleased to learn of Springer's interest in an authoritative and up-to-date textbook (and eBook) dedicated to the topic of cholangiocarcinoma, and together we sought to recruit a broad representation of world experts to provide a global perspective on this very matter. I am delighted to say that this effort has produced a unique, 26-chapter compendium of work authored by an impressive international group of leaders in the field. The chapters, organized into three parts, have been curated to recount the fundamental principles, evolving trends, and latest insights regarding cholangiocarcinoma across the spectrum of basic, translational, and clinical research as well as the state of the art of multidisciplinary patient care, including diagnosis, staging, treatment, surveillance, and beyond. On behalf of the authors, I believe this book will serve as a valuable contribution to the field and an important, unified, and practical resource for investigators and clinicians at all levels of expertise as well as trainees, patients, and patient advocates aspiring to learn more regarding this subject. Moreover, it is my sincere hope that this book will help cultivate greater collaboration among clinicians, scientists, patients, and industry to seek new knowledge to improve care for patients with these malignancies.

Los Angeles, CA, USA James H. Tabibian

Acknowledgment

To my family—most especially my wife and children—thank you for your patience, understanding, and support. My love for you is beyond measure.

To all the authors and co-authors of this book, thank you for the time, effort, and expertise you have invested not only in this textbook but also in the work you routinely do to advance the field.

To all my mentors and colleagues who have helped me throughout the years, thank you for your guidance, inspiration, and camaraderie. I aspire to return the favor and gestures of kindness.

To all the clinicians, researchers, and other biomedical professionals who help patients and families afflicted by cholangiocarcinoma, thank you and Godspeed.

To the Springer team, thank you for making this a smooth process and ensuring that we realize this endeavor to fruition, even in the midst of the COVID-19 pandemic.

I sincerely hope that, in sharing the collective experience and wisdom compiled herein, we will enhance fundamental understanding and clinical care of cholangiocarcinoma and encourage future collaborative efforts that illuminate ways to further improve the length and quality of life of our patients—the vital underpinning and focus of this book.

Contents

Contributors

Jad Abou-Khalil, MD, CM, MSc, FRCSC Department of Surgery, Division of General Surgery – Hepatobiliary and Pancreatic Surgery Unit, The Ottawa Hospital, Ottawa, ON, Canada

Pilar Acedo, Ph.D Institute for Liver & Digestive Health, University College London, Royal Free Hospital Campus, London, UK

Vatche G. Agopian, MD Division of Liver and Pancreas Transplantation, Department of Surgery, University of California, Los Angeles (UCLA), Los Angeles, CA, USA

Liver Transplantation and Hepatobiliary Surgery, General Surgery Residency Program, Department of Surgery, David Geffen School of Medicine at UCLA, Ronald Reagan Medical Center, Los Angeles, CA, USA

Ahmad Hassan Ali, MBBS Division of Gastroenterology and Hepatology, Mayo Clinic Rochester, Rochester, MN, USA

Department of Internal Medicine, Texas Tech University Health Sciences Center, Amarillo, TX, USA

Thomas J. An, MD Department of Radiology, Massachusetts General Hospital, Boston, MA, USA

Camila Bahamonde-Ovando, MD Department of Internal Medicine, Hospital Puerto Montt, Puerto Montt, Chile

Chiara Braconi, MD, Ph.D Institute of Cancer Sciences, Beatson West of Scotland Cancer Centre, University of Glasgow, Glasgow, UK

Giovanni Brandi, MD, Ph.D Department of Experimental, Diagnostic and Specialty Medicine, S. Orsola-Malpighi University Hospital, Bologna, Italy

John Bridgewater, MRCP, Ph.D Department of Medical Oncology, University College London Cancer Institute, London, UK

James R. Butler, MD, Ph.D Division of Liver and Pancreas Transplantation, Department of Surgery, University of California, Los Angeles (UCLA), Los Angeles, CA, USA

Silvia Cagnin, MD Department of Molecular Medicine, University of Padua School of Medicine, Padua, Italy

Elizabeth J. Carey, MD Division of Gastroenterology and Hepatology, Mayo Clinic Arizona, Phoenix, AZ, USA

Renato Carrasco-Farias, MD Digestive Endoscopy Unit, Hospital Puerto Montt, Puerto Montt, Chile

Roongruedee Chaiteerakij, MD, Ph.D Division of Gastroenterology, Department of Medicine, Chulalongkorn University, Bangkok, Thailand

Yaovalux Chamgramol, Ph.D Department of Pathology, Faculty of Medicine, Khon Kaen University, Khon Kaen, Thailand

Raksawan Deenonpoe, DVM, Ph.D Department of Pathology, Faculty of Medicine, Khon Kaen University, Khon Kaen, Thailand

Monica Deshmukh, MD Department of Radiology, Olive View-UCLA Medical Center, Sylmar, CA, USA

Robin L. Dietz Jr, MD Department of Pathology and Laboratory Medicine, David Geffen School of Medicine at UCLA, Olive View-UCLA Medical Center, Sylmar, CA, USA

L. M. J. W. van Driel, MD, Ph.D Department of Gastroenterology and Hepatology, Erasmus MC, Rotterdam, The Netherlands

Luca Fabris, MD, Ph.D Department of Molecular Medicine, University of Padua School of Medicine, Padua, Italy

Digestive Disease Section, Liver Center, Yale University, New Haven, CT, USA

Payman Fathizadeh, MD Department of Pathology and Laboratory Medicine, David Geffen School of Medicine at UCLA, Olive View-UCLA Medical Center, Sylmar, CA, USA

S. Franssen, DM Department of Surgery, Erasmus MC Cancer Institute, Rotterdam, The Netherlands

Andrés García-Sampedro, B.Sc, MSc Institute for Liver & Digestive Health, University College London, Royal Free Hospital Campus, London, UK

Sepideh Gholami, MD Division of Surgical Oncology, Department of Surgery, University of California, Davis, Sacramento, CA, USA

Timothy Gilbert, MBChB, MRes Department of Hepato-Biliary Surgery, Aintree University Hospital, Liverpool University Hospitals NHS Foundation Trust, Liverpool, UK

Mark D. Girgis, MD Department of Surgery, University of California, Los Angeles, Los Angeles, CA, USA

Christopher Goldring, BSc, Ph.D Sherrington Building, Institute of Translational Medicine, University of Liverpool, Liverpool, UK

Sonya Hessey, MRCP, MRes Department of Medical Oncology, University College London Hospital, London, UK

Dai Inoue, MD Department of Radiology, Kanazawa University Hospital, Kanazawa, Japan

D. M. de Jong, B.Sc Department of Gastroenterology and Hepatology, Erasmus MC, Rotterdam, The Netherlands

Sean J. Judge, MD, MS Department of Surgery, University of California, Davis, Sacramento, CA, USA

Russell C. Kirks, MD General, Thoracic, and Vascular Surgery, Virginia Mason Medical Center, Seattle, WA, USA

B. Groot Koerkamp, MD, Ph.D Department of Surgery, Erasmus MC Cancer Institute, Rotterdam, The Netherlands

Kazuto Kozaka, MD Department of Radiology, Kanazawa University Hospital, Kanazawa, Japan

Michael Levy, MD Division of Gastroenterology and Hepatology, Mayo Clinic, Rochester, MN, USA

Thomas W. Loehfelm, MD, Ph.D Department of Radiology, University of California, Davis, Sacramento, CA, USA

Sukanya Luang, Ph.D Department of Biochemistry, Faculty of Medicine, Khon Kaen University, Khon Kaen, Thailand

Hassan Malik, FRCS, MD Department of Hepato-Biliary Surgery, Aintree University Hospital, Liverpool University Hospitals NHS Foundation Trust, Liverpool, UK

Rodrigo Mansilla-Vivar, MD, MHA Digestive Endoscopy Unit, Hospital Puerto Montt, University San Sebastian, Puerto Montt, Chile

Luca Maroni, MD, Ph.D Department of Gastroenterology and Hepatology, Università Politecnica delle Marche, Ancona, Italy

Neil Marya, MD Division of Gastroenterology and Hepatology, Mayo Clinic, Rochester, MN, USA

Marco Marzioni, MD Department of Gastroenterology and Hepatology, Università Politecnica delle Marche, Ancona, Italy

Michael A. Mederos, MD Department of Surgery, University of California, Los Angeles, Los Angeles, CA, USA

Joachim C. Mertens, MD Gastroenterology and Hepatology, University Hospital Zürich, Zürich, Switzerland

Masahiko Minamiya, MD Gene Osaka Clinic Inc., Osaka, Japan

Shaden Mohammad, MD Department of Radiology, Olive View-UCLA Medical Center, Sylmar, CA, USA

Anja Moncsek Gastroenterology and Hepatology, University Hospital Zürich, Zürich, Switzerland

Nishant V. Munugala, MD, MPH Internal Medicine, University of Arizona, Tucson, AZ, USA

Yasuni Nakanuma, MD Department of Diagnostic Pathology, Shizuoka Cancer Center, Shizuoka, Japan

Department of Diagnostic Pathology, Fukui Prefecture Saiseikai Hospital, Fukui, Japan

Koushiro Ohtsubo, MD Division of Medical Oncology, Cancer Institute, Kanazawa University Hospital, Kanazawa, Japan

Masayuki Ohtsuka, MD Department of Hepatobiliary Pancreatic Surgery, Chiba University Hospital, Chiba, Japan

Anokh Pahwa, MD Department of Radiology, Olive View-UCLA Medical Center, Sylmar, CA, USA

Chawalit Pairojkul, MD Department of Pathology, Faculty of Medicine, Khon Kaen University, Khon Kaen, Thailand

Daniel Palmer, FRCP, B.Sc, Ph.D Sherrington Building, Institute of Translational Medicine, University of Liverpool, Liverpool, UK

Maitraya Patel, MD Department of Radiology, Ronald Reagan UCLA Medical Center, Los Angeles, CA, USA

Stephen P. Pereira, B.Sc, Ph.D, FRCP, FRCPE Institute for Liver & Digestive Health, University College London, Royal Free Hospital Campus, London, UK

Chatchai Phoomak, Ph.D Department of Therapeutic Radiology, Yale University School of Medicine, New Haven, CT, USA

Marc Quinn, MBChB Sherrington Building, Institute of Translational Medicine, University of Liverpool, Liverpool, UK

Flavio G. Rocha, MD, FACS General, Thoracic, and Vascular Surgery, Virginia Mason Medical Center, Seattle, WA, USA

Nobuo Sakaguchi, MD, Ph.D Department of Immunology, Graduate School of Medical Sciences, Kumamoto University, Kumamoto, Japan

Department of Microbiology and Cell Biology, Tokyo Metropolitan Institute of Medical Science, Kamikitazawa, Setagaya-ku, Tokyo, Japan

Prakasit Sa-ngiamwibool, MD Department of Pathology, Faculty of Medicine, Khon Kaen University, Khon Kaen, Thailand

Tarek Sawas, MD, MPH Division of Gastroenterology and Hepatology, Mayo Clinic, Rochester, MN, USA

Rachna T. Shroff, MD Hematology/Oncology, University of Arizona Cancer Center, Tucson, AZ, USA

Carlie Sigel, MD Department of Pathology, Memorial Sloan Kettering Cancer Center, New York, NY, USA

Atit Silsirivanit, Ph.D Department of Biochemistry, and Center for Translational Medicine, Faculty of Medicine, Khon Kaen University, Khon Kaen, Thailand

Amisha Singh, BS Internal Medicine, University of Arizona, Tucson, AZ, USA

James H. Tabibian, MD, Ph.D, FACP Division of Gastroenterology, Department of Medicine, Olive View-UCLA Medical Center, Sylmar, CA, USA

David Geffen School of Medicine at UCLA, Los Angeles, CA, USA

Simona Tavolari, B.Sc Division of Medical Oncology, IRCSS, Azienda Ospedaliero-Universitaria of Bologna, Bologna, Italy

Center for Applied Biomedical Research, S.Orsola-Malpighi University Hospital, Bologna, Italy

Katsuhiko Uesaka, MD Department of Hepatobiliary Pancreaetic Surgery, Shizuoka Cancer Center, Shizuoka, Japan

Karoly Viragh, MD Department of Radiology, Olive View-UCLA Medical Center, Sylmar, CA, USA

Hanlin L. Wang, MD, Ph.D Department of Pathology and Laboratory Medicine, David Geffen School of Medicine at UCLA, Ronald Reagan UCLA Medical Center, Los Angeles, CA, USA

Tao Wang, MD Department of Pathology and Molecular Medicine, Queen's University, Kingston, ON, Canada

Sakda Waraasawapati, MD Department of Pathology, Faculty of Medicine, Khon Kaen University, Khon Kaen, Thailand

Eric Wehrenberg-Klee, MD Division of Interventional Radiology, Department of Radiology, Massachusetts General Hospital, Boston, MA, USA

Sopit Wongkham, Ph.D Department of Biochemistry, and Center for Translational Medicine, Faculty of Medicine, Khon Kaen University, Khon Kaen, Thailand

Part I
Anatomy and Histology of the Biliary Tree and Cholangiocarcinoma

Chapter 1
Anatomy of the Biliary Tree: Normal, Anomalous, and Relationship to Cholangiocarcinoma

Jad Abou-Khalil

Abbreviations

CBD	Common bile duct
CCA	Cholangiocarcinoma
CHD	Common hepatic duct
LHD	Left hepatic bile duct
LLS	Left lateral section
RAD	Right anterior bile duct
RHD	Right hepatic bile duct
RPD	Right posterior bile duct

Overview

Cholangiocarcinoma (CCA), a malignancy of the biliary epithelium, can arise anywhere within the biliary system, from the intrahepatic ducts to the hepatopancreatic ampulla. Understanding biliary anatomy and the breadth of its variation finds particular importance in the treatment of CCA. This chapter will describe standard configurations of the left and right biliary tree, their confluence, the gallbladder, and common bile duct (CBD) and identify common variations on this standard anatomy as they relate to the treatment of CCA, especially surgical.

J. Abou-Khalil (✉)
Department of Surgery, Division of General Surgery – Hepatobiliary and Pancreatic Surgery Unit, The Ottawa Hospital, Ottawa, ON, Canada
e-mail: jaboukhalil@toh.ca

J. H. Tabibian (ed.), *Diagnosis and Management of Cholangiocarcinoma*,
https://doi.org/10.1007/978-3-030-70936-5_1

Anatomy of the Left Biliary System

The left bile duct (LHD) is formed by the confluence of segments 2, 3, 4a, and 4b. Four common anatomical variants of its formation are described [1]. In the most common configuration, the segments 2 and 3 bile ducts join to form a left lateral section (LLS) [2] duct close to the umbilical fissure. 55% of individuals share this configuration. This confluence occurs at the umbilical fissure, medial to the fissure, or lateral to it 5%, 50%, and 45% of the time, respectively, joining a single segment 4 duct to form the left hepatic duct (LHD). The second most common configuration, seen 30% of the time, finds two separate ducts from 4a and 4b, respectively, joining the LLS duct. In the third most common variant, the segments 3 and 4 ducts join to the right of the umbilical fissure and are joined by the segment 2 duct closer to the hilum; this occurs 10% of the time. In the fourth configuration, seen in 5% of individuals, segments 2, 3, and 4 join together at the umbilical fissure. Of note, in the second and fourth configuration, the segment 4 duct can join the LHD to the left of the umbilical fissure, exposing this duct to a risk of injury whenever a transection plane runs through the umbilical fissure, for example, during segments 2 and 3 resection for an intrahepatic CCA in segments 2 and 3 (Fig. 1.1).

Using corrosion casting, surgical anatomists of the mid-twentieth century, from Rex to Couinaud, described the anatomical relationship of the biliary tree to the portal vein and its segmental branches [3]. The LHD always lies superiorly

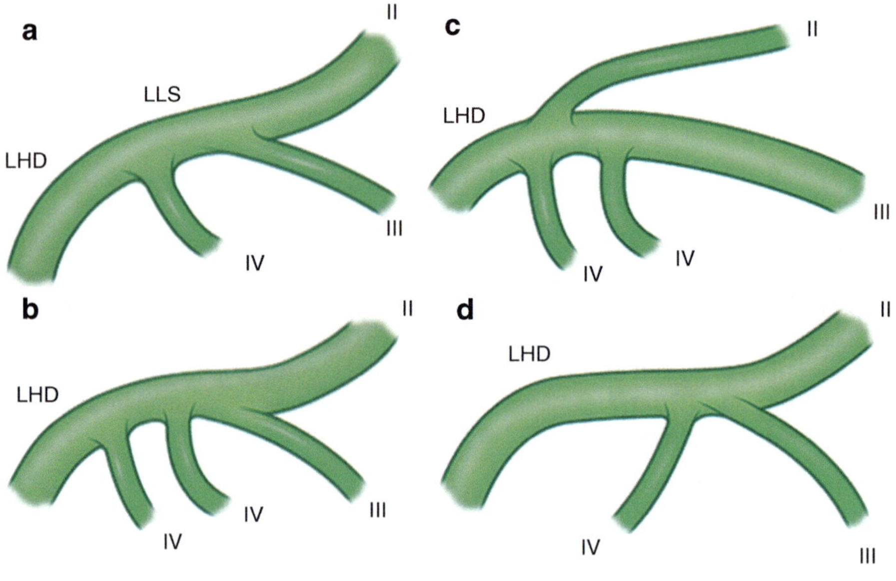

Fig. 1.1 Four common anatomical variants of the left viliary drainage system: (**a**) the segment 2 and 3 bile ducts join to form a left lateral section (LLS) duct close to the umbilical fissure, joining a single segment 4 duct to form the left hepatic duct (LHD). (**b**) two separate ducts from 4a and 4b, respectively, joining the LLS duct. (**c**) the segment 3 and 4 ducts join to the right of the umbilical fissure and are joined by the segment 2 duct closer to the hilum. (**d**) segments 2,3, and 4 join together at the umbilical fissure

(cephalad) to the portal vein, a relationship that allows access to the left hepatic duct during a "Hepp-Couinaud" maneuver, wherein the hilar plate is lowered to reveal the left hepatic duct behind the portal vein. This universal configuration is variably termed epiportal or supraportal. More distally towards the segmental branches of the biliary tree, this relationship is mostly maintained, except for a described hypoportal configuration of the segment 3 branches, occurring in 3.6% and up to 8% of livers [3, 4]. The presence of a parenchymal or fibrous bridge over the Rex's recess is a surface clue to the presence of a hypoportal segment 3 duct. This does not occur with segment 2 branches, due to the embryological origin of the ducts – with segments 3 and 4 arising together as an anteriomedial sector within the left lobe and segment 2 arising separately as a left posterior-lateral sector.

The LHD is longer than the right hepatic duct (RHD), measuring 2–5 cm, and courses more horizontally. The RHD, if present at all, usually measures 1 cm before it bifurcates into its anterior and posterior tributaries.

Anatomy of the Right Bile Ducts and the Biliary Confluence

Similarly to the left liver, the bile ducts draining segments 5, 6, 7, and 8 in the right liver join together in four commonly recognizable configurations [5, 6]. The most common configuration finds the right anterior bile duct (RAD) draining segments 5 and 8 meeting with the right posterior bile duct (RPD) draining segments 6 and 7 to become the RHD. This configuration, termed type 1, is found in 56% of livers (Fig. 1.2). Unlike in the left liver where the LHD is universally epiportal, the RHD can be hypoportal 20% of the time. Specifically, the RPD can lie in a hypoportal configuration, hooking behind the right anterior portal vein branch – a configuration described by Hjortsjö and eponymously named Hjortsjö's hook. The type 2 configuration (14% of livers) presents as a triple confluence of the LHD with the RAD and the RPD, with no distinct RHD. In types 3a and 3b, the RAD and RPD join the LHD, respectively, in 5% and 15% of livers. In types 4a and 4b, the RAD and RPD, respectively, join the CHD below the confluence – a pattern termed *convergence etagée*. The long-held belief that small bile ducts connect the gallbladder lumen to intrahepatic bile ducts, so-called ducts of Luschka, is disproven. There are nonetheless bile ducts lying in close proximity to the cystic plate which can be injured in the course of a cholecystectomy.

Every effort must be made to delineate biliary anatomy prior to embarking on a liver resection for the treatment of a CCA. Particular attention must be drawn to the anatomical variants mentioned above in planning hepatectomies for hilar CCA, as the anatomy determines the number and location of bile ducts that will be encountered at the planned transection line and that will need to be reconstructed. For example, a CCA involving the LHD may present with dilatation of both the LHD and the RPD if the RPD inserts into the LHD (Fig. 1.2).

Embryologically, the intrahepatic bile ducts form from the ductal plate, a thin layer of cells that surrounds the portal vein branches and that follow its branching

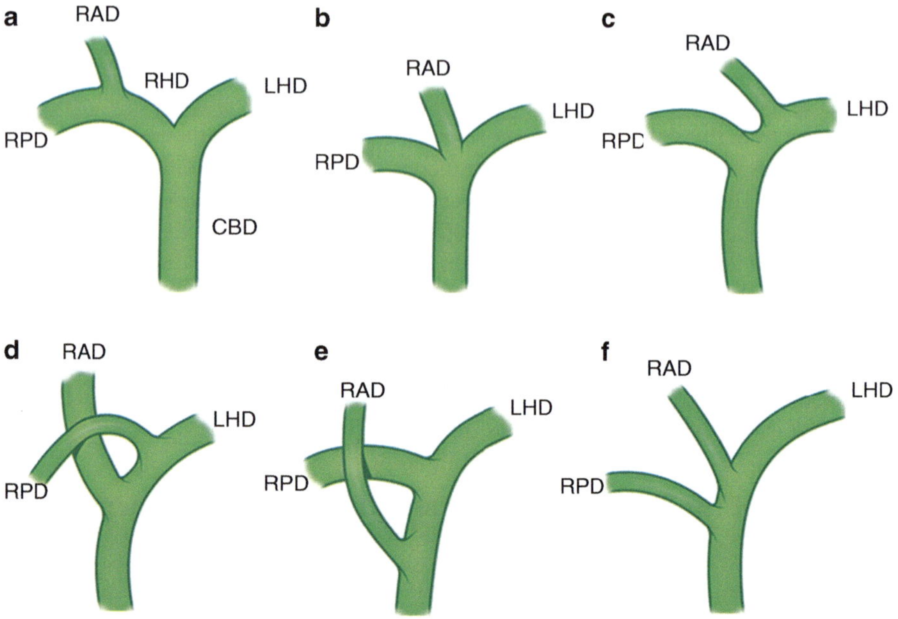

Fig. 1.2 Anatomic variation of the biliary confluence according to the Nakamura classification. (**a**) Type 1; (**b**) type 2; (**c**) type 3a; (**d**) type 3b; (**e**) type 4a; (**f**) type 4b. LHD, left hepatic duct; RAD, right anterior duct; RPD, right posterior duct. (Reproduced with permission from Elsevier. Source: https://doi.org/10.1016/j.suc.2018.12.005)

pattern within the developing liver [7]. Therefore, biliary anatomy typically tracks portal venous anatomy, and variants of portal venous anatomy should consequently raise suspicion of biliary ductal anatomical variation.

The Caudate Ducts

The Spigelian lobe (i.e., Couinaud's segment 1), the caudate process, and the paracaval caudate (described by Couinaud as a 9th segment but rarely referred to as such in contemporary nomenclature) form the caudate lobe. Each of these portions of the caudate lobe is drained by at least one duct, with up to five ducts draining the caudate. The Spigelian lobe drains into the LHD, with the remainder of the caudate draining into the left-right confluence, the RHD, or the RPD. But as elsewhere in the liver, this drainage pattern is highly variable, and this laterality is not universal. A third of Spigelian lobes drain into the RHD or the RPD, especially when the RPD inserts into the LHD. Conversely, a third of the paracaval and caudate process ducts insert into the LHD [8]. This explains the oncologic benefit observed when performing a caudate resection as part of the treatment of hilar CCAs; caudate resection in this context is associated with margin-negative resection and improved long-term survival [9]. Particular attention to dilatation of the caudate ducts in the context of hilar CCA can yield important clues as to their insertion in relationship to the obstructing tumor.

The Gallbladder and Extrahepatic Bile Ducts

The gallbladder lies at the equator between the right and left hemiliver, an imaginary line known as Cantlie's line or the Rex-Cantlie line coursing between segments 4b and 5, through the bed of the gallbladder towards the vena cava posteriorly. The gallbladder is mostly peritonealized, except for its posterior surface which lies on the cystic plate, a fibrous area on the underside of the liver. The proportion if its circumference varies, from a pedicled gallbladder with little to no contact with the cystic plate to a mostly intrahepatic gallbladder surrounded by liver parenchyma. The gallbladder carries no muscularis mucosa, no submucosa, and a discontinuous muscularis and only carries a serosa on the visceral peritonealized surface. These anatomical specificities facilitate the direct invasion of gallbladder cancer into the liver. This is why the surgical treatment of gallbladder cancer mandates a radical cholecystectomy, which includes resection of a wedge of segments 4b and 5, when the T stage is higher or equal to T1b [10].

From the body of the gallbladder, a conical infundibulum becomes a cystic duct that extends as the lower edge of the hepatocystic triangle towards the porta hepatis and joins with the common hepatic duct (CHD) to form the CBD. As in the rest of the biliary system, variation is the rule when it comes to the cystic duct confluence with the CHD. It can variably run parallel to it for a distance prior to inserting or spiral behind it and insert on its medial aspect. It can variably insert into the RHD or the RPD, the latter in 4% of livers and particularly when the RPD inserts into the CHD (i.e., below the left-right ductal confluence). This configuration is notorious for exposing the RPD to a risk of injury at the time of cholecystectomy. Rare variations of gallbladder anatomy, including gallbladder duplication and gallbladder agenesis, are also described but are rare [2, 11, 12].

The CBD courses anterolaterally within the hepatoduodenal ligament, usually to the right of the hepatic artery and anterolaterally to the portal vein. However, hepatic arterial anatomy can vary, and when an accessory or replaced hepatic artery is present arising from the superior mesenteric artery, the accessory or replaced vessel courses lateral to the CBD. In its conventional configuration, the right hepatic artery crosses posteriorly to the RHD as it heads towards the right liver, but 25% of the time it crosses anteriorly. These anatomical variants are all relevant to developing a sound surgical strategy to treat hilar CCA. Of note, while left hepatic artery anatomy can also be quite variable, rarely does it affect surgical decision-making in CCA to the same degree as right hepatic artery anatomy.

Distally, the CBD enters the head of the pancreas, joining the pancreatic duct to form the hepatopancreatic ampulla. Just distal to this is the sphincter of Oddi, which controls emptying of ampullary contents into the second portion of the duodenum. The treatment of CCAs of the distal, intrapancreatic portion of the bile duct involves a pancreaticoduodenectomy (Chap. 14, Judge et al.). When the junction of the CBD and the pancreatic duct occurs before the sphincter complex, reflux of pancreatic enzymes into the biliary tree can lead to chronic inflammatory changes and anatomical distortion resulting in choledochal cysts, known risk factors for the development of CCA (Chap. 5, Chaiteerakij).

Arterial Supply of the Biliary Tree and Its Implications for Resectability of Cholangiocarcinoma and Bilioenteric Reconstruction

Unlike the rest of the liver parenchyma, which receives dual supply from the arterial and portal venous circulation, the biliary tree is exclusively alimented by the arterial system. The LHD and RHD are alimented respectively by the left hepatic artery and right hepatic artery, which can frequently display replaced, accessory, and aberrant origins – the left artery arising conventionally from the hepatic artery proper but alternatively from the left gastric artery and the right hepatic artery arising from the hepatic artery proper but also variably from the superior mesenteric artery. In hilar CCA, variable combinations of hepatic arterial anatomy and tumor location can either favor resectability or make a tumor unresectable. For example, a CCA involving the confluence of the right and left bile ducts might have a higher chance of being resectable if the right liver is alimented by a replaced right hepatic artery distant from the tumor than if the right hepatic artery coursed in its conventional location in close proximity to the hilum, where it risks being involved by tumor.

Within the hilum of the liver, a plexus of arteries connects the right and left hepatic arteries. Termed the "hilar epicholedochal plexus," this vascular network provides collateral circulation that can maintain arterial supply to one side of the liver if the ipsilateral vessel is damaged [13]. The preservation of arterial blood supply to the liver remnant is crucial, particularly when creating an enterobiliary anastomosis. Its absence leads to ischemic cholangiopathy and liver abscesses that can be difficult to treat [14].

The CBD receives arterial supply inferiorly from paired arterioles arising from the gastroduodenal artery and the posterior superior pancreaticoduodenal artery, the most important and constant arterial supply to the distal CBD. Proximally the CBD is alimented by paired arterioles of the right hepatic artery. These vessels, known as the marginal arteries, run in parallel to the CBD, laterally and medially to it. Denuding the CBD of this arterial supply risks stricture formation after choledocho-enteric anastomosis.

Conclusion

CCA can arise anywhere along the biliary tree. A thorough understanding of the anatomy of the bile ducts, its common variant configurations, and its relationship to correspondingly variable vascular anatomy is necessary to allow for the safe surgical treatment of CCA.

References

1. Reichert PR, Renz JF, D'Albuquerque LAC, Rosenthal P, Lim RC, Roberts JP, et al. Surgical anatomy of the left lateral segment as applied to living-donor and split-liver transplantation: a clinicopathologic study. Ann Surg. 2000;232(5):658–64. PubMed PMID: PMC1421220.
2. Darnis B, Mohkam K, Cauchy F, Cazauran JB, Bancel B, Rode A, et al. A systematic review of the anatomical findings of multiple gallbladders. HPB (Oxford). 2018;20(11):985–91. PubMed PMID: 29887260. Epub 2018/06/12. eng.
3. Kitamura H, Mori T, Arai M, Tsukada K, Numata M, Kawasaki S. Caudal left hepatic duct in relation to the umbilical portion of the portal vein. Hepato-Gastroenterology. 1999;46(28):2511–4. PubMed PMID: 10522029. Epub 1999/10/16. eng.
4. Ozden I, Kamiya J, Nagino M, Uesaka K, Sano T, Nimura Y. Clinicoanatomical study on the infraportal bile ducts of segment 3. World J Surg. 2002;26(12):1441–5.
5. Nakamura T, Tanaka K, Kiuchi T, Kasahara M, Oike F, Ueda M, et al. Anatomical variations and surgical strategies in right lobe living donor liver transplantation: lessons from 120 cases. Transplantation. 2002;73(12):1896–903. PubMed PMID: 12131684. Epub 2002/07/20. eng.
6. Varotti G, Gondolesi GE, Goldman J, Wayne M, Florman SS, Schwartz ME, et al. Anatomic variations in right liver living donors11No competing interests declared. J Am Coll Surg. 2004;198(4):577–82.
7. Van Eyken P, Sciot R, Callea F, Van der Steen K, Moerman P, Desmet VJ. The development of the intrahepatic bile ducts in man: a keratin-immunohistochemical study. Hepatology. 1988;8(6):1586–95. PubMed PMID: 2461337. Epub 1988/11/01. eng.
8. Kitami M, Murakami G, Ko S, Takase K, Tuboi M, Saito H, et al. Spiegel's lobe bile ducts often drain into the right hepatic duct or its branches: study using drip-infusion cholangiography-computed tomography in 179 consecutive patients. World J Surg. 2004;28(10):1001–6.
9. Birgin E, Rasbach E, Reissfelder C, Rahbari NN. A systematic review and meta-analysis of caudate lobectomy for treatment of hilar cholangiocarcinoma. Eur J Surg Oncol. 2020;46(5):747–53. PubMed PMID: 31987703. Epub 2020/01/29. eng.
10. Hickman L, Contreras C. Gallbladder cancer: diagnosis, surgical management, and adjuvant therapies. Surg Clin North Am. 2019;99(2):337–55. PubMed PMID: 30846038. Epub 2019/03/09. eng.
11. Harlaftis N, Gray SW, Skandalakis JE. Multiple gallbladders. Surg Gynecol Obstet. 1977;145(6):928–34. PubMed PMID: 337542. Epub 1977/12/01. eng.
12. Tabibian JH, Tabibian N, Aguet JC. Choledochal cyst complications presenting as duodenal obstruction in an 82-year-old patient with gallbladder agenesis. Dig Dis Sci. 2009;54(1):184–7. PubMed PMID: 18478329. Epub 2008/05/15. eng.
13. Strasberg SM, Helton WS. An analytical review of vasculobiliary injury in laparoscopic and open cholecystectomy. HPB (Oxford). 2011;13(1):1–14. PubMed PMID: 21159098. PubMed Central PMCID: PMC3019536. Epub 2010/12/17. eng.
14. Deltenre P, Valla DC. Ischemic cholangiopathy. Semin Liver Dis. 2008;28(3):235–46. PubMed PMID: 18814077. Epub 2008/09/25. eng.

Chapter 2
Anatomic and Morphologic Classifications of Cholangiocarcinoma

Michael A. Mederos and Mark D. Girgis

Abbreviations

AJCC	American Joint Committee on Cancer
CCA	Cholangiocarcinoma
dCCA	Distal cholangiocarcinoma
iCCA	Intrahepatic cholangiocarcinoma
IG	Intraductal growing
LCSGJ	The Liver Cancer Study Group of Japan
MF	Mass-forming
MSKCC	Memorial Sloan Kettering Cancer Center
pCCA	Perihilar cholangiocarcinoma
PI	Periductal infiltrating
TNM	Tumor, lymph node, metastases

Introduction

Cholangiocarcinoma (CCA) originates from the bile duct epithelium at any aspect of the biliary tree. Contemporary anatomic classification separates CCA into three entities based on the location of origin: intrahepatic, perihilar, and distal CCA (Figs. 2.1, and 2.2). These three categories have different and sometimes overlapping risk factors, presentation, and outcomes. For example, while distal CCA often presents with jaundice and pruritus due to biliary obstruction, intrahepatic CCA might present with vague abdominal pain and sometimes jaundice often due to the mass effect of the tumor on other structures and ducts. Each anatomic category can be further subdivided by the tumor morphology and growth pattern (Fig. 2.2).

M. A. Mederos · M. D. Girgis (✉)
Department of Surgery, University of California, Los Angeles, Los Angeles, CA, USA
e-mail: mmederos@mednet.ucla.edu; mdgirgis@mednet.ucla.edu

J. H. Tabibian (ed.), *Diagnosis and Management of Cholangiocarcinoma*,
https://doi.org/10.1007/978-3-030-70936-5_2

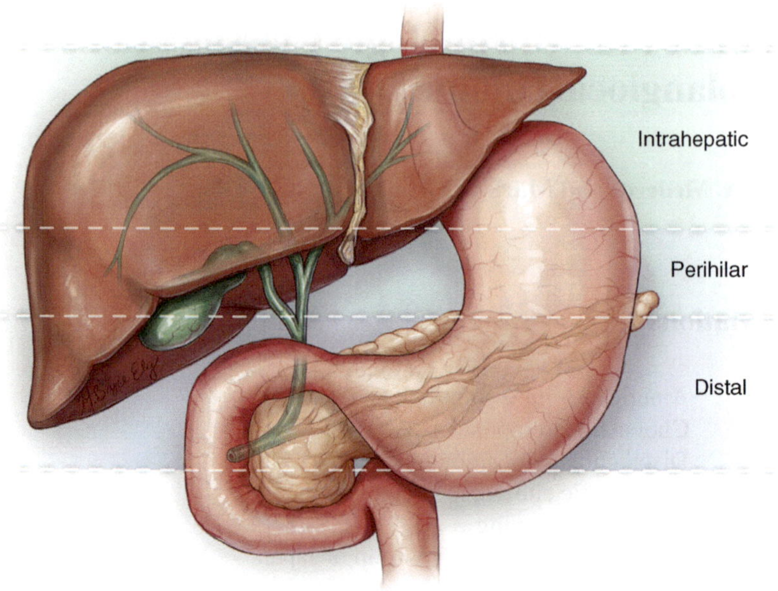

Fig. 2.1 Anatomic classification of cholangiocarcinoma. (Illustration by Hannah Bryce Ely, CMI)

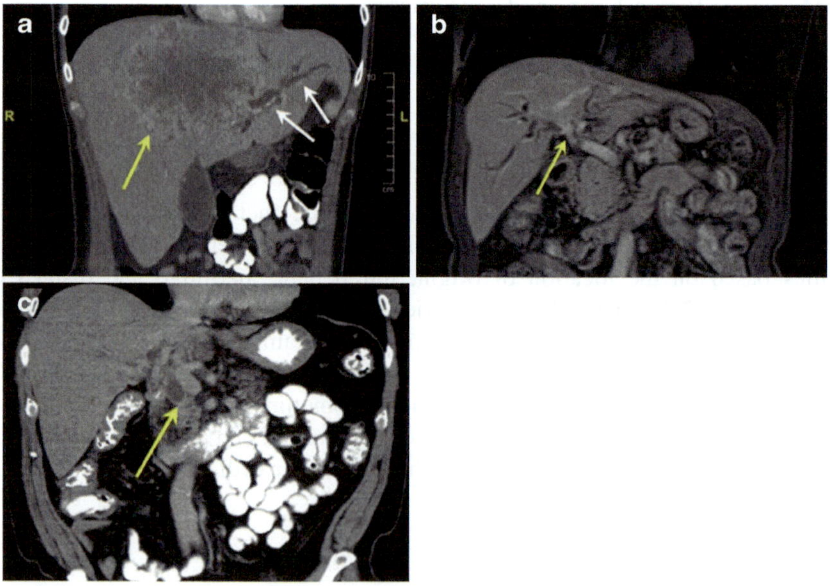

Fig. 2.2 Imaging of cholangiocarcinoma. (**a**) Computed tomography (CT) of mass-forming intrahepatic cholangiocarcinoma. The yellow arrow demonstrates the peripheral enhancement of the large tumor. The white arrows highlight associated biliary dilation; (**b**) MRI of perihilar cholangiocarcinoma (yellow arrow); (**c**) CT of distal cholangiocarcinoma. The yellow arrow demonstrates an abrupt filling defect of the dilated common bile duct

Intrahepatic Cholangiocarcinoma

Morphology

Intrahepatic CCA (iCCA) may originate anywhere from the microscopic bile ducts in the liver periphery to the second-order bile ducts. It is the least common of the three anatomic types of CCA (5–10% of all CCA) [1]; however, the incidence of this anatomic subtype has steadily increased in the USA from roughly 1200 new cases in 2004 to 3800 new cases in 2015 [2]. The Liver Cancer Study Group of Japan (LCSGJ) classifies iCCA into three distinct morphologic subtypes based on gross appearance: mass forming, periductal infiltrating, and intraductal growing. A 4th category includes tumors with more than one component of the three morphologic subtypes (e.g., mass forming + periductal infiltrating) (Fig. 2.3) [3]. These macroscopic growth patterns are likely associated with differences in risk factors, cellular origin, and biological progression [4]. The relationship between the morphologic subtype and prognosis has been debatable [5]. Previously, the 7th edition of the American Joint Committee on Cancer (AJCC 7) staging manual stipulated that iCCAs with a periductal-infiltrating component are designated as T4 lesions due to a perceived worse prognosis. This characterization was excluded in the 8th edition of the AJCC staging manual (AJCC 8) with the recommendation that morphology continues to be documented for data collection [6]. However, new data suggest morphologic subtype might indeed have long-term prognostic significance in those undergoing curative-intent resection [5, 7].

Mass Forming

The purely mass-forming (MF) growth pattern is the most common morphology of iCCA (60%) [6]. MF iCCA appears as a mass within the hepatic parenchyma, arising from small intrahepatic bile ducts or hepatic progenitor cells with no discernible invasion of a major branch of the portal triad [3]. Tumors of this morphologic subtype can grow to large sizes and are often greater than 5 cm in those who undergo surgical resection [8]. The tumor cells are typically at the periphery of the lesion, and the center is characterized by necrosis and scarring. Because of this radial growth configuration, peripheral arterial enhancement is a common imaging finding (Fig. 2.2a). Multiple intrahepatic lesions are common in MF iCCA, but it is difficult to distinguish if multiple tumors represent multifocal disease (multiple primary tumors) or intrahepatic metastasis from an index lesion (satellite lesions) [9]. Nevertheless, the presence of more than three lesions is associated with significantly worse disease-free and overall survival in those undergoing hepatic resection with curative intent [10].

Periductal Infiltrating

In contrast to the distinct borders of the MF subtype, periductal-infiltrating (PI) iCCA arises from large bile duct epithelium and peribiliary glands and is characterized by a diffuse longitudinal growth pattern along large intrahepatic bile ducts on both gross and microscopic examination [1]. This growth pattern often causes intrahepatic biliary dilatation due to stricture or obstruction, and there are no distinct borders or apparent invasion of the surrounding liver parenchyma. Often included in this subtype is the MF + PI mixed variant, which exhibits features of both subtypes (Fig. 2.3). Tumors with a PI component represent approximately 40% of iCCAs [6]. Compared to the mass-forming and intraductal growing subtypes, patients with PI or MF + PI tumors have more major vascular invasion, lymphovascular invasion, and perineural invasion [7].

Intraductal Growing

The intraductal-growth (IG) subtype of iCCA is characterized by the tumor's papillary growth toward or within the bile duct lumen (Fig. 2.3) [3]. The precursor lesion associated with intraductal growing tumors is termed intraductal papillary neoplasm of the bile duct and is discussed in detail elsewhere in this book (Chap. 3, Nakanuma et al. and Chap. 4, Fathizadeh et al.). On computed tomography (CT) imaging, this growth pattern often appears as biliary ectasia due to dilation of the bile duct proximal to the lesion. Because this morphology is intraductal, it may be confused for hepatolithiasis. The IG subtype of iCCA has been associated with a better prognosis compared to the MF and PI subtypes. However, data suggest that IG more frequently demonstrates adverse pathologic features, such as lymphovascular invasion, perineural invasion, and poor/undifferentiated tumors when compared to MF iCCA. Nevertheless, despite these features, the overall prognosis of the IG subtype appears more favorable than MF and PI iCCA [5].

Staging

The preferred system for staging CCA is the AJCC tumor, lymph node, and metastases (TNM) classification. Intrahepatic, perihilar, and distal CCA are staged independently [11]. Staging of iCCA has been significantly modified over the past two decades. Prior to 2010, the AJCC staged iCCA using data derived from HCC. However, iCCA has since been recognized as a separate entity given the several differences in clinical features, biology, and growth patterns, and a new staging system separate from HCC was developed in AJCC 7 (Table 2.1) [12]. In AJCC 7, the T stage focused on vascular invasion, number of tumors, and extension beyond the visceral peritoneum and/or penetration of other surrounding structures. Tumor size was initially excluded as it was not considered a significant adverse prognostic

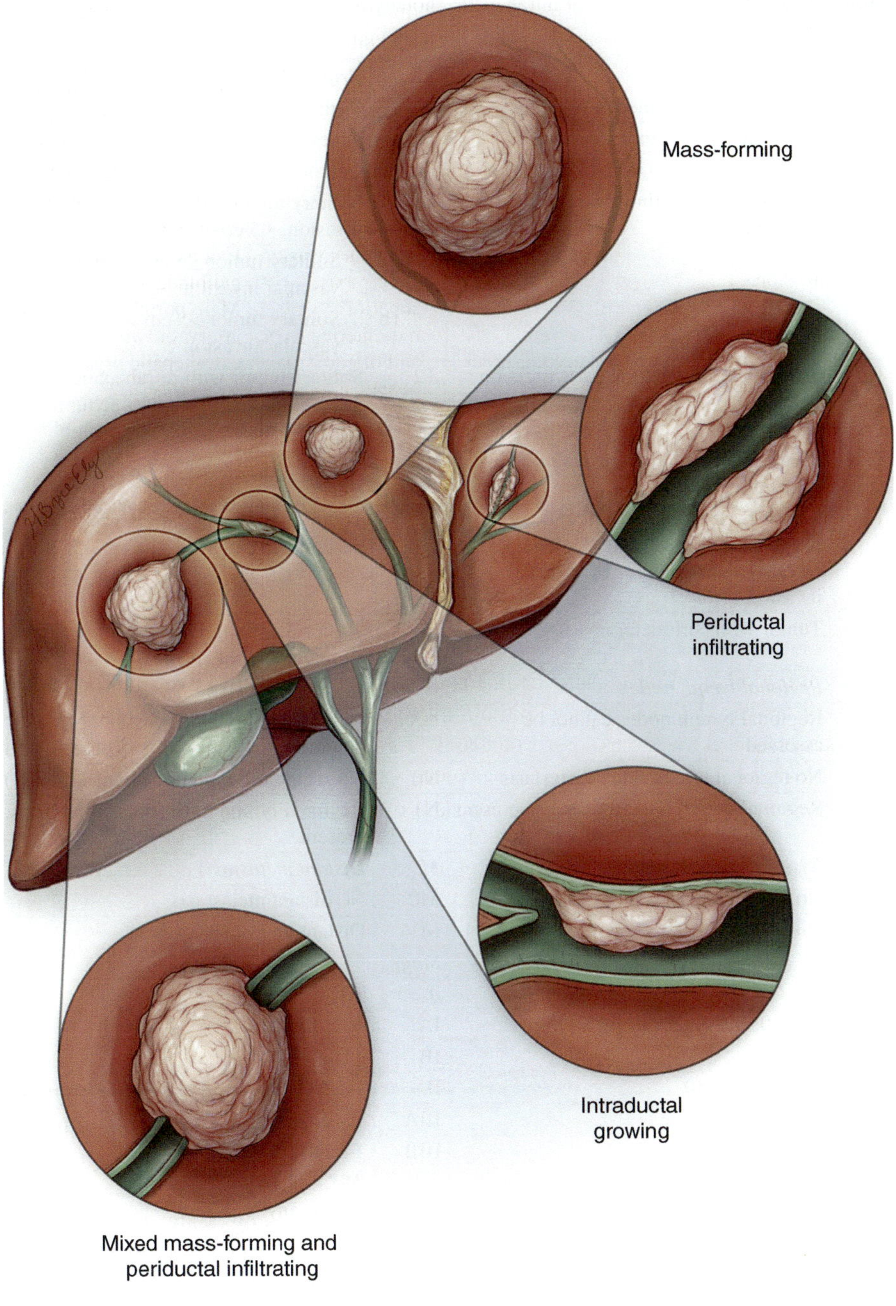

Fig. 2.3 Morphologic classification of intrahepatic cholangiocarcinoma. (Illustration by Hannah Bryce Ely, CMI)

Table 2.1 AJCC 7 and 8 staging of intrahepatic cholangiocarcinoma

AJCC 7th ed.		AJCC 8th ed.	
T	*Primary tumor*	*T*	*Primary tumor*
TX	Primary tumor cannot be assessed	TX	Primary tumor cannot be assessed
T0	No evidence of primary tumor	T0	No evidence of primary tumor
Tis	Carcinoma in situ (intraductal tumor)	Tis	Carcinoma in situ (intraductal tumor)
T1	Solitary tumor without vascular invasion	T1	Solitary tumor without vascular invasion, ≤5 cm or >5 cm
		T1a	Solitary tumor ≤5 cm without vascular invasion
		T1b	Solitary tumor >5 cm without vascular invasion
T2a	Solitary tumor with vascular invasion	T2	Solitary tumor with intrahepatic vascular invasion or multiple tumors, with or without vascular invasion
T2b	Multiple tumors, with or without vascular invasion		
T3	Tumor perforating the visceral peritoneum or involving the local extrahepatic structures by direct invasion	T3	Tumor perforating the visceral peritoneum
T4	Tumor with periductal invasion	T4	Tumor involving local extrahepatic structures by direct invasion
N	*Regional lymph nodes*	*N*	*Regional lymph nodes*
NX	Regional lymph nodes cannot be assessed	NX	Regional lymph nodes cannot be assessed
N0	No regional lymph node metastasis	N0	No regional lymph node metastasis
N1	Regional lymph node metastasis present	N1	Regional lymph node metastasis present
M	*Distant metastasis*	*M*	*Distant metastasis*
M0	No distant metastasis	M0	No distant metastasis
M1	Distant metastasis present	M1	Distant metastasis present
Stage		*Stage*	
0	Tis, N0, M0	0	Tis, N0, M0
I	T1, N0, M0	IA	T1a, N0, M0
		IB	T1b, N0, M0
II	T2a–b, N0, M0	II	T2, N0, M0
III	T3, N0, M0	IIIA	T3, N0, M0
		IIIB	T4, N0, M0 Any T, N1, M0
IVA	T4, N0, M0 Any T, N1, M0	IV	Any T, any N, M1
IVB	Any T, any N, M1		

indicator for iCCA [12, 13]. However, size was included in the current edition (AJCC 8) after several studies, and a meta-analysis demonstrated an association with tumor size and survival that was likely not seen in prior studies due to the limited number of patients with small tumors [8]. Additionally, tumors with a periductal-infiltrating growth pattern were classified at T4 lesions in AJCC 7 because this was thought to beget a worse prognosis. However, morphologic classification was omitted in AJCC 8 because the data regarding growth type and prognosis was inconsistent and no clear conclusion could be drawn [14, 15]. The AJCC 8 does recommend to document growth patterns for data collection.

Altogether, the T stage in AJCC 8 is now classified by tumor size, number of tumors, vascular invasion, extension beyond the visceral peritoneum, and invasion of extrahepatic structures. High-grade dysplasia that does not extend beyond the basement membrane are in situ tumors (Tis). Tumors that are ≤5 cm or >5 cm without vascular invasion are classified as T1a and T1b, respectively. This translates to a 5-year overall survival of 51.7% and 32.6% ($P < 0.001$), respectively. T2 tumors include solitary tumors with vascular invasion or multiple tumors with or without vascular invasion. Approximately one fifth of patients with iCCA have multiple tumors at the time of surgery [16, 17]. T3 tumors include any iCCA that perforates the visceral peritoneum, and T4 tumors directly invade extrahepatic structures (Table 2.1).

Lymph node metastasis is an important prognostic indicator and is common in iCCA, reported as high as 40% in those who underwent resection with regional lymphadenectomy. For right-sided tumors, the AJCC defines regional lymph nodes as hilar (common bile duct, hepatic artery, portal vein, and cystic duct), periduodenal, and peripancreatic lymph node areas. For left-sided tumors, these lymph node sites include the inferior phrenic, hilar, and gastrohepatic lymph nodes. Spread to these regional lymph nodes is associated with a worse overall survival compared to those with no nodal disease (median 18.0 vs. 45.0 months, $P < 0.001$) [18]. Anatomically, lymph node metastasis was identified in 38.4% of patients who had a lymphadenectomy of the hepatoduodenal ligament (lymph node station 12) compared to 57.8% in those who had a lymphadenectomy beyond station 12 ($P < 0.001$). AJCC 8 classifies nodal disease as N0 (no regional lymph node metastasis) or N1 (regional lymph node metastasis present) (Table 2.1). Spread to extra-regional lymph nodes (celiac, periaortic, and pericaval nodes) is considered M1 disease, however. M1 classification also includes extrahepatic sites, which most commonly includes the bone, peritoneum, lungs, and pleura.

Since the release of AJCC 8, several studies have challenged the current staging criteria and suggest that growth pattern should be reintroduced into the staging system. A multi-institutional study across 14 centers analyzed 1083 patients who underwent curative-intent resection of iCCA and found that patients with the PI or mixed (MF + PI) subtypes had higher rate of invasion of adjacent organs, positive margins, major vascular invasion, lymphovascular invasion, and perineural invasion. Overall 5-year survival in patients with a PI component was significantly worse, even after propensity matching for clinicopathologic variables (26.2% vs. 35.7%, respectively; $p = 0.03$) [7]. Further, the timing and pattern of disease recurrence seem to differ between the growth types.

Perihilar Cholangiocarcinoma

Perihilar CCA (pCCA) is the most common category among bile duct cancers (50–70%) [19]. In 1965, Gerald Klatskin published his series of 13 patients with adenocarcinoma of the hepatic duct confluence, outlining in great deal the distinctive manifestation of the disease [20]. These tumors eventually became known as the eponymous Klatskin tumor. By definition these tumors involve the extrahepatic bile ducts distal to the segmental hepatic ducts and proximal to the cystic duct (Figs. 2.1, and 2.2b). Risk factors associated with pCCA include male gender, advanced age, choledochal cysts, and inflammatory conditions that result in a high cellular turnover (e.g., primary sclerosing cholangitis, inflammatory bowel disease, and gallstone disease).

Perihilar CCA tends to have a sclerosing histologic growth pattern, which makes these tumors characteristically fibrotic and infiltrative, particularly along the ducts and surrounding structures. In contrast, the papillary histologic subtype is usually well-differentiated and characterized by an intraductal growth pattern [21].

Staging Systems

Bismuth-Corlette

Henri Bismuth and Marvin Corlette introduced a classification for pCCA in 1975 with modification in 1992 [22, 23]. The Bismuth-Corlette classification is frequently used to this day and focuses on the level and extension of tumor invasion along the proximal extrahepatic biliary tree (Table 2.2, Fig. 2.4). Type I lesions involve the common hepatic duct below the confluence of the right and left hepatic ducts, while type II lesions involve the confluence but does not extend to the right or left hepatic ducts. Type III tumors involve the confluence and extend to the right or left hepatic ducts, designated IIIa and IIIb, respectively. Type IV tumors involve the confluence and extend to both the right and left hepatic ducts. Although commonly used to classify pCCA tumors and help guide the surgical approach, the Bismuth-Corlette

Table 2.2 Bismuth-Corlette classification of perihilar cholangiocarcinoma

I	Tumor involves the common hepatic duct below the confluence of the right and left ducts
II	Tumor involves the hepatic duct confluence but does not extend above the confluence
IIIa	Tumor involves the confluence with extension to the *right* hepatic duct up to second-order ducts
IIIb	Tumor involves the confluence with extension to the *left* hepatic duct up to second-order ducts
IV	Tumor involves the confluence with extension to *bilateral* hepatic ducts up to second-order ducts

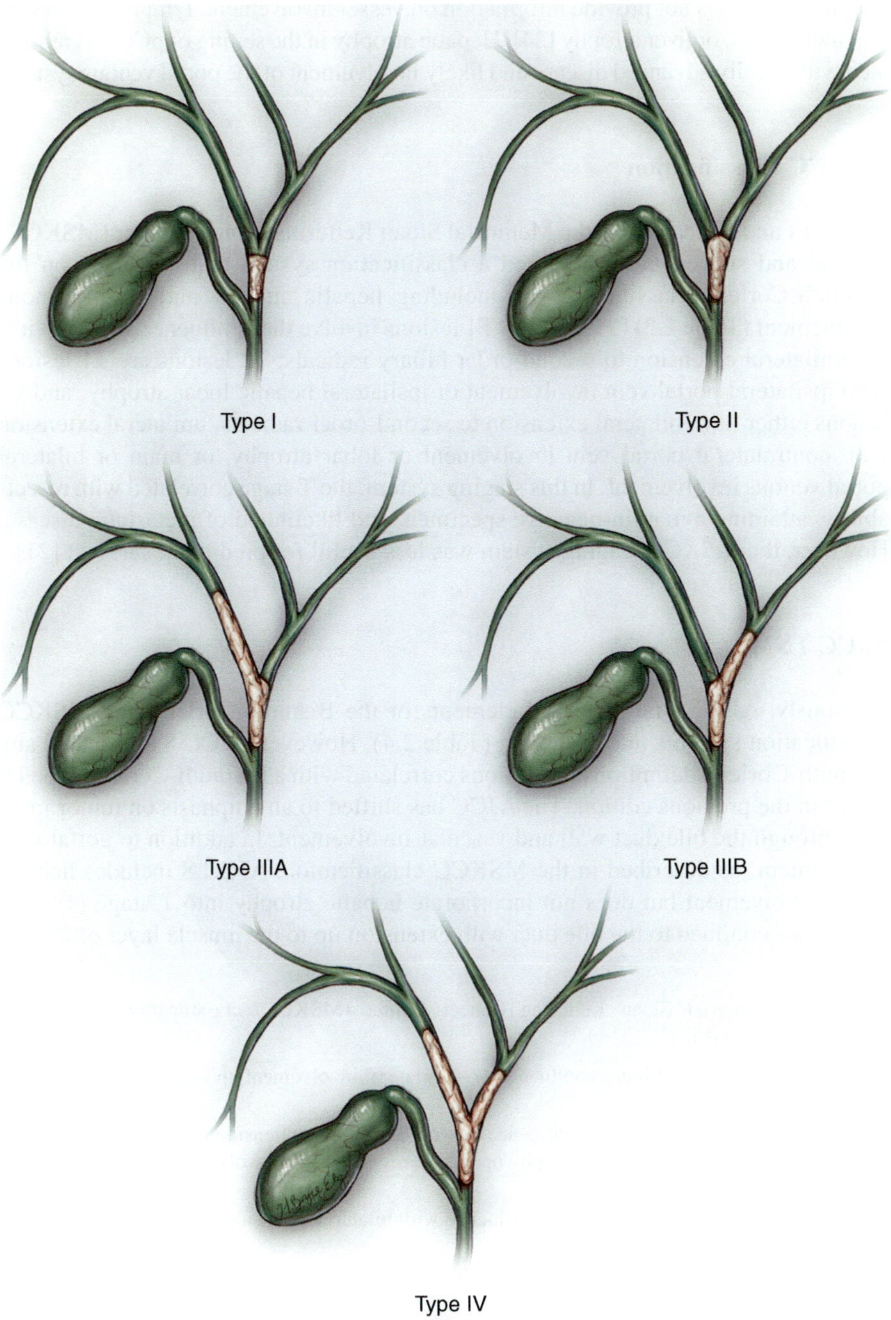

Fig. 2.4 Bismuth-Corlette classification of perihilar cholangiocarcinoma. (Illustration by Hannah Bryce Ely, CMI)

classification does not provide information on vessel involvement, lymph node or distant metastases, or liver atrophy [24]. Hepatic atrophy in the setting of pCCA is associated with locally advanced disease and likely involvement of the portal venous system.

MSKCC Classification

Blumgart and colleagues at the Memorial Sloan Kettering Cancer Center (MSKCC) devised and subsequently modified a classification system that expanded on the Bismuth-Corlette classification by including hepatic atrophy and portal venous involvement (Table 2.3) [21, 25, 26]. T1 lesions involve the confluence with or without unilateral extension to second-order biliary radicals; T2 lesions are T1 lesions with ipsilateral portal vein involvement or ipsilateral hepatic lobar atrophy; and T3 lesions either have bilateral extension to second-order radicals, unilateral extension with contralateral portal vein involvement or lobar atrophy, or main or bilateral portal venous involvement. In this staging system, the T stage correlated with resectability, attaining a margin-negative specimen, and likelihood of metastatic disease. However, the MSKCC staging system was less useful for predicting survival [21].

AJCC TNM

Previously, AJCC 7 incorporated elements of the Bismuth-Corlette and MSKCC classification systems into T staging (Table 2.4). However, AJCC 8 eliminated any Bismuth-Corlette definitions; T4 lesions correlated with a Bismuth-Corlette type IV tumor in the previous edition. The AJCC has shifted to an emphasis on tumor invasion through the bile duct wall and vascular involvement. In addition to portal vein involvement, as described in the MSKCC classification, AJCC 8 includes hepatic artery involvement but does not incorporate hepatic atrophy into T stage [19]. T1 tumors are confined to the bile duct with extension up to the muscle layer or fibrous

Table 2.3 Memorial Sloan Kettering Cancer Center (MSKCC) classification of perihilar cholangiocarcinoma [21]

I	Tumor involves the biliary confluence +/− unilateral involvement up to the second-order biliary radicals
II	Tumor involving the biliary confluence +/− unilateral duct extension to second-order biliary radicals **and** *ipsilateral* liver atrophy or *ipsilateral* portal vein involvement
III	Any of the following: I. Tumor involving the biliary confluence with bilateral extension to second-order biliary radicals II. Tumor involving the biliary confluence + unilateral extension to second-order biliary radicals with *contralateral* portal vein involvement III. Tumor involving the biliary confluence + unilateral extension to second-order biliary radicals with *contralateral* hepatic lobar atrophy IV. Tumor involving the biliary confluence with main or bilateral portal venous involvement

Table 2.4 AJCC 7 and8 staging of perihilar cholangiocarcinoma

AJCC 7th ed.		AJCC 8th ed.	
T	*Primary tumor*	*T*	*Primary tumor*
TX	Primary tumor cannot be assessed	TX	Primary tumor cannot be assessed
T0	No evidence of primary tumor	T0	No evidence of primary tumor
Tis	Carcinoma in situ	Tis	Carcinoma in situ/high-grade dysplasia
T1	Tumor confined to the bile duct, with extension up to the muscle layer or fibrous tissue	T1	Tumor confined to the bile duct, with extension up to the muscle layer or fibrous tissue
T2a	Tumor invades beyond the wall of the bile duct to surrounding adipose tissue	T2a	Tumor invades beyond the wall of the bile duct to surrounding adipose tissue
T2b	Tumor invades adjacent hepatic parenchyma	T2b	Tumor invades adjacent hepatic parenchyma
T3	Tumor invades unilateral branches of the portal vein or hepatic artery	T3	Tumor invades unilateral branches of the portal vein or hepatic artery
T4	Tumor invades main portal vein or its branches bilaterally, or the common hepatic artery, or the second-order biliary radicals bilaterally, or unilateral second-order biliary radicals with contralateral portal vein or hepatic artery involvement	T4	Tumor invades main portal vein or its branches bilaterally, or the common hepatic artery, or unilateral second-order biliary radicals with contralateral portal vein or hepatic artery involvement
N	*Regional lymph nodes*	*N*	*Regional lymph nodes*
NX	Regional lymph nodes cannot be assessed	NX	Regional lymph nodes cannot be assessed
N0	No regional lymph node metastasis	N0	No regional lymph node metastasis
N1	Regional lymph node metastasis (including nodes along the cystic duct, common bile duct, hepatic artery, and portal vein)	N1	One to three positive lymph nodes typically involving the hilar, cystic duct, common bile duct, hepatic artery, posterior pancreaticoduodenal, and portal vein lymph nodes
N2	Metastasis to periaortic, pericaval, superior mesenteric artery, and/or celiac artery lymph nodes	N2	Four or more positive lymph nodes from the sites described for N1
M	*Distant metastasis*	*M*	*Distant metastasis*
M0	No distant metastasis	M0	No distant metastasis
M1	Distant metastasis present	M1	Distant metastasis present
Stage		*Stage*	
0	Tis, N0, M0	0	Tis, N0, M0
I	T1, N0, M0	I	T1, N0, M0
II	T2a–b, N0, M0	II	T2a–b, N0, M0
IIIA	T3, N0, M0	IIIA	T3, N0, M0
IIIB	T1–3, N1, M0	IIIB	T4, N0, M0
		IIIC	Any T, N1, M0
IVA	T4, N0–1, M0	IVA	Any T, N2, M0
IVB	Any T, N2, M0 Any T, any N, M1	IVB	Any T, any N, M1

tissue. Tumors that invade beyond the bile duct to surrounding adipose tissue are T2a, and those that invade the hepatic parenchyma are T2b. Tumors that invade branches of the portal vein and hepatic artery unilaterally are T3. Perihilar tumors are T4 when there is invasion of the main portal vein and common hepatic artery or if there is unilateral extension to second-order biliary radicals with contralateral portal vein or hepatic artery involvement. In a multi-institutional study analyzing actual 5-year survival in patients who underwent resection with curative intent, none with T3 or T4 tumors were 5-year survivors [27].

pCCA frequently metastasizes to regional lymph node basins (hilar, cystic duct, choledochal, portal, hepatic arterial, and posterior pancreaticoduodenal lymph nodes) due to the extensive periductal lymphatics. Nodal metastases are as high as 50% in some series and are directly related to T stage. Furthermore, multiple positive lymph nodes is adversely related to survival (RR 1.61; 1.01–2.56) [28]. Accordingly, AJCC 8 updated the N stage and incorporated the number of positive lymph nodes: one to three regional lymph node metastases are designated N1 and greater than four lymph nodes is N2. Extra-regional lymph node metastases (outside the hepatoduodenal ligament) are considered distant and are designated M1. Other common sites of metastasis include the peritoneum, liver, lung, bone, brain, and skin.

Distal Cholangiocarcinoma

CCA that develops in common bile duct (between the ampulla of Vater and the confluence of the common hepatic duct and cystic duct) is categorized as distal CCA (dCCA) and comprises 20–30% of bile duct cancers (Figs. 2.1 and 2.2c) [29]. The distal most aspect of the common bile duct (CBD) sits within the pancreatic parenchyma at the head of the pancreas and is the most common site of dCCA. At this location, dCCA frequently presents with biliary obstructive symptoms: painless jaundice, pruritus, and acholic stools. Pancreatic ductal dilatation and evidence of pancreatitis may also be encountered during the workup. Tumors at this location are positioned near, and frequently involve, important structures, which confers prognostic significance and impacts surgical planning. Nearby organs that may be invaded directly include to the pancreas, stomach, duodenum, gallbladder, colon, and omentum. Arteries that may be involved include the superior mesenteric, celiac, splenic, and hepatic arteries. Veins involved include the portal, splenic, splenoportal confluence, and the superior mesenteric vein and its branch vessels. Differentiating dCCA from other periampullary tumors such as ampullary carcinoma and pancreatic neoplasms is often difficult to discern on imaging and endoscopic evaluation.

Staging

Unlike pCCA, which has multiple staging systems, dCCA is only staged by the AJCC TNM system and is used for both clinical and pathologic staging of dCCA. For clinical locoregional staging, high-quality cross-sectional imaging and/or evaluation via endoscopic ultrasound (EUS) is critical to delineate depth of invasion and involvement of surrounding structures and to identify pathologic lymph nodes. Previously, T stage was stratified by histologic invasion (i.e., confined to the bile duct or extends beyond the wall of the bile duct) (Table 2.5). This method for T staging was

Table 2.5 AJCC 7 and 8 staging of distal cholangiocarcinoma

AJCC 7th ed.		AJCC 8th Ed.	
T	*Primary tumor*	*T*	*Primary tumor*
TX	Primary tumor cannot be assessed	TX	Primary tumor cannot be assessed
T0	No evidence of primary tumor	T0	No evidence of primary tumor
Tis	Carcinoma in situ	Tis	Carcinoma in situ/high-grade dysplasia
T1	Tumor confined to the bile duct histologically	T1	Tumor invades the bile duct wall with a depth less than 5 mm
T2	Tumor invades beyond the wall of the bile duct	T2	Tumor invades the bile duct wall with a depth of 5–12 mm
T3	Tumor invades the gallbladder, pancreas, duodenum, or other adjacent organs without involvement of the celiac axis or the superior mesenteric artery	T3	Tumor invades the bile duct wall with a depth greater than 12 mm
T4	Tumor involves the celiac axis or the superior mesenteric artery	T4	Tumor involves the celiac axis, superior mesenteric artery, and/or common hepatic artery
N	*Regional lymph nodes*	*N*	*Regional lymph nodes*
NX	Regional lymph nodes cannot be assessed	NX	Regional lymph nodes cannot be assessed
N0	No regional lymph node metastasis	N0	No regional lymph node metastasis
N1	Regional lymph node metastasis	N1	Metastasis in one to three regional lymph nodes
		N2	Metastasis in four or more regional lymph nodes
M	*Distant metastasis*	*M*	*Distant metastasis*
M0	No distant metastasis	M0	No distant metastasis
M1	Distant metastasis present	M1	Distant metastasis present
Stage		*Stage*	
0	Tis, N0, M0	0	Tis, N0, M0
1A	T1, N0, M0	I	T1, N0, M0
IB	T2, N0, M0		
IIA	T3, N0, M0	IIA	T1, N1, M0 T2, N0, M0
IIB	T1–3, N1, M0	IIB	T2, N1, M0 T3, N0, M0 T3, N1, M0
III	T4, any N, M0	IIIA	T1–3, N2, M0
		IIIB	T4, any N, M0
IV	Any T, any N, M1	IV	Any T, any N, M1

problematic, however, because of the variable thickness along the common bile duct and the characteristic and marked desmoplastic reaction that often obscures the boundaries of the bile duct wall and the extent of tumor invasion from the basal lamina [30]. Further, this T-stage classification was not associated with survival outcome. Instead, the measured depth of invasion demonstrated a better correlation with survival [31]. Accordingly, AJCC 8 defines T stage by a measured depth of invasion into the bile duct wall: T1, <5 mm; T2, 5–12 mm; and T3, >12 mm. T4 is defined by invasion of the celiac axis, superior mesenteric artery, or common hepatic artery (Table 2.5). Unfortunately, for reasons listed above, dCCA is often misclassified as pancreatic adenocarcinoma or ampullary carcinoma, which have different staging classifications, tumor biology, and patient outcomes [29, 32]. Even after resection of a periampullary tumor, dCCA is often misdiagnosed on pathologic evaluation [33].

Lymph node metastasis occurs in approximately 40% of patients with dCCA who undergo surgical resection. Regional lymph nodes include those along the common bile duct and hepatic artery, the posterior and anterior pancreaticoduodenal nodes, and the nodes along the right lateral wall of the superior mesenteric artery. Similar to pCCA, the number of metastatic lymph nodes in dCCA appears to be useful in predicting patient outcomes. One study evaluating lymph node metastasis in 370 patients who underwent resection for dCCA found that patients with 4 or more involved nodes had a significantly shorter median survival compared to patients with only 1 to 3 involved nodes (1.3 vs. 2.2 years; $p = 0.001$) [34]. Accordingly, the N stage has been modified to reflect these outcomes (N1, one to three positive lymph nodes; N2, four or more positive nodes). Regarding distant metastases, the most common sites include the liver, peritoneum, and lungs [29].

Conclusion

CCA is a malignant tumor that can arise from any part of the biliary tree, anatomically separated into three categories based on the site of origin: intrahepatic, perihilar, and distal. The morphologies, risk factors, presentation, treatment, and outcomes for each anatomic category of CCA are often variable but sometimes overlap. The anatomic location of CCA is used to determine staging, as assessed by the AJCC, and is critical to deciding on treatment and determining prognosis for patients afflicted with these malignancies.

References

1. Bergquist A, von Seth E. Epidemiology of cholangiocarcinoma. Best Pract Res Clin Gastroenterol. 2015;29(2):221–32.
2. Wu L, Tsilimigras DI, Paredes AZ, Mehta R, Hyer JM, Merath K, et al. Trends in the incidence, treatment and outcomes of patients with intrahepatic cholangiocarcinoma in the USA:

facility type is associated with margin status, use of lymphadenectomy and overall survival. World J Surg. 2019;43(7):1777–87.
3. Yamasaki S. Intrahepatic cholangiocarcinoma: macroscopic type and stage classification. J Hepato-Biliary-Pancreat Surg. 2003;10(4):288–91.
4. Zhang XF, Lv Y, Weiss M, Popescu I, Marques HP, Aldrighetti L, et al. Should utilization of lymphadenectomy vary according to morphologic subtype of intrahepatic cholangiocarcinoma? Ann Surg Oncol. 2019;26(7):2242–50.
5. Bagante F, Weiss M, Alexandrescu S, Marques HP, Aldrighetti L, Maithel SK, et al. Long-term outcomes of patients with intraductal growth sub-type of intrahepatic cholangiocarcinoma. HPB (Oxford). 2018;20(12):1189–97.
6. Aloia TA, Pawlik TM, Taouli B, Rubbia-Brandt L, Vauthey JN. Intrahepatic bile ducts. In: Amin MB, editor. AJCC cancer staging manual. 8th ed. Chicago: American Joint Committee on Cancer; 2017. p. 295–302.
7. Bagante F, Spolverato G, Weiss M, Alexandrescu S, Marques HP, Aldrighetti L, et al. Impact of morphological status on long-term outcome among patients undergoing liver surgery for intrahepatic cholangiocarcinoma. Ann Surg Oncol. 2017;24(9):2491–501.
8. Mavros MN, Economopoulos KP, Alexiou VG, Pawlik TM. Treatment and prognosis for patients with intrahepatic cholangiocarcinoma: systematic review and meta-analysis. JAMA Surg. 2014;149(6):565–74.
9. Weber SM, Ribero D, O'Reilly EM, Kokudo N, Miyazaki M, Pawlik TM. Intrahepatic cholangiocarcinoma: expert consensus statement. HPB (Oxford). 2015;17(8):669–80.
10. Spolverato G, Bagante F, Weiss M, Alexandrescu S, Marques HP, Aldrighetti L, et al. Comparative performances of the 7th and the 8th editions of the American Joint Committee on Cancer staging systems for intrahepatic cholangiocarcinoma. J Surg Oncol. 2017;115(6):696–703.
11. Amin MB; American Joint Committee on Cancer, American Cancer Society. AJCC cancer staging manual. 8th ed. In: Amin MB, Editor-in-chief, Edge SB, et al., Gress DM, RHIT, CTR, Technical editor, Meyer LR, CAPM, Managing editor. Chicago: American Joint Committee on Cancer/Springer; 2017. xvii, 1024 p.
12. Edge SB; American Joint Committee on Cancer. AJCC cancer staging manual. 7th ed. New York: Springer; 2010. xiv, 648 p.
13. Nathan H, Aloia TA, Vauthey JN, Abdalla EK, Zhu AX, Schulick RD, et al. A proposed staging system for intrahepatic cholangiocarcinoma. Ann Surg Oncol. 2009;16(1):14–22.
14. Igami T, Ebata T, Yokoyama Y, Sugawara G, Takahashi Y, Nagino M. Staging of peripheral-type intrahepatic cholangiocarcinoma: appraisal of the new TNM classification and its modifications. World J Surg. 2011;35(11):2501–9.
15. Ronnekleiv-Kelly SM, Pawlik TM. Staging of intrahepatic cholangiocarcinoma. Hepatobiliary Surg Nutr. 2017;6(1):35–43.
16. Bagante F, Spolverato G, Merath K, Weiss M, Alexandrescu S, Marques HP, et al. Intrahepatic cholangiocarcinoma tumor burden: a classification and regression tree model to define prognostic groups after resection. Surgery. 2019;166(6):983–90.
17. Buettner S, Ten Cate DWG, Bagante F, Alexandrescu S, Marques HP, Lamelas J, et al. Survival after resection of multiple tumor foci of intrahepatic cholangiocarcinoma. J Gastrointest Surg. 2019;23(11):2239–46.
18. Zhang XF, Xue F, Dong DH, Weiss M, Popescu I, Marques HP, et al. Number and station of lymph node metastasis after curative-intent resection of intrahepatic cholangiocarcinoma impact prognosis. Ann Surg. 2020. Ahead of print.
19. Nagorney DM, Pawlik TM, Chun YS, Ebata T, Vauthey JN. Perihilar bile ducts. In: Amin MB, editor. AJCC cancer staging manual. 8th ed. Chicago: American Joint Committee on Cancer; 2017. p. 311–6.
20. Klatskin G. Adenocarcinoma of the hepatic duct at its bifurcation within the porta hepatis. An unusual tumor with distinctive clinical and pathological features. Am J Med. 1965;38:241–56.

21. Matsuo K, Rocha FG, Ito K, D'Angelica MI, Allen PJ, Fong Y, et al. The Blumgart preoperative staging system for hilar cholangiocarcinoma: analysis of resectability and outcomes in 380 patients. J Am Coll Surg. 2012;215(3):343–55.
22. Bismuth H, Corlette MB. Intrahepatic cholangioenteric anastomosis in carcinoma of the hilus of the liver. Surg Gynecol Obstet. 1975;140(2):170–8.
23. Bismuth H, Nakache R, Diamond T. Management strategies in resection for hilar cholangiocarcinoma. Ann Surg. 1992;215(1):31–8.
24. Deoliveira ML, Schulick RD, Nimura Y, Rosen C, Gores G, Neuhaus P, et al. New staging system and a registry for perihilar cholangiocarcinoma. Hepatology. 2011;53(4):1363–71.
25. Burke EC, Jarnagin WR, Hochwald SN, Pisters PW, Fong Y, Blumgart LH. Hilar Cholangiocarcinoma: patterns of spread, the importance of hepatic resection for curative operation, and a presurgical clinical staging system. Ann Surg. 1998;228(3):385–94.
26. Jarnagin WR, Fong Y, DeMatteo RP, Gonen M, Burke EC, Bodniewicz BJ, et al. Staging, resectability, and outcome in 225 patients with hilar cholangiocarcinoma. Ann Surg. 2001;234(4):507–17; discussion 17–9.
27. Tran TB, Ethun CG, Pawlik TM, Schmidt C, Beal EW, Fields RC, et al. Actual 5-year survivors after surgical resection of hilar cholangiocarcinoma. Ann Surg Oncol. 2019;26(2):611–8.
28. Aoba T, Ebata T, Yokoyama Y, Igami T, Sugawara G, Takahashi Y, et al. Assessment of nodal status for perihilar cholangiocarcinoma: location, number, or ratio of involved nodes. Ann Surg. 2013;257(4):718–25.
29. Krasinskas A, Pawlik TM, Mino-Kenudson M, Vauthey JN. Distal bile duct. In: Amin MB, editor. AJCC cancer staging manual. 8th ed. Chicago: American Joint Committee on Cancer; 2017. p. 317–25.
30. Hong SM, Presley AE, Stelow EB, Frierson HF Jr, Moskaluk CA. Reconsideration of the histologic definitions used in the pathologic staging of extrahepatic bile duct carcinoma. Am J Surg Pathol. 2006;30(6):744–9.
31. Hong SM, Pawlik TM, Cho H, Aggarwal B, Goggins M, Hruban RH, et al. Depth of tumor invasion better predicts prognosis than the current American Joint Committee on Cancer T classification for distal bile duct carcinoma. Surgery. 2009;146(2):250–7.
32. Bledsoe JR, Shinagare SA, Deshpande V. Difficult diagnostic problems in pancreatobiliary neoplasia. Arch Pathol Lab Med. 2015;139(7):848–57.
33. Pomianowska E, Grzyb K, Westgaard A, Clausen OP, Gladhaug IP. Reclassification of tumour origin in resected periampullary adenocarcinomas reveals underestimation of distal bile duct cancer. Eur J Surg Oncol. 2012;38(11):1043–50.
34. Kiriyama M, Ebata T, Aoba T, Kaneoka Y, Arai T, Shimizu Y, et al. Prognostic impact of lymph node metastasis in distal cholangiocarcinoma. Br J Surg. 2015;102(4):399–406.

Chapter 3
Intraductal Tumors of the Biliary Tract: Precursor Lesions and Variants

Yasuni Nakanuma, Katsuhiko Uesaka, Masayuki Ohtsuka, Koushiro Ohtsubo, Dai Inoue, and Kazuto Kozaka

Abbreviations

AUS	Abdominal ultrasonography
BilIN	Biliary intraepithelial neoplasm
CA19-9	Carbohydrate antigen 19-9
CCA	Cholangiocarcinoma
CEA	Carcinoembryonic antigen
CT	Computed tomography
ERC	Endoscopic retrograde cholangiography
EST	Endoscopic sphincterotomy
EUS	Endoscopic ultrasonography
gIPNB	Gastric intraductal papillary neoplasm of the bile duct
HE staining	Hematoxylin and eosin staining
iCCA	Intrahepatic cholangiocarcinoma

Y. Nakanuma (✉)
Department of Diagnostic Pathology, Shizuoka Cancer Center, Shizuoka, Japan

Department of Diagnostic Pathology, Fukui Prefecture Saiseikai Hospital, Fukui, Japan

K. Uesaka
Department of Hepatobiliary Pancreaetic Surgery, Shizuoka Cancer Center, Shizuoka, Japan
e-mail: k.uesaka@scchr.jp

M. Ohtsuka
Department of Hepatobiliary Pancreatic Surgery, Chiba University Hospital, Chiba, Japan
e-mail: otsuka-m@faculty.chiba-u.jp

K. Ohtsubo
Division of Medical Oncology, Cancer Institute, Kanazawa University Hospital, Kanazawa, Japan
e-mail: ohtsubo@staff.kanazawa-u.ac.jp

D. Inoue · K. Kozaka
Department of Radiology, Kanazawa University Hospital, Kanazawa, Japan
e-mail: d-inoue@lake.ocn.ne.jp

J. H. Tabibian (ed.), *Diagnosis and Management of Cholangiocarcinoma*,
https://doi.org/10.1007/978-3-030-70936-5_3

ICPN	Intracholecystic papillary neoplasm
IDUS	Intraductal ultrasonography
iIPNB	Intestinal intraductal papillary neoplasm of the bile duct
IPMN	Intraductal papillary mucinous neoplasm
IPNB	Intraductal papillary neoplasm of bile duct
ITPN	Intraductal tubulopapillary neoplasm of the bile duct
MCN	Mucinous cystic neoplasm
MDCT	Multidetector computed tomography
MR	Magnetic resonance imaging
MRC	Magnetic resonance cholangiography
MUC	Mucin core protein
NBI	Narrow-band imaging
oIPNB	Oncocytic intraductal papillary neoplasm of the bile duct
PanIN	Pancreatic intraepithelial neoplasm
pbIPNB	Pancreatobiliary intraductal papillary neoplasm of the bile duct
POCS	Peroral cholangioscopy
WHO	World Health Organization

Introduction

In our experience, there are generally at least two types of tumors involving the biliary tree. One is characterized by a nodular or sclerosing lesion affecting the bile duct wall and periductal tissue and the other by tumors that mainly grow in the intraductal lumen and usually show no or slight stromal invasion [1–3]. In the latter type, several diseases are included (Table 3.1), and they present unique

Table 3.1 Intraductal tumors of the biliary tract, related lesions, and mimickers

Primary intraductal neoplasm
Intraductal papillary neoplasm of the bile duct
Biliary intraepithelial neoplasm
Intraductal tubulopapillary neoplasm
Pyloric gland adenoma
Other rare benign intraductal neoplasms
Tubular adenoma or neoplasm [142, 143]
Tubulovillous adenoma [144]
Villous adenoma [145]
Undifferentiated carcinoma
Carcinosarcoma
Related neoplasms
Mucinous cystic neoplasm (MCN)
Intracystic papillary neoplasm (ICPN)
Mimickers
Conventional CCA with intraluminal lesions
Metastatic carcinoma of the bile duct
Hepatocellular carcinoma emboli in the bile duct

clinicopathological features that differ from nodular sclerosing *cholangiocarcinoma (CCA)* [4, 5]. Among them, *intraductal papillary neoplasms of the bile duct (IPNBs)* are a representative intraductal neoplasm. The affected bile ducts are dilated and filled with a grossly visible exophytic tumor and histologically neoplastic biliary epithelia [2, 6–8].

IPNBs have been studied in comparison to *intraductal papillary mucinous neoplasms (IPMNs)* of the pancreas, which are also a preinvasive intraductal papillary neoplasm associated with invasive carcinoma and intramucosal spread of neoplastic epithelia [9–14].

Another well-known intraductal tumor of the biliary tract is biliary intraepithelial neoplasm (BilIN) [1, 2, 8, 15–20]. This lesion is microscopically identifiable as a flat or micropapillary lesion. BilINs are reportedly an important precursor or preinvasive lesion of conventional nodular/sclerosing CCA, and there are also other categories of intraductal neoplasms [8, 21–23]. Metastatic carcinoma growing in the bile duct lumen also shows similar gross and imaging characteristics [24].

Recently, the World Health Organization (WHO) published the Classification of Digestive System Tumours 5th edition (2019), in which the new term, "benign and precursor lesions," was proposed based on recent progress in this field [4, 7, 10, 15, 25]. We herein review the pathological features of benign and prcursor lesions of the bile duct, particularly IPNB, based on this WHO classification, with reference to the molecular and genetic features, imaging, diagnosis, and management. Other types of benign and precursor lesions of the bile duct are also briefly reviewed.

Intraductal Papillary Neoplasms of the Bile Duct (IPNBs)

IPNB is characterized by intraductal neoplastic growth of biliary epithelia covering fine fibrovascular stalks that lack an ovarian-mesenchymal-type stroma, mainly involving the extrahepatic and intrahepatic bile ducts [7]. IPNBs are associated with variable intramucosal (lateral) spread of neoplastic epithelia around the main papillary tumor, and multifocal occurrence is also reported [2, 3, 7, 21, 26, 27]. The cell of origin of a majority of IPNBs is believed to be the biliary lining cells, while some IPNBs might be derived from the cells in peribiliary glands, which are distributed along the extrahepatic and intrahepatic bile ducts [28–31]. IPNBs are thought to be premalignant lesions with the potential to progress invasive tumors. IPNBs may develop through a multistep process or sequence, eventually followed by invasion [27, 32]. Consequently, IPNBs, particularly those without invasion, usually progress slowly, and patients appear to have better survival in comparison to patients with conventional CCA [27, 33].

Since the first report of IPNBs in the English literature [6], IPNBs have been further studied, and data are now accumulating [12, 27]. IPNBs show variable gross and histopathological features, molecular and genetic features, and biological behavior [6, 32–42]. IPNBs are regarded as preinvasive biliary lesions that are not frequently associated with stromal invasion (IPNB associated with invasive

Table 3.2 Proposed, accepted, and unrecommended terms for intraductal tumors and related lesion by WHO Classification of Tumours (2019)

WHO proposed terms (2019)	WHO accepted terms	WHO unrecommended terms
IPNB (intraductal papillary neoplasm of the bile duct)	Biliary papilloma and papillomatosis	Biliary adenoma Intestinal adenoma Papillary (villous) adenoma Tubulopapillary (tubule-villous) adenoma Noninvasive papillary neoplasm (carcinoma) Papillary carcinoma Mucin-secreting biliary tumor
MCN (mucinous cystic neoplasm)		Hepatobiliary cystadenoma; adenocarcinoma
Low-grade BilIN (biliary intraepithelial neoplasm) High-grade BilIN (biliary intraepithelial neoplasm)	Dysplasia Carcinoma in situ	

carcinoma) [7]. The incidence of invasion and the histological features in fact differ among several proposed subcategories (or several synonymous names) of IPNB [39, 42, 43]. This heterogeneity and complexity lead to controversy in relation to the clinicopathological recognition and diagnosis of IPNB, suggesting that IPNBs are not a homogeneous disease [44–46]. Several nomenclatures have previously been applied to these tumors according to the dominant feature(s) [36, 45–49]; however, the use of these obsolete terms is not recommended at the present time (Table 3.2) [7].

Epidemiology and Risks

Epidemiology

IPNBs are reported worldwide and affect typically middle-aged to elderly adults (50–80 years of age) and show a male predominance [7, 27, 40, 50–56]. IPNBs account for 9–38% of all bile duct carcinomas [33, 40, 46, 53, 57]. The highest incidence of IPNB is reported in Far Eastern countries [46, 50, 51, 55, 58].

The pathobiology of IPNB may present geographic variation between Asian and Western populations. Cordon-Weeks et al. reported that IPNBs identified in centers from Asia were more likely to be intrahepatic and were less frequently invasive in comparison to those from Western centers [27, 32, 33, 52]. IPNBs account for 10–38% of all bile duct tumors in East Asian populations but only 7–12% of all bile duct tumors in Western populations [32, 33, 50, 51, 55]. The pooled prevalence in Asian populations was more than twice that in Western populations [27], and IPNBs in Western centers showed higher rates of invasive disease and were less frequently associated with mucus production and more frequently of the pancreatobiliary subtype [7, 27, 32, 33].

Risk Factors

Hepatolithiasis and liver fluke infection (*Clonorchis sinensis* in Korea or *Opisthorchis viverrini* infection in South East Asia) are believed to be major risk factors for IPNB [50, 51, 53–56, 59]. In addition, approximately 30% of patients have a previous history or concomitant existence of biliary stones, as shown in the reports from Far Eastern countries [36, 60, 61], but not from Western countries [32, 33]. IPNBs also reportedly develop in primary sclerosing cholangitis [62] and congenital biliary tract disease [63]. Interestingly, these etiologic factors are also known as major risk factors for nodular sclerosing perihilar/distal CCA and mass-forming and periductal *intrahepatic cholangiocarcinoma* (*iCCA*) [1, 4, 5], suggesting that chronic biliary tract irritation and inflammation may be causally related to the development of IPNB in addition to other types of CCA. Recently, an outbreak of IPNB was reported among young adult workers in the offset color proof-printing department at a printing company in Japan [64]. They were chronically exposed to chlorinated organic solvents, including dichloromethane and 1,2-dichloropropane. Interestingly, IPNB or IPNB associated with invasive carcinoma was observed in various sites of the intrahepatic large bile ducts, perihilar bile ducts and distal bile ducts in these patients [65].

A significant proportion of IPNB cases are completely asymptomatic in endemic and non-endemic areas [27]. Imaging modalities (see below) appear to have some value in screening and detecting IPNB in asymptomatic patients who are at a high risk of developing IPNB [62, 63, 66].

Pathology

Gross Features

Location Along the Biliary Tree

While the locations of IPNBs have varied in several reports, the majority of IPNBs (67%) were located at the intrahepatic bile ducts in Asian countries, while in Western countries, they were more common in the extrahepatic bile ducts [8, 27, 54, 55] or hepatic hilum [32, 33] (Table 3.3). Some cases simultaneously involved the intrahepatic and extrahepatic bile ducts [27, 67, 68]. Despite these variable locations, when IPNB exists in the intrahepatic bile ducts, it tends to be found in the left-sided biliary ductal system [27, 46, 61], for reasons which remain uncertain.

Table 3.3 Pathologic characteristics of intraductal papillary neoplasm of the bile duct (IPNB)

Tumor location	Intrahepatic: More than half in East Asian countries Extrahepatic[a]: More than half in Western countries	
Tumor number	Single Conglomerate Multiple	60% 40% Occasional
Tumor size (including height of IPNB)	1–6.6 cm (larger than 0.5 cm in almost all cases)	
Mucus overproduction	Present 40% (particularly in intrahepatic IPNB) Absent 60%	
Tumor grade	Low grade High grade High grade with invasion	10% 50% 40%
Subtype	Intestinal subtype Gastric subtype PB[b] subtype Oncocytic subtype	45% 30% 15% 10%

[a]Including perihilar bile duct
[b]Pancreatobiliary, cited from Refs. [4, 27]

Main Tumors and the Surrounding Bile Duct Mucosa

Generally, IPNBs present as papillary or villous, exophytic growth (range, 1–6 cm) (Fig. 3.1) [13, 27, 46, 69]; height, at least 5 mm from the adjacent biliary mucosa) in the dilated bile ducts are typical; however, some papillary neoplasms with a similar histopathology that are <5 mm but >3 mm in height are occasionally encountered [42]. These exophytic lesions are usually conglomerates of smaller or higher polypoid lesions but are not infrequently single or isolated.

Gross features and anatomical location The gross features of IPNBs depend on their anatomical location, state of excessive mucin secretion, or macro-invasion of the liver [7, 50, 51]. IPNBs located in the intrahepatic bile ducts tend to be larger inboth mass and length than those inthe extrahepatic bile ducts [13,42,70]. Some IPNBs, particularly those arising in the extrahepatic bile ducts, are associated with cylindrical or fusiform morphology with moderate dilatation of the affected bile ducts and appear as a cast-like structures, while other IPNBs, particularly those in the intrahepatic bile duct, present with marked macroscopic dilatation or unilocular or multilocular cystic changes [2, 3, 7, 35]. These cystic changes represent cystic dilatation of the bile ducts and usually show luminal communication with the adjacent bile duct, so they are not true cysts. However, such anatomic communication with the bile duct is sometimes difficult to confirm. The proportion of neoplastic components to mucinous fluid in these cystic IPNBs is variable in individual cases. The internal surfaces of the cystic lesions are smooth or finely granular, and papillary mural nodules are commonly observed.

Surrounding bile duct mucosa A variable proportion of the mucosa around the main papillary conglomerate lesions shows visible granular or small papillary lesions (Fig. 3.1d), suggesting neoplastic mucosal changes that are continuous with the main lesion [2, 3, 7, 26]. The extent of these lesions is variable, and in some

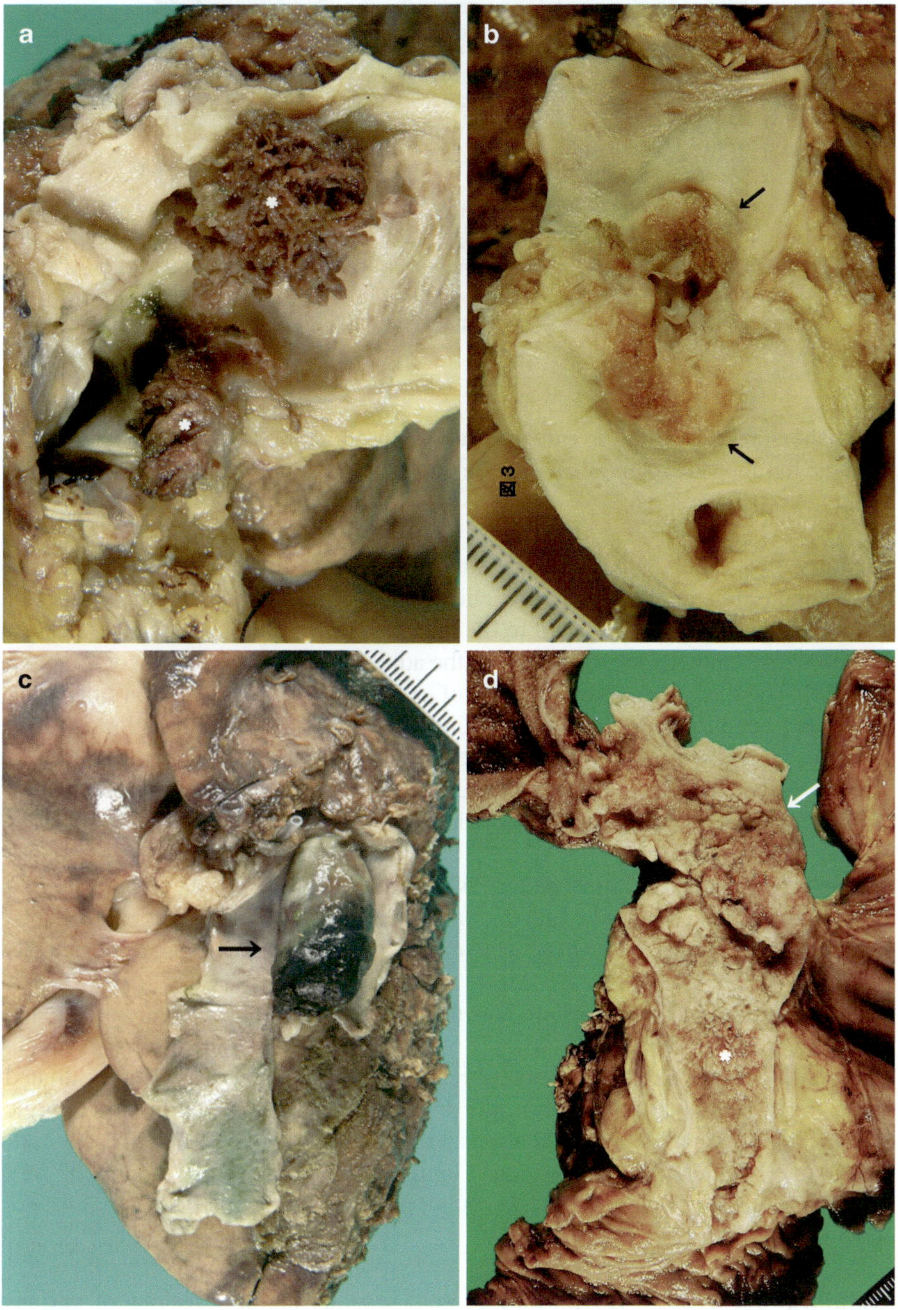

Fig. 3.1 Gross features of intraductal papillary neoplasm of bile duct. (**a**) Papillary lesion in the distal bile duct. Two parts (*) are from a single lesion. (**b**) Congromelate polypoid lesions (→) in the perihilar bile duct. (**c**) Single polypoid tumor (→) in the perihilar bile duct. (**d**) Conglomerate polypoid lesions (→) and surrounding granular or rough mucosa (*) in the perihilar and distal bile duct. (**e**) Papillary lesions in the wall of cystically dilated intrahepatic bile ducts (*) and invasion (→)

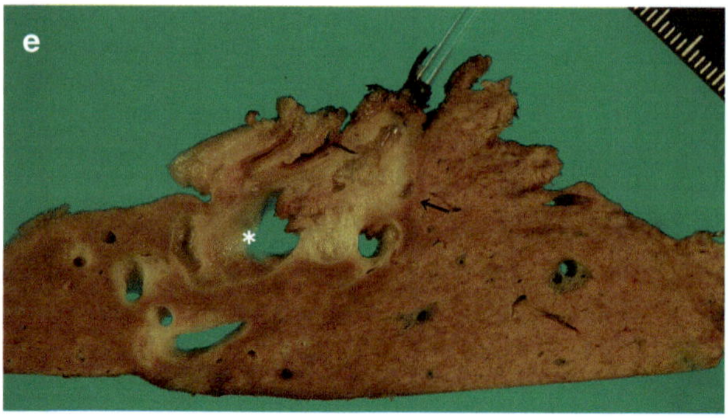

Fig. 3.1 (continued)

cases, the spread is wide or extensive along the biliary tree, randing extensively from the intrahepatic to extrahepatic bile duct; such cases deserve to be classified as a subtype of IPNB [55]/

Variants In addition, IPNBs that are suspected to arise in the peribiliary glands or in the smaller bile ducts directly branching from the hilar bile ducts show saccular or aneurismal dilatations attached to the hilar bile duct [28, 29, 31]. In these cases, the neoplastic epithelia are extending to the adjacent bile duct through communication [28]. There are also several reports of extensive bile duct dilatation filled with mucin and lined by superficially spreading, microscopically identifiable, noninvasive biliary neoplasm, but grossly visible papillary neoplasms were not identifiable [45, 71]. It remains to be clarified whether or not cases with an unusual presentation of IPNB or related lesions should be included as variants of IPNB.

Parenchymal invasion Intrahepatic IPNBs in the intrahepatic bile ducts occasionally show invasion outside the bile duct and then into the surrounding parenchyma, occasionally presenting massive parenchymal lesions that are radiologically detectable.

Excessive mucin hypersecretion This is more frequently observed in intrahepatic IPNBs than in extrahepatic IPNBs [7, 69, 70]. Bile ducts with excessive mucin secretion located upstream and downstream from IPNBs are significantly dilated due to the large amount of mucin in the duct lumen. The most common radiologic findings in IPNB are bile duct dilatation and intraductal masses [51, 61]. Early studies classified the bile duct tumors based on their ability to produce mucin [46, 49]. However, excessive mucin production is not pathognomonic of IPNB and does not occur in all cases of IPNB [7].

Multifocal occurrence IPNBs may present separate multiple lesions of various stages along the biliary tree, both synchronously and dyssynchronously [27, 71]. Some may represent multiple occurrence of IPNB in the bile duct mucosa with a neoplastic predisposition, while others are due to intraluminal implantation or dissemination of neoplastic cells of the main papillary tumor along the biliary tree [72]. Recurrence of IPNB or CCA after surgical resection of IPNB may occur due to the implantation or cancerization of neoplastic cells [73].

Histological Features

Main Tumors

IPNBs are characterized by preinvasive papillary, villous, and/or tubular biliary neoplasms covering or associated with fine fibrovascular stalks or stroma in variably dilated bile ducts (Fig. 3.2). Some cases of IPNB, particularly oncocytic subtype,

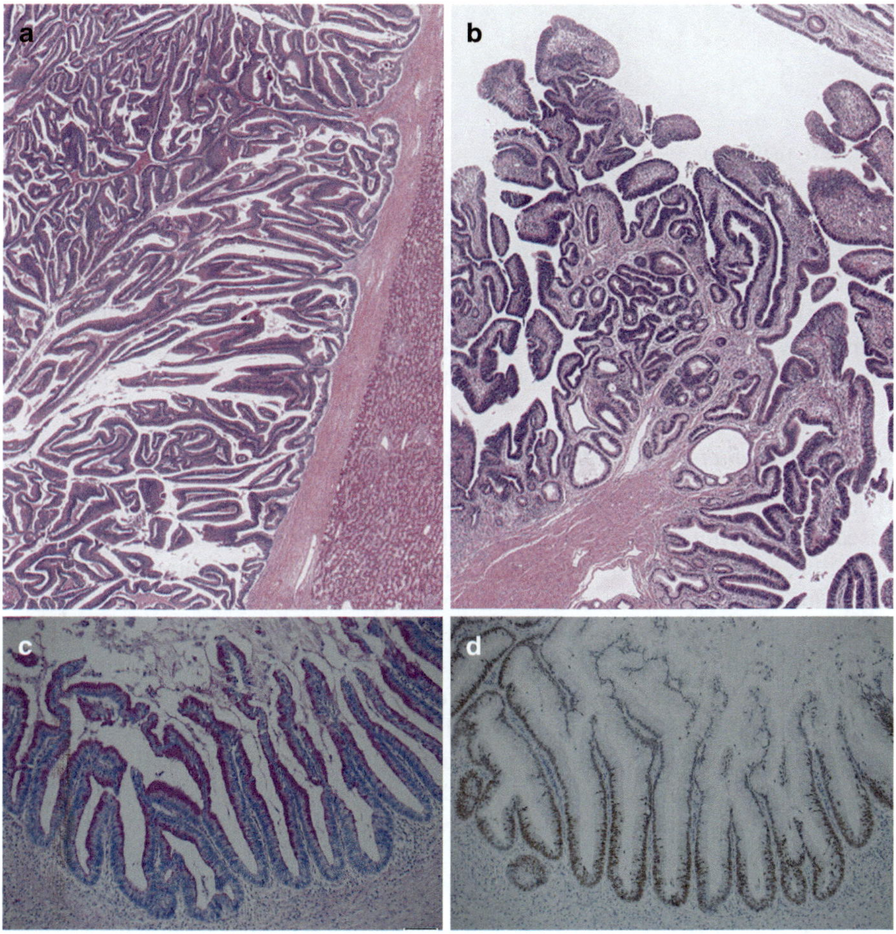

Fig. 3.2 Histological features of intraductal papillary neoplasm of bile duct. (**a**) In the dilated bile duct, papillary lesions with fine fibrovascular stalks (intestinal phenotype) are seen. H&E staining. (**b**) Papillotubular neoplasm (intestinal subtype) with fibrovascular stalks in the distal bile duct resembling tubular neoplasm of the colorectum. H&E staining. (**c**) Villous/papillary epithelia of intraductal papillary neoplasmof bile duct are positive for mucin. PAS staining after diastase digestion. (**d**) Villous/papillary epithelia of intraductal papillary neoplasm of bile duct are positive for CDX2, intestinal marker. Immunostaining for CDX2. (**e**) Papillary neoplasm in the bile duct (pancreatobiliary subtype, *) is associated with flat or micropapillary intraepithelial neoplastic lesion (→) in the surrounding mucosa. HE staining

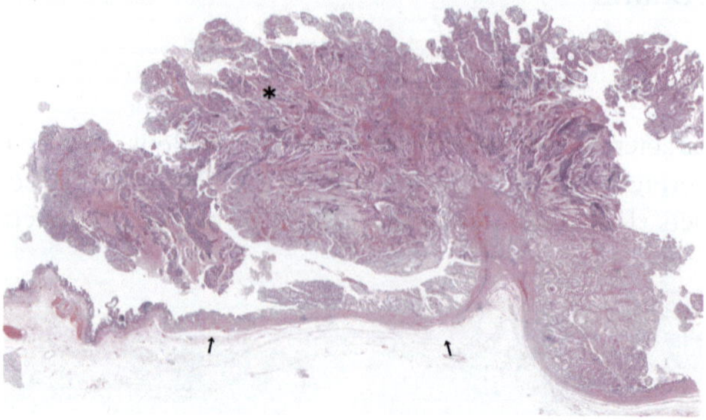

Fig. 3.2 (continued)

show mildly widened stroma due to edema with inflammatory cell infiltration. The histology of IPNB is heterogeneous and variable among cases: surface epithelia are single-layered or stratified, and the cytoplasm is mucinous in some cases but not in others. IPNBs show variable atypia of lining epithelial cells and structural alterations [2, 3, 7, 38]. The histology of IPNBs can be assessed by consideration of four subtypes and also the degree of atypia of the lining epithelia.

Degree of Atypia of Intraepithelial Neoplasia (Dysplasia)

IPNBs are traditionally graded into low-grade and high-grade dysplasia, mainly based on the cellular atypia and structural changes, particularly nuclear atypia and alteration, as is observed in IPMN [2, 3, 7, 43]. For example, the latter shows hyperchromatic nuclei, nucleoli, nuclear and cellular pleomorphism, and a loss of polarity, while the former does not. Some IPNBs totally belong to low-grade dysplasia, while others belong to high-grade dysplasia or high-grade dysplasia with foci of low-grade dysplasia. With respect to the four subtypes (see below), more than 90% of pancreatobiliary IPNBs and intestinal IPNBs belong to high-grade dysplasia, while approximately two-tenth of gastric IPNBs and oncocytic IPNBs belong to low-grade dysplasia, with the remainder belonging to high-grade dysplasia. Characteristically, the four subtypes show unique features of low- and high-grade dysplasia, individually [3].

Four Subtypes of IPNBs

IPNBs are histologically classifiable into four subtypes based on their cell lineages, and they are practically subtyped based on the lining epithelial cells and architecture: *intestinal IPNB* (*iIPNB*), *gastric IPNB* (*gIPNB*), *pancreatobiliary IPNB* (*pbIPNB*), and *oncocytic IPNB* (*oIPNB*) [2, 3, 7, 38]. Main characters of four subtypes are shown in Tables 3.4a, 3.4b, 3.4c, 3.4d. While many cases are predominantly composed of an individual subtype, admixtures of foci of other subtypes and cases

Table 3.4a Characteristics of intestinal subtype of IPNB (iIPNB)

Histological features	Defined by neoplastic epithelia lining the fibrovascular cores showing columnar cells with pseudostratified, cigar-shaped nuclei and basophilic or amphophilic cytoplasm with variable amounts of supranuclear mucin, resembling colorectal mucosal epithelia and neoplasms thereof and admixed with goblet-like cells in the lining epithelia Presenting mainly villous structures, papillovillous, or mixed papillotubular or tubular patterns reminiscent of tubular or villotubular neoplasms of the colorectum
Immunohistochemistry	Positive for CK20 and/or CDX2 in their cytoplasm. Positive for MUC2 in goblet cells

Table 3.4b Characteristics of gastric subtype of IPNB (gIPNB)

Histological features	Composed of tall columnar lining cells with basally oriented nuclei and abundant pale mucinous cytoplasm, reminiscent of the gastric foveolar epithelium, intermingling with glandular areas reminiscent of gastric pyloric glands High-grade dysplasia showing columnar epithelia with more complicated structures including irregular papillary or tubular or microcystic changes with atypical features
Immunohistochemistry	Positive for MUC5AC in the foveolar areas and for MUC6 in the pyloric gland portions

Table 3.4c Characteristics of pancreatobiliary subtype of IPNB (pbIPNB)

Histological features	Defined by ramifying fine and thin branches and papillae covered by cuboidal to low columnar epithelia with round, hyperchromatic nuclei, prominent nucleoli, and acidophilic or amphophilic or pale cytoplasm and by a less mucinous appearance Including the cases with irregular papillary architecture with more stratified nuclei and solid or comedo-like structures with atypical structures and cells and nuclei
Immunohistochemistry	Positive for S100P and MUC1 and negative for MUC5AC in these neoplastic cells

Table 3.4d Characteristics of oncocytic subtype of IPNB (oIPNB)

Histological features	Defined by complex and arborizing papillae with delicate fibrotic and edematous stroma, lined by one to several stratified layers of cuboidal to columnar cells with abundant eosinophilic granular cytoplasm and occasional hyaline globules, with hyperchromatic, round, large, and fairly uniform nuclei and with intraepithelial lumina
Immunohistochemistry	Positive for MUC5AC

with controversial subtyping are sometimes observed [3, 4]. This subtyping is facilitated by immunohistochemistry to detect mucus core proteins and cytokeratins [2, 7, 38]. As for the incidence, iIPNB is the most common subtype, followed by gIPNB, pbIPNB and oIPNB. There are no apparent differences in sex or age among the four subtypes of IPNB.

The Surrounding Mucosa

IPNBs consistently accompany intraepithelial neoplasia spreading in the surrounding bile duct mucosa around the main grossly visible papillary or polypoid lesion(s) (Fig. 3.1d). Histologically, almost all lesions of such surrounding intraepithelial neoplasia present the same phenotype as the main papillary or polypoid lesions (Fig. 3.2e), while the gastric neoplasm can be seen in the surrounding mucosa around the main papillary lesions belonging to other subtypes. Their atypia is the same or more atypical or milder in comparison to the main lesion. In addition, in some cases of IPNB, invasion predominantly develops at the site of lateral-spreading flat or non-papillary neoplastic areas immediately around as well as remote from the main IPNB tumor [3, 26]. Similar phenomena have also been reported in IPMN cases in which carcinoma develops in the non-papillary flat neoplastic area around the IPMN [11].

While this lesion is a constant and integrated component of IPNB, its significance or mechanism remains speculative. Some may reflect intraductal spread of carcinoma associated with IPNBs or a preceding biliary epithelial lesion from which the main papillary lesion arises as multifocal tumorigenesis.

Stromal Invasion

IPNB may progress from low-grade to high-grade dysplasia and then to invasive adenocarcinoma (IPNB associated with invasive carcinoma) [2, 3, 7, 26, 55], as is observed in IPMN [11]. IPNBs are not infrequently invasive at the time of surgical resection [7]. Surgical series demonstrate high rates of invasive cancer arising from IPNB, with rates ranging from 40% to 70% [27]. The time lag between the development of IPNB in hepatolithiasis is 6–8 years, and high-grade dysplasia can take 1–2 years to develop into an invasive lesion [74]. Microinvasive carcinoma was the most common level of invasiveness in a previously reported series. Stromal invasion into the duct wall occurs at the main papillary or polypoid lesions and also at the spreading neoplastic lesion in the surrounding mucosa [2, 3, 7, 26]. Stromal invasion in the surrounding spreading intraepithelial neoplastic lesion occurs in IPNB cases in which the main lesion(s) does not show such stromal invasion [26], suggesting that in the clinical setting, physicians should be careful of such spreading and invasion. Extensive sampling may be required to identify small foci of invasion, particularly in tumors with extensive flat or non-papillary neoplastic spreading around the papillary tumors, as is observed in IPMN [9, 11]. Invasion into the fibrovascular stalks near the bile duct wall is also identifiable, resulting in wide fibrovascular stalks. However, the incidence of invasion differs according to the anatomical location of IPNB. That is, approximately 30% of cases of intrahepatic IPNBs are invasive, while many extrahepatic IPNBs show at least focal stromal invasion at the time of surgical resection [3, 70], implying that intrahepatic IPNBs are less aggressive than extrahepatic IPNBs.

Invasive parts of IPNBs usually show tubular adenocarcinoma with a desmoplastic reaction and only occasionally show foci of colloid carcinoma with or without tubular adenocarcinoma components [75]. The oncocytic subtype shows invasion of oncocytic adenocarcinoma.

As may be expected, IPNBs with invasion show a significantly worse prognosis in comparison to those with no evidence of invasion. Pancreatobiliary IPNB expresses MUC1 and is more frequently associated with invasive disease than other IPNB subtypes [2, 3, 27].

Genetic and Molecular Alterations

Recently, several molecular genetic changes have been reported in IPNB, but the molecular pathogenesis remains to be clarified [27, 32, 39, 43, 76–85]. Recently, using targeted next-generation sequencing, Yang et al. identified frequent mutations of *KRAS* (49%), *GNAS* (32%), *RNF43* (24%), *APC* (24%), *TP53* (24%), and *CTNNB1* (11%) in IPNBs [39, 43]. These molecular genetic changes are evaluated below with respect to progression and also subtyping.

Noninvasive and Invasive IPNBs

The development of IPNB follows a sequential progression in association with the stepwise acquisition of molecular alterations affecting common oncogenic pathways [32, 78]. Progression of dysplasia and invasion is accompanied by the accumulation of genetic alterations. *KRAS* and *p16* alterations occur early and in tumors with low-grade dysplasia and precede the increased expression of *PT53*. *SMAD-4* mutations have only been identified in tumors from patients with invasion [27, 76]. The overexpression of EZH2 may be associated with malignant behavior [79]. The expression of IPM3 and DNMT1 is significantly increased in invasive IPNB [80].

Subtyping and Type 1 and Type 2 Subclassifications

(i) *Four subtypes*: In eastern Asia, *GNAS* mutations were detected in less than half of all cases of IPNB, and all cases with *GNAS* mutations had intestinal differentiation with villous architecture and mucus hypersecretion [43, 74, 82, 83]. Mutations of RNF43, a tumor suppressor gene, were also frequent in the intestinal IPNB [39]. When divided into the intrahepatic and extrahepatic classifications, in intestinal IPNBs arising in the intrahepatic bile ducts, *GNAS* and *KRAS* mutations are frequent, as is observed in intestinal IPMN [74]. As for non-intestinal IPNBs, mutations in *APC* or *CTNNB1* both of which belong to the Wnt/β-catenin pathway, were observed in one-fourth of IPNBs and were mutually exclusive [84]. In immunohistochemistry, the aberrant cytoplasmic and/or nuclear expression of β-catenin was found in not only IPNBs with *APC* or *CTNNB1* mutations but also IPNBs with wild-type *APC* and *CTNNB1*. Interestingly, *APC* and *CTNNB1* alterations were unique to IPNB and exceptional in non-papillary CCA [84]. Mutations of genes, such as *SMAD4*, *PIK3CA*, *APC*, and *CTNNB1*, which are also seen in colorectal neoplasms [86, 87], were frequent in intestinal IPNBs of the extrahepatic bile ducts [74], and the pancreatobiliary subtype arising in the extrahepatic bile ducts also showed *CTNNB1* mutation [39, 84]. iIPNB arising in the extrahepatic bile ducts also undergoes a similar pathway [74]. Thus, at present, the activation of the Wnt/β-catenin signaling pathway may be relevant to the development and progression of non-intestinal-type IPNBs, as well as iIPNBs arising in the extrahepatic bile ducts.

(ii) *Type 1 and type 2 subclassifications*: Type 1 IPNBs present frequent *KRAS*, *GNAS*, and *RNF43* mutations, while type 2 IPNBs show frequent *TP53*, *SMAD4*, and *KMT2C* mutations but rarely show *GNAS* mutations [39, 43].

New Subclassification of IPNBs

IPNBs have been studied historically in comparison to IPMNs [2, 12–14, 16, 34, 87]. Thus, firstly, the comparisons of IPNB and IPMN are described. Then, the new subclassification of IPNB into types 1 and 2 is described based on this comparison [2, 3, 38, 41, 42].

Comparison of IPNB and Pancreatic IPMN

There are several biliary and pancreatic diseases that share many clinical and pathological features and which can be regarded as a spectrum of "biliary diseases with pancreatic counterparts" [2, 3, 38, 70, 87]. In fact, the pathological and clinical similarities between IPMN and some IPNB cases have been reported [2, 6, 12, 38], suggesting that IPMNs and some IPNB cases can be included in this spectrum. For example, IPNBs are also divided into four subtypes, as is observed in IPMN [3, 7], and IPNBs also frequently show excessive intraductal mucin hypersecretion. In addition, there have been several reports of synchronous and dyssynchronous occurrence of IPNB and IPMN in the same patient [26, 67, 68].

However, other IPNBs are variably different from IPMN [13, 14, 42]. The following are some examples of differences. IPMNs can involve the main pancreatic duct (main duct type), branch duct (branch duct type), or both ducts (combined type). The branch duct type of IPMN is usually multicystic and usually of the gastric subtype. While IPNBs involving the extrahepatic bile ducts and intrahepatic large bile duct may correspond to the main pancreatic duct type, the counterparts of branch-type IPMN in the biliary tract remain speculative. Cystic micropapillary neoplasms in the peribiliary glands, which usually show gastric immunophenotypes [38, 88, 89], could be counterparts of branch-type IPMN.

While four subtypes are recognizable in IPNB and IPMN [9–11], the histology of the subtypes of IPNBs and IPMNs are not the same in all cases. The excessive mucin hypersecretion from the neoplastic epithelium into the ductal lumen is a highly characteristic and consistent finding in IPMN [9, 11], while mucus hypersecretion is a frequent but not consistent finding in IPNB [11]. Thus, IPNB with excessive mucin hypersecretion may be a real counterpart of IPMN, while IPNB without mucin hypersecretion may be another category [14, 82, 83, 90]. Both IPNBs and IPMNs show various grades of dysplasia, ranging from low- to high-grade dysplasia, while the proportion of high-grade dysplasia is high in IPNB. As for the gastric subtype, a majority of these IPNBs are the branch duct type with low-grade dysplasia and foveola type is predominant. However, the gastric subtype of IPNB consists of predominantly high-grade dysplasia, and pyloric type is not infrequent. The intestinal subtype of IPNB presents villous, papillary, and also tubular components, as is observed in intestinal adenoma in the intestine, while the intestinal subtype of IPMN shows only villous components [9, 11, 74]. Together, these findings suggest that some IPNBs resemble the four prototypic subtypes of IPMN, while the histology of others differs to varying degrees from the four prototypical IPMNs.

There are many anatomical, embryological, and experimental data and backgrounds that support the occurrence of similar diseases in the biliary tract and pancreas [2, 3, 87, 91–95]. Interestingly, the bile ducts may show variable pancreatic features, including peribiliary glands containing pancreatic acini [96–98], which makes it plausible for diseases with similar features to develop in the pancreas as well as the biliary tract [2, 87]. However, embryologically, the origin and development of the several compartments of biliary tree are thought to differ, with the bile ducts proximal to the right and left bile ducts derived from the ductal plates and remodeled bile ducts around the hepatic parenchyma, which are derived from albumin-positive hepatoblasts in the hepatic diverticulum, and the bile ducts distal from the extrahepatic bile ducts derived from the albumin-negative hepatoblasts in the hepatic diverticulum [87–94, 99]. These embryological and anatomic differences and characteristics along the biliary tree may be related to the development of IPNBs with different pathobiologies, some of which are similar to IPMNs. Based on our recent studies, approximately half of IPNBs showed similar histopathological features to IPMNs, while the other half did not [2, 3, 70].

Type 1 and 2 Subclassifications

The low-grade and high-grade dysplasias are mainly graded on cellular and nuclear characteristics and architectural changes of the intraepithelial neoplasm. It is well-known that IPNBs show structural changes or alterations: some cases show regular papillary, villous, or tubular structures and a relatively homogeneous appearance, while others show irregular papillary, villous, or tubular structures and a heterogeneous appearance. Mainly based on these structural alterations, Japan-Korea expert biliary pathologists proposed a new subclassification of IPNB into types 1 and 2 [38, 39, 41–43, 100]. Interestingly, IPNBs with low-grade dysplasia (about 10% of all IPNBs) belong to type 1 (Fig. 3.3a), while IPNBs with high-grade dysplasia

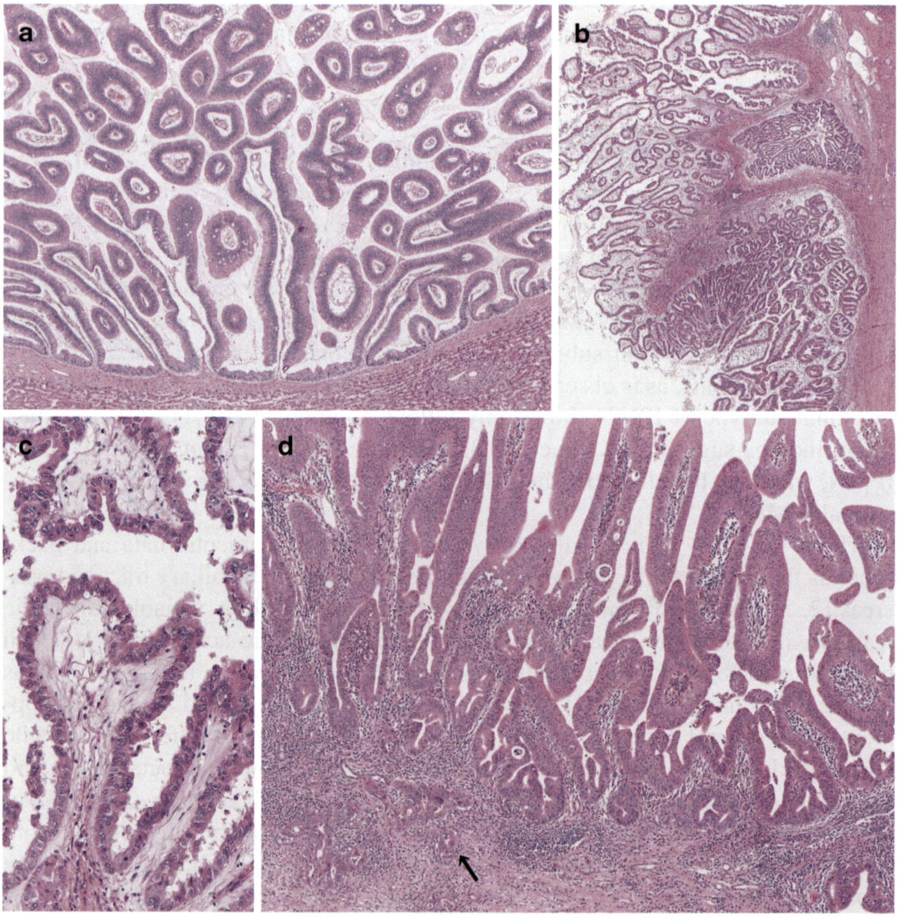

Fig. 3.3 (**a**) Intestinal subtype showing regular villous growth with low grade dysplasia. Type 1. H&E staining. (**b**, **c**) Oncocytic subtype show regular papillary growth (**b**). Cellular and nuclear changes are of high grade dysplasia (**c**). Type 2. H&E staining. (**d**) Intestinal subtype showing irregular villous and papillary patterns with complicated histologies and high grade dysplasia. Arrow shows stromal invasion. Type 2. H&E staining

(30%) also belong to type 1 (Fig. 3.3b, c), while the remaining IPNBs with high-grade dysplasia (60%) belong to type 2 (Fig. 3.3d). In addition, type 2 also not infrequently shows foci of complicated lesions, such as cribriform and solid components, and relatively large cystic changes and foci of bizarre cells and nuclear changes. Coagulative necrosis is also experienced in type 2. Neuroendocrine differentiation has been reported in type 2 IPNB [101]. However, such features are absent in type 1. In type 1, papillary fibrovascular stalks are generally thin (depending on the subtype), while fibrovascular stalks are variably widened at the basal side in some cases. Interestingly, type 1 more or less resembles or shares features of any of the four prototypic subtypes of IPMNs (depending on subtype), while type 2 differs variably from the prototypic subtypes of IPMNs (depending on subtype) [2, 9, 10]. The main differential features between types 1 and 2 are shown in Table 3.5.

As for other characteristics, type 1 tends to arise in the intrahepatic bile ducts, while type 2 develops similarly in the extrahepatic and intrahepatic bile ducts. However, some cases show type 1 and 2 IPNBs synchronously and/or asynchronously in different part(s) of the intrahepatic and extrahepatic bile ducts, suggesting that type 1 and 2 IPNBs could be part of the spectrum of IPNBs along the biliary tree.

Furthermore, according to recent studies, types 1 and 2 show other clinicopathological and molecular-genetic differences [3, 39, 42, 43, 100]: Type 1 IPNBs were

Table 3.5 Type 1 and 2 intraductal papillary neoplasms of the bile duct (IPNB)

	Type 1 IPNB	Type 2 IPNB
Structures	Regular villous, papillary or tubular structures Homogeneous appearance	Irregular and complicated villous, papillary, or tubular structures Heterogeneous appearance
Atypia of intraepithelial neoplasm	Low-grade dysplasia High-grade dysplasia with foci of low-grade dysplasia	High-grade dysplasia with minimal foci of low-grade dysplasia High-grade dysplasia
Location at the biliary tree	Usually intrahepatic bile duct	Intrahepatic and extrahepatic bile duct
Mucin overproduction	Frequent	Infrequent
Stromal invasion	Infrequent	Common
Subtypes		
Intestinal subtype	Equal	Equal
Gastric subtype	Frequent	Infrequent
PB subtype	Equal	Equal
Oncocytic subtype	Frequent	Infrequent
Similarities to prototypic subtypes of IPMN	Similar (depending on subtype)	Different variably (depending on subtype)
Complicated lesions such as solid or cribriform pattern, coagulative necrosis, and cystic changes	Almost absent	Frequent
Bizarre cellular and nuclear changes	Absent	Infrequent
Fibrovascular stalks	Thin to slightly widened (depending on subtype)	Thin to widened (depending on subtype)

associated with a noninvasive phenotype, gastric and oncocytic subtypes, development in the intrahepatic bile ducts, mucin hypersecretion, a relatively good prognosis, and old age, while type 2 IPNBs were associated with an invasive phenotype, the pancreatobiliary subtype, relatively develop frequently within the extrahepatic bile ducts, and present a worse prognosis in comparison to type 1 IPNBs. As for postoperative survival, both types showed a relatively good prognosis in comparison to conventional CCA. However, type 1 is known to be associated with a favorable prognosis, and type 2 is associated with a worse prognosis [42], and recent studies validated the significance [43, 100].

This new subclassification could be promising in the preoperative evaluation and management and in assessing the prognosis. This could be applicable in preoperative imaging and endoscopy, and valuable preoperative information may be obtained [102]. However, its application in biopsies and cytology is limited at the moment.

Diagnosis

Main Clinical Features and Laboratory Data

Intermittent or recurrent, right upper quadrant abdominal pain (85%) and acute cholangitis or jaundice are the most common clinical manifestations, but a certain percentage (5–29%) of patients has no symptoms at diagnosis [27, 39, 46, 50, 52, 103–106].

Alkaline phosphatase was the most dysregulated enzyme [14, 46, 54]. CEA and CA19-9, tumor markers, were elevated in 42% of IPNB patients [27], though they are unlikely to have high sensitivity or specificity for the diagnosis of IPNB [29, 105]. It is likely that traditional tumor markers will be of low sensitivity and specificity for the diagnosis of IPNB or its differentiation from other biliary tumors, as their serum levels vary widely among IPNB patients [27].

Imaging Findings

US, CT/MRI, cholangiography, IDUS, and cholangioscopy are main imaging modalities. Their representative findings of IPNB are shown in Fig. 3.4.

Ultrasonography (US)

Abdominal ultrasonography (*AUS*) is often performed as a first-line modality in patients with some symptom or any hematological abnormality, as well as just screening, to detect both bile duct dilatation and intraductal masses [27]. Biliary tract dilatation is the most common finding in patients with IPNB, while intraductal tumors themselves are not always detected by AUS [27].

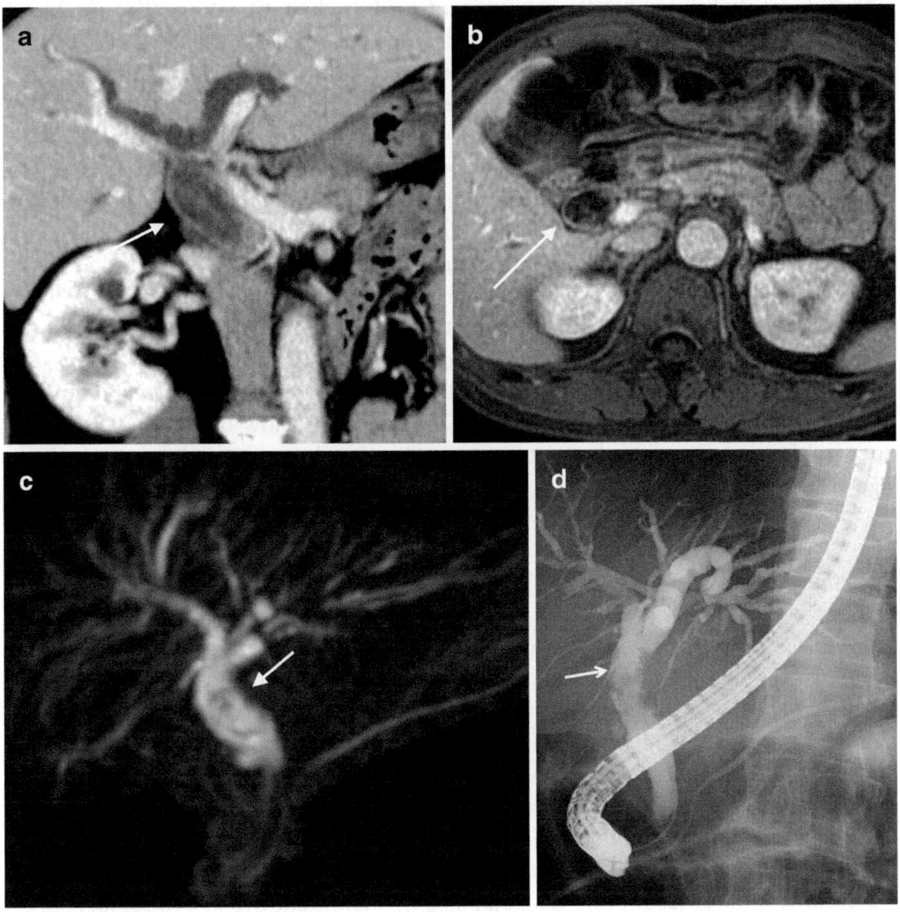

Fig. 3.4 Imagings of intraductal papillary neoplasmof bile duct (IPNB) (60 year-old man with IPNB in common hepatic duct). (**a**) Contrast-enhanced computed tomography (CT) showing enhanced papillary tumor (arrow). (**b**) Magnetic resonance cholangiography (MRC) showing irregular filling defects with dilatation of up- and downstream of biliary duct (arrow). (**c**) Endoscopic retrograde cholangiography (ERC) showing irregular filling defects (arrow). (**d**) Cholangioscopic (CHF-B260; Olympus Corporation) findings showing papillary tumor located in common hepatic duct (arrows)

Endoscopic ultrasonography (*EUS*) was used after other modalities to obtain tissue samples [45, 107].

Cross-Sectional Imaging

Computed tomography (*CT*) including *multidetector CT* (*MDCT*) and *magnetic resonance imaging* (MRI) are the most imaging modalities frequently reported to have been used for the diagnosis of IPNB [27, 69, 107, 108]. The most important morphological changes are the presence of (a) bile duct dilatation, (b) intraductal mass(es), (c) cystic lesion(s), and (d) macro-invasion of the liver [27, 51]. The patterns of bile duct dilatation are diffuse duct ectasia, localized duct dilatation, and cystic dilatation (Fig. 3.1). Intraductal or intracystic masses can be also detected by these modalities, although its sensitivity is reported to be in the range of 41.2–97% [48, 108, 109]. MRI reveals IPNB as isointense to hypointense masses on T1-weighted images and hyperintense masses on T2-weighted images [108]. On CT, the enhancement pattern of IPNB is isodense or hyperdense during the late arterial phase and not hyperdense during the portal venous and delayed phase, in comparison to the normal hepatic parenchyma [109]. Other findings obtained by CT are infiltration of the neoplasm along the duct wall and intense rim enhancement at the base of the lesion [21]. Excessive mucin, even if it exists, cannot be detected on CT or MRI. The addition of diffusion-weighted MRI was superior for evaluating the invasiveness of tumors [108]. Some IPNBs may only show dilatation of the bile ducts without visible intraductal tumors on imaging because of their microscopic size [110, 111].

Cholangiography

Endoscopic retrograde cholangiography (*ERC*) and *magnetic resonance cholangiography* (*MRC*) are useful for showing the entire bile duct to define the extent of IPNB [111, 112]. ERC is useful for the detection of mucobilia, which is seen in nearly one-third of patients with IPNB, as evidenced by diffuse dilatation of the bile duct with an irregular or amorphous filling defect [36, 112]. *Duodenoscopy* frequently shows a dilated papillary orifice with mucin. However, the existence of the thick mucin filling the dilated biliary tree often prevents the visualization of intraductal tumors [105, 111–113]. The luminal communication of IPNB with cystic changes with the adjacent bile duct can also be identified. Brush cytological specimens and even tissue specimens are available during ERC.

MRC is also a standard, noninvasive method for demonstrating the extent of narrowing or dilatation of the bile duct and multifocal intraductal tumors, but it cannot detect the presence of mucin overproduction in the bile duct [114]. IPNB usually shows a signal defect against bile juice, which shows a high signal intensity. The affected bile duct in IPNB does not usually demonstrate stricture or sometimes demonstrates localized bile duct dilatation due to the mucin production of the tumor [110].

Intraductal Ultrasonography (IDUS)

IDUS is reportedly useful for the evaluation of the lateral spread of CCA [120–122] and is a simple method for diagnosing the location of IPNB and assessing the depth and extent of invasion, even in the presence of thick mucin.

Cholangioscopy

Peroral cholangioscopy (*POCS*) can visualize the bile duct directly and assess the extent of the tumor [74, 114] (Fig. 3.5). POCS was recently improved by the introduction of newly developed equipment, such as high-resolution video-cholangiography [115], and can be performed immediately after ERC with endoscopic sphincterotomy (EST). After the sufficient removal of mucin [116, 117], POCS can approach the bile duct directly and can assess the surface and other characteristics of intraductal tumors and the surrounding biliary mucosa [118]. Characteristic findings of IPNB by cholangioscopy include papillary projections with or without the surrounding fish-egg-like or granular mucosa. In the observation of the fine mucosal structure, narrow-band imaging (NBI) is reported to be better than light imaging [119–122]. NBI shows the fine mucosal structure and microvessels in the tumor. PCS allows for tissue and cytology samples to be obtained.

The CHF-B260 and *CHF-B290 scopes* are reported to have a higher capability with regard to making an accurate diagnosis of features such as lateral spread and extent [123, 124]. *SpyGlass DS* (*SpyDS*) is a newly developed peroral digital cholangioscope [118, 125–128]. The SpyDS shows dramatic improvements in several aspects, particularly the newly added injection and suction functions through a two-port adaptor [129].

Pathological Diagnosis

Tissue and Cytology Sampling

ERC and cholangioscopy allow for tissue and cytology samples to be obtained from the intraductal tumor and the surrounding mucosa [112, 128, 129]. SpyGlass-guided forceps biopsy is also a hopeful possibility [126], because it improves maneuverability.

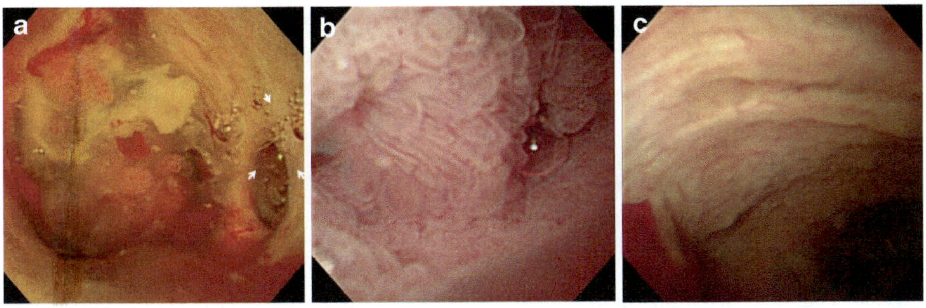

Fig. 3.5 Cholangioscopic features of intraductal papillary neoplasm of bile duct (IPNB). (**a**) Cholangioscopic (CHF-B260; Olympus Corporation) findings showing papillary tumor located in common hepatic duct (arrows). (**b, c**) IPNB visualized by peroral cholangioscopy. Papillary projections in the bile duct (**b**) with the surrounding granular mucosa (**c**)

Findings in Tiny Tissue Specimens

An accurate diagnosis cannot be always made by biopsy because of the existence of mixed pathologic findings, including coexisting or admixing inflammatory and other reactive changes in the same lesion [7, 27]. In addition, the size of specimens is not always adequate, and contamination and other artificial changes are also superimposed.

Structural alterations, such as villous or papillary structures, particularly the villous pattern, and excessive mucin may be helpful in the diagnosis of IPNBs (Fig. 3.6). Typical cells with a cellular specimen composed of papillary groups and linear strips of mostly cuboidal/columnar cells with mild atypia and vacuolated cytoplasm may reflect the pathology of IPNB [7, 103]. However, a pathological diagnosis made using a preoperative biopsy specimen does not always reflect the maximum degree of atypia, because IPNBs are often composed of varying degrees of cytoarchitectural atypia (low-/high-grade dysplasia).

Cytological Findings

Prominent papillary proliferation with often broad, double-cell layered sheets of an atypical columnar epithelium suggests IPNB but may not be specific [7, 126, 127, 130–132]. Fibrovascular cores are sometimes observed. Dysplastic but not frankly malignant nuclear features are often seen in IPNB.

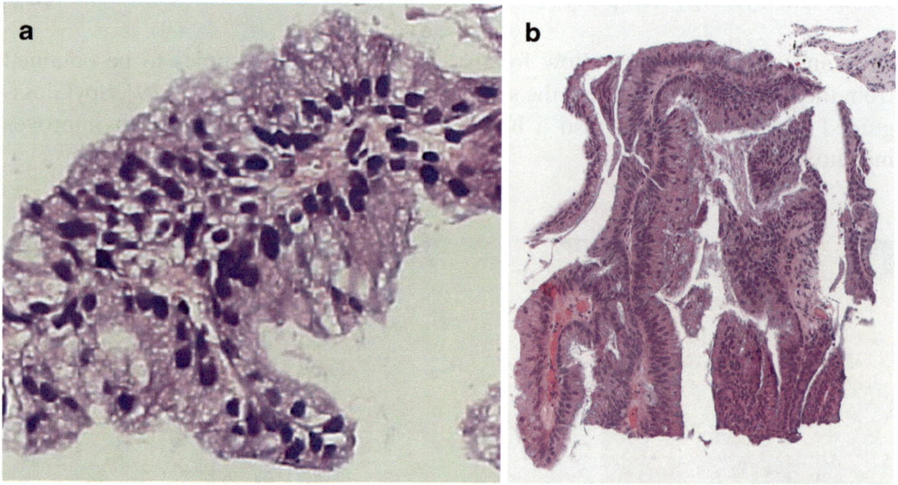

Fig. 3.6 Pathological findings of biopsies from intraductal papillary neoplasm of bile duct (IPNB). (**a**) Papillary cellular proliferation with oval nuclei and abundant cytoplasmic mucin, suggesting high grade IPNB. H&E staining. (**b**) Papillary cellular proliferation with hyperchromatic and stratified nuclei, suggesting low grade IPNB. H&E staining

Preoperative Assessment, Treatment, and Prognosis

Published studies examining the management and long-term postoperative outcomes of IPNB are still limited based on their design as retrospectively collected case series from single centers or due to relatively small numbers of patients from some multicenter studies [27, 46, 55].

Preoperative Assessment

Patients without distant metastasis are eligible for surgical treatment. In order to choose an appropriate surgical procedure, an exact preoperative assessment of IPNB, including the tumor location, histological atypia, extension of tumor spread, and lymph node metastasis, is important [27, 68]. Imaging assessment plays a major role in not only the diagnosis but also the management strategy that is employed [69].

AUS, MDCT, MRI, and cholangiography are usually performed to assess tumor location [27]. However, the existence of abundant mucin often makes a precise diagnosis difficult, and POCS can overcome this obstacle by the removal of mucin [133]. Tissue and cytology specimens obtained during ERCP, POCS, and EUS provide information on the presence of neoplastic or malignant cells, the grade of atypia, and possibly the subtype. The depth of invasion of the tumor is usually investigated by CT, cholangiography, and IDUS [27]. Intramural extension along the bile duct, which is not uncommon in IPNB, can be assessed by MDCT and cholangiography, whereas evaluating the extent of the superficial (intraepithelial) spread is difficult with these modalities. Instead, mucosal observation of the tumor and the adjacent bile duct mucosa with tissue sampling by POCS might be essential [27, 108, 110, 133, 134], although these assessments have some limitations in sensitivity and specificity. Lymph node involvement is estimated by MDCT, EUS, and fluorodeoxyglucose-positron emission tomography.

The preoperative determination of the type 1 and type 2 subclassifications of IPNB is strongly weighted, and it is possible in imaging [102] but is difficult in tiny tissue or cytology specimens.

Treatment

All patients with IPNB should be considered for treatment for two reasons [27, 51, 69, 132]. First, high-grade dysplasia with minimal invasion is frequently seen in IPNB, and the examination of preoperative biopsy specimens shows relatively low sensitivity in determining the maximum degree of cytoarchitectural atypia and the diagnosis of invasive disease [27], as mentioned above. Second, papillary tumors and associated mucin often cause recurrent cholangitis and obstructive jaundice, even if the tumors exhibit low-grade dysplasia.

The major treatment of IPNB is surgical resection, which—in principle—is performed in the same manner as surgical resection for CCA (e.g., major hepatectomy with or without bile duct resection, or pancreaticoduodenectomy). Regional lymphadenectomy should also be performed. On the other hand, in cases of IPNB with low- to high-grade dysplasia and limited superficial spread, limited resection preserving the organ functions (e.g., extensive extrahepatic bile duct resection) can be selected [27, 103, 127]. In such cases, a precise preoperative diagnosis is essential but is often difficult. The subclassification of IPNB may be helpful for making the decision to perform limited resection, because type 1 IPNB usually shows less aggressive behavior than type 2 IPNB [38, 42, 43, 100]. Intraoperative frozen sections of the bile duct stump are needed to confirm a cancer-free surgical margin.

In contrast, in cases of IPNB with extensive superficial spread that may have positive margins, even after extensive resection, resection for the whole biliary tree by liver transplantation with or without pancreaticoduodenectomy is theoretically regarded as the only curative treatment [107, 131, 132, 135, 136]. However, the efficacy of this procedure remains unclear, and the indication of liver transplantation for patients with IPNB is very limited at present [137].

When major surgery is not possible, some palliative treatments such as cholangioscopic electrocoagulation, iridium-192 intraluminal therapy [136], and argon plasma coagulation [137, 138] have been reported.

Survival and Prognostic Factors

While the median postoperative survival of IPNB patients is favorable in comparison to conventional nodular/sclerosing perihilar/distal CCA or periductal/mass-forming iCCA [4, 27, 46, 61], few reports have demonstrated the outcomes after the surgical resection of IPNB. Luvira et al. reported that the median postoperative survival of 102 IPNB patients was 1728 days with 1-, 3-, and 5-year overall survival rates of 86.3%, 63.7%, and 44.8%, respectively [50]. Similarly, a meta-analysis showed pooled random effect estimates of postoperative survival to the time point were 96% at 1 year, 79% at 3 years, and 65% at 5 years [27], although the results varied dramatically among studies.

Factors that have been reported to be associated with adverse outcomes include high serum CA19-9, lymph node metastasis, R0 or R1/2 resection, invasive IPNB, tumor multiplicity, and the high expression of MUC1, a hepatobiliary marker, in the tumor tissue [27, 50]. The gross classification of IPNBs proposed by Luvira et al. also predicted survival very well [51]. According to this report, the survival of IPNB patients with cystic variant and micropapillary lesions was favorable, with no tumor-related deaths within 3 years after surgery, whereas the respective median survival times for IPNBs with unilateral intrahepatic duct dilatation (intrahepatic IPNB), bilateral intrahepatic duct dilatation (extrahepatic IPNB), and macro-invasion were 1888 days, 673 days, and 578 days, respectively. Intrahepatic IPNB shows a favorable prognosis in comparison to IPNBs arising in the extrahepatic bile ducts [139]. At present, the histologic subtypes are not necessarily associated with survival, and there have been no reports on prognostic differences between IPNBs with low-grade and high-grade dysplasia. With respect to the type 1 and type 2 subclassifications of IPNB [42], Aoki et al. reported that type 1 showed a favorable prognosis in comparison to type 2 [43, 100].

Biliary Intraepithelial Neoplasms (BilINs)

BilINs are an another intraductal neoplasm of the bile duct and are found on the mucosa of the bile duct and gallbladder [1, 15]. They are regarded as premalignant and preinvasive lesions, while their exact significance remains to be clarified [16–20]. While gross identification of BilINs is difficult, they may be recognized based on the identification of a subtle and nonspecific granular or rough bile duct mucosa. A histological examination shows flat or micropapillary biliary epithelial changes occasionally with the continuous involvement of the intramural peribiliary glands.

Conventional CCAs are presumed to follow BilIN; however, the exact sequence and progression remain to be elucidated [1, 76]. Occasionally, early invasive adenocarcinoma is found in the foci of BilINs. They are graded as low-grade BilIN (previously termed BilIN-1/BilIN-2) and high-grade BilIN (previously termed BilIN-3 (Fig. 3.7). The former correspond to low-grade dysplasia and the latter to high-grade dysplasia (carcinoma in situ). Their main differential features are shown in Table 3.6 [1, 16]. High-grade BilIN usually forms a field of various extents of lesional spread on the biliary mucosa [1, 16]. Interestingly, some BilINs present with pseudopapillary- or micropapillary-like lesions (micropapillary BilINs), but their heights are less than 3 mm, which differentiates them from IPNB [1–3, 17, 42].

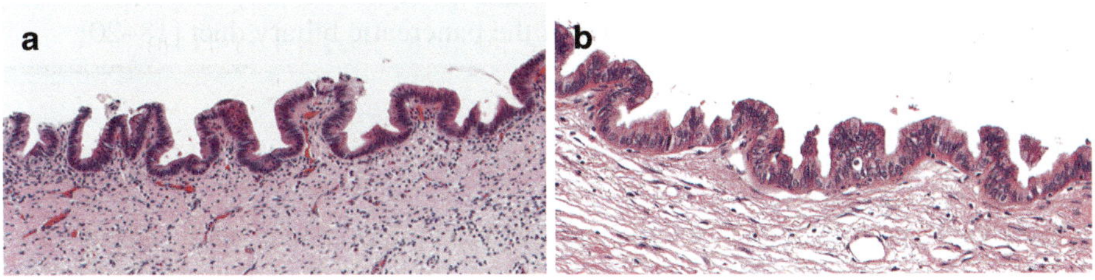

Fig. 3.7 Pathological findings of biliary intraepithelial neoplasm (BilIN). (**a**) Low-grade BilIN. H&E staining. (**b**) High-grade BilIN. H&E staining

Table 3.6 Comparison between low-grade and high-grade biliary intraepithelial neoplasm (BilIN)

Characters	Low-grade BilIN (BilIN-1/ BilIN-2)	High-grade BilIN (BilIN-3)
Histology	Flat/pseudopapillary/ micropapillary Hyperchromatic nuclei Increased N/C ratio Nuclear stratification	Flat/pseudopapillary/micropapillary Hyperchromatic and irregular nuclei Increased N/C ratio, pleomorphic, and bizarre nuclei Disordered nuclear polarity
Involvement of biliary mucosa	Relatively small foci or area	Relatively extensive area

High-grade BilINs are constantly positive for S100P, a differential point from reactive changes [18].

Three cellular phenotypes, including the pancreatobiliary, gastric, and intestinal subtypes, are recognized in BilIN [15]. When BilIN is associated with invasive carcinoma, the phenotype of BilIN does not correspond to that of carcinoma [15, 17].

Similarities to pancreatic intraepithelial neoplasm (PanIN), particularly between high-grade BilIN and high-grade PanIN, have been reported [16]. However, genetic changes could differ between the BilINs and PanIN.

Clinical Features

BilINs are typically found incidentally in bile duct and gallbladder specimens that are resected for other reasons [1, 15–17].

Risk Factors or Background Lesions

In addition to hepatolithiasis, BilINs are often encountered in the mucosa adjacent to conventional CCA and can also be found in patients with hepatolithiasis, PSC, choledochal cyst, and anomalous union of the pancreatic biliary duct [18–20].

Pathogenesis

It has been suggested that chronic biliary inflammation may induce neoplastic changes of the biliary epithelia [17]. *KRAS* mutations occur in approximately 40% of BilIN cases and are identified as an early molecular event during the progression of BilIN, while *PT53* mutation appears to be a late molecular event [76, 77, 140].

Other Intraductal Tumors of Biliary Tract

Several intraductal biliary tumors other than IPNB and BilINs are also reported (Table 3.1), as follows. Some may be a precursor of CCA.

Primary Intraductal Neoplasm of the Bile Duct

1. *Intraductal Tubulopapillary Neoplasms of the Bile Duct (ITPNs)*
   The most important microscopic characteristics of ITPNs are as follows [23]: (i) the tumor is mainly composed of tubular configurations with abortive papillary components, and the tumor cells contain no cytoplasmic mucin, and (ii) uniform high-grade dysplasia is observed throughout the tumor, and no low-grade areas are seen. The expression of MUC5AC is consistently negative. These features contrast with those of IPNBs. The histological subtyping used for IPNBs is not applicable to ITPNs. This may also be a biliary counterpart of pancreatic ITPN [22].
2. *Pyloric Gland Adenoma*
   Pyloric gland adenoma, which resembles a pyloric gland and expresses MUC6, has been reported in the bile duct [141].
3. *Other Benign Neoplasms*
   Benign intraductal epithelial neoplasms are reported under several names [8, 16, 142–145]. They will be categorized into several types or incorporated in other types of intraductal neoplasm in the future.

   (a) Tubular adenoma or neoplasm of the bile duct
   (b) Tubulovillous adenoma of the bile duct
   (c) Villous adenoma of the bile duct

4. *Undifferentiated Carcinoma*
   Undifferentiated carcinoma is occasionally associated with osteoclastic giant cells.
5. *Carcinosarcomas*

Related Neoplasms

1. *Mucinous Cystic Neoplasm (MCN)*
   MCN shows unilocular or multilocular cystic lesions covered by biliary epithelia and subepithelial ovarian-like stroma [25, 146, 147]. MCN is another type of intraepithelial neoplasm of the hepatobiliary system but fails to communicate

with the adjoining bile duct lumen; thus, it differs from IPNB with cystic changes [34, 35].

2. *Intracholecystic Papillary Neoplasm (ICPN)*

   ICPN is a grossly visible, mass-forming, noninvasive neoplasm arising in the mucosa [148, 149] and projecting into the lumen of the gallbladder. Some ICPNs arise in the Rokitansky-Aschoff sinus [150], while some grow through the cystic duct into the extrahepatic bile duct [151].

Mimickers

1. *Conventional CCAs with Intraductal Growth*

   Conventional perihilar and distal CCAs are associated with the following findings: nodular/sclerosing growth affecting the bile duct wall and periductal tissue; and the luminal side of the bile duct from which the CCA might have arisen is obliterated and erosive or shows remnants of flat/micropapillary carcinoma [1, 4, 5]. Occasionally, conventional CCA presents with intraductal growth composed of invasive carcinoma with desmoplasia continuous with invasive ductal and periductal invasive carcinoma [1, 42]. Papillary components, usually microscopic and less than 5 mm in height, have occasionally been encountered on the luminal surface or the mucosa adjoining these invasive conventional CCAs [1, 15–21]. The clinical and pathologic differentiation of these nodular sclerosing CCAs with micropapillary components from IPNB associated with invasive carcinoma are occasionally controversial [152, 153]. At present, "papillary or villous components comprising >50% of the intraductal tumor and papillary growth typically >5 mm in height" are the proposed diagnostic criteria for IPNB, particularly type 2 IPNB associated with invasive carcinoma [42] in differentiation from conventional CCA.
2. *Metastasis from Colon Carcinoma*

   Metastatic carcinomas, particularly those from colorectal adenocarcinoma, also show grossly visible intraluminal growth in the bile duct [24]. They present a cast-like growth, and a histological examination shows colorectal adenocarcinoma.
3. *Hepatocellular Carcinoma Emboli in the Bile Duct*

Conclusions

In conclusion, IPNBs are characterized by grossly exophytic growth in the dilated bile duct and histologically fine fibrovascular stalks covered by villous, papillary, or tubular epithelial neoplastic epithelia. They are divided into the intestinal, gastric, pancreatobiliary, and oncocytic subtypes; the intestinal subtype is the most common followed by other subtypes. IPNBs show low-grade dysplasia and high-grade dysplasia with regular structures and a homogeneous appearance and with irregular and complicated structures and a heterogeneous appearance. The former two are regarded as type 1, while the last is regarded as type 2. Type 1 IPNBs may share features of the prototypic subtypes of pancreatic IPMN, while type 2 variably differs from the prototypic subtypes of pancreatic IPMN. Type 1 and 2 IPNBs showed different clinicopathological features, including mucus overproduction and postoperative survival, and unique genetic alterations. Characteristic exophytic growth in the duct and associated ductal lesions are delineated by cross-sectional imaging and the observation of an intraductal tumor and mucus hypersecretion by cholangiography and cholangioscopy. Surgical intervention is recommended for all patients with suspected IPNB. A further study with a large study population is required to elucidate the characteristics of IPNB and other intraductal neoplasms of the bile duct and to improve early detection and prevention of invasion in patients with these neoplasms.

Conflicts of Interest The authors declare no conflicts of interest in association with the present study.

References

1. Nakanuma Y, Kakuda Y. Pathologic classification of cholangiocarcinoma: new concepts. Best Pract Res Clin Gastroenterol [Internet]. 2015;29(2) [Cited 2020 Mar 1]:277–93. https://doi.org/10.1016/j.bpg.2015.02.006.
2. Nakanuma Y, Sudo Y. Biliary tumors with pancreatic counterparts. Semin Diagn Pathol [Internet]. 2017 [Cited 2020 Mar 3];34(2):167–75. https://doi.org/10.1053/j.semdp.2016.12.013.
3. Nakanuma Y, Kakuda Y, Uesaka K. Characterization of intraductal papillary neoplasm of the bile duct withrespect to the histopathologic similarities to pancreatic intraductal papillary mucinous neoplasm. Gut Liver [Internet]. 2019 [Cited 2020 Mar 2];13(6):617–27. https://doi.org/10.5009/gnl18476.
4. Nakanuma Y, Klimstra DS, Komuta M, Zen Y. Intrahepatic cholangiocarcinoma. In: The WHO Classification of Tumours Editoral Board. WHO classification of tumors, digestive system tumours [Internet]. 5th ed. Lyon: International Agency for Research on Cancer; 2019. p. 254–9. [Cited 2020 Mar 1].
5. Roa JC, Adsay NV, Arola J, Tuis WM, Zen Y. Carcinoma for the extrahepatic bile duct. In: The WHO Classification of Tumours Editoral Board. WHO classification of tumors, digestive system tumours [Internet]. 5th ed. Lyon: International Agency for Research on Cancer; 2019. p. 289–91. [Cited 2020 Mar 1].
6. Chen TC, Nakanuma Y, Zen Y, Chen MF, Jan YY, Yeh TS, Chiu CT, Kuo TT, Kamiya J, Oda K, Hamaguchi M, Ohno Y, Hsieh LL, Nimura Y. Intraductal papillary neoplasia of the liver associated with hepatolithiasis. Hepatology [Internet]. 2001 [Cited 2020 Mar 2];34(4 Pt 1):651–8.
7. Nakanuma Y, Basturk O, Esposito I, Klimstra DS, Komuta M, Zen Y. Intraductal papillary neoplasm of the bile duct. In: The WHO Classification of Tumours Editoral Board. WHO

classification of tumors, digestive system tumours [Internet]. 5th ed. Lyon: International Agency for Research on Cancer; 2019. p. 279–8. [Cited 2020 Mar 1].
8. Hucl T. Precursors to cholangiocarcinoma. Gastroenterol Res Pract [Internet]. 2019;2019:1389289. https://doi.org/10.1155/2019/1389289. eCollection 2019.
9. Basturk O, Esposito I, Fukushima N, Furukawa T, Hong SM, Kloppel G, Maitra A, Zamboni G. Pancreatic intraductal papillary mucinous neoplasm. In: The WHO Classification of Tumor Editorial Board. WHO classification of tumors, digestive system tumours. 5th ed. [Internet] ed. Lyon: International Agency for Research on Cancer; 2019. p. 315–6. [Cited 2020 Mar 3].
10. Basturk O, Esposito I, Fukushima N, Furukawa T, Hong SM, Kloppel G, Maitra A, Zamboni G. Pancreatic intraductal oncocytic papillary neoplasm. In: The WHO Classification of Tumor Editorial Board. WHO classification of tumors, digestive system tumours. 5th ed. [Internet] ed. Lyon: International Agency for Research on Cancer; 2019. p. 310–4 [Cited 2020 Mar 3].
11. Adsay NV, Kloppel G, Fukushima N, Hruban RH, Klimstra DS, Kloppel G, Offerhaus GJA, Pitman MB, Shimizu M, Zamboni G. In: Bosman FT, Carneiro F, Hruban RH, Theise ND, editors. Intraductal neoplasm of the pancreas. World Health Organization classification of tumours of the digestive system. Lyon: International Agency for Research on Cancer; 2010. p. 217–24 [Cited 2020 Mar 3].
12. Kloek JJ, van der Gaag NA, Erdogan D, Rauws EA, Busch OR, Gouma DJ, ten Kate FJ, van Gulik TM. A comparative study of intraductal papillary neoplasia of the biliary tract and pancreas. Hum Pathol [Internet]. 2011 [Cited 2020 Mar 3];42(6):824–32. https://doi.org/10.1016/j.humpath.2010.09.017.
13. Fukumura Y, Nakanuma Y, Kakuda Y, Takase M, Yao T. Clinicopathological features of intraductal papillary neoplasms of the bile duct: a comparison with intraductal papillary mucinous neoplasm of the pancreas with reference to subtypes. Virchows Arch [Internet]. 2017 [Cited 2020 Mar 2];471(1):65–76. https://doi.org/10.1007/s00428-017-2144-9.
14. Minagawa N, Sato N, Mori Y, Tamura T, Higure A, Yamaguchi K. A comparison between intraductal papillary neoplasms of the biliarytract (BT-IPMNs) and intraductal papillary mucinous neoplasms of the pancreas (P-IPMNs) reveals distinct clinical manifestations and outcomes. Eur J Surg Oncol [Internet]. 2013 [Cited 2020 Mar 3];39(6):554–8. https://doi.org/10.1016/j.ejso.2013.02.016.
15. Basturk O, Aishima S, Esposito I. Biliaray intraepithelial neoplasia. In: The WHO Classification of Tumours Editoral Board. WHO classification of tumors, digestive system tumours [Internet]. 5th ed. Lyon: International Agency for Research on Cancer [Internet]; 2019. p. 273–5 [Cited 2020 Mar 1].
16. Sato Y, Sasaki M, Harada K, Aishima S, Fukusato T, Ojima H, Kanai Y, Kage M, Nakanuma Y, Tsubouchi H, Hepatolithiasis Subdivision of Intractable Hepatobiliary Diseases Study Group of Japan (Chairman, Hirohito Tsubouchi). Pathological diagnosis of flat epithelial lesions of the biliary tract with emphasis on biliary intraepithelial neoplasia. J Gastroenterol [Internet]. 2014 [Cited 2020 Mar 3];49(1):64–72. https://doi.org/10.1007/s00535-013-0810-5.
17. Aishima S, Iguchi T, Fujita N, Taketomi A, Maehara Y, Tsuneyoshi M, Oda Y. Histological and immunohistological findings in biliary intraepithelial neoplasia arising from a background of chronic biliary disease compared with liver cirrhosis of non-biliary aetiology. Histopathology [Internet]. 2011 [Cited 2020 Mar 3];59(5):867–75. https://doi.org/10.1111/j.1365-2559.2011.04011.x.
18. Nakanuma Y, Uchida T, Sato Y, Uesaka K. An S100P-positive biliary epithelial field is a preinvasive intraepithelial neoplasm in nodular-sclerosing cholangiocarcinoma. Hum Pathol [Internet]. 2017 [Cited 2020 Mar 3];60:46–57. https://doi.org/10.1016/j.humpath.2016.10.003.

19. Aishima S, Kubo Y, Tanaka Y, Oda Y. Histological features of precancerous and early cancerous lesions of biliary tract carcinoma. J Hepatobiliary Pancreat Sci [Internet]. 2014 [Cited 2020 Mar 9];21(7):448–52.
20. Zen Y, Adsay NV, Bardadin K, Colombari R, Ferrell L, Haga H, Hong SM, Hytiroglou P, Klöppel G, Lauwers GY, van Leeuwen DJ, Notohara K, Oshima K, Quaglia A, Sasaki M, Sessa F, Suriawinata A, Tsui W, Atomi Y, Nakanuma Y. Biliary intraepithelial neoplasia: an international interobserver agreement study and proposal for diagnostic criteria. Mod Pathol [Internet]. 2007 [Cited 2020 Mar 9];20(6):701–9.
21. Nakanuma Y, Uesaka K, Miyayama S, Yamaguchi H, Ohtsuka M. Intraductal neoplasms of the bile duct. A new challenge to biliary tract tumor pathology. Histol Histopathol [Internet]. 2017 [Cited 2020 Mar 9];32(10):1001–15. https://doi.org/10.14670/HH-11-892.
22. Yamaguchi H, Shimizu M, Ban S, Koyama I, Hatori T, Fujita I, Yamamoto M, Kawamura S, Kobayashi M, Ishida K, Morikawa T, Motoi F, Unno M, Kanno A, Satoh K, Shimosegawa T, Orikasa H, Watanabe T, Nishimura K, Ebihara Y, Koike N, Furukawa T. Intraductal tubulopapillary neoplasms of the pancreas distinct from pancreatic intraepithelial neoplasia and intraductal papillary mucinous neoplasms. Am J Surg Pathol [Internet]. 2009 [Cited 2020 Mar 3];33(8):1164–72. https://doi.org/10.1097/PAS.0b013e3181a162e5.
23. Schlitter AM, Jang KT, Klöppel G, Saka B, Hong SM, Choi H, Offerhaus GJ, Hruban RH, Zen Y, Konukiewitz B, Regel I, Allgäuer M, Balci S, Basturk O, Reid MD, Esposito I, Adsay V. Intraductal tubulopapillary neoplasms of the bile ducts: clinicopathologic, immunohistochemical, and molecular analysis of 20 cases. Mod Pathol [Internet]. 2015 [Cited 2020 Mar 9];28(9):1249–64. https://doi.org/10.1038/modpathol.2015.61.
24. Yamao T, Hayashi H, Higashi T, Takeyama H, Kaida T, Nitta H, Hashimoto D, Chikamoto A, Beppu T, Baba H. Colon cancer metastasis mimicking intraductal papillary neoplasm of the extra-hepatic bile duct. Int J Surg Case Rep [Internet]. 2015[Cited 2020 Mar 2];10:91–3. https://doi.org/10.1016/j.ijscr.2015.01.053.
25. Basturk O, Nakanuma Y, Aishima S, Esposito I, Klimstra DS, Komuat M, Zen Y. Mucinous cystic neoplasm of the liver and biliary system. In: The WHO Classification of Tumor Editorial Board. WHO classification of tumors, digestive system tumours. 5th ed. [Internet] ed. Lyon: International Agency for Research on Cancer; 2019. p. 250–3 [Cited 2020 Mar 9].
26. Nakanuma Y, Miyata T, Uchida T, Uesaka K. Intraductal papillary neoplasm of bile duct is associated with a unique intraepithelial spreading pattern. Int J Clin Exp Pathol [Internet]. 2016 [Cited 2020 Mar 9];9(11):11129–38. Available from: www.ijcep.com/ISSN:1936-2625/ UCEP0037052.
27. Gordon-Weeks AN, Jones K, Harriss E, Smith A, Silva M. Systematic review and meta-analysis of current experience in treating IPNB: clinical and pathological correlates. Ann Surg [Internet]. 2016 [Cited 2020 Mar 9];263(4):656–63. https://doi.org/10.1097/ SLA.0000000000001426.
28. Nakanuma Y, Sato Y. Cystic and papillary neoplasm involving peribiliary glands: a biliary counterpart of branch-type intraductal papillary mucinous [corrected] neoplasm? Hepatology [Internet]. 2012 [Cited 2020 Mar 9];55(6):2040–1. https://doi.org/10.1002/hep.25590.
29. Lim JH, Zen Y, Jang KT, Kim YK, Nakanuma Y. Cyst-forming intraductal papillary neoplasm of the bile ducts: description of imaging and pathologic aspects. AJR Am J Roentgenol [Internet]. 2011 [Cited 2020 Mar 9];197(5):1111–20. https://doi.org/10.2214/ AJR.10.6363.
30. Miyazaki M, Kimura F, Shimizu H, Yoshidome H, Otsuka M, Kato A, Hideyuki Y, Nozawa S, Furukawa K, Mituhashi N, Takeuchi D, Suda K, Takano S. Extensive hilar bile duct resection using a transhepatic approach for patients with hepatic hilar bile duct diseases. Am J Surg [Internet]. 2008 [Cited 2020 Mar 9];196(1):125–9. https://doi.org/10.1016/j. amjsurg.2007.04.020.
31. Nakanishi Y, Zen Y, Hirano S, Tanaka E, Takahashi O, Yonemori A, Doumen H, Kawakami H, Itoh T, Nakanuma Y, Kondo S. Intraductal oncocytic papillary neoplasm of the bile duct:

the first case of peribiliary gland origin. J Hepatobiliary Pancreat Surg [Internet]. 2009 [Cited 2020 Mar 9];16(6):869–73. https://doi.org/10.1007/s00534-009-0070-1.
32. Schlitter AM, Born D, Bettstetter M, Specht K, Kim-Fuchs C, Riener MO, Jeliazkova P, Sipos B, Siveke JT, Terris B, Zen Y, Schuster T, Höfler H, Perren A, Klöppel G, Esposito I. Intraductal papillary neoplasms of the bile duct: stepwise progression to carcinoma involves common molecular pathways. Mod Pathol [Internet]. 2014 [Cited 2020 Mar 9];27(1):73–86. https://doi.org/10.1038/modpathol.2013.112.
33. Rocha FG, Lee H, Katabi N, DeMatteo RP, Fong Y, D'Angelica MI, Allen PJ, Klimstra DS, Jarnagin WR. Intraductal papillary neoplasm of the bile duct: a biliary equivalent to intraductal papillary mucinous neoplasm of the pancreas? Hepatology [Internet]. 2012 [Cited 2020 Mar 2];56(4):1352–60. https://doi.org/10.1002/hep.25786.
34. Zen Y, Fujii T, Itatsu K, Nakamura K, Minato H, Kasashima S, Kurumaya H, Katayanagi K, Kawashima A, Masuda S, Niwa H, Mitsui T, Asada Y, Miura S, Ohta T, Nakanuma Y. Biliary papillary tumors share pathological features with intraductal papillary mucinous neoplasm of the pancreas. Hepatology [Internet]. 2006 [Cited 2020 Mar 2];44(5):1333–43.
35. Zen Y, Fujii T, Itatsu K, Nakamura K, Konishi F, Masuda S, Mitsui T, Asada Y, Miura S, Miyayama S, Uehara T, Katsuyama T, Ohta T, Minato H, Nakanuma Y. Biliary cystic tumors with bile duct communication: a cystic variant of intraductal papillary neoplasm of the bile duct. Mod Pathol [Internet]. 2006 [Cited 2020 Mar 2];19(9):1243–54. Epub 2006 Jun 2.
36. Yeh TS, Tseng JH, Chen TC, Liu NJ, Chiu CT, Jan YY, Chen MF. Characterization of intrahepatic cholangiocarcinoma of the intraductal growth-type and its precursor lesions. Hepatology [Internet]. 2005 [Cited 2020 Mar 2];42(3):657–64.
37. Ying S, Ying M, Liang W, Wang Z, Wang Q, Chen F, Xiao W. Morphological classification of intraductal papillary neoplasm of the bile duct. Eur Radiol [Internet]. 2018 [Cited 2020 Mar 2];28(4):1568–78. https://doi.org/10.1007/s00330-017-5123-2.
38. Nakanuma Y, Uesaka K, Miyayama S, Yamaguchi H, Ohtsuka M. Intraductal neoplasms of the bile duct. A new challenge to biliary tract tumor pathology. Histol Histopathol [Internet]. 2017 [Cited 2020 Mar 2];32(10):1001–15. https://doi.org/10.14670/HH-11-892.
39. Yang CY, Huang WJ, Tsai JH, Cheng A, Chen CC, Hsu HP, Jeng YM. Targeted next-generation sequencing identifies distinct clinicopathologic and molecular entities of intraductal papillary neoplasms of the bile duct. Mod Pathol [Internet]. 2019 [Cited 2020 Mar 2];32(11):1637–45. https://doi.org/10.1038/s41379-019-0306-9.
40. Ohtsuka M, Kimura F, Shimizu H, Yoshidome H, Kato A, Yoshitomi H, Furukawa K, Takeuchi D, Takayashiki T, Suda K, Takano S, Kondo Y, Miyazaki M. Similarities and differences between intraductal papillary tumors of the bile duct with and without macroscopically visible mucin secretion. Am J Surg Pathol [Internet]. 2011 [Cited 2020 Mar 2];35(4):512–21. https://doi.org/10.1097/PAS.0b013e3182103f36.
41. Park HJ, Kim SY, Kim HJ, Lee SS, Hong GS, Byun JH, Hong SM, Lee MG. Intraductal papillary neoplasm of the bile duct: clinical, imaging, and pathologic features. AJR Am J Roentgenol [Internet]. 2018 [Cited 2020 Mar 2];211(1):67–75. https://doi.org/10.2214/AJR.17.19261.
42. Nakanuma Y, Jang KT, Fukushima N, Furukawa T, Hong SM, Kim H, Lee KB, Zen Y, Jang JY, Kubota K. A statement by the Japan-Korea expert pathologists for future clinicopathological and molecular analyses toward consensus building of intraductal papillary neoplasm of the bile duct through several opinions at the present stage. J Hepatobiliary Pancreat Sci [Internet]. 2018 [Cited 2020 Mar 2];25(3):181–7. https://doi.org/10.1002/jhbp.532. Epub 2018 Feb 12.
43. Aoki Y, Mizuma M, Hata T, Aoki T, Omori Y, Ono Y, Mizukami Y, Unno M, Furukawa T. Intraductal papillary neoplasms of the bile duct are consisted of two distinct types specifically associated with clinicopathological features and molecular phenotypes. J Pathol [Internet]. 2020 [Cited 2020 May 22];251(1):38–48. https://doi.org/10.1002/path.5398. Epub 2020 Mar 10. J Pathol. 2020. PMID: 32100878.

44. Fujikura K, Fukumoto T, Ajiki T, Otani K, Kanzawa M, Akita M, Kido M, Ku Y, Itoh T, Zen Y. Comparative clinicopathological study of biliary intraductal papillary neoplasms and papillary cholangiocarcinomas. Histopathology [Internet]. 2016 [Cited 2020 Mar 2];69(6):950–61. https://doi.org/10.1111/his.13037.
45. Lim JH, Jang KT. Mucin-producing bile duct tumors: radiological-pathological correlation and diagnostic strategy. J Hepatobiliary Pancreat Sci [Internet]. 2010 [Cited 2020 Mar 9];17(3):223–9. https://doi.org/10.1007/s00534-009-0154-y.
46. Kubota K, Nakanuma Y, Kondo F, Hachiya H, Miyazaki M, Nagino M, Yamamoto M, Isayama H, Tabata M, Kinoshita H, Kamisawa T, Inui K. Clinicopathological features and prognosis of mucin-producing bile duct tumor and mucinous cystic tumor of the liver: a multi-institutional study by the Japan Biliary Association. J Hepatobiliary Pancreat Sci [Internet]. 2014 [Cited 2020 Mar 9];21(3):176–85. https://doi.org/10.1002/jhbp.23.
47. Onoe S, Shimoyama Y, Ebata T, Yokoyama Y, Igami T, Sugawara G, Nakamura S, Nagino M. Prognostic delineation of papillary cholangiocarcinoma based on the invasive proportion: a single-institution study with 184 patients. Surgery [Internet]. 2014 [Cited 2020 Mar 3];155(2):280–91. https://doi.org/10.1016/j.surg.2013.08.011.
48. Lee SS, Kim MH, Lee SK, Jang SJ, Song MH, Kim KP, Kim HJ, Seo DW, Song DE, Yu E, Lee SG, Min YI. Clinicopathologic review of 58 patients with biliary papillomatosis. Cancer [Internet]. 2004 [Cited 2020 Mar 9];100(4):783–93.
49. Shibahara H, Tamada S, Goto M, Oda K, Nagino M, Nagasaka T, Batra SK, Hollingsworth MA, Imai K, Nimura Y, Yonezawa S. Pathologic features of mucin-producing bile duct tumors: two histopathologic categories as counterparts of pancreatic intraductal papillary-mucinous neoplasms. Am J Surg Pathol [Internet]. 2004 [Cited 2020 Mar 9];28(3):327–38.
50. Luvira V, Pugkhem A, Bhudhisawasdi V, Pairojkul C, Sathitkarnmanee E, Luvira V, Kamsa-Ard S. Long-term outcome of surgical resection for intraductal papillary neoplasm of the bile duct. J Gastroenterol Hepatol [Internet]. 2017 [Cited 2020 Mar 9];32(2):527–33. https://doi.org/10.1111/jgh.13481.
51. Luvira V, Somsap K, Pugkhem A, Eurboonyanun C, Luvira V, Bhudhisawasdi V, Pairojkul C, Kamsa Ard S. Morphological classification of intraductal papillary neoplasm of the bile duct with survival correlation. Asian Pac J Cancer Prev [Internet]. 2017 [Cited 2020 Mar 9];18(1):207–13.
52. Barton JG, Barrett DA, Maricevich MA, Schnelldorfer T, Wood CM, Smyrk TC, Baron TH, Sarr MG, Donohue JH, Farnell MB, Kendrick ML, Nagorney DM, Reid Lombardo KM, Que FG. Intraductal papillary mucinous neoplasm of the biliary tract: a real disease? HPB (Oxford) [Internet]. 2009 [Cited 2020 Mar 3];11(8):684–91. https://doi.org/10.1111/j.1477-2574.2009.00122.x.
53. Yeh CN, Jan YY, Yeh TS, Hwang TL, Chen MF. Hepatic resection of the intraductal papillary type of peripheral cholangiocarcinoma. Ann Surg Oncol [Internet]. 2004 [Cited 2020 Mar 3];11(6):606–11.
54. Kim KM, Lee JK, Shin JU, Lee KH, Lee KT, Sung JY, Jang KT, Heo JS, Choi SH, Choi DW, Lim JH. Clinicopathologic features of intraductal papillary neoplasm of the bile duct according to histologic subtype. Am J Gastroenterol [Internet]. 2012 [Cited 2020 Mar 9];107(1):118–25. https://doi.org/10.1038/ajg.2011.316.
55. Jung G, Park KM, Lee SS, Yu E, Hong SM, Kim J. Long-term clinical outcome of the surgically resected intraductal papillary neoplasm of the bile duct. J Hepatol [Internet]. 2012 [Cited 2020 Mar 3];57(4):787–93. https://doi.org/10.1016/j.jhep.2012.05.008.
56. Yang J, Wang W, Yan L. The clinicopathological features of intraductal papillary neoplasms of the bile duct in a Chinese population. Dig Liver Dis [Internet]. 2012 [Cited 2020 Mar 9];44(3):251–6. https://doi.org/10.1016/j.dld.2011.08.014.
57. Patel N, Goodman A. Utility of endoscopic retrograde cholangiopancreatography in the treatment of intraductal papillary neoplasm of the bile duct. ACG Case Rep J [Internet]. 2019

[Cited 2020 Mar 9];6(7):e00122. https://doi.org/10.14309/crj.0000000000000122. eCollection 2019 July.
58. Chan-On W, Nairismägi ML, Ong CK, Lim WK, Dima S, Pairojkul C, Lim KH, McPherson JR, Cutcutache I, Heng HL, Ooi L, Chung A, Chow P, Cheow PC, Lee SY, Choo SP, Tan IB, Duda D, Nastase A, Myint SS, Wong BH, Gan A, Rajasegaran V, Ng CC, Nagarajan S, Jusakul A, Zhang S, Vohra P, Yu W, Huang D, Sithithaworn P, Yongvanit P, Wongkham S, Khuntikeo N, Bhudhisawasdi V, Popescu I, Rozen SG, Tan P, Teh BT. Exome sequencing identifies distinct mutational patterns in liver fluke-related and non-infection-related bile duct cancers. Nat Genet [Internet]. 2013 [Cited 2020 Mar 9];45(12):1474–8. https://doi.org/10.1038/ng.2806.
59. Jang KT, Hong SM, Lee KT, Lee JG, Choi SH, Heo JS, Choi DW, Choi D, Lim JH. Intraductal papillary neoplasm of the bile duct associated with Clonorchis sinensis infection. Virchows Arch [Internet]. 2008 [Cited 2020 Mar 9];453(6):589–98. https://doi.org/10.1007/s00428-008-0682-x.
60. Kim KM, Lee JK, Shin JU, Lee KH, Lee KT, Sung JY, Jang KT, Heo JS, Choi SH, Choi DW, Lim JH. Clinicopathologic features of intraductal papillary neoplasm of the bile duct according to histologic subtype. Am J Gastroenterol [Internet]. 2012 [Cited 2020 Mar 3];107(1):118–25. https://doi.org/10.1038/ajg.2011.316.
61. Paik KY, Heo JS, Choi SH, Choi DW. Intraductal papillary neoplasm of the bile ducts: the clinical features and surgical outcome of 25 cases. J Surg Oncol [Internet]. 2008 [Cited 2020 Mar 9];97(6):508–12. https://doi.org/10.1002/jso.20994.
62. Hachiya H, Kita J, Shiraki T, Iso Y, Shimoda M, Kubota K. Intraductal papillary neoplasm of the bile duct developing in a patient with primary sclerosing cholangitis: a case report. World J Gastroenterol [Internet]. 2014 [Cited 2020 Mar 9];20(42):15925–30. https://doi.org/10.3748/wjg.v20.i42.15925.
63. Kim BS, Joo SH, Lim SJ, Joo KR. Intrahepatic biliary intraductal papillary mucinous neoplasm with gallbladder agenesis: case report. Surg Laparosc Endosc Percutan Tech [Internet]. 2012 [Cited 2020 Mar 9];22(5):e277–80. https://doi.org/10.1097/SLE.0b013e31824a7e6c.
64. Kubo S, Nakanuma Y, Takemura S, Sakata C, Urata Y, Nozawa A, Nishioka T, Kinoshita M, Hamano G, Terajima H, Tachiyama G, Matsumura Y, Yamada T, Tanaka H, Nakamori S, Arimoto A, Kawada N, Fujikawa M, Fujishima H, Sugawara Y, Tanaka S, Toyokawa H, Kuwae Y, Ohsawa M, Uehara S, Sato KK, Hayashi T, Endo G. Case series of 17 patients with cholangiocarcinoma among young adult workers of a printing company in Japan. J Hepatobiliary Pancreat Sci [Internet]. 2014 [Cited 2020 Mar 9];21(7):479–88. https://doi.org/10.1002/jhbp.86.
65. Sato Y, Kubo S, Takemura S, Sugawara Y, Tanaka S, Fujikawa M, Arimoto A, Harada K, Sasaki M, Nakanuma Y. Different carcinogenic process in cholangiocarcinoma cases epidemically developing among workers of a printing company in Japan. Int J Clin Exp Pathol [Internet]. 2014 [Cited 2020 Mar 9];7(8):4745–54. eCollection 2014.
66. Kinoshita M, Takemura S, Tanaka S, Shinkawa H, Hamano G, Ito T, Koda M, Aota T, Nakanuma Y, Sato Y, Nakamori S, Arimoto A, Yamamoto T, Toyokawa H, Kubo S. The clinical significance of fluorine-18 fluorodeoxyglucose positron emission tomography in patients with occupational cholangiocarcinoma. Asian Pac J Cancer Prev [Internet]. 2018 [Cited 2020 Mar 9];19(7):1753–9.
67. Luvira V, Pugkhem A, Tipwaratorn T, Chamgramol Y, Pairojkul C, Bhudhisawasdi V. Simultaneous extensive intraductal papillary neoplasm of the bile duct and pancreas: a very rare entity. Case Rep Surg [Internet]. 2016 [Cited 2020 Mar 9];2016:1518707. https://doi.org/10.1155/2016/1518707. Epub 2016 Jan 26.
68. Ren X, Zhu CL, Qin XF, Jiang H, Xia T, Qu Y-P. Co-occurrence of IPMN and malignant IPNB complicated by a pancreatobiliary fistula: a case report and review of the literature. World J Clin Cases [Internet]. 2019;7(1):102–8. https://doi.org/10.12998/wjcc.v7.i1.102.

69. Ohtsuka M, Shimizu H, Kato A, Yoshitomi H, Furukawa K, Tsuyuguchi T, Sakai Y, Yokosuka O, Miyazaki M. Intraductal papillary neoplasms of the bile duct. Int J Hepatol [Internet]. 2014 [Cited 2020 Mar 3];2014 [Cited 2020 Mar 9]:459091. https://doi.org/10.1155/2014/459091.
70. Nakanuma Y, Kakuda Y, Uesaka K, Miyata T, Yamamoto Y, Fukumura Y, Sato Y, Sasaki M, Harada K, Takase M. Characterization of intraductal papillary neoplasm of bile duct with respect to histopathologic similarities to pancreatic intraductal papillary mucinous neoplasm. Hum Pathol [Internet]. 2016 [Cited 2020 Mar 2];51:103–13. https://doi.org/10.1016/j.humpath.2015.12.022. Epub 2016 Jan 19.
71. Nanashima A, Sumida Y, Tamaru N, Nakanuma Y, Abo T, Tanaka K, Sawai T, Yasutake T, Nagayasu T, Hayashi T, Fukuda Y. Intraductal papillary neoplasm of the bile duct extending superficially from the intrahepatic to extrahepatic bile duct. J Gastroenterol [Internet]. 2006 [Cited 2020 Mar 9];41(5):495–9.
72. Yokode M, Yamashita Y, Zen Y. Biliary intraductal papillary neoplasm with metachronous multiple tumors – true multicentric tumors or intrabiliary dissemination: a case report and review of the literature. Mol Clin Oncol [Internet]. 2017;6(3) [Cited 2020 Mar 9]:315–20. https://doi.org/10.3892/mco.2017.1139. Epub 2017 Jan 23.
73. Kinoshita M, Asaoka T, Eguchi H, Hanaki T, Iwagami Y, Akita H, Noda T, Gotoh K, Kobayashi S, Mori M, Doki Y. A case of intraductal papillary neoplasm of the bile duct that developed 38 years after choledochoduodenostomy with invasive adenocarcinoma and lymph node metastasis. Surg Case Rep [Internet]. 2019 [Cited 2020 Mar 9];5(1):93. https://doi.org/10.1186/s40792-019-0651-4.
74. Nakanuma Y, Kakuda Y, Fukumura Y, Sugino T, Uesaka K, Serizawa M, Terada T, Ohnishi Y. The pathologic and genetic characteristics of the intestinal subtype of intraductal papillary neoplasms of the bile duct. Am J Surg Pathol [Internet]. 2019 [Cited 2020 Mar 1];43(9):1212–20. https://doi.org/10.1097/PAS.0000000000001295.
75. Wan XS, Xu YY, Qian JY, Yang XB, Wang AQ, He L, Zhao HT, Sang XT. Intraductal papillary neoplasm of the bile duct. World J Gastroenterol [Internet]. 2013 [Cited 2020 Mar 9];19(46):8595–604. https://doi.org/10.3748/wjg.v19.i46.8595.
76. Nakanishi Y, Zen Y, Kondo S, Itoh T, Itatsu K, Nakanuma Y. Expression of cell cycle-related molecules in biliary premalignant lesions: biliary intraepithelial neoplasia and biliary intraductal papillary neoplasm. Hum Pathol [Internet]. 2008 [Cited 2020 Mar 9];39(8):1153–61. https://doi.org/10.1016/j.humpath.2007.11.018.
77. Zen Y, Sasaki M, Fujii T, Chen TC, Chen MF, Yeh TS, Jan YY, Huang SF, Nimura Y, Nakanuma Y. Different expression patterns of mucin core proteins and cytokeratins during intrahepatic cholangiocarcinogenesis from biliary intraepithelial neoplasia and intraductal papillary neoplasm of the bile duct--an immunohistochemical study of 110 cases of hepatolithiasis. J Hepatol [Internet]. 2006 [Cited 2020 Mar 2];44(2):350–8.
78. Abraham SC, Lee JH, Boitnott JK, Argani P, Furth EE, Wu TT. Microsatellite instability in intraductal papillary neoplasms of the biliary tract. Mod Pathol [Internet]. 2002 [Cited 2020 Mar 9];15(12):1309–17.
79. Sasaki M, Matsubara T, Yoneda N, Nomoto K, Tsuneyama K, Sato Y, Nakanuma Y. Overexpression of enhancer of zeste homolog 2 and MUC1 may be related to malignant behaviour in intraductal papillary neoplasm of the bile duct. Histopathology [Internet]. 2013 [Cited 2020 Mar 9];62(3):446–57. https://doi.org/10.1111/his.12016.
80. Sasaki M, Sato Y. Insulin-like growth factor II mRNA-binding protein 3 (IMP3) is a marker that predicts presence of invasion in papillary biliary tumors. Hum Pathol [Internet]. 2017 [Cited 2020 Mar 9];62:152–9. https://doi.org/10.1016/j.humpath.2016.12.028.
81. Sasaki M, Matsubara T, Nitta T, Sato Y, Nakanuma Y. GNAS and KRAS mutations are common in intraductal papillary neoplasms of the bile duct. PLoS One [Internet]. 2013 [Cited 2020 Mar 9];8(12):e81706. https://doi.org/10.1371/journal.pone.0081706. eCollection 2013.

82. Tsai JH, Liau JY, Yuan CT, Cheng ML, Yuan RH, Jeng YM. RNF43 mutation frequently occurs with GNAS mutation and mucin hypersecretion in intraductal papillary neoplasms of the bile duct. Histopathology [Internet]. 2017 [Cited 2020 Mar 9];70(5):756–65. https://doi.org/10.1111/his.13125.
83. Tsai JH, Yuan RH, Chen YL, Liau JY, Jeng YM. GNAS is frequently mutated in a specific subgroup of intraductal papillary neoplasms of the bile duct. Am J Surg Pathol [Internet]. 2013 [Cited 2020 Mar 2];37(12):1862–70. https://doi.org/10.1097/PAS.0b013e3182986bb5.
84. Fujikura K, Akita M, Ajiki T, Fukumoto T, Itoh T, Zen Y. Recurrent mutations in APC and CTNNB1 and activated Wnt/β-catenin signaling in intraductal papillary neoplasms of the bile duct: a whole exome sequencing study. Am J Surg Pathol [Internet]. 2018 [Cited 2020 Mar 9];42(12):1674–85. https://doi.org/10.1097/PAS.0000000000001155.
85. Lee SH, Jung SH, Kim TM, Rhee JK, Park HC, Kim MS, Kim SS, An CH, Lee SH, Chung YJ. Whole-exome sequencing identified mutational profiles of high-grade colon adenomas. Oncotarget [Internet]. 2017 [Cited 2020 Mar 9];8(4):6579–88. https://doi.org/10.18632/oncotarget.14172.
86. Cancer Genome Atlas Network. Comprehensive molecular characterization of human colon and rectal cancer. Nature [Internet]. 2012;487(7407):330–7. https://doi.org/10.1038/nature11252.
87. Nakanuma Y. A novel approach to biliary tract pathology based on similarities to pancreatic counterparts: is the biliary tract an incomplete pancreas? Pathol Int [Internet]. 2010 [Cited 2020 Mar 9];60(6):419–29. https://doi.org/10.1111/j.1440-1827.2010.02543.x.
88. Miyata T, Uesaka K, Nakanuma Y. Cystic and papillary neoplasm at the hepatic hilum possibly originating in the peribiliary glands. Case Rep Pathol [Internet]. 2016 [Cited 2020 Mar 9];2016:9130754. https://doi.org/10.1155/2016/9130754.
89. Uchida T, Yamamoto Y, Ito T, Okamura Y, Sugiura T, Uesaka K, Nakanuma Y. Cystic micropapillary neoplasm of peribiliary glands with concomitant perihilar cholangiocarcinoma. World J Gastroenterol [Internet]. 2016 [Cited 2020 Mar 9];22(7):2391–7. https://doi.org/10.3748/wjg.v22.i7.2391.
90. Kim JR, Jang KT, Jang JY, Lee K, Kim JH, Kim H, Kim SW, Kwon W, Choi DW, Heo J, Han IW, Hwang S, Kim WJ, Hong SM, Kim DS, Yu YD, Kim JY, Nah YW, Park HW, Choi HJ, Han HS, Yoon YS, Park SJ, Hong EK, Seo HI, Park DY, Kang KJ, Kang YN, Yu HC, Moon WS, Lim CS, Bae JM, Jo S, Lee W, Roh YH, Jeong JS, Jeong CY, Lee JS, Song IS, Kim KH, Kim HG, Cho CH, Joo SH, Won KY, Kim HJ, Choi JH, Chu CW, Lee JH, Park IY, Lee H, Lee SE, Kim HS, Lee HK, Cho MS, Kim H, Han KM. Clinicopathologic analysis of intraductal papillary neoplasm of bile duct: Korean multicenter cohort study. HPB (Oxford) [Internet]. 2019 [Cited 2020 Mar 1]. https://doi.org/10.1016/j.hpb.2019.11.007. pii: S1365-182X(19)33200-9. [Epub ahead of print].
91. Sumazaki R, Shiojiri N, Isoyama S, Masu M, Keino-Masu K, Osawa M, Nakauchi H, Kageyama R, Matsui A. Conversion of biliary system to pancreatic tissue in Hes1-deficient mice. Nat Genet [Internet]. 2004 [Cited 2020 Mar 9];36(1):83–7.
92. Shiojiri N. Development and differentiation of bile ducts in the mammalian liver. Microsc Res Tech [Internet]. 1997 [Cited 2020 Mar 9];39(4):328–35.
93. Spence JR, Lange AW, Lin SC, Kaestner KH, Lowy AM, Kim I, Whitsett JA, Wells JM. Sox17 regulates organ lineage segregation of ventral foregut progenitor cells. Dev Cell [Internet]. 2009 [Cited 2020 Mar 9];17(1):62–74. https://doi.org/10.1016/j.devcel.2009.05.012.
94. Carpino G, Renzi A, Franchitto A, Cardinale V, Onori P, Reid L, Alvaro D, Gaudio E. Stem/progenitor cell niches involved in hepatic and biliary regeneration. Stem Cells Int [Internet]. 2016 [Cited 2020 Mar 9];2016:3658013. https://doi.org/10.1155/2016/3658013.
95. Wang Y, Lanzoni G, Carpino G, Cui CB, Dominguez-Bendala J, Wauthier E, Cardinale V, Oikawa T, Pileggi A, Gerber D, Furth ME, Alvaro D, Gaudio E, Inverardi L, Reid LM. Biliary tree stem cells, precursors to pancreatic committed progenitors: evidence for possible life-long pancreatic organogenesis. Stem Cells [Internet]. 2013 [Cited 2020 Mar 9];31(9):1966–79. https://doi.org/10.1002/stem.1460.

96. Zen Y, Hubscher SG, Nakanuma Y. Bile duct diseases. In: Burt AD, Ferrell LD, Hubscher SG, editors. MacSween's pathology of the liver. Elsever; 2018 [Cited 2020 March 6]. Chapter 9. ISBN: 978-0-7020-6697.9. Available from www.elsevier.com/permissons.
97. Nakanuma Y, Hoso M, Sanzen T, Sasaki M. Microstructure and development of the normal and pathologic biliary tract in humans, including blood supply. Microsc Res Tech [Internet]. 1997 [Cited 2020 Mar 9];38(6):552–70.
98. Terada T, Nakanuma Y, Kakita A. Pathologic observations of intrahepatic peribiliary glands in 1000 consecutive autopsy livers. Heterotopic pancreas in the liver. Gastroenterology [Internet]. 1990 [Cited 2020 Mar 9];98(5 Pt 1):1333–7.
99. Enomoto K, Nishikawa Y. Development and anatomy of the bile duct. In: Nakanuma Y, editor. Pathology of the bile duct. Elsevier; 2017 [Cited 2020 March 6]. https://doi.org/10.1007/978-981-10-3500-5. Chapter 1. ISBN 978-981-10-3500-. Library of Congress Control Number: 2017938880.
100. Kubota K, Jang JY, Nakanuma Y, Jang KT, Haruyama Y, Fukushima N, Furukawa T, Hong SM, Sakuraoka Y, Kim H, Matsumoto T, Lee KB, Zen Y, Kim J, Miyazaki M, Cho DWi, Heo JS, Endo I, Hwang S, Nakamura M, Han HS, Uemoto S, Park SJ, Hong EK, Nanashima A, Kim DS, Kim JY, Ohta T, Kang KJ, Fukumoto T, Nah YW, Seo HI, Inui K, Yoon DS, Unno M. Clinicopathological characteristics of intraductal papillary neoplasm of the bile duct: a Japan-Korea collaborative study. J Hepatobiliary Pancreat Sci [Internet]. 2020 [Cited 2020 June 23]. https://doi.org/10.1002/jhbp.785. Online ahead of print. J Hepatobiliary Pancreat Sci. 2020. PMID: 32511838.
101. Onishi I, Kitagawa H, Harada K, Maruzen S, Sakai S, Makino I, Hayashi H, Nakagawara H, Tajima H, Takamura H, Tani T, Kayahara M, Ikeda H, Ohta T, Nakanuma Y. Intraductal papillary neoplasm of the bile duct accompanying biliary mixed adenoneuroendocrine carcinoma. World J Gastroenterol [Internet]. 2013 [Cited 2020 Mar 9];19(20):3161–4. https://doi.org/10.3748/wjg.v19.i20.3161.
102. Komori T, Inoue D, Zen Y, Yoneda N, Kitao A, Kozaka K, Yokka A, Toshima F, Matsubara T, Kobayashi S, Gabata T. CT imaging comparison between intraductal papillary neoplasms of the bile duct and papillary cholangiocarcinomas. Eur Radiol [Internet]. 2019 [Cited 2020 Mar 9];29(6):3132–40.
103. Nanashima A, Imamura N, Hiyoshi M, Hamada T, Yano K, Wada T, Kawakami H, Ban T, Kubota Y, Sato Y, Harada K. Planned limited resection of the extrahepatic bile duct in a case of intraductal papillary neoplasm of the bile duct based on preoperative examinations. Clin J Gastroenterol [Internet]. 2019 [Cited 2020 Mar 9]. https://doi.org/10.1007/s12328-019-01049-8.
104. Choi SC, Lee JK, Jung JH, Lee JS, Lee KH, Lee KT, Rhee JC, Jang KT, Choi SH, Heo JS, Choi DW, Lim JH. The clinicopathological features of biliary intraductal papillary neoplasms according to the location of tumors. J Gastroenterol Hepatol [Internet]. 2010 [Cited 2020 Mar 9];25(4):725–30. https://doi.org/10.1111/j.1440-1746.2009.06104.x.
105. D'souza MA, Isaksson B, Löhr M, Enochsson L, Swahn F, Lundell L, Arnelo U. The clinicopathological spectrum and management of intraductal papillary mucinous neoplasm of the bile duct (IPMN-B). Scand J Gastroenterol [Internet]. 2013 [Cited 2020 Mar 9];48(4):473–9. https://doi.org/10.3109/00365521.2012.722672. Epub 2013 Jan 21.
106. Sánchez Rodríguez E, Caminoa Lizarralde A, Foruny Olcina JR, Vázquez Sequeiros E. Intraductal papillary mucinous neoplasm of the biliary tract: a lesion of the bile duct lumen. Rev Esp Enferm Dig [Internet]. 2019 [Cited 2020 Mar 9];111(10):796–7. https://doi.org/10.17235/reed.2019.6186/2019.
107. Patel A, Sonnenday CJ, Schulman AR. Recurrent extrahepatic cholangiocarcinoma after bile duct resection for intraductal papillary mucinous neoplasm of the bile duct. VideoGIE [Internet]. 2019 [Cited 2020 Mar 9];4(11):519–21. https://doi.org/10.1016/j.vgie.2019.07.008. eCollection 2019 Nov.
108. Yoon HJ, Kim YK, Jang KT, Lee KT, Lee JK, Choi DW, Lim JH. Intraductal papillary neoplasm of the bile ducts: description of MRI and added value of diffusion-weighted

MRI. Abdom Imaging [Internet]. 2013 [Cited 2020 Mar 9];38(5):1082–90. https://doi.org/10.1007/s00261-013-9989-4.
109. Ogawa H, Itoh S, Nagasaka T, Suzuki K, Ota T, Naganawa S. CT findings of intraductal papillary neoplasm of the bile duct: assessment with multiphase contrast-enhanced examination using multi-detector CT. Clin Radiol [Internet]. 2012 [Cited 2020 Mar 9];67(3):224–31. https://doi.org/10.1016/j.crad.2011.08.015.
110. Lim JH, Jang KT, Choi D. Biliary intraductal papillary-mucinous neoplasm manifesting only as dilatation of the hepatic lobar or segmental bile ducts: imaging features in six patients. AJR Am J Roentgenol [Internet]. 2008 [Cited 2020 Mar 9];191(3):778–82. https://doi.org/10.2214/AJR.07.2091.
111. Tsuyuguchi T, Sakai Y, Sugiyama H, Miyakawa K, Ishihara T, Ohtsuka M, Miyazaki M, Yokosuka O. Endoscopic diagnosis of intraductal papillary mucinous neoplasm of the bile duct. J Hepatobiliary Pancreat Sci [Internet]. 2010 [Cited 2020 Mar 9];17(3):230–5. https://doi.org/10.1007/s00534-009-0153-z.
112. Yeh TS, Tseng JH, Chiu CT, Liu NJ, Chen TC, Jan YY, Chen MF. Cholangiographic spectrum of intraductal papillary mucinous neoplasm of the bile ducts. Ann Surg [Internet]. 2006 [Cited 2020 Mar 9];244(2):248–53.
113. Tsou YK, Liu NJ, Wu RC, Lee CS, Tang JH, Hung CF, Jan YY. Endoscopic retrograde cholangiography in the diagnosis and treatment of mucobilia. Scand J Gastroenterol [Internet]. 2008 [Cited 2020 Mar 9];43(9):1137–44. https://doi.org/10.1080/00365520802029856.
114. Hyodo T, Kumano S, Kushihata F, Okada M, Hirata M, Tsuda T, Takada Y, Mochizuki T, Murakami T. CT and MR cholangiography: advantages and pitfalls in perioperative evaluation of biliary tree. Br J Radiol [Internet]. 2012 [Cited 2020 Mar 9];85(1015):887–96. https://doi.org/10.1259/bjr/21209407. Epub 2012 Mar 14.
115. Bill JG, Chaterjee D, Mullady DK. Using peroral cholangioscopy to diagnose an intraductal papillary neoplasm of the bile duct. VideoGIE [Internet]. 2017 [Cited 2020 Mar 9];3(2):55–7. https://doi.org/10.1016/j.vgie.2017.10.006. eCollection 2018 Feb.
116. Ogawa T, Ito K, Koshita S, Kanno Y, Masu K, Kusunose H, Sakai T, Murabayashi T, Hasegawa S, Noda Y. Usefulness of cholangioscopic-guided mapping biopsy using SpyGlass DS for preoperative evaluation of extrahepatic cholangiocarcinoma: a pilot study. Endosc Int Open [Internet]. 2018 [Cited 2020 Mar 9];6(2):E199–204. https://doi.org/10.1055/s-0043-117949.
117. Kung JWC, Parks RW, Ireland HM, Kendall TJ, Church NI. Intraductal papillary neoplasm of the bile duct: the role of single-operator cholangioscopy. VideoGIE [Internet]. 2017 [Cited 2020 Mar 9];3(2):55–7. https://doi.org/10.1016/j.vgie.2017.10.006. eCollection 2018 Feb.
118. Park MS, Kim TK, Kim KW, Park SW, Lee JK, Kim JS, Lee JH, Kim KA, Kim AY, Kim PN, Lee MG, Ha HK. Differentiation of extrahepatic bile duct cholangiocarcinoma from benign stricture: findings at MRCP versus ERCP. Radiology [Internet]. 2004 [Cited 2020 Mar 9];233(1):234–40.
119. Itoi T, Sofuni A, Itokawa F, Tsuchiya T, Kurihara T. Evaluation of peroral videocholangioscopy using narrow-band imaging for diagnosis of intraductal papillary neoplasm of the bile duct. Dig Endosc [Internet]. 2009 [Cited 2020 Mar 9];21(Suppl 1):S103–7. https://doi.org/10.1111/j.1443-1661.2009.00849.x.
120. Itoi T, Sofuni A, Itokawa F, Tsuchiya T, Kurihara T, Ishii K, Tsuji S, Moriyasu F, Gotoda T. Peroral cholangioscopic diagnosis of biliary-tract diseases by using narrow-band imaging (with videos). Gastrointest Endosc [Internet]. 2007 [Cited 2020 Mar 9];66(4):730–6.
121. Igarashi Y, Okano N, Ito K, Suzuki T, Mimura T. Effectiveness of peroral cholangioscopy and narrow band imaging for endoscopically diagnosing the bile duct cancer. Dig Endosc [Internet]. 2009 [Cited 2020 Mar 9];21(Suppl 1):S101–2. https://doi.org/10.1111/j.1443-1661.2009.00871.x.
122. Itoi T, Sofuni A, Itokawa F, Tsuchiya T, Kurihara T. Evaluation of peroral videocholangioscopy using narrow-band imaging for diagnosis of intraductal papillary neoplasm of the bile duct. Dig Dig Endosc [Internet]. 2009 [Cited 2020 Mar 9];21(Suppl 1):S103–7. https://doi.org/10.1111/j.1443-1661.2009.00849.x.

123. Kawaguchi Y, Kawashima Y, Maruno A, Ito H, Ogawa M, Izumi H, Furukawa D, Yazawa N, Nakagori T, Hirabayashi K, Mine T. An intraductal papillary neoplasm of the bile duct at the duodenal papilla. Case Rep Oncol [Internet]. 2014 [Cited 2020 Mar 9];7(2):417–21. https://doi.org/10.1159/000364999. eCollection 2014 May.
124. Kanno Y, Koshita S, Ogawa T, Masu K, Kusunose H, Sakai T, Murabayashi T, Haegawa S, Kozakai F, Yonamine K, Kawakami Y, Fujii Y, Horaguchi J, Noda Y, Ito K. Peroral cholangioscopy by SpyGlass DS versus CHF-B260 for evaluation of the lateral spread of extrahepatic cholangiocarcinoma. Endosc Int Open [Internet]. 2018 [Cited 2020 Mar 9];6(11):E1349–54. https://doi.org/10.1055/a-0743-5283.
125. Nishikawa T, Tsuyuguchi T, Sakai Y, Sugiyama H, Miyazaki M, Yokosuka O. Comparison of the diagnostic accuracy of peroral video-cholangioscopic visual findings and cholangioscopy-guided forceps biopsy findings for indeterminate biliary lesions: a prospective study. Gastrointest Endosc [Internet]. 2013 [Cited 2020 Mar 9];77(2):219–26. https://doi.org/10.1016/j.gie.2012.10.011.
126. Kalaitzakis E, Webster GJ, Oppong KW, Kallis Y, Vlavianos P, Huggett M, Dawwas MF, Lekharaju V, Hatfield A, Westaby D, Sturgess R. Diagnostic and therapeutic utility of single-operator peroral cholangioscopy for indeterminate biliary lesions and bile duct stones. Eur J Gastroenterol Hepatol [Internet]. 2012 [Cited 2020 Mar 9];24(6):656–64. https://doi.org/10.1097/MEG.0b013e3283526fa1.
127. Miyazaki M, Kimura F, Shimizu H, Yoshidome H, Otsuka M, Kato A, Hideyuki Y, Nozawa S, Furukawa K, Mituhashi N, Takeuchi D, Suda K, Takano S. Surgical strategy for mucin-producing bile duct tumor. J Hepatobiliary Pancreat Sci [Internet]. 2010 [Cited 2020 Mar 9];17(3):236–40. https://doi.org/10.1007/s00534-009-0152-0.
128. Sakai Y, Tsuyuguchi T, Ishihara T, Sugiyama H, Miyakawa K, Yasui S, Eto R, Fujimoto T, Ohtsuka M, Miyazaki M, Yokosuka O. Usefulness of peroral cholangioscopy in preoperative diagnosis of intraductal papillary neoplasm of the bile duct. Hepatogastroenterology [Internet]. 2010 [Cited 2020 Mar 9];57(101):691–3.
129. Ogura T, Imanishi M, Kurisu Y, Onda S, Sano T, Takagi W, Okuda A, Miyano A, Amano M, Nishioka N, Yamada T, Masuda D, Takenaka M, Kitano M, Higuchi K. Prospective evaluation of digital single-operator cholangioscope for diagnostic and therapeutic procedures (with videos). Dig Endosc [Internet]. 2017 [Cited 2020 Mar 9];29(7):782–9. https://doi.org/10.1111/den.12878.
130. Tsui WM, Lam PW, Mak CK, Pay KH. Fine-needle aspiration cytologic diagnosis of intrahepatic biliary papillomatosis (intraductal papillary tumor): report of three cases and comparative study with cholangiocarcinoma. Diagn Cytopathol [Internet]. 2000 [Cited 2020 Mar 9];22(5):293–8.
131. Canepa M, Yao R, Nam GH, Patel NR, Pisharodi L. Cytomorphology of intraductal papillary neoplasm of the biliary tract. Diagn Cytopathol [Internet]. 2019 [Cited 2020 Mar 9];47(9):922–6. https://doi.org/10.1002/dc.24212.
132. Ohtsuka M, Kimura F, Shimizu H, Yoshidome H, Kato A, Yoshitomi H, Furukawa K, Mitsuhashi N, Takeuchi D, Takayashiki T, Suda K, Miyazaki M. Surgical strategy for mucin-producing bile duct tumor. J Hepatobiliary Pancreat Sci [Internet]. 2010 [Cited 2020 Mar 9];17(3):236–40. https://doi.org/10.1007/s00534-009-0152-0.
133. Vibert E, Dokmak S, Belghiti J. Surgical strategy of biliary papillomatosis in Western countries. J Hepatobiliary Pancreat Sci [Internet]. 2010 [Cited 2020 Mar 9];17(3):241–5. https://doi.org/10.1007/s00534-009-0151-1.
134. Hacihasanoglu E, Memis B, Pehlivanoglu B, Avadhani V, Freedman AA, Goodman MM, Adsay NV, Reid MD. Factors impacting the performance characteristics of bile duct brushings: a clinico-cytopathologic analysis of 253 patients. Arch Pathol Lab Med [Internet]. 2018;142(7) [Cited 2020 Mar 9]:863–70. https://doi.org/10.5858/arpa.2017-0150-OA.
135. Charre L, Boillot O, Goffette P, Geubel A, Gigot JF, Sempoux C, Lerut J. Long-term survival after isolated liver transplantation for intrahepatic biliary papillomatosis. Transpl Int [Internet]. 2006 [Cited 2020 Mar 9];19(3):249–52.

136. Gunven P, Gorsetman J, Ohlsen H, Ruden BI, Lundell G, Skoog L. Six-year recurrence free survival after intraluminal iridium-192 therapy of human bilobar biliary papillomatosis. A case report. Cancer [Internet]. 2000 [Cited 2020 Mar 9];89(1):69–73.
137. Brauer BC, Fukami N, Chen YK. Direct cholangioscopy with narrow-band imaging, chromoendoscopy, and argon plasma coagulation of intraductal papillary mucinous neoplasm of the bile duct. Gastrointest Endosc [Internet]. 2008 [Cited 2020 Mar 9];67(3):574–6. https://doi.org/10.1016/j.gie.2007.07.031. Epub 2008 Jan 22.
138. Cha B, Park JS, Jeong S, Lee DH, Kim JM. Direct cholangioscopy with argon plasma coagulation of an intraductal papillary mucinous neoplasm of the bile duct. Korean J Intern Med [Internet]. 2019 [Cited 2020 Mar 9];34(4):940–1. https://doi.org/10.3904/kjim.2017.301.
139. Matsumoto T, Kubota K, Hachiya H, Sakuraoka Y, Shiraki T, Shimizu T, Mori S, Iso Y, Kato M, Yamagishi H, Imai Y, Aoki T. Impact of tumor location on postoperative outcome of intraductal papillary neoplasm of the bile duct. World J Surg [Internet]. 2019 [Cited 2020 Mar 9];43(5):1313–22. https://doi.org/10.1007/s00268-019-04913-3.
140. Hsu M, Sasaki M, Igarashi S, Sato Y, Nakanuma Y. KRAS and GNAS mutations and p53 overexpression in biliary intraepithelial neoplasia and intrahepatic cholangiocarcinomas. Cancer [Internet]. 2013 [Cited 2020 Mar 9];119(9):1669–74. https://doi.org/10.1002/cncr.27955.
141. Hatzibougias DI, Fouzas I, Bobos M, Papanikolaou V, Daoudaki M, Kotoula V, Hytiroglou P, Albores-Saavedra J. Tubular pyloric gland adenoma of the left and right hepatic ducts: report of a unique case with immunohistochemical and molecular studies. Int J Surg Pathol [Internet]. 2016 [Cited 2020 Mar 9];24(4):347–52. https://doi.org/10.1177/1066896915625110.
142. Katabi N, Torres J, Klimstra DS. Intraductal tubular neoplasms of the bile ducts. Am J Surg Pathol [Internet]. 2012 [Cited 2020 Mar 9];36(11):1647–55. https://doi.org/10.1097/PAS.0b013e3182684d4f.
143. Sato Y, Osaka H, Harada K, Sasaki M, Nakanuma Y. Intraductal tubular neoplasm of the common bile duct. Pathol Int [Internet]. 2010;60(7):516–9. https://doi.org/10.1111/j.1440-1827.2010.02550.x.
144. Akaydin M, Ersoy YE, Erozgen F, Ferlengez E, Kaplan R, Celik A, Memmi N, et al. Tubulovillous adenoma in the common bile duct causing obstructive jaundice. Acta Gastroenterol Belg [Internet]. 2009 [Cited 2020 May 22];72(4):450–4. PMID: 20163042.
145. Čekas K, Rudaitis V, Beiša V, Jotautas V, Rutkauskaitė D, Meškauskas R, Stratilatovas E. Common bile duct villous adenoma: a case report and review of the literature. J Med Case Rep [Internet]. 2016 [Cited 2020 May 22];10:18. https://doi.org/10.1186/s13256-015-0789-z.
146. Quigley B, Reid MD, Pehlivanoglu B, Squires MH 3rd, Maithel S, Xue Y, Hyejeong C, Akkas G, Muraki T, Kooby DA, Sarmiento JM, Cardona K, Sekhar A, Krasinskas A, Adsay V. Hepatobiliary mucinous cystic neoplasms with ovarian type stroma (so-called "Hepatobiliary cystadenoma/cystadenocarcinoma"): clinicopathologic analysis of 36 cases illustrates rarity of carcinomatous change. Am J Surg Pathol [Internet]. 2018 [Cited 2020 Mar 9];42(1):95–102. https://doi.org/10.1097/PAS.0000000000000963.
147. Fujikura K, Akita M, Abe-Suzuki S, Itoh T, Zen Y. Mucinous cystic neoplasms of the liver and pancreas: relationship between KRAS driver mutations and disease progression. Histopathology [Internet]. 2017 [Cited 2020 Mar 9];71(4):591–600. https://doi.org/10.1111/his.13271.
148. Basturk O, Aishima S, Esposito I. Intracholecystic papillary neoplasm. In: The WHO Classification of Tumor Editorial Board. WHO classification of tumors, digestive system tumours. 5th ed. [Internet] ed. Lyon: International Agency for Research on Cancer; 2019. p. 276–8 [Cited 2020 Mar 9].
149. Albores-Saavedra J, Adsay NV, Crawford JM, et al. Carcinoma of the gallbladder and extrahepatic bile ducts. In: Bosman FT, Carneiro F, Hruban RH, Theise ND, editors. World Health Organization classification of tumours of the digestive system [Internet]. Lyon: International Agency for Research on Cancer; 2010 [Cited 2020 Mar 9]. p. 266–73 [Cited 2020 Mar 4].
150. Sato R, Ando T, Tateno H, Rikiyama T, Furukawa T, Ebina N. Intracystic papillary neoplasm with an associated mucinous adenocarcinoma arising in Rokitansky-Aschoff sinus

of the gallbladder. Surg Case Rep [Internet]. 2016 [Cited 2020 Mar 9];2(1):62. https://doi.org/10.1186/s40792-016-0189-7.
151. Yokode M, Hanada K, Shimizu A, Minami T, Hirohata R, Abe T, Amano H, Yonehara S, Zen Y. Intracholecystic papillary neoplasm of the gallbladder protruding into the common bile duct: a case report. Mol Clin Oncol [Internet]. 2019 [Cited 2020 Mar 9];11(5):488–92. https://doi.org/10.3892/mco.2019.1919.
152. Albores-Saavedra J, Murakata L, Krueger JE, Henson DE. Noninvasive and minimally invasive papillary carcinomas of the extrahepatic bile ducts. Cancer [Internet]. 2000 [Cited 2020 Mar 2] [Cited 2020 Mar 9];89(3):508–15.
153. Hoang MP, Murakata LA, Katabi N, Henson DE, Albores-Saavedra J. Invasive papillary carcinomas of the extrahepatic bile ducts: a clinicopathologic and immunohistochemical study of 13 cases. Mod Pathol [Internet]. 2002 [Cited 2020 Mar 2];15(12):1251–8.

Chapter 4
Pathologic Basis and Classification of Biliary Epithelial Neoplasms

Payman Fathizadeh, Hanlin L. Wang, and Robin L. Dietz Jr

Abbreviations

AC	Adenocarcinoma
AJCC	American Joint Committee on Cancer
ASC	Adenosquamous carcinoma
BAF	Biliary adenofibroma
BilIN	Biliary intraepithelial neoplasm
C	Combined
CA 19-9	Carbohydrate antigen 19-9
CA	Carcinoma
CC	Clear cell
CD	Cluster of differentiation
CEA	Carcinoembryonic antigen
c-HCC-CCA	Combined hepatocellular-cholangiocarcinoma
CK	Cytokeratin
D	Distal
DPM	Ductal plate malformation
EHBD	Extrahepatic bile duct
EMA	Epithelial membrane antigen
FISH	Fluorescent in situ hybridization
GB	Gallbladder

P. Fathizadeh (✉) · R. L. Dietz Jr
Department of Pathology and Laboratory Medicine, David Geffen School of Medicine at UCLA, Olive View-UCLA Medical Center, Sylmar, CA, USA
e-mail: Pfathizadeh@dhs.lacounty.gov

H. L. Wang
Department of Pathology and Laboratory Medicine, David Geffen School of Medicine at UCLA, Ronald Reagan UCLA Medical Center, Los Angeles, CA, USA
e-mail: HanlinWang@mednet.ucla.edu

J. H. Tabibian (ed.), *Diagnosis and Management of Cholangiocarcinoma*,
https://doi.org/10.1007/978-3-030-70936-5_4

HCC	Hepatocellular carcinoma
HCV	Hepatitis C virus
IC	Infiltrative class
iCAA	Intrahepatic cholangiocarcinoma
ICD-O	*International Classification of Diseases for Oncology*
ICPN	Intracholecystic papillary neoplasm
IHC	Immunohistochemical staining
IPNB	Intraductal papillary neoplasm of the bile duct
ISH	In situ hybridization
ITPNB	Intraductal tubulopapillary neoplasm of the bile duct
LD	Large duct
MANEC	Mixed adenoneuroendocrine carcinoma
MCN	Mucinous cystic neoplasm
MEN	Multiple neuroendocrine neoplasia
MiNEN	Mixed neuroendocrine-non-neuroendocrine neoplasm
MUC	Mucin
NEC	Neuroendocrine carcinoma
NEN	Neuroendocrine neoplasm
NES	Neuron-specific enolase
NET	Neuroendocrine tumor
P	Peripheral
PanIn	Pancreatic intraepithelial neoplasm
PC	Proliferative class
PGA-GB	Pyloric gland adenoma of the gallbladder
PSC	Primary sclerosing cholangitis
SCC	Squamous cell carcinoma
SC-GB	Sarcomatoid carcinoma of the gallbladder
SD	Small duct
VHL	Von Hippel-Lindau
VMC	von Meyenburg complex
WHO	World Health Organization
ZE	Zollinger-Ellison

Introduction

Bile duct carcinomas (BD-CAs) may occur anywhere in the biliary tract from the canals of Hering to the ampulla of Vater and gallbladder. There have been inconsistencies in the classification and nomenclature used to describe these neoplasms, which to some extent have impeded their understanding from a clinical and research perspective. Historically, BD-CAs have been categorized on the bases of location, growth patterns on gross examination, and histological features. Advancements in genetic, epigenetic, and molecular studies have explored individual characteristics of this heterogeneous group and contributed to the current World Health Organization (WHO) histological classification. This chapter focuses on the pathologic classification of carcinomas of the biliary epithelium (cholangiocytes) and their precursor lesions.

Overview

Anatomically, BD-CAs are categorized as small duct intrahepatic cholangiocarcinoma (SD-iCCA), large duct intrahepatic cholangiocarcinoma (LD-iCCA), perihilar (or proximal) extrahepatic bile duct carcinoma (P-EHBD-CA), distal extrahepatic bile duct carcinoma (D-EHBD-CA), and gallbladder adenocarcinoma (GB-AC). LD-iCCA, EHBD-CA, and GB-AC emerge from epithelial precursors, while no definite precursor lesion has been elucidated for SD-iCCA to date. Adopted from pancreatic counterparts, precursors of BD-CAs are divided into biliary intraepithelial neoplasia (BilIN) and intraductal papillary neoplasms of the bile duct (IPNB). Intracholecystic papillary neoplasms (ICPN) are counterparts of IPNB in the gallbladder (Table 4.1).

Morphologically, the main growth patterns of BD-CA have been categorized as mass forming (MF), periductal/peripheral infiltrating (PI), and intraluminal growth (IG). The SD-iCCAs are exclusively mass forming, in contrast to the rest of BD-CAs which may display one or more than one growth pattern (Table 4.2). Perihilar tumors may also show a periductal nodular growth.

Histologically, invasive carcinomas, IPNB, and ICPN are often categorized based on the overall architecture of the mass and the predominant histological composition. The main fibrovascular/stromal architectures on which the epithelial cells are arranged include papillary, villous, tubular, and cystic. The epithelial composition is often a mixture of biliary and gastrointestinal differentiation with scattered neuroendocrine cells. The most commonly encountered epithelial phenotypes are biliary, gastric foveolar, intestinal, gastric pyloric gland, and oncocytic. The final histological classification is based on the predominant population (Fig. 4.1). In the histological landscape of BD-CA, a range of benign hyperplastic, metaplastic, reactive, and regenerative epithelial changes are frequently present in the background, which adds to the complexity of histological and cytological diagnosis (Fig. 4.2).

In this chapter, we follow the most recent WHO classification of tumors, the AJCC staging manual, and the College of American Pathologists protocols for examination of tumors (Table 4.3). The histological grading of BD-CA is adopted from other gastrointestinal carcinomas and determined by the percentage of gland formation, with >95% as grade 1 or well differentiated, 50–95% as grade 2 or moderately differentiated, and <50% as grade 3 or poorly differentiated. Conventionally, the highest degree of atypia determines the final histological grade of a precursor lesion. The diagnosis of "undifferentiated carcinoma" is applied to those tumors

Table 4.1 General categories of biliary epithelial neoplasms

Benign
Bile duct adenoma
Adenofibroma
Noninvasive/preinvasive precursors
Microscopic
Biliary intraepithelial neoplasia (BilIN)
Low grade
High grade
Macroscopic polypoid
Intraductal papillary neoplasm of the bile duct (IPNB)
Low grade
High grade
Intracholecystic papillary neoplasm (ICPN)
Low grade
High grade
Macroscopic cystic
Mucinous cystic neoplasm (MCN)
Low grade
High grade
Invasive carcinoma
Intrahepatic cholangiocarcinoma (iCCA)
Small duct iCCA (SD-iCCA)
Large duct iCCA (LD-iCCA)
Extrahepatic bile duct carcinoma (EHBD-CA)
Perihilar (P-EHBD-CA)
Distal (D-EHBD-CA)
Gallbladder (GB-AC)
Combined hepatocellular-cholangiocarcinoma (c-HCC-CCA)

without any apparent glandular, squamous, or neuroendocrine differentiation by morphology or immunohistochemistry (IHC). The clinical and prognostic significance of the adjacent vital structures and the predominant growth patterns have also been applied to the pathological staging of these tumors (Table 4.4).

A unified classification based on the biology of these tumors is critical in the era of targeted therapies and individualized medicine. Prolonged inflammation appears to have a central role in the pathogenesis of BD-CA, although the specific etiology or risk factors remain unclear in many cases. The overall pathogenic events involve

Table 4.2 Classification of BD-CA based on location, growth pattern, and precursor

Anatomical location			Cell of origin	Growth pattern	Precursor lesion
iCCA	SD	Peripherally located	Canals of Hering	MF	Not well-known
	LD	Centrally located	BE, PDG	PI, MF, IG, nodular, cystic	BilIN, IPNB
EHBD	P	Hepatic ducts	BE, PDG	PI, MF, IG, nodular, cystic	BilIN, IPNB
	D	Common bile duct	BE, PDG	PI, MF, IG, cystic	BilIN, IPNB
Gallbladder		Gallbladder	BE, PDG	PI, MF, IG, cystic	BilIN, ICPN

SD-iCCA presents as a MF tumor infiltrating liver parenchyma. MF pattern can be seen in conjunction with other patterns anywhere from intrahepatic large ducts to extrahepatic biliary system. In PI pattern, tumor infiltrates around large bile ducts with direct invasion of the adjacent structures. A longitudinal PI extension along EHBDs can present as a biliary stricture. IG may be seen in the large intrahepatic bile ducts or extrahepatic biliary system. Tumors with IG pattern exhibit an intraluminal mass or polypoid projections

BilIN is a grossly invisible noninvasive epithelial lesion. IPNB is a noninvasive mass-forming polypoid intraluminal projection. ICPN is a >1 cm noninvasive sessile or pedunculated polyp within the gallbladder lumen. The concept and nomenclature of biliary precursors have been adopted from their pancreatic counterparts. BE from canals of Hering to distal EHBD varies in shape and function. Epithelial cells lining the small intrahepatic bile ducts are cuboidal with small amounts of cytoplasm. Cytoplasmic contents gradually increase towards large ducts and EHBDs. PDGs are the plausible origin of cystic tumors

iCCA intrahepatic cholangiocarcinoma, *EHBD* extrahepatic bile duct, *SD* small duct, *LD* large duct, *P* periductal/peripheral, *D* distal, *BE* biliary epithelium, *PDG* periductal glands, *MF* mass forming, *PI* periductal infiltration, *IG* intraductal growth, *BilIN* biliary intraepithelial neoplasia, *IPNB* intraductal papillary neoplasm of the bile duct, *ICPN* intracholecystic papillary neoplasm

activation of inflammatory and/or proliferative pathways with progressive accumulation of oncogenic alterations [1–4]. BD-CAs in the large bile ducts and gallbladder generally seem to involve inflammatory pathways resulting in escalating malignant transformation of the epithelial cells lining the bile duct lumen or periductal glands. Conversely, SD-iCCA appears to arise from hepatic progenitor cells in the canals of Hering or bile ductules by accumulation of proliferative genetic and epigenetic alterations [5–7].

The development of high-throughput molecular technologies has led to an increased understanding of the highly heterogeneous nature of genomic and epigenetic alterations in BD-CAs. This heterogeneity may be due to the different background in which these tumors arise and, also, partially attribute to the inconsistency in classifications, terminologies, and study populations. The increase in knowledge about the biology of biliary carcinomas in the past decade has contributed to the evolution towards molecular categorization for potential targeted therapies, which hold promise, as discussed elsewhere in this book (Chap. 21, Munugala N et al.).

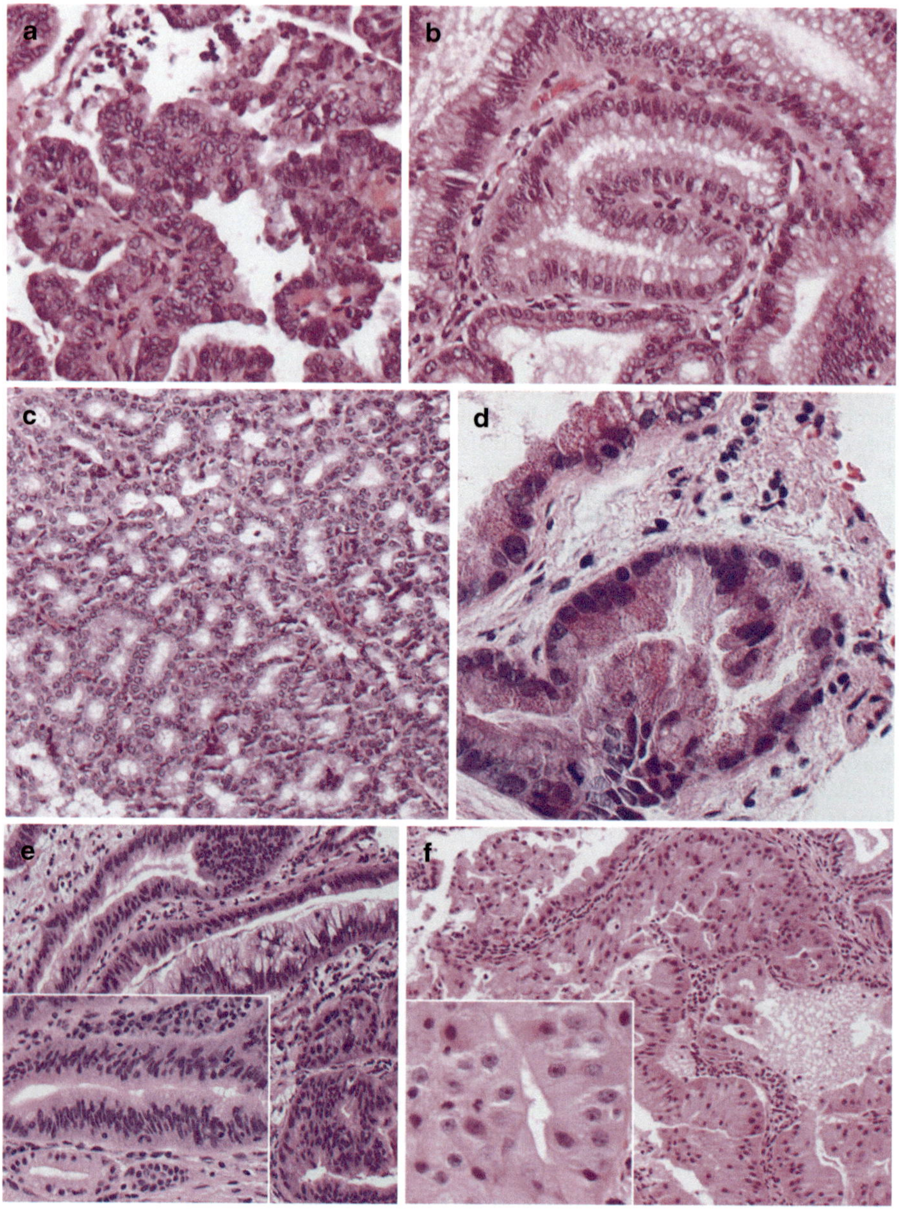

Fig. 4.1 Spectrum of epithelial differentiation phenotypes. (**a**) Biliary differentiation: cuboidal or low columnar cells with round to void nuclei and small amounts of cytoplasm. (**b–d**) Various types of gastric differentiation. (**b**) Foveolar differentiation resembles gastric foveolar epithelium characterized by columnar to low columnar epithelial cells with large to moderate amounts of apical cytoplasm and basally located ovoid or round nuclei. (**c**) Pyloric gland differentiation resembles gastric pyloric gland or duodenal Brunner glands. (**d**) Gastric differentiation may demonstrate a range of morphologies with scattered Paneth cells (**d**). (**e**) Intestinal differentiation may show a range of columnar cells with pseudostratified cigar-shaped nuclei and foci of goblet cell differentiation. A spectrum of epithelial differentiation with overlap phenotypes may be present. (**f**) Oncocytic differentiation is rare and characterized by large cells with abundant granular cytoplasm and centrally located round nuclei with prominent nucleoli

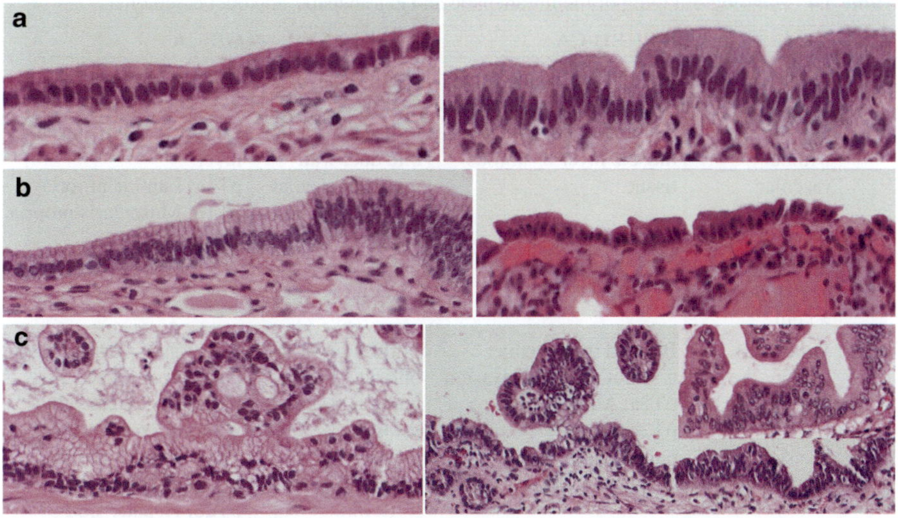

Fig. 4.2 Benign, reactive, and neoplastic epithelia. (**a**) Normal biliary epithelium. Morphology of the normal biliary epithelium ranges from cuboidal in proximal intrahepatic bile ducts (upper) to low columnar in the large intrahepatic ducts and extrahepatic biliary system (lower). (**b**) Reactive biliary epithelium. Under inflammatory influence, the biliary epithelium may undergo hyperplastic (upper) or regenerative (lower) changes characterized by increased or decreased cytoplasmic contents. Nuclear changes are minimal in benign epithelial lesions. (**c**) Neoplastic biliary epithelium. Biliary intraepithelial neoplasia (BilIN) is microscopic noninvasive malignant transformation of the biliary lining ranging from low-grade (upper) to high-grade BilIN (lower). High-grade BilIN is characterized by large nuclei displaced towards the luminal surface (loss of basal polarity) and conspicuous mitotic figures

Table 4.3 Histologic classification and histologic types of bile duct carcinoma

P-EHBD, D-EHBD, and gallbladder	iCCA
Adenocarcinoma	*Adenocarcinoma*
Biliary type Intestinal type Mucinous adenocarcinoma Clear cell adenocarcinoma Signet-ring cell (poorly cohesive) carcinoma Adenosquamous carcinoma Mucinous cystic neoplasm with an associated invasive carcinoma	LD-iCCA SD-iCCA c-HCC-CCA IPNB with an associated invasive carcinoma MCN with an associated invasive carcinoma
Other carcinoma types	*Other carcinoma types*
Squamous cell carcinoma Undifferentiated carcinoma Large cell neuroendocrine carcinoma Small cell neuroendocrine carcinoma MiNEN Carcinoma, type cannot be determined	Undifferentiated carcinoma Large cell neuroendocrine carcinoma Small cell neuroendocrine carcinoma MiNEN Carcinoma, type cannot be determined

P-EHBD perihilar (or proximal) extrahepatic bile duct, *D-EHBD* distal extrahepatic bile duct, *MiNEN* mixed neuroendocrine-non-neuroendocrine neoplasm, *LD-iCCA* large bile duct intrahepatic cholangiocarcinoma, *SD-iCCA* small duct intrahepatic cholangiocarcinoma, *c-HCC-CCA* combined hepatocellular-cholangiocarcinoma, *IPNB* intraductal papillary neoplasm of the bile duct, *MCN* mucinous cystic neoplasm

Table 4.4 Pathologic staging of the intrahepatic and extrahepatic bile duct carcinomas

	iCCA	P-EHBD-CA	D-EHBD-CA	GB-CA
pTis	Intraductal tumor	High-grade dysplasia	High-grade dysplasia	High-grade dysplasia
pT1	Solitary without vascular invasion pT1a: Solitary <5 cm pT1 b: Solitary >5 cm	Confined to the bile duct muscle layer or fibrous tissue	Infiltration of the bile duct wall without vascular invasion Depth of infiltration <5 mm	Confined to the muscular layer pT1a: Lamina propria pT1b: Muscularis propria
pT2	Multifocal and/or intrahepatic vascular invasion	Beyond the bile duct without vascular invasion pT2a: Adipose tissue pT2b: Hepatic parenchyma	Infiltration of the bile duct wall without vascular invasion Depth of infiltration 5–12 mm	Invasion to perimuscular connective tissue pT2a: Peritoneal side without serosal surface (visceral peritoneum) invasion pT2b: Hepatic side without extension into the liver
pT3	Visceral peritoneal perforation	Invasion to unilateral branches of the portal vein or hepatic artery	Infiltration of the bile duct wall without vascular invasion Depth of infiltration >12 mm	Extension beyond gallbladder Serosal perforation, hepatic parenchyma, and/or one other adjacent organ/structure such as extrahepatic bile ducts, omentum, pancreas, or gastrointestinal tract
pT4	Extrahepatic invasion	Invasion to main portal vein or its branches bilaterally, or common hepatic artery, or unilateral second-order biliary radicals with contralateral portal vein or hepatic artery involvement	Vascular invasion Celiac axis, superior mesenteric artery, and/or common hepatic artery	Extension beyond gallbladder Main portal vein, hepatic artery, or two or more extrahepatic organs/structures

iCCA intrahepatic cholangiocarcinoma, *P-EHBD-CA* perihilar extrahepatic bile duct carcinoma, *D-EHBD-CA* distal extrahepatic bile duct carcinoma, *GB-CA* gallbladder carcinoma

Biliary Intraepithelial Neoplasia (BilIN)

Biliary intraepithelial neoplasia (BilIN) is a microscopic, preinvasive, flat, or micropapillary neoplasm of the biliary epithelium [8, 9]. BilIN is a precursor lesion of carcinomas of the extrahepatic, perihilar, and large hilar bile ducts. The concept and terminology of BilIN are adopted from pancreatic intraepithelial neoplasia (PanIN) and represent the noninvasive/preinvasive steps of carcinogenesis in the flat epithelium.

Epidemiology and Clinical Presentation of BilIN

BilIN is an asymptomatic microscopic finding in surgical specimens removed for other reasons; therefore, the real incidence of these lesions has not been accurately determined [10]. Most data are collected in association with other conditions (cholelithiasis, primary sclerosing cholangitis (PSC), cirrhosis, etc.). The overall incidence of and risk factors for BilIN seem to parallel invasive carcinoma and IPNB. In Asian countries, BilIN is more frequently intrahepatic and associated with flukes and hepatolithiasis, whereas in the United States and Western countries, these lesions are often extrahepatic and related to PSC, cholelithiasis, choledochal maljunction or cysts, and chemicals such as Thorotrast [11, 12]. In regions where cholelithiasis is endemic, low-grade and high-grade BilINs are present in 15% and up to 3.5% of cholecystectomy specimens, respectively, compared to 5% and 0.1% as reported in other countries [8]. BilIN has been reported in hilar and extrahepatic biliary carcinomas (58%) and carcinomas arising in the setting of PSC (83%), hepatitis C (HCV) cirrhosis (92%), and alcoholic cirrhosis (95%). In one study, the incidence of BilIN in the setting of PSC with and without carcinoma was 83% and 37%, respectively [13]. Multifocal BilIN (≥10 ducts) has been reported in most biliary carcinomas occurring in the setting of cirrhosis (alcoholic 91%, alcoholic + HCV 92%, HCV 61%) [13–15].

Macroscopy and Microscopy of BilIN

On gross examination, the mucosa may appear unremarkable, thickened, or finely granular. The gold standard of diagnosis and classification of BilIN rests on the severity of architectural and cytological atypia by routine histological examination. Ancillary studies have limited utility [9, 10]. The fifth edition of the WHO classification reduced the traditional three-tiered BilIN system to a two-tiered system, where the former BilIN-1 (low-grade), BilIN-2 (intermediate-grade), and BilIN-3 (high-grade) categories are now simply low-grade BilIN (BilIN-1 and BilIN-2) and high-grade BilIN (BilIN-3). Improved diagnostic reproducibility, understanding of BilIN biological nature (including formation, progression, and behavior), and clinical management were the primary drivers of this revision [8, 13, 16, 17].

Low-grade BilIN is typically focal with a flat or low micropapillary configuration. Epithelial cells are cuboidal or low columnar with hyperchromatic round to ovoid nuclei and high N:C ratio. Nuclei are confined to the basal or mid-portion of the cytoplasm. Elongated nuclei with focal nuclear pseudostratification (formerly BilIN-2) are currently categorized in this group (Fig. 4.2). The proliferative index, highlighted by Ki67, may be mildly to moderately increased.

High-grade BilIN (carcinoma in situ) may be flat or form complex micropapillary architecture. In denuded mucosa, clinging high-grade epithelium may be the only microscopic finding. Epithelial cells arranged in micropapillary configuration contain large hyperchromatic nuclei with irregular nuclear contour and nuclear pleomorphism (Fig. 4.2). Loss of basal nuclear orientation with displacement to the luminal side of the cytoplasm, conspicuous nuclear pseudostratification, and markedly increased Ki67 labeling are characteristic findings. Neoplastic changes commonly extend to the peribiliary glands. When mitoses are present in the BilIN, it suggests a high-grade lesion [8–10, 14, 16, 17]; mitoses may be seen in the reactive, non-dysplastic epithelium, however.

Inflammatory conditions and procedural interventions (such as stent placement) often result in significantly atypical, yet benign, epithelial changes. The distinction between low-grade BilIN and non-neoplastic atypical epithelial changes (hyperplastic and regenerative) is a common diagnostic challenge. Benign lesions are flat, low papillary, or focally low micropapillary, and the epithelial lining may be mildly crowded compared to the normal surrounding mucosa. Benign epithelial changes characteristically exhibit a gradual transition to the normal epithelium, whereas the transition between neoplastic and normal epithelium is abrupt. The hyperplastic biliary epithelium is columnar with increased apical cytoplasm and basally aligned small round nuclei. Regenerative atypia is characterized by attenuated epithelium, cytoplasmic basophilia, prominent intercellular clefts, isomorphic nuclei, smooth nuclear contour, and evenly dispersed fine chromatin (Fig. 4.2) [9, 10, 16]. Occasional mitosis with normal configuration, necrosis, and inflammatory infiltration may be present in the regenerative/reactive biliary epithelium and, in the absence of other neoplastic features, is not adequate for the diagnosis of intraepithelial neoplasia.

In cytologic preparations, high-grade BilIN and invasive carcinoma may share features. The most consistent findings are a "two-cell (benign and neoplastic) population," three-dimensional arrangement, cellular discohesion, nuclear pleomorphism, high N:C ratio, irregular nuclear contour, unevenly distributed nuclear chromatin, and single cytoplasmic mucin vacuoles. Hypercellularity, necrosis, inflammation, and mitosis are not definitive cytological criteria. Low-grade BilIN shows milder cytological changes, often difficult to distinguish from benign epithelial changes [8, 16, 18].

Ancillary studies generally have limited value in the diagnosis of BilIN. The Ki67 proliferative index in the malignant neoplastic biliary epithelium is significantly higher than in non-neoplastic reactive epithelium. Overexpression of *p53* is present in a subset of lesions and is a late event in the high-grade and invasive stage. Overexpression of *p53* and S100P supports neoplastic change and has not been described in benign epithelial changes [16, 19–21]. A recent study described CD15 expression in neoplastic biliary epithelium with a sensitivity and specificity of 80% and 90%, respectively [22]. In some instances, with marked inflammation or other significant confounding factors, a diagnosis of "indeterminate for dysplasia" has been proposed.

Pathogenesis and Molecular Pathology of BilIN

The pathogenesis of BilIN involves prolonged inflammation followed by sequential accumulation of genetic and epigenetic alterations and malignant transformation of the biliary epithelium. *KRAS* and *p53* mutations are the most common alterations in the progression of normal epithelium to BilIN and invasive carcinoma. *KRAS* mutation is an early event detected in BilIN (30%), non-neoplastic large duct epithelium (41%), and periductal glands (44%). As mentioned earlier, *p53* overexpression is a late event and is identified in invasive carcinoma of extrahepatic (38%) and large intrahepatic (18%) ducts [16, 23–25]. Progression of low-grade BilIN to high-grade BilIN and biliary-type adenocarcinoma is associated with an increased expression of MUC1 (EMA). Except for the intestinal phenotype, BilINs are typically negative for MUC2 [16, 26–28].

Intraductal Papillary Neoplasm of the Bile Duct (IPNB)

Intraductal papillary neoplasms of the bile duct (IPNBs) are grossly visible, noninvasive neoplasms of the bile duct epithelium. They grossly appear as sessile or pedunculated intraluminal projections. The WHO classification uses the term "IPNB" as a substitute for other diagnostic terminologies such as biliary papilloma, biliary papillomatosis, biliary adenoma, noninvasive papillary neoplasm, and mucin-secreting biliary tumor.

Epidemiology and Clinical Presentation of IPNB

The incidence, risk factors, and location (i.e., distribution) of IPNB as well as the rate of association with invasive carcinoma vary in different regions of the world [29, 30]. The overall peak incidence is in the 60th and 70th decades of life, with a slight male predominance [31]. The prevalence of IPNB in Korea, Japan, and China is significantly higher than in Western countries. Furthermore, in Asian countries, IPNB accounts for 10–30% of bile duct tumors compared to 7–11% in Western countries [30, 31]. In most cases, the etiology of IPNBs is unclear. Flukes and lithiasis are common risk factors in Asian patients, whereas in the Western hemisphere, most IPNBs are associated with conditions such as PSC [31–34]. The clinical and radiologic features of IPNB vary in different patient populations [29, 30]. In the United States, most IPNBs are in the perihilar region (60%), followed by distal common bile duct (30%) and liver (10%). Invasive carcinoma is more frequently present in IPNBs arising in distal bile ducts (93%), compared to the hilar (65%), and the intrahepatic (25%) lesions [30]. Abdominal pain, jaundice, weight loss, cholangitis, and fever are the most common symptoms. Serum bilirubin levels and liver function tests are abnormal in most patients [31, 35]. Radiographic studies reveal biliary dilatation (>80%), intraluminal mass, and biliary stones.

IPNBs are heterogeneous neoplasms with different survival rates. Theoretically, complete excision of IPNBs without an invasive component is curative. However, recurrence (local or remote) 5 years after surgery with invasive carcinoma has been reported in these patients, albeit rarely [30]. Invasive carcinoma is present in 40–80% of IPNBs at the time of diagnosis, which adversely affects disease-free survival; however, the overall prognosis is better than ordinary biliary adenocarcinoma [33, 34, 36–38]. In IPNBs with invasive carcinoma, depth of invasion more than 0.5 cm, an invasive component of more than 10%, poorly differentiated histology, expression of MUC1, and lymphovascular invasion are all significant prognostic factors [30, 33, 39]. Radiologic appearance of IPNB as a predictor of survival has been investigated [36]. Based on radiologic patterns, IPNB can be categorized into five classes: class 1, "classic intrahepatic" IPNB with intraductal mass and unilateral intrahepatic duct dilatation; class 2, "classic extrahepatic" IPNB with intraluminal mass and bilateral intrahepatic dilatation; class 3, "cystic variant" characterized by a cystic lesion with visible internal papillary projections and communication with the bile duct; class 4, "micropapillary" lesion without discernible tumor but with disproportionate bile duct dilatation; and class 5, "macroinvasive tumor" with grossly visible infiltrative tumor arising from IPNB. In a large series of Asian patients, class 1 was the most frequent (46%), followed by classes 5, 4, 2, and 3. All patients with class 3 and class 4 patterns survived through the 3 years postoperative follow-up, while the median survival time was significantly shorter in class 1 (63 months), class 2 (63 months), and class 5 (19 months) [36]. It is plausible that class 4 pattern represents a cystic variant of the IPNB and is regarded as development of IPNB within the periductal gland. Many authorities consider the cystic IPNB as the biliary counterparts of the branching duct-type IPMN of the pancreas, which can explain the comparable behavior of these tumors and long-term survival in these patients [39, 40].

Macroscopy and Microscopy of IPNB

Regardless of location, IPNBs present as sessile or pedunculated polyps with papillary, tubulopapillary, or villous architecture. The majority of IPNBs are papillary (80%), followed by villous and tubulopapillary. "Biliary papillomatosis" is a rare condition characterized by several papillary lesions along the bile ducts [41]. The location and quantity of mucin secretion play essential roles in the macroscopic and radiologic appearance of IPNBs. Non-mucinous extrahepatic IPNBs cause dilatation of the proximal bile duct lumen; in contrast, IPNBs with mucin hypersecretion result in a fusiform pattern due to distention of the proximal and distal ductal segments. Intrahepatic IPNBs more often appear as a unilocular or multilocular cystic mass, which can be confused with mucinous cystic neoplasm (MCN) of the bile duct [8]. Similarly, IPNBs arising from peribiliary glands may form cystic or saccular lesions around large bile ducts [32, 39]. Periductal nodularity may represent intramural involvement. Invasive carcinoma associated with IPNBs is difficult to appreciate on gross examination. Thus, complete sampling and careful microscopic examination of the entire exophytic lesion and the grossly unremarkable adjacent wall are required.

IPNBs usually display a mixture of biliary (pancreaticobiliary), intestinal, gastric foveolar, gastric pyloric gland-like, and oncocytic phenotypes. Conventionally, the predominant proportion determines the histological type (Fig. 4.3). The most common epithelial type in the United States is the biliary type (70%), followed by gastric foveolar, oncocytic, and intestinal types [30]. In Asian countries, the intestinal type is more common. It has been suggested that predominant or substantial gastric-type differentiation is a prognostically favorable histological finding [30].

Based on their similarities to pancreatic intraductal papillary mucinous neoplasm (IPMN), Nakanuma et al. proposed to classify IPNBs into type 1 IPNB, with features similar to IPMN, and type 2 IPNB, incompatible with IPMN [42]. According to their study, type 1 IPNBs are likely to occur in the large intrahepatic (hilar) or proximal extrahepatic (perihilar) hepatic ducts. Histologically, type 1 IPNBs display a regular and homogenous architecture with mild cytological atypia and rare complex cellular configurations (i.e., solid, cribriform, or crowded). They are typically mucin-producing and associated with stromal invasion in less than 50% of

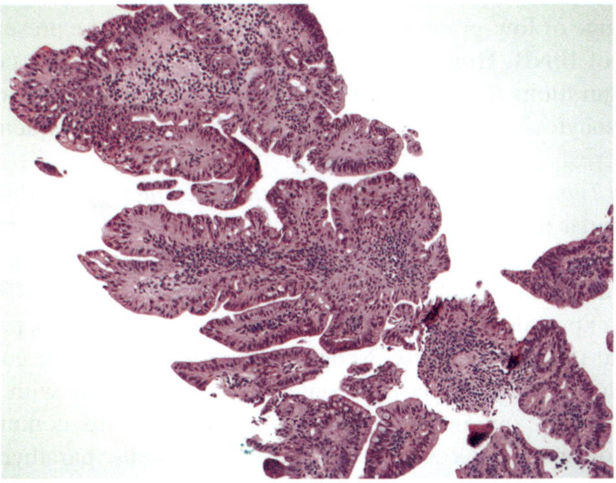

Fig. 4.3 Intraductal papillary neoplasm of the common bile duct showing papillary proliferation of dysplastic biliary-type epithelial cells (intraductal biopsy specimen). The patient presented with biliary obstruction. Endoscopic retrograde cholangiopancreatography showed a papillary lesion in the common bile duct that partially obstructed the duct lumen. Endoscopic ultrasound showed no evidence of infiltrative growth in the duct wall or surrounding tissue

cases. Type 2 IPNBs are more diverse and may arise in any location, from the large proximal to distal extrahepatic bile ducts. Complex configurations, high-grade dysplasia, and stromal invasion are common in this group. Papillary and villous architecture, crowded tubules, cribriform and solid epithelial configurations, and overt malignant cytologic features are typically present. More than 80% of type 2 IPNBs are associated with stromal invasion. In addition to the location and architecture, Nakanuma et al. also categorized IPNBs based on their lineage of epithelial differentiation into intestinal (47.8%), gastric (23.2%), biliary (15.9%), and oncocytic (1.6%).

Intestinal IPNBs with papillary or tubulopapillary architectures are more common in type 2 IPNBs than type 1. Histologically, the intestinal-type epithelium is columnar with pseudostratified cigar-shaped nuclei, variable amounts of cytoplasmic mucin contents, and scattered goblet cells. *Intrahepatic* intestinal-type IPNBs predominantly show villous architecture, resembling colorectal villous adenomas and intestinal-type IPMNs of the pancreas, and harbor *GNAS* and *KRAS* mutations comparable to those seen in intestinal-type IPMNs; by contrast, *extrahepatic* intestinal-type papillary and tubulopapillary IPNBs show genetic mutations in the *SMAD4*, *PIK3CA*, *APC*, and *CTNNB1* genes, like colorectal neoplasms [42]. In gastric-type IPNBs, the epithelial lining is predominantly foveolar with abundant pale apical mucinous cytoplasm and intersperses with scattered goblet- and pyloric gland-type epithelial cells. Biliary-type IPNBs display thin, branching, fibrovascular cores lined by a single layer of non-mucinous, small cuboidal, or low-columnar epithelial cells with scant eosinophilic or amphophilic cytoplasm. Oncocytic-type IPNBs exhibit a conspicuous complex architecture by arborizing fibrovascular core lined by one to several layers of oncocytic cells with abundant granular cytoplasm, centrally located large nuclei, and prominent nucleoli. A range of low-grade to high-grade dysplasia can be present in all histological types of IPNB. High-grade dysplasia is characterized by complex histological configurations (solid and cribriform) and marked cytological atypia, including anisocytosis, high N:C ratio, pleomorphic nuclei, frequent mitosis, and tumor cell necrosis.

Intraductal Tubulopapillary Neoplasm of the Bile Duct (*ITPNB*) (also known as intraductal tubular neoplasm of the bile duct) is a rare non-mucin-producing neoplasm comprised of small, back-to-back tubules with minimal intervening stroma, minor abortive papillae, and foci of solid growth pattern (Fig. 4.4). The tumor presents as an expansile "cast-like" mass in the intrahepatic (70%), perihilar (20%), or extrahepatic (10%) bile ducts. Neoplastic epithelial cells are cuboidal or low columnar with variable cytoplasmic contents. Epithelial cells with intracytoplasmic mucin without any intraluminal mucin secretion are commonly present. Scattered oncocytes, clear cells, thyroid follicle-like cells, parathyroid-like cells, microcalcifications and psammoma bodies (15%), and Mallory-like hyaline globules (5%) have been described in these lesions. Diffuse high-grade dysplasia, tumor necrosis (85%), and absence of intraluminal mucin are characteristic findings. Invasive carcinoma is present in 80% of cases and morphologically is indistinguishable from ordinary biliary adenocarcinoma. Despite the high incidence of

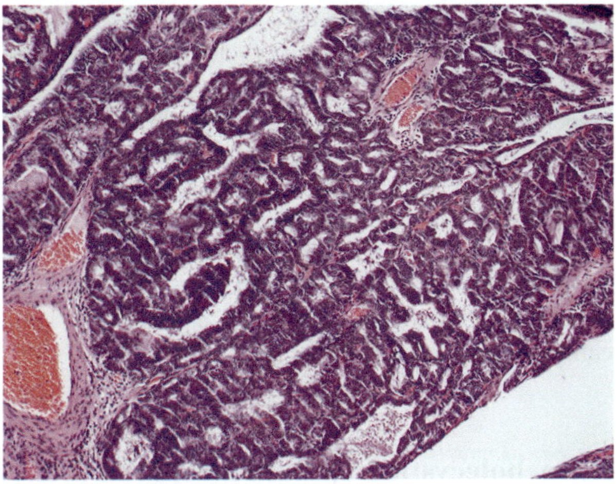

Fig. 4.4 Intraductal tubulopapillary neoplasm of the common bile duct showing polypoid proliferation of dysplastic biliary-type epithelial cells that form small back-to-back tubules

invasive carcinoma, the overall prognosis of ITPNB is favorable with a 1-, 3-, and 5-year survival rate of 100%, 90%, and 90%, respectively [43]. The IHC profile and genetic alteration of ITPNB and IPNB are different. Approximately 80% of IPNBs are positive for MUC5AC, but ITPNBs are negative for MUC5AC and positive for MUC1 (~80%) and MUC6 (~30%). Mutation in *p16* is the most common genetic alteration found in ITPNBs. Other common genetic alterations seen in IPNBs are not found in ITPNBs.

Pathogenesis and Molecular Pathology of IPNB

Hepatolithiasis and *Clonorchis* infection (see Chap. 11, Waraasawapati et al.) are the major known risk factors of IPNB in Asia, but there is no such association consistently found in Western countries [29, 30, 44]. Evidence supports the presence of progenitor cells in the biliary epithelium and periductal glands which may play a fundamental role [39, 45]. Like other precursors, it is plausible that under the influence of a given etiopathogenic insult, the progenitor cells may undergo a progressive accumulation of oncogenic mutations and eventually evolve to IPNB. In the setting of hepatolithiasis, the development of IPNB and transformation to high-grade dysplasia (carcinoma in situ) and invasive carcinoma may take 6–8 and 1–2 years, respectively [46].

A common mechanism linking carcinogenesis has been described for several molecular pathways [38, 47]. The stepwise progression of molecular alterations includes mutated *KRAS*, loss of *p16*, and *TP53* overexpression in low-grade lesions, whereas *SMAD4* loss is seen in later phases of tumor development [38]. Overexpression of *EZH2* is associated with malignant behavior in IPNB, with upregulated MUC1 and downregulated MUC6 expression [48]. Studies that have been conducted on IPNB have shown some conflicting results, such as in the frequency of *GNAS* mutations [47]. *GNAS* mutations have been associated with mucin hypersecretion and villous architecture, although some larger studies have shown no association between mucin secretion and *GNAS* mutations [48, 49]. A case series of tubulopapillary neoplasms were found to have *CDKN2A/p16* mutations and very low rates or absent mutations in *KRAS*, *PIK3CA*, or *SMAD4/DPC* loss [43]. The development of carcinoma in cases with pancreaticobiliary maljunction occurs in association with intracholecystic tubulopapillary neoplasm. Pancreatic maljunction involves a supra-Oddi union of the pancreatic duct and common bile duct, dubbed "reflux-associated cholecystopathy" and causes a chemical inflammation-dysplasia-carcinoma sequence [50].

Intracholecystic Papillary Neoplasm (ICPN)

Intracholecystic papillary neoplasms (ICPNs) are mass-forming, noninvasive neoplastic epithelial proliferations in the gallbladder lumen conventionally >1 cm. ICPNs are often solitary, but one-third of the cases can be multifocal. In the WHO classification, "ICPN" substitutes other terms such as adenoma, noninvasive papillary neoplasm, papillomatosis, intracystic papillary neoplasm, and noninvasive papillary carcinoma [51].

Epidemiology and Clinical Features of ICPN

ICPNs are present in 0.6% of cholecystectomy specimens and comprised approximately 5% of all gallbladder polyps. Although more than half of ICPNs are associated with invasive carcinoma, only about 6% of primary adenocarcinomas of the gallbladder arise in ICPNs. With an overall mean age of 61 years, ICPNs have been reported in the third to tenth decades of life with a female-to-male ratio of 2:1 [51, 52]. Rare cases of ICPN in pediatric patients with metachromatic leukodystrophy have been reported [51, 53]. Radiologic studies fail to detect approximately 10% of ICPNs, and in about 50% of cases, these lesions are reported as cancer. When symptomatic, patients mostly present with right upper quadrant pain or biliary colic and less frequently with obstructive jaundice and hemobilia [51, 54–56]. At the time of diagnosis, approximately 20% of the patients have concurrent neoplasms, most commonly of gastrointestinal origin. The prognosis of ICPNs with and without invasion is favorable with a 3-year survival rate of 60% and 90%, respectively. Deaths several years after resection of ICPNs without invasive foci have been reported, which may be explained by the multifocal emergence of neoplastic precursors elsewhere in the biliary tract under influence of the initial risk factors [51, 52, 57, 58].

Macroscopy and Microscopy of ICPN

ICPNs are intraluminal polyps ranging in size between 1 and 8 cm, with a median size of 2.2 cm. They often arise in the fundus, followed by the body and neck of the gallbladder. ICPNs can be sessile or pedunculated or rarely present as a mass (Fig. 4.5a). Seventy percent of ICPNs are solitary, and approximately one-third are multifocal with skipped non-neoplastic epithelium within the mass or in the surrounding flat mucosa. Large lesions may be necrotic or hemorrhagic, and those with a thin pedicle often detach from the wall and float in the gallbladder lumen and may be mistaken as sludge [51, 57, 58].

Histologically, on low magnification, ICPNs display a papillary epithelial proliferation with fibrovascular cores (Fig. 4.5b, c). Fibrosis and chronic inflammation can be seen in ICPN, which may be primary or secondary to an inflammatory process in the gallbladder. The histological classification of ICPNs is based on the dominant (>75%) architecture and the epithelial lineage. The most common and largest ICPNs are papillary (43%; mean: 2.8 cm), followed by tubulopapillary

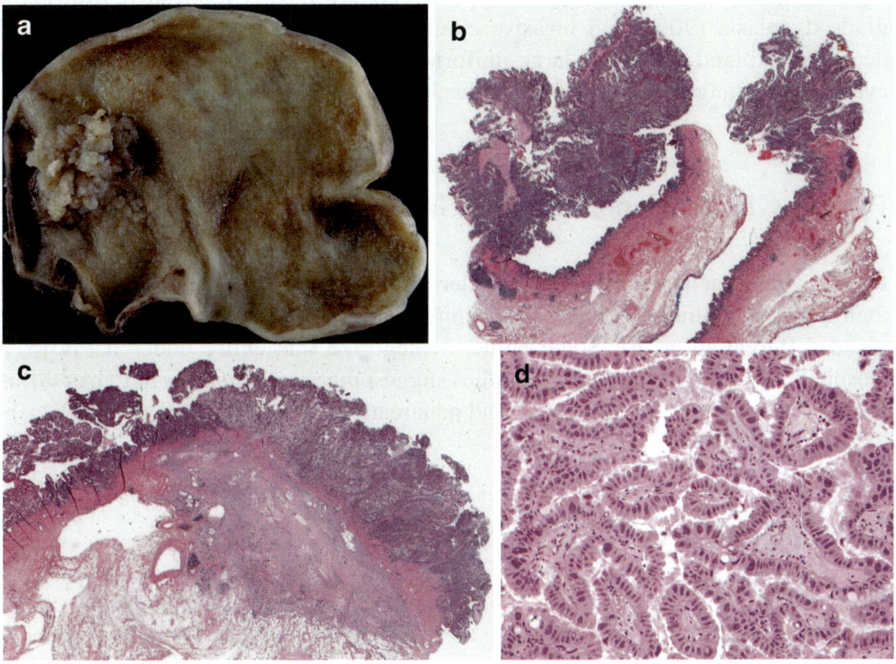

Fig. 4.5 Intracholecystic papillary neoplasm. (**a**) Gross examination of a cholecystectomy specimen revealing a 4.3 cm polypoid mucosal lesion with a lobulated and villous configuration in the gallbladder body near the neck region. (**b**) Low magnification of the lesion showing pedunculated exophytic papillary neoplastic proliferation. (**c**) Sessile intracholecystic papillary neoplasm with invasion into the underlying wall and adipose tissue. (**d**) Higher magnification view showing biliary-type neoplastic cells that form a papillary architecture with fibrovascular cores

(31%; mean: 2.7 cm) and tubular (26%; mean: 2.0 cm). The main histological types are biliary (50%), gastric pyloric gland (20%), gastric foveolar (16%), intestinal (8%), and oncocytic (6%). In addition to the predominant cellular population, most ICPNs (90%) contain secondary, unclassified, or hybrid epithelial phenotypes. Typically, a spectrum of neoplastic transformation ranging from normal appearing to highly atypical morphology can be seen in a given polyp.

High-grade dysplasia is recognized by complex architecture, such as solid sheet and cribriform arrangements, and cytological findings including single-cell necrosis or apoptotic bodies, cellular pleomorphism, markedly enlarged nuclei, anisocytosis, loss of basal nuclear polarity, and centrally located nuclei with clear cell features. Stromal invasion can be detected in overall more than half of ICPNs. The most common site of invasion is the polyp base (70%), but invasive foci in both base and head, head only, and invasion separate from the ICPN mass are also possible. In half of the cases, BilIN is present in the flat gallbladder mucosa surrounding the mass. An occasional extension of the epithelial proliferation into the Rokitansky-Aschoff sinuses is a diagnostic pitfall that may be mistaken as invasive carcinoma. Histological findings most frequently associated with invasive carcinoma include papillary architecture, extensive high-grade dysplasia, and biliary or foveolar histological type. Gastric pyloric gland-type ICPNs are mostly associated with high-grade dysplasia (90%) and invasive carcinoma (20%); however, they consist of deceptively bland-appearing large uniform epithelial cells with small amounts of cytoplasm, arranged in small, back-to-back glands without intervening stroma.

Pyloric Gland Adenoma of the Gallbladder (PGA-GB)

Pyloric gland adenoma of the gallbladder (PGA-GB) is a noninvasive polyp larger than 1 cm in diameter comprised of epithelial cells with gastric pyloric/Brunner gland differentiation [8]. Some authors categorize this entity under ICPN [51]. Despite morphologic similarities, studies suggest that tumorigenesis of PGAs-GB is distinct from the gastric, duodenal, and pancreatic counterparts [59].

Epidemiology and Clinical Presentation of PGA-GB

PGAs-GB are found in up to 0.5% of the gallbladders removed for chronic cholecystitis or cholelithiasis and comprise the vast majority (~80%) of gallbladder adenomas. They are seen equally in both genders with a mean age of 63 years [59]. Gallstones are present in at least 50% of cases [60]. PGA-GB is not associated with multifocal biliary precursors and carries a minimal risk of carcinoma of the gallbladder. The incidence of high-grade dysplasia and invasive carcinoma in PGA-GB is 27% and 1%, respectively. Polyps with high-grade dysplasia are considered pTis (carcinoma in situ) and cured by cholecystectomy. Invasive carcinoma arising in PGA-GB is usually intestinal type with a favorable prognosis [51, 60].

Macroscopy and Histology of PGA-GB

PGAs-GB are sessile or pedunculated polyps and may occur in any part of the gallbladder. Those pedunculated polyps with thin stalk may detach from the wall and appear as a floating mass. A rare case of PGA-GB in the cystic duct with invasive carcinoma has been reported [61]. Histologically, the polyp is composed of packed back-to-back glands with minimal intervening stroma (Fig. 4.6). Neoplastic epithelial cells have small, round, basally located nuclei and abundant foamy cytoplasmic mucin akin to pyloric gland and Brunner gland epithelial cells. Scattered Paneth cells and neuroendocrine cells are usually present. Focal cholesterolosis or squamous morules can also be seen in 10–30% of the cases [59]. Complex, back-to-back glandular architecture is a characteristic feature of PGA-GB and not a criterion for high-grade dysplasia in these polyps. Pyloric metaplasia and small mucosal projections <0.5 cm with pyloric metaplasia are common in cholecystectomy specimens, which differ from PGA-GB. Metaplasia, like other reactive epithelial changes, is ill-demarcated and typically displays a gradual transition from metaplastic to normal epithelium. Mucosal projections less than 0.5 cm arising in a background of pyloric metaplasia are not categorized as PGA-GB. PGA-GB is strongly positive for MUC6 and beta-catenin and may be focally positive for MUC2, MUC5AC, and CDX2. An association between high nuclear beta-catenin expression, mucin-poor morphology, and high-grade dysplasia has been described in these lesions [60].

Molecular Pathology of PGA-GB

The limited investigations performed on PGA-GB suggest a molecular pathogenesis distinct from ordinary adenocarcinoma of the gallbladder. GPA-GB is significantly associated with mutation of *CTNNB1* and nuclear expression of beta-catenin protein but negative for *TP53*, *CDKN2A*, and *GNAs* mutations and rarely positive for *KRAS* mutation [59, 61].

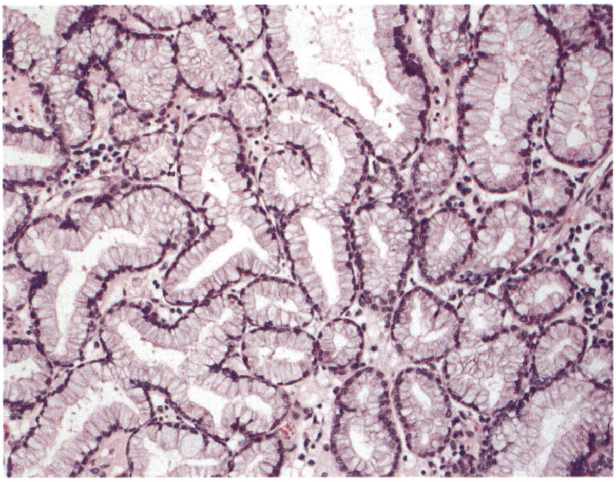

Fig. 4.6 Pyloric gland adenoma of the gallbladder showing packed back-to-back small glands resembling mucous glands of the gastric pylorus or Brunner glands of the duodenum. This example was a 1 cm polyp found in a cholecystectomy specimen

Gallbladder Carcinoma (GB-CA)

Gallbladder carcinoma (GB-CA) represents 80–95% of biliary tract carcinomas worldwide. According to global statistics in 2018, gallbladder carcinoma is the 22nd most frequent cancer and the 17th cause of death from cancer worldwide [62]. The highest prevalence of GB-CA is seen in the South American Indians of Chile [63]. In the United States, American Indians and Alaska Natives have the highest GB-CA incidence and death rates. Overall, GB-CA is approximately twice more common in women. Nearly half of GB-CAs are detected incidentally at cholecystectomy, and approximately 35% are diagnosed at advanced stages with lymph node and/or distant metastasis, with a 5-year survival of only 5% [64]. The most common risk factors for GB-CA include cholelithiasis, prolonged inflammatory conditions, family history of gallstones, older age, poor diet, obesity, and certain ethnicities (e.g., American Indian, Alaska Native), or abnormal anatomy of the biliary tract causing an abnormal flow of bile (e.g., PSC) or reflux of the pancreatic juice into the biliary tract [65–68]. Gallbladder adenocarcinoma (GB-AC) comprises approximately 95% of all GB-CAs and most commonly arise in the fundus (70%), followed by the body and neck. In a large series of GB-ACs, more than half of the tumors were not apparent by gross examination. Clinically unexpected tumors are often in the neck. Even with careful inspection, more than 30% of pT2 and 70% of pT1 cancers may be missed on gross examination (Fig. 4.7). Diagnosis of occult early GB-CAs (intramucosal or intramuscular) in clinically and grossly unexpected cases is important, as patients are significantly younger and may develop extrahepatic biliary carcinoma several years after cholecystectomy, with a 5- and 10-year survival rates of approximately 90%.

Cholecystectomy specimens from patients with risk factors for biliary tract carcinoma, and those with any suspicious finding on gross examination (e.g., hyalinizing cholecystitis), must be thoroughly examined and sampled with a high index of suspicion [69–71]. Porcelain gallbladder (diffuse calcification) is associated with an increased risk of GB-CA with a clinical course at least as aggressive as regular GB-CA. Interestingly, partial mucosal calcifications (also known as incomplete porcelain gallbladder or hyalinizing cholecystitis) are more likely to be associated with invasive carcinoma than diffuse calcification [69]. Hyalinizing cholecystitis is known for a deceptively smooth lumen with occult microscopic carcinoma concealed in the fibrotic wall, warranting microscopic examination of the entire specimen (Fig. 4.8).

GB-AC: Biliary Type

GB-AC of biliary (pancreaticobiliary) type is the most common type, comprising more than 70% of all GB-CAs. "Adenocarcinoma, NOS," and "gallbladder adenocarcinoma" have also been used to describe these tumors. Biological, histological, and IHC features of this type are analogous to the adenocarcinoma of the pancreatic duct [72]. Macroscopically, tumors are typically fibrotic, firm, and infiltrative,

Fig. 4.7 Microscopic anatomy of the gallbladder and its importance in pathologic staging. Unlike the gastrointestinal tract, the gallbladder wall lacks a distinct muscularis mucosa, submucosal soft tissue, and muscularis propria. Muscular tissue in the gallbladder wall consists of a single layer of intersecting circular, longitudinal, and oblique smooth muscle bundles close to the mucosal lamina propria and surface epithelium. The muscular layer separates the mucosa from adventitial connective tissue. p: pathologic; T: tumor staging. pT: pathologic tumor staging

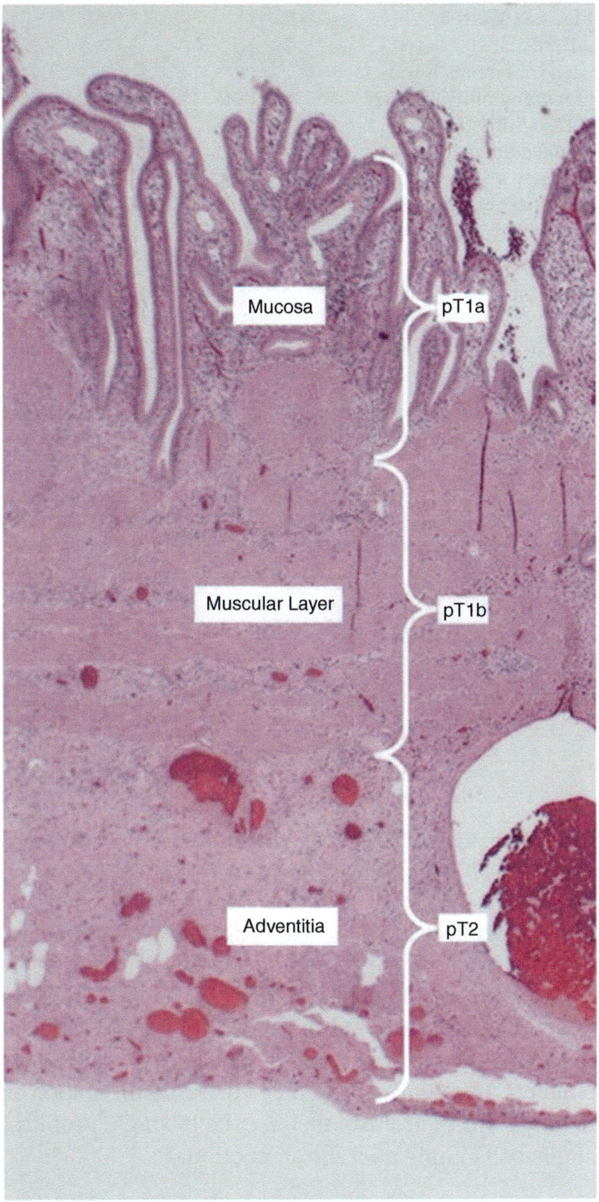

based on precursor lesions, and may be flat or exophytic. Advanced tumors emerging from BilIN appear as a white, firm, infiltrative mass with or without intraluminal projection. Early stage of flat tumors arising from BilIN may be inapparent on gross examination of the gallbladder lumen and cross sections of the wall. These tumors may appear as white flat or finely granular surface with ill-defined firm white cut surfaces which is often difficult to distinguish from the surrounding

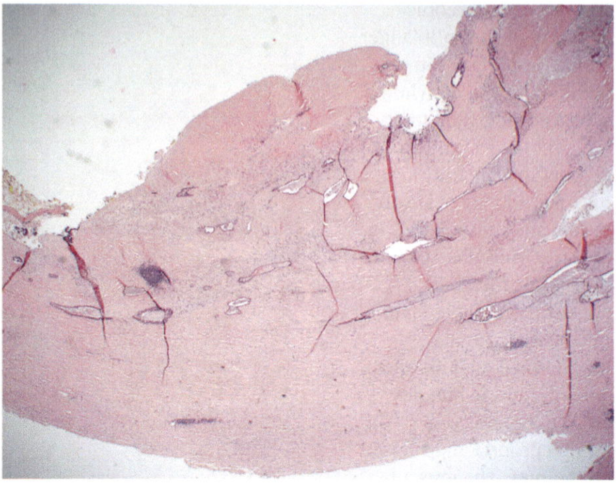

Fig. 4.8 Well-differentiated adenocarcinoma arising in the setting of hyalinizing cholecystitis. The gallbladder wall is diffusely fibrotic, and neoplastic glands are deceptively bland

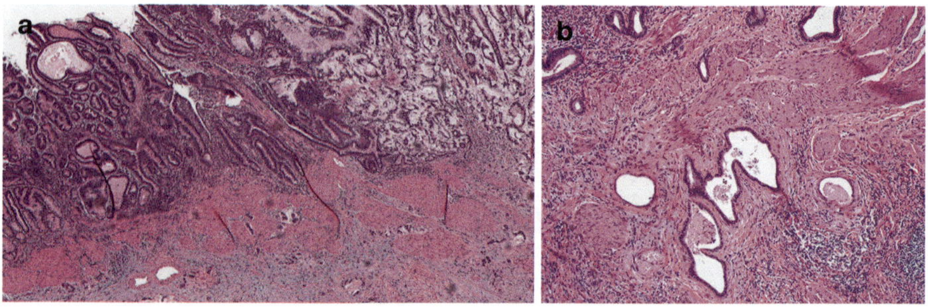

Fig. 4.9 (**a**) Intraepithelial neoplasia involving gallbladder mucosa and invasion of the underlying wall (**b**) Gallbladder wall infiltrated by adenocarcinoma

chronic cholecystitis. Invasive carcinomas arising in ICPNs in advanced stages show an intraluminal component and invasion of the underlying wall in an infiltrating pattern. Histologically, biliary-type adenocarcinoma shows irregular glands and ducts of variable size and shape, infiltrating the gallbladder wall (Fig. 4.9). Epithelial cells may vary from cuboidal to columnar with variable amounts of cytoplasmic contents. Intratumoral variations in the configuration and morphology of the epithelial cells are typical. Epithelial cells in single profiles, sheets, nested patterns or in single cells imply poor differentiation.

GB-AC: Papillary and Micropapillary Types

The "papillary" and "micropapillary" types are two deceptively similar terms that define significantly distinct entities with striking differences in morphology, biology, and behavior. Histologically, papillary and villous lesions are recognized by their fibrovascular cores, a structure not present in micropapillary architecture. In papillary and villous architectures, epithelial cells are attached to fibrovascular projections

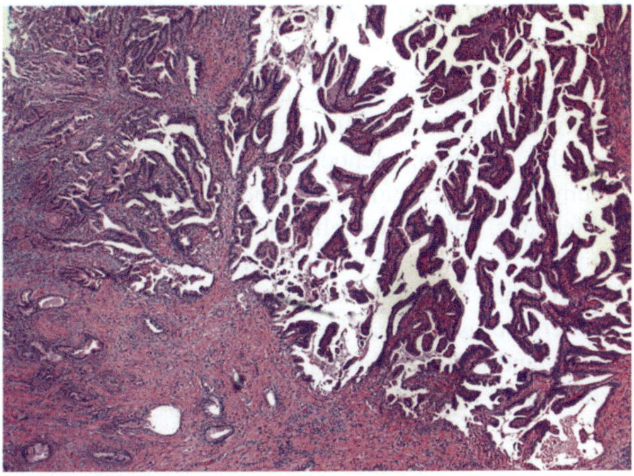

Fig. 4.10 Papillary adenocarcinoma of the gallbladder showing a papillary or villous configuration. A component of conventional invasive adenocarcinoma with a tubular morphology is also present (lower left)

(Fig. 4.10). Instead, in "micropapillary" tumors, one can imagine that the epithelial cells are aggregates or adhered along an arbitrary line without any fibrous or vascular component or a basement membrane [71]. Microscopically, micropapillary tumors infiltrating a fibrous stroma exhibit small clusters of cohesive tumor cells floating in lacunar spaces scattered in the fibrous stroma. A particular functional orientation of the epithelial cells is seen in the micropapillary tumors described as "reversed polarity" or "inside-out" growth pattern. It means that the cytoplasmic membrane facing the stroma (lacuna wall) displays secretory properties analogous to the apical surface of the normal glandular epithelial cells. This feature can be highlighted by strong MUC1 immunostain of the stroma-facing part of the cell membrane. It has been suggested that this feature, coupled with an absence of the gel-forming mucin MUC2, may be one of the key reasons for the distinct morphology of this tumor type by separating the tumor cells from stroma (lacuna formation) and facilitating their spread and early metastasis [73]. In approximately 20% of GB-ACs, a micropapillary pattern is noted and may comprise up to 10% of the tumor mass. The presence of the micropapillary pattern in GB-ACs is an adverse histological prognostic findings and an independent predictor of nodal metastasis [74, 75].

Papillary architecture is common in ICPNs and GB-ACs. Papillary GB-AC arising in papillary ICPNs is a slow-growing tumor with a favorable prognosis compared to the ordinary GB-AC. The true incidence of pure papillary GB-AC is unclear because in most data papillary ICPNs, carcinoma arising in papillary ICPNs, and pure papillary GB-AC have been lumped together. Unlike ordinary GB-CAs, liver function tests and serum tumor markers are often unremarkable in papillary GB-AC. Macroscopic examination of the gallbladder shows sessile polypoid nodules or cauliflower-like projections into the gallbladder lumen. Histologically, the intraluminal tumor and invasive glands exhibit papillary fibrovascular cores lined by malignant epithelial cells [76, 77]. GB-AC with an invasive papillary pattern is considered a well-differentiated histological grade. The percentage of the papillary or micropapillary patterns in an ordinary GB-AC is mentioned in the pathology report; however, the final histological classification is based on the predominant histological type.

GB-AC: Intestinal Type

Pure intestinal-type GB-AC is rare and usually associated with cholelithiasis and intestinal metaplasia in the uninvolved benign mucosa. Histologically, tumor cells resemble intestinal adenocarcinoma with irregular tubules and glands lined by tall columnar cells containing pseudostratified cigar-shaped nuclei, mixed scattered goblet cells, absorptive cells, and Paneth cells [76, 78]. Essentially it is much more common to see intestinal-type differentiation as a minor component in an ordinary GB-AC, than a predominantly intestinal-type GB-AC. Moreover, authorities believe that certain histological findings such as central necrosis, goblet cell-like intestinal mucin, and cellular basophilia are unusual in intestinal-type GB-AC and warrant exclusion of extrabiliary origin.

Mucinous Adenocarcinoma of the Gallbladder

Mucinous carcinoma of the gallbladder (MC-GB) conventionally refers to the tumors with more than 50% extracellular mucin. Only 2% of GB-CAs fit for this diagnosis, although approximately 10% of GB-ACs contain variable amounts of mucin. Cholecystitis is the most common clinical presentation of the MC-GB. These tumors are diagnosed at a more advanced stage (87% pT3) with a significantly worse outcome compared to the ordinary GB-CA. On gross examination, MC-GB displays wall thickening and gelatinous gray-white cut surfaces. Microscopically, the tumor is composed of abundant extracellular mucin pools with floating clusters of tumor cells or with tumor cells lining the borders of mucin pools (Fig. 4.11). Unlike its gastrointestinal counterpart, MC-GB is microsatellite stable. Tumor cells are positive for MUC2 and CK7 and negative for CK20, CDX2, and MUC6, which distinguishes this tumor from ordinary GB-AC and other gastrointestinal mucinous

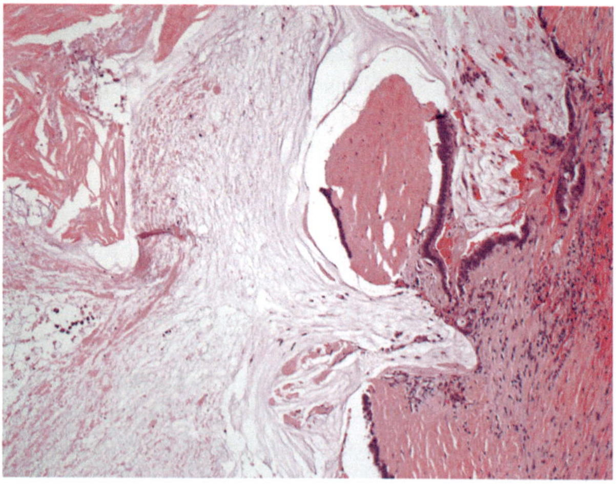

Fig. 4.11 Mucinous adenocarcinoma of the gallbladder showing the presence of abundant mucin. Tumor cells line the borders of mucin pools or float in mucin pools

tumors [78]. Colloid carcinoma of the gallbladder is exceedingly rare and is recognized by more than 90% intramural mucin with rare scattered tumor cells confined to the mucin pools.

Signet-Ring Cell (Poorly Cohesive) Carcinoma of the Gallbladder

The pure form of signet-ring cell GB-AC is a rare and aggressive tumor with a female-to-male ratio of 4:1. It is more common to see foci of signet-ring histology in other types as a minor component. Pure forms are often found in the gallbladders removed for cholelithiasis. In most reported cases, the serosal surface is unremarkable on gross examination. The gallbladder lumen often contains gallstone and/or mucin. On gross examination, the mucosa is ulcerated in some cases, and in others, it may appear velvety without a discernible lesion. Cut surfaces of the wall are usually thickened, but the fibrotic consistency seen in other GB-CAs may not be present, as tumor cells only minimally provoke desmoplastic reaction [79–82]. Characteristic microscopic feature is numerous poorly cohesive small epithelial cells in single or arranged in short single profiles or small nests, infiltrating the microscopic tissue planes (Fig. 4.12). Desmoplasia response, and therefore tumor fibrosis, is typically minimal to none. Signet-ring cells are small epithelial cells containing single cytoplasmic mucin vacuole displacing nucleus to the side. Nevertheless, in many instances, the tumor cells are mucin-poor with scant cytoplasm and no cytoplasmic vacuole. Therefore, in the WHO classification, the former "signet ring" has been substituted by "poorly cohesive" nomenclature to incorporate both cytomorphologies in this category [8].

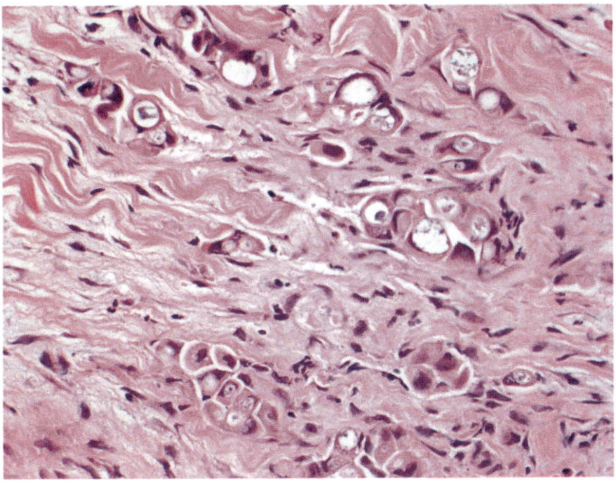

Fig. 4.12 Signet-ring cell carcinoma of the gallbladder showing small nests of poorly cohesive tumor cells or single individual tumor cells infiltrating the gallbladder wall

Clear Cell Adenocarcinoma of the Gallbladder

Primary clear cell (hypernephroid) adenocarcinoma of the gallbladder (CC-GB) is exceedingly rare and named after the histological resemblance to the clear cell renal cell carcinoma (Fig. 4.13). When encountered in the biliary tract, metastasis from the kidney must be excluded [49, 83]. The reported cases of primary CC-GB are more common than clear cell carcinoma (CC) of the extrahepatic bile ducts (70% vs 30%). Patients with CC-GB are in their 30s to 40s which is 20 years younger than those with extrahepatic CC counterparts. In all cases, foci of adenocarcinoma (90%) or squamous cell carcinoma (10%) are identified to support the primary nature of these tumors versus renal primary.

Microscopically, clear cells are in alveolar arrangements separated by delicate vessels or form large sheets. Cellular configuration in small cords, trabeculae, nests, and papillary configurations has also been described [84]. Tumor cells exhibit well-defined cytoplasmic border and clear cytoplasmic contents positive for diastase-labile PAS-positive granules and negative for mucin [85]. They are also positive for MUC1, AE1/AE3, CK7, CK8, and p53 and negative for CK19 and CK20. Focal hepatoid differentiation, positive for AFP and canalicular CEA, has been described in some cases [85, 86].

Squamous and Adenosquamous Carcinoma of the Gallbladder

Pure squamous cell carcinoma (SCC) is exclusively comprised of cells with squamous differentiation without any recognizable adenocarcinomatous component (Fig. 4.14). BilIN may be present in the surrounding mucosa and by itself does not exclude the diagnosis. Most SCC patients are in their 60s with cholelithiasis

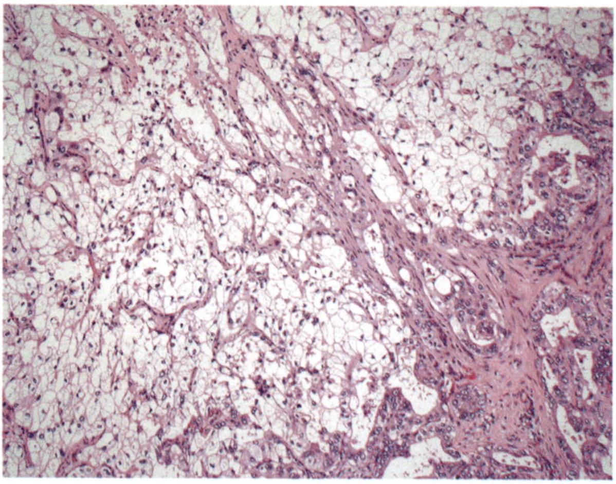

Fig. 4.13 Clear cell adenocarcinoma of the gallbladder showing sheets of neoplastic cells with abundant clear cytoplasm and delicate fibrovascular septa, resembling clear cell renal cell carcinoma. Focal conventional gland-forming adenocarcinoma is also present (lower right)

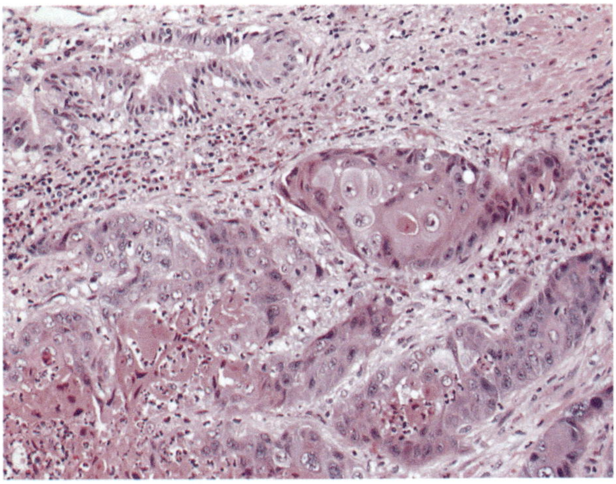

Fig. 4.14 Squamous cell carcinoma of the gallbladder showing nests of neoplastic cells with keratinizing cytoplasm. Residual gallbladder mucosa is present (upper left)

but without other known risk factors for biliary carcinomas. Tumors are mostly in the fundus (40%) and may occupy more than two-thirds of the gallbladder (30%). The most common clinical presentation is abdominal pain, and the overall clinical presentation is mainly like ordinary GB-AC [87, 88]. Adenosquamous carcinoma (ASC) is arbitrarily categorized as a tumor with 25–99% squamous differentiation [87]. Focal squamous differentiation is found in 5% of the ordinary GB-AC. This finding is of uncertain biological significance and generally is not mentioned in pathology reports [2]. Primary SCC and ASC comprise <1% and up to 4% of the gallbladder carcinomas, respectively. SCC and ASC are four times more common in women than men and are associated with a worse prognosis than ordinary GB-AC. Approximately 85% of the patients are not found to have clinical suspicion for malignancy prior to surgery. In approximately 60% of cases, tumors may not be noticeable by gross examination, where tumor appears as a plaque-like mural thickening and an induration indistinguishable from cholecystitis. When macroscopically visible, tumors appear as ulcerated hemorrhagic flat lesions or exophytic masses infiltrating underlying tissue with gray-white cut surfaces. Microscopically, a range of well to poor differentiation can be seen. Keratinization is more common in SCC than ASC (88% vs 65%). In ASC, distinct IHC phenotypes of squamous differentiation (e.g., p40, p63, CK5/6) and glandular differentiation (e.g., BerEP4, CK7, CEA) are expressed.

Hepatoid Adenocarcinoma of the Gallbladder

Hepatoid adenocarcinoma is characterized by prominent hepatocellular differentiation. Foci of adenocarcinoma mixed with hepatoid differentiation are almost always present and support gallbladder origin. Hepatoid adenocarcinomas described in different organs generally have phenotypes and behaviors analogous to hepatocellular carcinoma (HCC) of the liver [89, 90]. Gross appearance of the tumor is solid white to yellow mass infiltrating the adjacent structures. The diagnosis of hepatoid adenocarcinoma is essentially based on the histological findings that resemble those of HCC in the absence of a liver lesion (Fig. 4.15). On microscopic examination, hepatoid cells are large polygonal cells that are arranged in trabeculae, solid sheets, or nests. Akin to hepatocytes, they contain abundant eosinophilic cytoplasm, intracellular bile pigments, and large centrally located round nuclei with prominent nucleoli. The hepatoid component of the tumor is positive for Hep Par-1 and arginase-1 and demonstrates histological and IHC phenotypes of HCC. In challenging cases, the presence of CK7-positive epithelial cells supports adenocarcinoma, while CD10 and polyclonal CEA highlight canalicular structures in hepatoid component. Serum AFP may be elevated in tumors from both origins [91].

Sarcomatoid Carcinoma of the Gallbladder

Sarcomatoid carcinoma of the gallbladder (SC-GB) is defined as a carcinoma with foci of sarcomatous differentiation. This tumor has also been described by other terms such as "spindle cell carcinoma," "malignant mixed tumor," or "carcinosarcoma." However, "sarcomatoid carcinoma" seems to be more applicable, as both cell types are thought to be from a common epithelial origin and sarcomatous cells exhibit a mixed epithelial and mesenchymal phenotype. SC-GB is an exceedingly rare tumor of elderly women in the seventh decade of life and associated with a grave outcome. An abdominal mass, pain, and jaundice are the most common clinical presentations. Most gallbladders are distended by an intraluminal mass infiltrating the adjacent structures. On gross examination, unlike ordinary GB-AC, these tumors are soft and

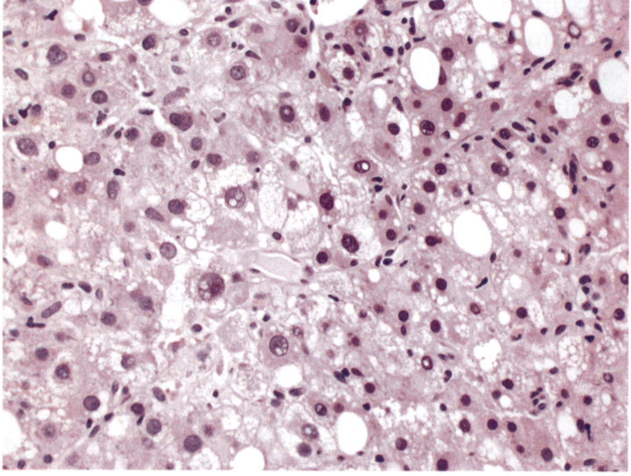

Fig. 4.15 Hepatoid adenocarcinoma of the gallbladder showing sheets of polygonal tumor cells with abundant eosinophilic cytoplasm, morphologically resembling hepatocellular carcinoma. A liver primary must be ruled out in such cases before the diagnosis can be made

fleshy without desmoplastic fibrosis [92]. Histologically, SC-GB is recognized by sarcomatous tumor cells mixed with adenocarcinomatous component or composed predominantly or entirely of sarcomatous component (Fig. 4.16). The transition between the two components may be subtle or distinct. The sarcomatous cells may display a wide range of mesenchymal differentiation from bland-appearing spindle cells to pleomorphic cells, giant cells, bone, cartilage, or rhabdoid cells [92]. Malignant cells are connected by desmosome-like junctions, positivity for pankeratin and vimentin, and contain cytoplasmic intermediate filaments [8, 92, 93].

Undifferentiated Carcinoma of the Gallbladder

Undifferentiated carcinomas are malignant epithelial tumors without any glandular or squamous differentiation. The presence of undifferentiated foci in other histological types changes the histological grade, but not the histological type. Undifferentiated carcinoma of the gallbladder is rare with approximately 100 reported cases. This tumor is more common in women (7:1.6) with a median age of 57–60 years, in different series. The median survival of the patients is less than 9 months [94]. Tumors manifest as a mass with nonspecific firm whitish cut surfaces. Various cellular morphologies such as large round, polygonal, multinucleated, pleomorphic, and spindle-shaped cells, as well as medullary-type growth (syncytial growth with inflammatory cell infiltrates), have been described [95, 96]. All tumors are positive for MUC1, pankeratin (AE1/AE3), and CEA, supporting the epithelial nature of the neoplastic cells. Vimentin may be expressed in some tumor cells. Many tumors show foci of endocrine differentiation and IHC reaction to somatostatin, gastrin, serotonin, pancreatic polypeptide, and HCG [96].

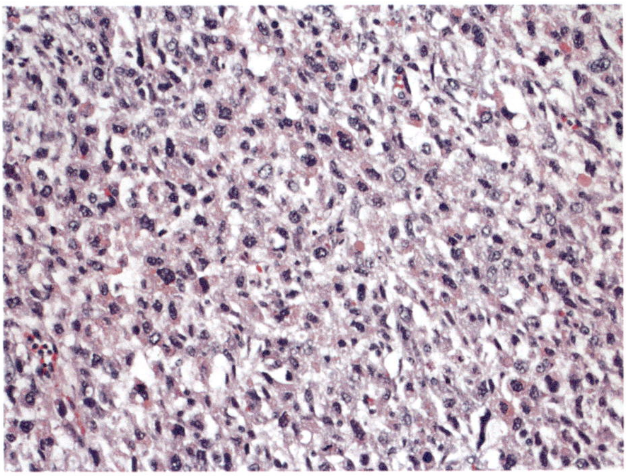

Fig. 4.16 Sarcomatoid carcinoma of the gallbladder showing a sarcomatous component characterized by poorly cohesive short spindled or round epithelioid tumor cells. These cells are immunohistochemically positive for pankeratin

Pathogenesis and Molecular Pathology of GB-CA

Data about GB-CA is limited due to a paucity of cases and heterogeneity of the available data. The overall most frequently mutated genes in GB-CA are TP53, *CDKN2A*, *ARID1A*, and *ERBB2* [97–99]. Zuo et al. described the importance of the liver X receptor (LXR)/retinoid X receptor (RXR) and farnesoid X receptor (FXR)/RXR pathways in GB-CA. The *LXR* and *FXR* genes are important in lipid metabolism and function as tumor suppressors, and their downregulation appears to be critical for GB-CA pathogenesis. In the series presented by this group, the key genes involved in these pathways were *SERPINB3* and *KLK*. They demonstrated overexpression of these genes, especially in female patients, and suppression of *APO1* gene [100]. Park et al. suggested that estrogen receptor genes and other hormone-associated genes could play a role in the etiology of biliary tract cancers, especially in men [101]. Some investigators have underscored the value of epithelial growth factor (EGFR) in HER2-positive tumors in targeted therapies [102]. Moreover, akin to the colorectal cancer, the presence of *KRAS* mutations may preclude gallbladder cancer patients to respond to anti-EGFR treatment [103]. Microsatellite instability has also been found in up to 10% of GB-CA and the premalignant lesions and has been considered in targeted therapies. Inactivation of the mismatch repair genes early in carcinogenesis of certain GB-CAs has been demonstrated; however, it has not been found to be associated with survival or a clinicopathological feature [100, 104]. Several different single nucleotide pleomorphisms (SNP) have shown to be associated with GB-CA, although larger validation studies are needed [105].

Extrahepatic Bile Duct Carcinoma (EHBD-CA)

Extrahepatic bile ducts carcinomas (EHBD-CAs) comprise a heterogeneous group of tumors arising in the perihilar (P-EHBD) or distal biliary tract (D-EHBD). In the second version of the WHO's International Classification of Diseases for Oncology (ICD-O-2) coding system, which was used between 1992 and 2000, perihilar tumors (Klatskin tumor) were classified as intrahepatic instead of extrahepatic. This classification at least partially contributed to the variation in incidence and features of biliary carcinomas reported in the literature [106–109]. In the third version (ICD-O-3), perihilar tumors (Klatskin tumor) were classified as extrahepatic tumors. Perihilar tumors are defined as those involving the main lobar extrahepatic bile ducts distal to segmental bile ducts and proximal to the cystic duct. Tumors located between the junction of the cystic duct-common hepatic duct and the ampulla of Vater are considered distal bile duct tumors [110, 111]. The most common location of bile duct carcinoma is perihilar (50%), followed by distal (40%) and intrahepatic (10%) [111, 112]. Perihilar and distal bile duct carcinomas share common pathogenesis and preinvasive epithelial precursors [113]. Mucin-secreting epithelial cells lining bile duct or periductal glands have been suggested as the possible cells of origin in the vast majority of EHBD-CAs [39, 45, 114–116].

Epidemiology and Clinical Presentation of the EHBD-CA

EHBD-CA equally affects men and women in the sixth to seventh decades of life, with the pyloric gland type seen in the early sixth decade. Predisposing factors of EHBD-CAs are analogous to BilIN and IPNB. Clinically, small tumors can cause biliary obstruction and present in the early stages of disease. The most common clinical presentations, similar to IPNB, are jaundice, abdominal pain, pruritus, nausea, vomiting, anorexia, weight loss, and cholangitis. Prolonged bile duct inflammation is a common finding in most cases. Risk factors include infestation with *Clonorchis sinensis* and *Opisthorchis viverrini*, PSC (especially with long-standing ulcerative colitis) [117], choledochal cysts, Caroli disease, congenital hepatic fibrosis, pancreaticobiliary maljunction, and any primary or iatrogenic condition associated with prolonged deranged bile duct flow or regurgitation of the pancreatic juice into the biliary tract. Pancreaticobiliary maljunction with bile duct dilatation and PSC are risk factors for biliary tract cancer. Pancreaticobiliary maljunction, particularly without bile duct dilatation, is a risk factor for gallbladder cancer. There are no evident risk factors for ampullary carcinoma.

Macroscopy and Histology of the EHBD-CA

EHBD-CA may appear as intraluminal nodular or papillary, periductal infiltrative, or longitudinal infiltrative sclerotic lesions (Fig. 4.17a–c). Cut surfaces of the tumor are firm pale-gray-white with irregular ill-defined borders infiltrating the surrounding tissue. Fibrotic borders may not accurately correspond to the infiltrating tumor cells. The histological and IHC phenotypes of EHBD-CA are similar to those of GB-CA, LD-iCCA, and pancreatic ductal adenocarcinoma (Table 4.3). The vast majority of EHBD-CAs are well to moderately differentiated biliary-type adenocarcinomas (~77%), comprised of irregular and angulated glands or tumor nests infiltrating a markedly fibrotic stroma with frequent perineural and lymphovascular invasions. Tumor cells are atypically mucin-producing but may vary in size, shape, and cytoplasmic contents. Conventionally, histological grade is analogous to other BD-CAs, and similarly signet-ring cell (poorly cohesive) adenocarcinomas are grade 3. Squamous cell carcinoma is rare in EHBDs and graded based on the highest grade present in the tumor as grade 1 (well differentiated), grade 2 (moderately differentiated), and grade 3 (poorly differentiated). These systems are not applicable to neuroendocrine tumors. Undifferentiated carcinomas are, by definition, high-grade tumors and lack any specific morphologic or IHC differentiation phenotype. The overall histomorphology of adenocarcinomas of the pancreatic duct and intrapancreatic common bile duct is usually similar. The primary site is determined based on the macroscopic and microscopic localization of the tumor origin and detection of epithelial precursor lesions in the corresponding anatomical structure (Fig. 4.18a–c). Poor histological prognostic factors include deep invasion (high

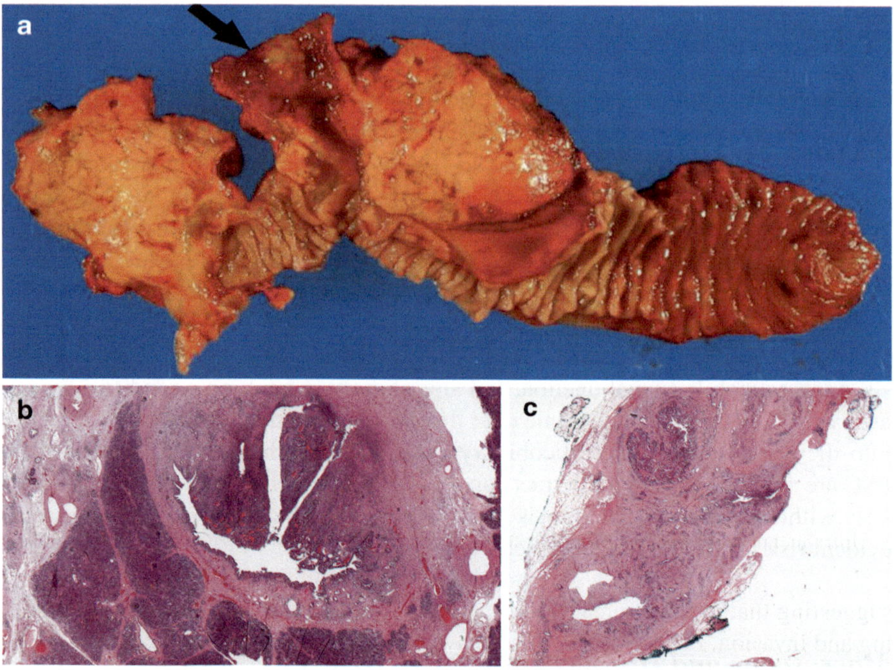

Fig. 4.17 Adenocarcinoma of the extrahepatic bile duct. (**a**) Whipple resection specimen showing a markedly dilated common bile duct (arrow) with a nodular mucosal surface. (**b**) Intrapancreatic common bile duct with intraluminal tumor projection and tumor cells infiltrating underlying stroma. (**c**) Extrahepatic bile duct with infiltrative tumor

stage), involvement of resection margin, flat configuration, high histological grade, vascular invasion, and perineural invasion [111, 118–121].

A rare pyloric gland phenotype has been described in carcinomas of the hilar region in younger patients. This tumor consists of more than 80% well-differentiated pyloric-type columnar cells with abundant mucin and basally located small hyperchromatic nuclei. Tumor cells are arranged in small- to medium-sized ducts or large dilated glands infiltrating fibrous stroma. Deceptively benign-appearing glands, foci of large complex glandular structures with micropapillae (stellar pattern), and frequent perineural invasions are characteristic findings. IHC stain highlights diffuse expression of MUC5AC and MUC6 and negative expression of MUC2 and CDX2 [122].

Tumor staging of the perihilar carcinomas (P-EHBD-CAs) has been a subject of debate and controversy. These tumors are in the proximity of vital vasculature in an anatomically complex and surgically challenging location. Different staging systems have been proposed to guide surgical management. The Bismuth-Corlette classification has been the most traditionally used system, based on the involved segments of EHBDs without considering other factors such as extrabiliary extension and anatomical variants. Blumgart et al. from Memorial Sloan Kettering Cancer Center (MSKCC) proposed the MSKCC staging system according to the location of bile duct involvement, local extension, presence of portal vein involvement, or

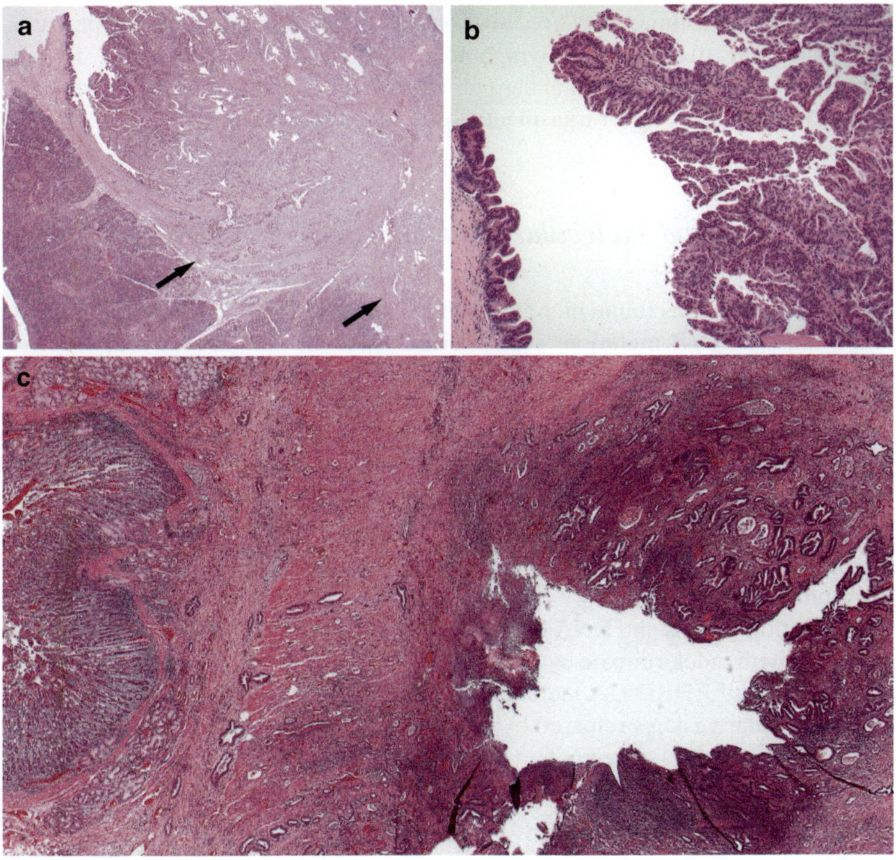

Fig. 4.18 Adenocarcinoma of the intrapancreatic common bile duct. (**a**) Low magnification showing adenocarcinoma invading the bile duct wall into the adjacent pancreatic parenchyma (arrows). The main bulk of the tumor is intraductal. (**b**) High magnification showing intraductal papillary neoplasm with high-grade dysplasia (right) and high-grade biliary intraepithelial neoplasia (left) as precursor lesions. (**c**) Intrapancreatic common bile duct with adenocarcinoma infiltrating surroundnig parenchyma

hepatic lobar atrophy, without considering the size of residual hepatic parenchyma [64, 123]. This system was studied on 225 patients based on the criteria of resectability at MSKCC, which was later challenged by changes in the surgical methods and criteria for resectability [64, 123, 124]. In the eighth edition of the American Joint Committee on Cancer (AJCC) and the Union for International Cancer Control (UICC) system, EHBD-CAs are divided into "perihilar" and "distal EHBD" tumors. In this system, the pathological staging of perihilar tumors is based on confinement to the bile duct wall or extension to the extrabiliary structure, whereas for distal tumors, in addition to the extrabiliary extension, microscopic measurement of the intramural infiltration is also considered in the pathological staging (Table 4.4) [110]. DeOliveira et al. proposed a new staging system with more detailed information about tumor location, size, vascular invasion, residual hepatic parenchymal volume after resection, lymph node status, and distant metastasis. The aim of this system is to provide a standard report with relevant information about resectability, indications for liver transplantation, and prognosis [124].

Pathogenesis and Molecular Pathology of the EHBD-CA

Molecular alterations found more frequently in EHBD-CA are *PRKACA/PRKACB*, *ELF3*, and *ARID1B* mutations [125]. EHBD-CAs also show the similar heterogenic molecular pattern as LD-iCCA [47]. The altered genes include *KRAS*, *TP53*, *CDKN2A*, and *SMAD4* [97]. Perihilar EHBD-CA and LD-iCCA have a higher frequency of *KRAS* mutations than SD-iCCA [126]. However, *MDM2* is not found to be amplified in distal EHBD-CA [127]. Biliary brushing cytology specimens are the gold standard of diagnosis of EHBD-CAs but, despite high specificity, are known to have low sensitivity. Molecular techniques have been developed that can increase the sensitivity of biliary brushings while maintaining a high specificity. Polysomy of CEP 3, 7, and 17 and 9p21 deletion, detected by fluorescence in situ hybridization (FISH) and DNA flow cytometry, can improve sensitivity in bile duct strictures with indeterminate cytology [128]. Techniques being developed to aid in the diagnosis of EHBD-CA include next-generation sequencing (NGS), the study of extracellular vesicles released by cells, proteomics, and liquid biopsy [129].

Mucinous Cystic Neoplasm (MCN) of the Liver and Biliary System

In the WHO classification, mucinous cystic neoplasms (MCN) have "ovarian-like stoma" (OLS) versus intraductal papillary neoplasms of the biliary tract (IPNB), which lack OLS [8]. Accordingly, MCN must meet all the following criteria: female gender, visually visible cystic neoplasm not arising in the biliary ducts, at least partial mucinous differentiation of the epithelial lining, and at least focal presence of the OLS. OLS is defined by spindle cells akin to the ovarian stroma aberrantly present in the stroma of the mixed epithelial and stromal tumor of the kidney and MCNs of the pancreas and liver. The spindle cells present in OLS are positive for ER, PR, alpha-inhibin, and FOXL2 (forkhead box L2) analogous to the ovarian stroma. FOXL2 is expressed in the early stages of female gonadal development and granulosa cell differentiation and is strongly expressed in granulosa cells throughout life. Some investigators argue that OLS can be seen in hepatobiliary development; thus, it is not restricted to women. In summary, based on the current WHO classification, a subset of formerly called "cystadenoma" or "cystadenocarcinoma" that do not have OLS cannot be classified as MCN [130, 131]. Authorities propose that cystic tumors lacking OLS could represent IPNBs with marked cystic changes [8].

Epidemiology and Clinical Presentation of MCN

Hepatic MCNs are very rare accounting for less than 5% of all hepatic cysts, with an incidence of 1 in 20,000–100,000. Most data in the literature do not clearly separate MCNs and cystic IPNBs. In large series of all benign and malignant "mucinous cysts," 88% of the patients were white female, and the mean age of patients was 54 years (14–83 years of age) [132]. The etiology and pathogenesis of MCN are unclear. Some investigators suggest that the presence of OLS and pick incidence in middle-aged women may indicate the role of female reproductive hormones. MCNs are often solitary, multilocular, and intrahepatic (80%) and often in the left lobe [132]. MCNs are rare in the gallbladder [133].

Abdominal pain and fullness, early satiety, jaundice, and weight loss are the most common symptoms; however, approximately 40% of the patients may be asymptomatic at the time of diagnosis [134]. Liver function tests and serum levels of CA19-9 and CEA tumor markers are within the normal range for most patients. Nevertheless, elevated tumor markers in the serum are uncommon in non-neoplastic cysts. Cyst fluid typically shows high levels of CEA and CA19-9, and in some cases, CA19-9 level in the cyst fluid may correlate with high-grade dysplasia and the proportion of invasive component [132]. Radiologic imaging reveals a multilocular cystic mass and biliary duct dilatation, which may mimic the radiological features of a hydatid cyst [135]. The overall prognosis of MCNs is excellent. Evidence supports clinicopathological similarities between MCNs of the liver and pancreas. Even invasive adenocarcinoma arising in MCN has a significantly better prognosis compared to the ordinary biliary adenocarcinoma. Despite its benign nature, globally, 18% of all benign mucinous cystic lesions of the liver (MCN and IPNB combined) recur after surgery. The high rate of recurrence is mainly attributed to certain interventions such as unroofing and fenestration and positive surgical margin. Many authors emphasize the importance of complete excision to prevent recurrence or malignant transformation. Some studies show invasive carcinoma to be more common in larger tumors, but in other large series, the size was not a predictor of malignancy. The presence of mural nodules, solid component, papillary projections, irregular thickening of the cyst wall, calcifications, hypervascularity, and enhancement after contrast has a high negative predictive value and a low positive predictive value. In other words, the absence of all these findings strongly suggests benignity, but their presence does not necessarily support malignancy [132]. No single predictive radiographic feature is identified.

Macroscopy and Histology of MCN

Tumors are well demarcated with a fibrous band and may range in size from 5 to 29 cm (mean size 11 cm). Benign tumors are usually larger at the time of diagnosis. The tumor is typically separated from the bile ducts; however, rarely polypoid protrusion into the bile duct lumen can be present. Sections of the benign tumor reveal multilocular cystic mass filled with mucinous or hemorrhagic fluid. Cysts are separated by thin fibrous septa and exhibit pale gray-white smooth or slightly trabeculated inner surface. Irregular wall thickening, large papillary projections, and solid fibrotic areas warrant a thorough sampling to exclude invasive carcinoma [131, 132].

Histologically, the vast majority of MCNs of the liver are benign and well delineated by a fibrous capsule. Cysts are lined by a single layer of flat, cuboidal, or columnar epithelial cells. Many MCNs display bland-appearing histology, resembling benign biliary cysts, lined by cuboidal to low columnar biliary-type epithelial cells with round to ovoid basally oriented nuclei. Different proportions of goblet cell, gastric foveolar, and intestinal differentiation can be seen. By definition, at least a minor population of mucin-producing cells is required for diagnosis. In challenging cases with scant mucin-producing cells, mucicarmine special stain is helpful to highlighting cytoplasmic mucin. The OLS appears as a subepithelial hypercellular spindle cell stroma, while the rest of the wall shows hypocellular collagenized ordinary fibrous tissue. In half of the cases, the OLS can be diffusely (>75%) dispersed in the fibrous tissue separating the cysts. The cyst wall and the OLS may undergo hemorrhagic or necrotic degeneration, dystrophic calcification, hyalinization, or luteinization (Fig. 4.19). Sometimes, especially in the large benign cysts, OLS is scant and difficult to discover [132]. At least focal OLS is required for the diagnosis of MCN. The OLS spindle cells are positive for alpha-inhibin, PR, ER and FLOX2 and negative for CD10 (an endometrial stromal marker) [136, 137]. The IHC profile of the epithelial cells is consistent with their lineage of differentiation and does not play a diagnostic role. Low-grade dysplasia is a common finding. High-grade dysplasia is rare and depicted by cellular crowding, cribriform arrangement, solid sheets, marked cytological atypia, nuclear pleomorphism, and conspicuous mitosis and occasionally by anaplastic cells. Invasive carcinoma associated with MCN displays classic morphologic features of an ordinary biliary adenocarcinoma.

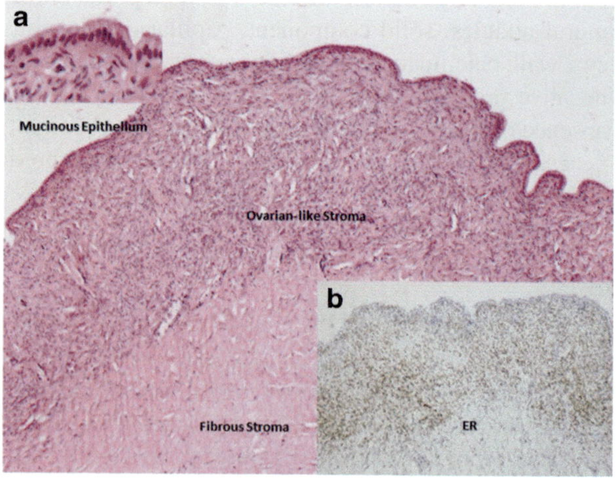

Fig. 4.19 Mucinous cystic neoplasm of the hepatobiliary system. (**a**) The cystic lesion is lined by a single layer of epithelial cells showing low-grade histology. Ovarian-type stroma is characterized by bland, relatively uniform short-spindled cells. (**b**) Stromal cells are positive for progesterone receptor by immunohistochemistry

Pathogenesis and Molecular Pathology of MCN

KRAS mutations have been found to be a major driver genetic alteration in the pathogenesis of MCN and may be one of the mutations that leads to high-grade dysplasia [138, 139]. MCN of the liver has a lower incidence of *KRAS* mutations, which may explain a lower rate of invasion compared to the extrahepatic mucinous cystic tumors [138]. *KRAS* mutations in MCN are associated with multilocular-cystic appearance and positivity for MUC1, MUC2, and MUC5AC [8]. All cases of MCN have wild-type *GNAS*, *RNF-43*, and *PIK3CA*, which are usually altered in other neoplasms of the hepatobiliary system [8].

Intrahepatic Cholangiocarcinoma (iCCA)

Primary liver carcinomas encompass malignant neoplasms with a range of differentiation from primitive progenitor cells to cholangiocytic or hepatocellular lineage. Tumors may be monomorphic or a mixture of different components. Classification of these tumors is merely based on routine histological examination. IHC studies play a supplemental role and should not ultimately determine the final diagnosis. Interpretation of IHC findings requires an in-depth understanding of specific and nonspecific immunophenotypes [121]. iCCA comprises a heterogeneous group of malignant primary liver carcinomas recognized by cholangiocytic differentiation, variable desmoplastic reaction, and absence of extrahepatic biliary or pancreatic adenocarcinoma [8].

Epidemiology and Clinical Presentation of iCCA

iCCA is the 2nd most common primary liver cancer, after HCC, and is responsible for 10–20% of primary live cancers and up to 10% of all bile duct carcinomas [140, 141]. Most patients are men in the fifth to seventh decade of life. The incidence, etiology, biology, and risk factors of iCCA vary worldwide. The overall prevalence of iCCA in East Asia is higher than that in the Western countries (71–80 vs 0.2–2 cases per 100,000 person-year). Between 1973 and 2012, the incidence of iCCA in the United States raised from 0.44 to 1.18 cases per 100,000, which corresponded to the increased prevalence of chronic liver diseases [141, 142]. The major global risk factors of iCCA are biliary parasitic infestations (*Clonorchis sinensis* and *Opisthorchis viverrini*), hepatolithiasis, PSC, exposure to the radiopaque medium thorium dioxide (Thorotrast), abnormal anatomy of the biliary tract, viral hepatitis B and C, alcoholic liver disease, hemochromatosis, and metabolic syndrome (including obesity). A definitive risk factor cannot be identified in many patients [140, 143–152]. The most common clinical presentations of iCCA in the large bile ducts include jaundice, malaise, abdominal pain, weight loss, and increased serum alkaline phosphatase level. Large duct iCCA with intraductal growth may present with complications of biliary obstruction, such as acute cholangitis. Small duct iCCA, however, is usually mass forming and presents at advanced sages with mass effect [126, 149].

Macroscopy and Histology of iCCA

In WHO classification, iCCAs are classified into "small duct" (SD) and "large duct" (LD) CCA. Other terms used in the literature to describe different variants of iCCA (e.g., peripheral CCA, cholangiocellular carcinoma, and cholangiolocellular carcinoma) fall into one of these two categories [8].

Large duct iCCAs (*LD-iCCA*) (also known as hilar CCA) arise in the large intrahepatic bile ducts proximal to the hepatic ducts. The precursor lesions and growth patterns of these tumors are similar to those for carcinomas of the extrahepatic bile ducts. The most common risk factors in Asian countries are liver flukes and hepatolithiasis, while in the Western countries, PSC and anatomical abnormalities of the extrahepatic biliary tract are the most reported risk factors. Precursors of LD-iCCA are BilIN and IPNBs, both of which may arise in the bile duct lumen or in the periductal glands [140, 144, 145, 148, 150, 152, 153]. LD-iCCAs are typically fibrotic whitish tumors with periductal infiltrative pattern, with or without intrahepatic mass-forming or intraluminal growth patterns [154, 155]. Histological features of LD-iCCA are identical to the perihilar EHBD-CA. Tumor cells are usually columnar to low columnar, forming irregular and angulated glands, which infiltrate an abundant desmoplastic stroma (Fig. 4.20). Variable amounts of cytoplasmic and extracellular mucin are characteristic findings, a feature that typically is not seen in the SD-iCCA. Perineural invasion is frequently present [156–158].

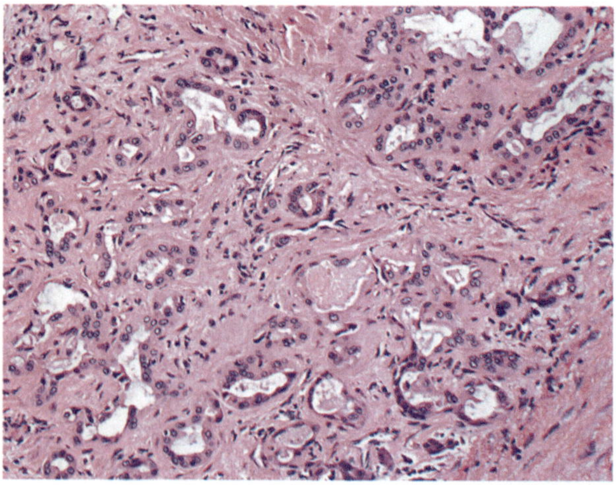

Fig. 4.20 Intrahepatic cholangiocarcinoma, large duct type, showing irregular glandular structures infiltrating a fibrotic stroma. Intraluminal mucin production is noted

Small duct iCCA (SD-iCCA) grows in a mass-forming pattern and appears as a mass in the periphery of the liver. These tumors originate from transdifferentiation of the hepatic progenitor cells or transformed mature hepatocytes under similar risk factors for HCC and c-HCC-CCA. No intraepithelial or intraductal precursor lesion has been described in the small bile ducts or ductules [143, 149, 151]. Rare associations with biliary adenofibroma and bile duct hamartoma (von Meyenburg complex) have been described [159–162]. Histologically, SD-iCCA is characterized by a mass-forming non-mucinous tumor infiltrating between hepatocytes at the interface (hepatic interface infiltrative pattern). Tumor cells are small cuboidal epithelial cells with scant cytoplasm, round nuclei, and fine chromatin. They form small ducts, tubules, or ductules with slit-like lumens or cord-like patterns. Desmoplastic (fibrotic) stroma is typically present.

According to the WHO classification, "cholangiolocarcinoma" and "iCCA with predominant ductal plate malformation (DPM) pattern" are two subtypes of SD-iCCA [8]. Cholangiolocarcinoma is a distinct malignant tumor, characterized by small cuboidal cells with more than 80% ductular configuration infiltrating a hyalinized fibrous stroma (Fig. 4.21). It has been suggested that this tumor arises from canal of Hering. IHC and molecular features of this tumor are analogous to well-differentiated SD-iCCA [5, 163]. Histological diagnosis of this entity is made based on the small and bland-appearing tumor cells arranged in anastomosing trabeculae, cords, or ill-formed ductules, embedded in a striking desmoplastic stroma. A rare spindle cell pattern has also been reported. The clinical and radiological features of this subtype are nonspecific. The iCCA with predominant DPM pattern shows desmoplastic stroma infiltrated by irregularly dilated ducts lined by a single layer of non-mucinous small cuboidal cells with occasional inspissated bile. This histological type is defined by intraluminal epithelial buddings and projections, resembling ductal plate malformation [164].

In summary, diagnosis and classification of the iCCA types are currently based on routine histological examination. Intracellular and extracellular mucin, a

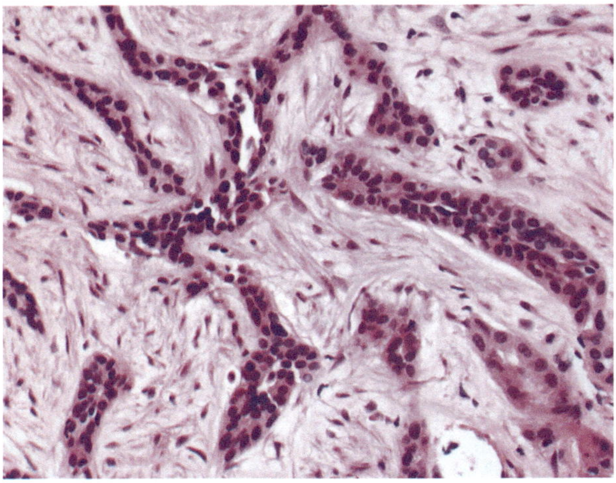

Fig. 4.21 Intrahepatic cholangiocarcinoma, small duct type, showing ductule-like structures lined by cuboidal tumor cells infiltrating a fibrotic stroma

characteristic finding in LD-iCCA, has not been described in SD-iCCA. LD-iCCA has a higher rate of desmoplasia and perineural invasion, whereas infiltration between hepatocytes at the interface (hepatic interface infiltrative pattern) and hepatoid phenotype are typical features of SD-iCCA [165]. In general, iCCAs and EHBD-CAs are immunoreactive to CK7, CK19, and MUC1. The LD-iCCA epithelial cells are positive for MUC5CA and MUC6 and negative for CD56, which is opposite to the IHC profile seen in the SD-iCCA [165]. Histological grading of LD-iCCA and SD-iCCA is determined by the proportion of gland formation like EHBD-CAs.

Pathogenesis and Molecular Pathology of iCCA

iCCAs have heterogeneous pathogeneses with diverse molecular and genetic alterations. Furthermore, due to limited understanding of pathogenesis and molecular data, there is no unanimous fundamental pathophysiologic classification for these tumors. Therefore, no molecular targeted agents have been approved for these tumors, and surgical resection is the only hope for effective treatment to date. Advanced molecular technologies have recently led to an increased understanding of iCCA, which has shown highly heterogeneous genomic and epigenetic aberrations [47]. This heterogeneity may be due to the different backgrounds in which iCCA arises and also partially because of inconsistencies in diagnosis and reporting [47]. Despite these challenges, the LD-iCCA and SD-iCCA have been found to have certain unique characteristic molecular features.

LD-iCCAs have *KRAS* and *TP53* mutations and mutations of other tumor suppressor genes and oncogenes while lacking the *IDH1/2* mutations and *FGFR2* fusions seen in SD-iCCA [8, 47, 126]. These molecular features are similar to those seen in hilar EHBD-CA [126]. *SMAD4* mutations are more commonly found in LD-iCCA versus SD-iCCA [158]. *MDM2* amplification is found to be present in 12% of LD-iCCA, which seems to be related to *SMAD4* loss and has been associated with an overall shorter survival [127]. Using molecular testing to differentiate between SD-iCCA and LD-iCCA may be useful in difficult borderline cases and may soon be used for determining targeted therapy [47].

SD-iCCA has been postulated to be derived from liver progenitor cells but may also transdifferentiate from mature hepatocytes into biliary-like cells [163, 166, 167]. SD-iCCA characteristically has *IDH1/2* mutations and *FGFR2* fusions more frequently than LD-iCCA and EHBD carcinomas [47, 126]. *FGFR2* and *IDH1/2* mutations are mutually exclusive and mostly limited to iCCA [97]. *FGFR2* mutations have been found to be associated with an improved overall survival, younger age of onset, and female gender, while *IDH1/2* mutations are not prognostic [97]. A lymphoepithelioma-like carcinoma, which by some authors has been described as a subtype of SD-iCCA, was found to be positive for Epstein-Barr virus by in situ hybridization in one study [126].

Similar to HCC, the risk factors of iCCA influence the genetic alterations. For example, COX2 and mPGES-1 were found to be highly expressed in tumors associated with PSC [168]. Liver fluke-associated iCCA has an increased rate of microsatellite instability (MSI), which is associated with response to MSI blockade and a better prognosis [47]. Liver fluke-associated iCCA also tends to not have *IDH1/2* or *BAP1* mutations and instead has been found to be enriched in *ERBB2* amplifications and *TP53* mutations [169, 170]. Liver fluke-negative iCCA was found to have high copy number alteration and expression of PD-1/PD-L2, or epigenetic abnormalities of the *IDH1/2* and *BAP1* genes, and *FGFR/PRKA*-related gene rearrangements, while EHBD-CA more often has *PRKACB* mutations [156, 170]. *BAP1* loss is more associated with SD-iCCA than adenocarcinoma of the EHBD or pancreas and is also associated with higher histological grade and interestingly a lack of lymphatic invasion [171]. The fact that *BAP1* mutations have been identified in iCCA, HCC, and cHCC-CCA suggests a common cell of origin for these malignancies [47, 172]. *BAP1* mutations have been recently described in a genetic syndrome. This autosomal-dominant tumor predisposition syndrome shows heterozygous germline *BAP1* mutations at 3p21 that have been found to be related to uveal melanoma, cutaneous melanocytic proliferations, renal cell carcinoma, basal cell carcinoma, and iCCA [171].

In terms of prognosis, patients with tumors harboring *FGFR2* mutations had a longer median cancer-specific survival, whereas *CDKN2A/B* and *ERBB2* alterations showed a worse prognosis [173, 174]. It has also been proposed that a subset of patients with *KRAS* mutations and increased levels of *EGFR* and *HER2* signaling could benefit from dual-target tyrosine kinase inhibitors using a secondary target downstream of *KRAS* [175]. The *FGFR2* fusions and *IDH1/2* mutations seen in ~60% of cases have also been suggested as therapeutic targets [173, 176].

BRAF V600E mutation, used in targeted therapy, is rare in bile duct carcinomas, found in only 1% of iCCA and none of the EHBD-CA [177].

The iCCAs can be categorized based on their pathogenic pathways [8]. Sia et al. performed a whole-genome expression profiling, chromosomal aberration, and signal pathway activation in a cohort of 149 iCCA cases from Europe and the United States. They identified two main biological classes of iCCA: proliferative class (PC) and inflammation class (IC) comprising 62% and 38% of all their tumors, respectively. Each class was further subclassified into three distinct categories. Tumors in the PC show genetic resemblance to the poor prognostic HCC such as cluster A, G3 proliferation, and S1 signature, which support a common progenitor cell origin. PC tumors evolve from activation of oncogenic signaling pathways including *RAS*, mitogen-activated protein kinase (*MAPK*), and *MET*; mutations in *KRAS* and *BRAF*; and significant enrichment of the signatures related to *EGFR*, *HER2*, and *MET* without amplification of these receptors. These tumors also demonstrated chromosomal alterations at 11q13.2 and 14q22.1. Tumors in the IC group emerge in a background of prolonged humoral immune response with imbalance of cytokines such as interleukins (IL) and are associated with a more favorable prognosis. These tumors are characterized by induction of immune response-related pathways; activation of *STAT3* oncogene (STAT family is a key transducer of cytokine signaling); overexpression of IL-4, IL-6, IL-10, and IL-17; and downregulation of TH1 cytokines. The PC tumors show poor to moderate histological differentiation, poor survival, and high rate of recurrence. In contrast, the IC tumors are well differentiated and associated with a better survival and lower recurrence rates.

Combined Hepatocellular-Cholangiocarcinoma (c-HCC-CCA)

The diagnosis of cHCC-CCA is based on unequivocal histological evidence of mixed hepatocellular and biliary differentiation accompanied by transition zones with intermediate morphology. The histological variants, degree of differentiation, percentage of each component, and architecture of the tumor mixture are not included in the diagnostic criteria (Table 4.1) [121, 178]. Approximately 2% of the primary liver carcinomas are qualified for the diagnosis of cHCC-CCA [121].

Epidemiology and Clinical Presentation of cHCC-CCA

cHCC-CCA is a rare tumor comprising 1–4.7% of all primary liver carcinomas [179]. Patients are mostly white men older than 65 years. In general, cHCC-CAA shows an overlap of the epidemiological, clinical, radiological, histological, and serological features of both HCC and iCCA [180–182]. The clinical features and behavior of cHCC-CCA vary in different regions of the world in a range between HCC and iCCA. This may be partially attributed to the variables such as ethnicity, risk factors, and pathogenesis. The commonly reported risk factors of cHCC-CCA include hepatitis B and C infection, hepatic cirrhosis, male gender, and transarterial chemoembolization [183]. Although prognostic factors vary in different study populations, the most commonly reported adverse risk factors include male gender, African-American race, tumor size >3 cm, multifocality, lymph node metastasis, vascular invasion, advanced stage, resection margin <2 cm from tumor, high levels of CA19-9 (>37 U/L), and GGT serum level >60 U/L [184–186]. The 5-year overall survival in the United States with and without liver transplantation is approximately 41% and 18%, respectively [184]. Studies on the South Korean population showed 1- and 3-year disease-free survival rates of 38% and 25%, respectively [185]. In a large population of HBV-related cHCC-CCA in China, 84% of the patients were male with a median age of 49 years. The post-resection 2-, 5-, and 10-year disease-free survival rates were 22%, 15%, and 11%, respectively.

Macroscopy and Histology of cHCC-CCA

The cHCC-CCA tumors typically present as an expansile solitary mass, which may grow up to 16 cm. Gross examination of the cut surfaces is nonspecific and is variably pale tan to green with areas of fibrosis, hemorrhage, or necrosis. Histologically, presence of hepatocytic, cholangiocytic, and intermediate (transitional) phenotypes are necessary for diagnosis (Fig. 4.22). The HCC component demonstrates hepatocytic phenotypes such as bile production, Mallory bodies, and bile canaliculi. Malignant hepatocytes typically grow in trabecular and/or

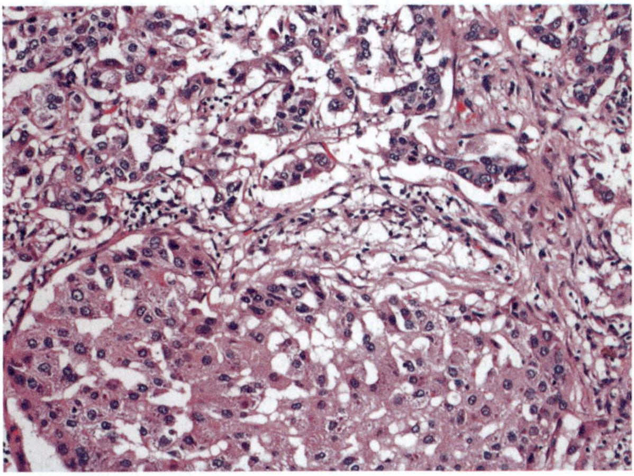

Fig. 4.22 Combined hepatocellular-cholangiocarcinoma showing both components of hepatocellular carcinoma (lower) and cholangiocarcinoma (upper)

pseudoglandular patterns or widened hepatic plates highlighted by reticulin stain. The iCCA component typically consists of mucin-producing biliary epithelium arranged in irregular angulated glands, trabeculae, cords, or single cells infiltrating a markedly fibrotic stroma. A range of well- to poorly differentiated morphology of each component can be seen. Variable amounts of intermediate tumor component without distinct hepatocytic or cholangiocytic differentiation, scattered between the well-formed HCC and iCAA components, are present. The intermediate tumor cells evolve from hepatic progenitor cells that are originally located in the canal of Hering and bile ductules. The hepatic progenitor cells are small epithelial cells with scant cytoplasm and positive for several stem cell IHC markers. The intermediate tumor cells show morphologic and IHC features of both cholangiocytes and hepatocytes. A range of histological patterns have been described in the intermediate zone. Tumor cells are often small with scant cytoplasm and round to ovoid nuclei arranged in trabeculae, solid nests, single profiles, or antler-like anastomosing patterns embedded in fibrous stroma or show abrupt glandular formation. A predominant spindle cells morphology has also been reported [187, 188]. The hepatocyte progenitor cells express progenitor markers such as CK7, CK19, CD56, EpCAM (BerEP4 and MOC31), and CD117 [189–191]. All tumor cells in the intermediate zone express at least one of these markers [187].

Intermediate cell carcinoma is a tumor entirely comprised of monotonous malignant intermediate cells with morphologic features between hepatocytes and cholangiocytes. Other primary liver tumors containing foci of intermediate cell carcinoma are not qualified for this diagnosis [192]. Tumor cells are monotonous small cuboidal or oval with scant pale cytoplasm arranged in trabeculae, cords, nests, or single profiles infiltrating abundant fibrous background. They lack cytoplasmic mucin and express a dual HCC and iCAA IHC profile. Intermediate cell carcinoma shares the clinical behavior of both HCC and iCCA [192].

Pathogenesis and Molecular Pathology of cHCC-CCA

The pathogenesis of cHCC-CCA involves a monoclonal liver progenitor cell origin with translineage differentiation [183, 193–195]. A recent comprehensive molecular study suggests subtypes of cHCC-CCA based on cells of origin: (1) Classical mixed subtype with intermingled typical HCC and iCCA differentiation. These tumors are derived from stem cells or a more mature progenitor with typical HCC or iCCA mutations such as *TERT* promoter or *TP53* mutations and show immunoreactivity to CK7, CK19, Hep Par-1, and glypican-3. (2) Hepatocyte progenitor/stem cell subtype derived from progenitor/stem cells with poorly differentiated morphology. These tumors share activation of proliferation signatures such as MYC, IGF2, mTOR, and NOTCH. Most of these tumors are immunoreactive to progenitor-like marker SALL4 (75%). This phenotype is not seen in the classical mixed type. The SALL4-positive tumors show biphenotypic gene expression and mutations in *TP53*, *BRAF*, and *FGFR2*. Approximately 25% of tumors with poorly differentiated morphology are comprised of SALL4-negative stem cells and exhibit hepatocyte-like gene expression and mutation in *TRET* and *TP53* [196].

Classical cHCC-CCA and undifferentiated carcinoma are aggressive tumors with poor prognosis. Prognosis of cHCC-CAA is worse than HCC and better than iCCA. A therapeutic biomarker has not been identified in these tumors [184, 197, 198].

Von Meyenburg Complex (VMC)

First described by von Meyenburg in 1918, VMCs, or bile duct microhamartomas, are usually subcapsular hepatic lesions resulting from ductal plate malformation due to incomplete involution of embryonic bile duct remnants [199]. VMCs are more common in men and can be seen in all ages. Uncomplicated VMCs are usually asymptomatic and without any effect on liver function tests. The clinical importance of VMC is its distinction from other lesions on imaging studies and core biopsies and the possibility of associated complications such as cholangitis and malignant transformation [159, 200–202].

On gross examination, MVCs are often multifocal, fibrotic gray-white nodules with irregular contours measuring <1.5 cm. Histologically, VMCs are directly adjacent to portal tracts and consist of numerous biliary ducts, ductules, and many irregularly dilated and branched biliary spaces, lined by bland-appearing biliary epithelium. Bile duct production or intraluminal eosinophilic material is typically present. Bile duct proliferation is embedded in conspicuous fibrocollagenous stroma with ill-demarcated irregular contour (Fig. 4.23).

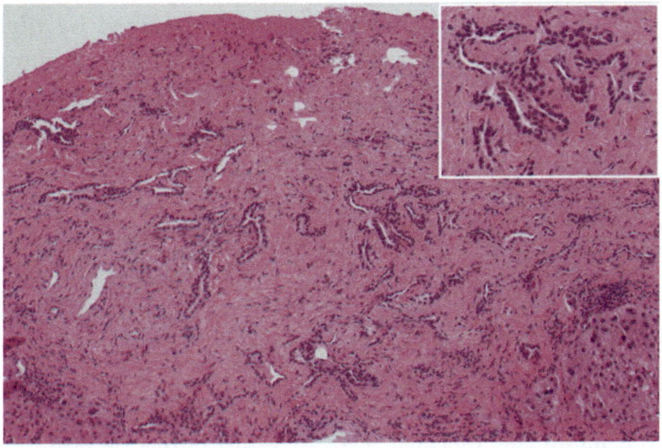

Fig. 4.23 von Meyenburg complex. Bile duct proliferation is embedded in conspicuous fibrocollagenous stroma with an ill-demarcated, irregular contour. Bile ducts are lined by benign cuboidal epithelium

Pathogenesis and Molecular Pathology of VMC

Pathogenesis of VMCs are related to ductal plate malformation and association with autosomal dominant polycystic kidney disease, Caroli disease, and hepatic fibrosis [203]. A stepwise transformation of the VMC to CCA associated with *p16IK4a* inactivation and loss of heterozygosity at foci harboring key oncogenes have been demonstrated [202, 204].

Biliary Adenofibroma

Biliary adenofibroma (BAF) is an unencapsulated, non-mucinous, solid microcystic biliary proliferation embedded in a fibrous stroma. BAF is a very rare benign tumor, with approximately 30% malignant potential, reported in the third to ninth decades of life with a 2:1 female preponderance [205–207]. In most patients, BAF has an indolent growth and overall being behavior with a very long disease-free survival. Incomplete excision is followed by local recurrence [207]. BAF presents as a solitary mass ranging between 1.5 and 16 cm, with well-circumscribed round to ovoid mass. Cut surfaces may show variable proportions of solid and microcystic or spongy appearing components. Histologically, the epithelial cells form tubular, acini, microcysts, and macrocysts. Occasionally larger cyst spaces contain complex polypoid and papillary intraluminal projections. The benign epithelial cells are small cuboidal to low columnar biliary epithelium with non-mucinous amphophilic cytoplasm, uniform small round to ovoid nuclei, and inconspicuous nuclei. The intervening stroma consists of fibrocollagenous tissue with occasional lymphoplasmacytic infiltration [205–208]. BAF may undergo a spectrum of preinvasive to invasive malignant transformation recognized by high-grade epithelial dysplasia and areas of stroma invasion with or without lymphovascular invasion [205, 208]. Epithelial cells in BDA are positive for CEA, MUC1, CK7, CK19, CA19-9 and CD10. Unlike BDA and peribiliary glands, BAF is negative for IF6 and acid mucin [208]. Benign epithelium and stroma always show a Ki67 of less than 10% and 1%, respectively.

Pathogenesis of BAF

Evidence shows that similar to von Meyenburg complex, BAF is a primary epithelial neoplasm that arises from interlobular or large bile ducts with a secondarily induced stroma [207, 208]. Amplification of CCND1 and ERBB2 and overexpression of P53 support the malignant nature of BAF and explain the potential for aggressive behavior and distant metastasis in some cases [207–209].

Bile Duct Adenoma (BDA)

Bile duct adenoma or peribiliary gland hamartoma is a bile duct tumor of unknown etiology, which is thought to originate from peribiliary glands with benign behavior, although rare malignant transformation has been reported [210, 211]. BDA is frequently an incidental finding with an incidence of 1.3% and reported in 50 out of 50,000 autopsies. In the largest series reported by Allaire et al., 103 out of 152 total cases were asymptomatic and detected incidentally, while 49 cases were found at autopsy [212]. BDA has been reported equally in both genders in a wide range of age from 1.5 to 99 years but mostly seen in the third to eighth decades of life (mean: 55 years). Macroscopically, tumor often appears as a single non-encapsulated subcapsular nodule of less than 2 cm in diameter with white fibrotic-appearing cut surfaces. The mean size is 1.3 cm [213]. An exceptionally large case measuring 9 cm in diameter has been reported [214]. Histologically, tumor is unencapsulated without infiltration into the adjacent hepatic parenchyma. Tumor cells are bland-appearing uniform small cuboidal biliary epithelial cells, similar to bile ductules, forming compact network of noncystic small ductal arrangements with no or small lumens (Fig. 4.24a–c). Non-biliary differentiation of undetermined significance such as clear cell, oncocytic, and signet-ring features has been described in BDA [215–217]. Bile duct proliferation is embedded in a fibrous stroma with hyalinized collagen and variable degrees of lymphoplasmacytic infiltration and possible microcalcification and non-necrotizing granulomatous reaction. Cytological atypia, lymphovascular invasion, bile productions, cystic change, and bile duct production are not present. The tumor cells express MUC1, CEA, CK7, CK19, CD56, and p16 in addition to foregut phenotype such as MUC5AC, MUC6, CD10, IF6, and TFF2

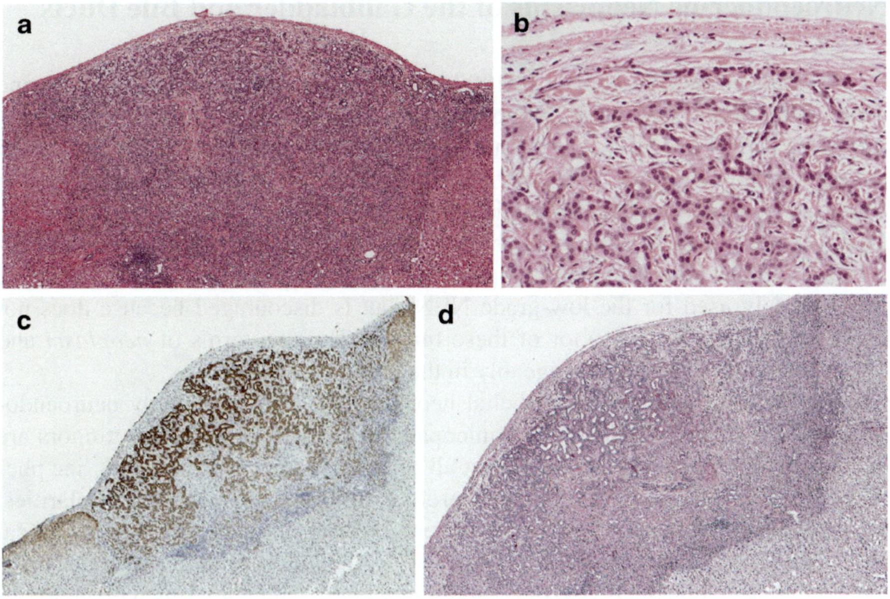

Fig. 4.24 Bile duct adenoma. (**a**, **b**) Tumor cells are bland-appearing uniform small cuboidal biliary epithelial cells, similar to bile ductules, forming compact network of noncystic small ductal arrangements with no or small lumens. (**c**, **d**) Structure of biliary proliferation and stroma highlighted by pankeratin immunohistochemical stain and periodic acid-Schiff (PAS) special stain

[210, 218, 219]. BDA is negative for AFP and p53 and shows a less than 10% (usually less than 2%) proliferative index by Ki67.

Reactive ductular proliferation, cholangiolocarcinoma, and von Meyenburg complex are important histological differential diagnoses of BDA. Configuration of the reactive ductular reaction is not nodular or well circumscribed. Cholangiolocarcinoma is larger, invasive, and cytologically atypical. A Ki67 >10%, positive EZH2 and p53, and negative CD10, CD56, and p16 are helpful to recognize cholangiolocarcinoma from BDA [220]. Von Meyenburg complex shows cystic changes and bile production that are not seen in BDA.

Pathogenesis

A focal reaction to physical or inflammatory stimulus and peribiliary glandular origin has been proposed in the pathogenesis of BDA. Analogous to the periductal glands, the epithelial cells in BDA co-express 1F6 and CD10, which is not seen in the bile ductules and interlobular bile duct epithelium [210]. BRAFp.V600E mutation has been demonstrated in many of BDA, suggesting neoplastic nature of these tumors [221].

Neuroendocrine Neoplasms of the Gallbladder and Bile Ducts

First introduced by Oberndorfer in 1907 as *karzinoide* (carcinoid), neuroendocrine neoplasms (NENs) were initially thought to be indolent and uncommon. However, they were later proved to be common, potentially aggressive, and heterogeneous in nature. The nomenclature of *neuroendocrine* was changed by some authorities to *endocrine* to underscore the epithelial, and not neural crest, origin of tumor cells. However, since tumor cells display both epithelial and neural phenotypes, the *neuroendocrine* has been currently adopted. Another controversial term is *carcinoid*, which widely used for the low-grade NENs but is discouraged because does not convey the malignant behavior of these tumors. The two terms of *neoplasm* and *tumor* have been used interchangeably in the literature [222].

The NENs are defined as epithelial neoplasm with predominantly neuroendocrine differentiation. Some of the clinicopathological features of these tumors are characteristic of the organ of origin, yet all share the common neuroendocrine phenotypes regardless of location [222]. Therefore, despite the phenotypic similarities, NENs of different site have distinct pathogenesis, molecular alterations, and clinical outcomes. According to the WHO classification, the NENs of the gallbladder (GB) and extrahepatic bile ducts (EHBDs) are biliary epithelial neoplasms with neuroendocrine differentiation [8]. NENs are further subclassified to neuroendocrine tumors (NEN) grade 1, 2, and 3, large neuroendocrine carcinoma (LC-NEC), small neuroendocrine carcinoma (SC-NEC), and mixed neuroendocrine-non-neuroendocrine neoplasm (MiNEN) (Table 4.5).

Epidemiology and Clinical Presentation of NENs

Approximately 0.2–2% and 0.2% of all NENs of the digestive system occur in the GB and EHBD, respectively [223, 224]. Most NENs of the biliary tract are in the GB. EHBD NENs are less common and tend to occur in the junctional zones. In GB and EHBD, NECs are significantly more common than NETs [225]. NENs of the GB and EHBD have been reported in the third to ninth decades of life (mean: sixth and seventh decades), with a female preponderance [225, 226]. The etiology of NENs of GB and EHBD remains unclear in many cases. Cholelithiasis and

Table 4.5 Grading classification of the neuroendocrine neoplasms

NEN	Mitosis per 10 HPF	Ki67 index
NET grade 1	<2	<2%
NET grade 2	2–20	3–20%
NEC grade 3	>20	>20%
LC-NEC	>20	>20%
SC-NEC	>20	>20%
MiNEN	>20	>20%

NEN neuroendocrine neoplasm, *LC* large cell, *SC* small cell, *NEC* neuroendocrine carcinoma, *HPF* high-power field abnormal bile duct flow due to maljunction are risk factors for GB NENs [227, 228]. Some NENs of the biliary system are associated with von Hippel-Lindau (VHL) syndrome and Multiple Endocrine Neoplasia (MEN) type 1.

The nature of GB and EHBD NENs are taught to be different [225]. The most common clinical presentation of the EHBD NEN is biliary obstruction, while gallbladder NENs are usually detected. The clinical presentations of the GB NECs are similar to GB adenocarcinoma [229]. Rarely, patients present with Zollinger-Ellison syndrome (ZE), which is often sporadic, and von Recklinghausen. In MEN1-associated ZE, gastrinomas are multifocal in the first three portions of the duodenum, with clinically notable and rare ectopic tumors in the EHBD [230]. Patients are usually women younger than under 50 years of age. Lymph node metastasis is noted in about 50% of cases [230, 231]. NEC of the GB and EHBD are aggressive tumors with a prognosis worse than adenocarcinoma, while low-grade NENs (grade 1 and 2) have a better outcome [225].

Macroscopy and Histology of NENs

Macroscopically, NENs of the biliary system usually appear as a solitary submucosal sessile or pedunculated polypoid mass. Low-grade NENs are usually less than 2 cm, but NECs may grow larger and invade surrounding tissues [232]. Cut surfaces of the tumor are with-gray or pale yellow and often firm in low-grade tumors due to fibrosis, while NECs may be soft [224, 226, 227, 229, 230]. Histologically, the low-grade NETs are comprised of monotonous cells arranged in nests (insular pattern), rosettes, acini, trabeculae, or sheets and embedded in a noticeable homogenous collagenized fibrous stroma, which contribute to the firm consistency (Fig. 4.25a). Tumor cells are monomorphous round, with small amounts of eosinophilic cytoplasm, round smooth centrally located nuclei, and fine dispersed so-called "salt-and-pepper" chromatin, with rare mitosis (Fig. 4.25b). In cytologic preparations, low-grade NETs are loosely cohesive and display the characteristic nuclear features mentioned above. In general, NENs share cytological features of round blue cells tumors, distinction of which involves ancillary studies such as IHC or in situ hybridization. NEN tumor cells are positive for synaptophysin, neuron-specific enolase (NES), CD56, and chromogranin (Fig. 4.25c, d). Chromogranin is a highly specific marker, although lack sensitivity of synaptophysin. CD56 is sensitive but also stains a wide range of leukocytes and other tumors. NES is positive in many neural crest tumors. Histologic grading of NENs is based on mitotic count or Ki67 index in ten high-power microscope fields (HPF). The low-grade NENs have a <20% Ki67 index. Analogous to the lung, NECs of the GB and EHBD are categorized as SC-NEC and LC-NEC. SC-NEC tumor cells are small with scant cytoplasm, hyperchromatic nuclei, homogenous chromatin, and characteristic nuclear molding (Fig. 4.25e). LC-NEC tumor cells may be monomorphous or pleomorphic with variable amounts of cytoplasm. Nuclei are large and contain prominent nucleoli. Tumor cells necrosis is typically present. In cytologic preparations, tumor cells are

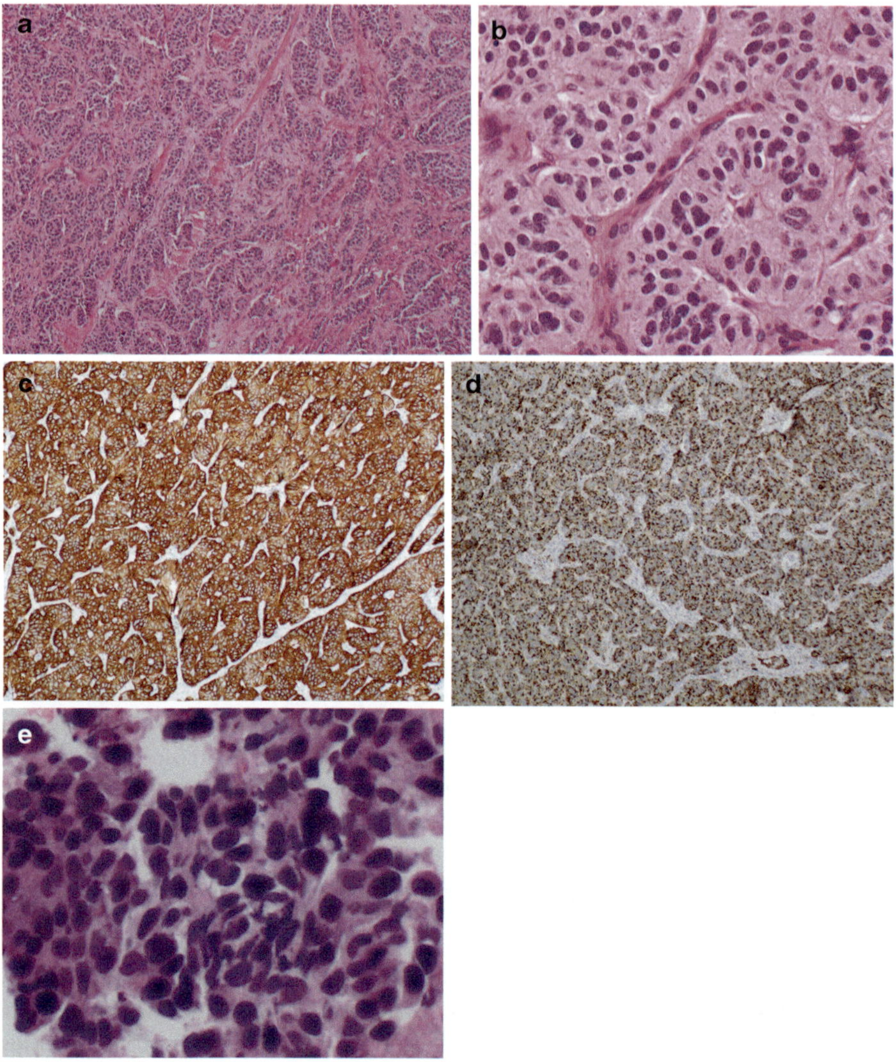

Fig. 4.25 Low-grade neuroendocrine tumor. (**a**) The tumor is comprised of monotonous cells in different arrangements interspersed with collagenized fibrous stroma. (**b**) Monomorphous tumor cells with round nuclei and fine dispersed so-called "salt-and-pepper" chromatin, rare mitosis, and small amounts of eosinophilic cytoplasm. Synaptophysin (**c**) and chromogranin (**d**) are highly sensitive and highly specific immunohistochemical marker for neuroendocrine differentiation, respectively. (**e**) Small cell neuroendocrine carcinoma consists of mitotically active small fragile calls with hyperchromatic nuclei. Nuclear molding with inconspicuous intervening cytoplasm is a helpful diagnostic histologic and cytologic finding

poorly cohesive small round blue cells with very high N:C ratio, hyperchromatic nuclei, nuclear molding, frequent mitosis, apoptotic bodies, and tumor necrosis in the background. LC-NEC is recognized by large nuclei and prominent nucleoli. NECs express common neuroendocrine phenotype and a Ki67 index >20%. They are also commonly positive for p53 and may show aberrant expression of TTF1, which may mislead to an impression of pulmonary primary. MiNEN is defined by combination of neuroendocrine and non-neuroendocrine phenotypes [8].

MiNENs of the GB and EHBD are exceedingly and a composite of NEN and adenocarcinoma, also known as *mixed adenoneuroendocrine carcinoma (MANEC).* Intestinal metaplasia is a frequent finding and is thought to be involved in the development of these tumors through a metaplasia-dysplasia-carcinoma sequence [233–235]. Tumors are more common in men (3.5:1), located in the common bile duct or common hepatic duct and range between 1 and 5 cm [233]. Histologically, adenocarcinoma and NECs are mixed but separate and can be recognized clearly. Adenocarcinoma is usually intestinal type, mucin producing, and poorly differentiated with common signet-ring-like tumor clusters. Adenocarcinoma is positive for CDX2, MUC2, CK19, and MUC5AC. In all reported cases, the neuroendocrine cells are strongly positive for synaptophysin, while other markers are positive in most but not all cases [233].

Pathogenesis and Molecular Pathology of the GB and EHBD NENs

Because of paucity of NEN in GB and EHBD and limited data, the pathogenesis of these tumors is unclear. Very small number of enterochromaffin cells in the biliary system is the plausible reason for very low incidence of NEN in this location. It has been postulated that following chronic inflammation or cholestasis biliary epithelium undergoes neuroendocrine metaplastic changes to engage in a number of autocrine and paracrine pathways, which over time increases number of neuroendocrine cells and risk of malignant transformation [236–238]. A EHBD carcinoid tumor found to have loss of heterozygosity with opposite allelic and IHC patterns signifying possibility of emergence of a new clone within the same tumor [239].

SC-NEC of the GB show large frequency of *p53* and *p16INK4a* and low frequency of *SMAD4* and *KRAS* mutations [232]. However, *KRAS*, *p53*, p16, and *SMAD4* do not appear to play a role in the pathogenesis or clinical course of the low-grade biliary NENs (carcinoids) [232, 240, 241]. Analysis of an advanced GB SC-NEC revealed gene enrichment associated with axon guidance, ERBB signaling sulfur metabolism, and calcium signaling. Somatic coding damage in *HMCN1*, *CDH10*, and *NCAM2-SGCZ* and *BTG3-CCDC40* gene fusions, with multiple chromosomal deletions, tandem duplications, and inversion, was also detected. This tumor also showed microsatellite instability and genome-wide copy number variations [242].

An EHBD carcinoid tumor found to have loss of heterozygosity with opposite allelic and IHC patterns signifying possibility of emergence of a new clone within the same tumor [239].

Summary

The biliary system gives rise to a heterogeneous group of epithelial neoplasms with different cells of origins and remarkable diversity in epidemiology, etiology, pathophysiology, genetic signature, morphological features, location, treatment approaches, and prognosis. Chronic inflammation triggers the majority of these neoplasms through a sequential progression from reactive changes to in situ malignant transformation and eventually invasive carcinoma. The pathological basis of neoplastic precursors and invasive lesions plays an essential role in multidisciplinary management of these challenging tumors. Historically, several factors have contributed to inconsistencies in the nomenclature used to describe these neoplasms and their classification. Advancements in genetic and molecular investigations have improved understanding of the pathophysiology and behavior of these neoplasms as well as their categorization. Further genetic and molecular investigations are required for proper categorization, early detection, effective treatment, and novel targeted therapy of these malignant neoplasms.

References

1. Roy S, Glaser S, Chakraborty S. Inflammation and progression of cholangiocarcinoma: role of angiogenic and lymphangiogenic mechanisms. Front Med (Lausanne). 2019;6:293.
2. Braconi C, Patel T. Cholangiocarcinoma: new insights into disease pathogenesis and biology. Infect Dis Clin N Am. 2010;24(4):871–84, vii.
3. Leyva-Illades D, McMillin M, Quinn M, Demorrow S. Cholangiocarcinoma pathogenesis: role of the tumor microenvironment. Transl Gastrointest Cancer. 2012;1(1):71–80.
4. Rizvi S, Gores GJ. Molecular pathogenesis of cholangiocarcinoma. Dig Dis. 2014;32(5):564–9.
5. Balitzer D, Joseph NM, Ferrell L, Shafizadeh N, Jain D, Zhang X, et al. Immunohistochemical and molecular features of cholangiolocellular carcinoma are similar to well-differentiated intrahepatic cholangiocarcinoma. Mod Pathol. 2019;32(10):1486–94.
6. Bragazzi MC, Ridola L, Safarikia S, Matteo SD, Costantini D, Nevi L, et al. New insights into cholangiocarcinoma: multiple stems and related cell lineages of origin. Ann Gastroenterol. 2018;31(1):42–55.
7. Roskams T. Liver stem cells and their implication in hepatocellular and cholangiocarcinoma. Oncogene. 2006;25(27):3818–22.
8. IARC. WHO Classification of tumours. Digestive system tumours. 5th ed. In: Board TWCoTE, editor. Maestro Gestion D'Edition, Villeurbanne, France: International Agency for Research of Cencer (IARC); 2019 June 2019. 635 p.

9. Zen Y, Adsay NV, Bardadin K, Colombari R, Ferrell L, Haga H, et al. Biliary intraepithelial neoplasia: an international interobserver agreement study and proposal for diagnostic criteria. Mod Pathol. 2007;20(6):701–9.
10. Ainechi S, Lee H. Updates on precancerous lesions of the biliary tract: biliary precancerous lesion. Arch Pathol Lab Med. 2016;140(11):1285–9.
11. Chan KW. Review of 253 cases of significant pathology in 7,910 cholecystectomies in Hong Kong. Pathology. 1988;20(1):20–3.
12. Roa I, Araya JC, Villaseca M, De Aretxabala X, Riedemann P, Endoh K, et al. Preneoplastic lesions and gallbladder cancer: an estimate of the period required for progression. Gastroenterology. 1996;111(1):232–6.
13. Lewis JT, Talwalkar JA, Rosen CB, Smyrk TC, Abraham SC. Precancerous bile duct pathology in end-stage primary sclerosing cholangitis, with and without cholangiocarcinoma. Am J Surg Pathol. 2010;34(1):27–34.
14. Wu TT, Levy M, Correa AM, Rosen CB, Abraham SC. Biliary intraepithelial neoplasia in patients without chronic biliary disease: analysis of liver explants with alcoholic cirrhosis, hepatitis C infection, and noncirrhotic liver diseases. Cancer. 2009;115(19):4564–75.
15. Kim KH, Dhupar R, Ueki S, Cardinal J, Pan P, Cao Z, et al. Donor graft interferon regulatory factor-1 gene transfer worsens liver transplant ischemia/reperfusion injury. Surgery. 2009;146(2):181–9.
16. EASL-EORTC clinical practice guidelines: management of hepatocellular carcinoma. J Hepatol. 2012;56(4):908–43.
17. Adsay NV, Basturk O, Cheng JD, Andea AA. Ductal neoplasia of the pancreas: nosologic, clinicopathologic, and biologic aspects. Semin Radiat Oncol. 2005;15(4):254–64.
18. Avadhani V, Hacihasanoglu E, Memis B, Pehlivanoglu B, Hanley KZ, Krishnamurti U, et al. Cytologic predictors of malignancy in bile duct brushings: a multi-reviewer analysis of 60 cases. Mod Pathol. 2017;30(9):1273–86.
19. Bergquist A, Glaumann H, Stal P, Wang GS, Broome U. Biliary dysplasia, cell proliferation and nuclear DNA-fragmentation in primary sclerosing cholangitis with and without cholangiocarcinoma. J Intern Med. 2001;249(1):69–75.
20. Nakanuma Y, Uchida T, Sato Y, Uesaka K. An S100P-positive biliary epithelial field is a preinvasive intraepithelial neoplasm in nodular-sclerosing cholangiocarcinoma. Hum Pathol. 2017;60:46–57.
21. Tsokos CG, Krings G, Yilmaz F, Ferrell LD, Gill RM. Proliferative index facilitates distinction between benign biliary lesions and intrahepatic cholangiocarcinoma. Hum Pathol. 2016;57:61–7.
22. Walter D, Herrmann E, Winkelmann R, Albert JG, Liese J, Schnitzbauer A, et al. Role of CD15 expression in dysplastic and neoplastic tissue of the bile duct – a potential novel tool for differential diagnosis of indeterminate biliary stricture. Histopathology. 2016;69(6):962–70.
23. Hruban RH, Maitra A, Kern SE, Goggins M. Precursors to pancreatic cancer. Gastroenterol Clin N Am. 2007;36(4):831–49, vi.
24. Hsu M, Sasaki M, Igarashi S, Sato Y, Nakanuma Y. KRAS and GNAS mutations and p53 overexpression in biliary intraepithelial neoplasia and intrahepatic cholangiocarcinomas. Cancer. 2013;119(9):1669–74.
25. Hucl T. Precursors to cholangiocarcinoma. Gastroenterol Res Pract. 2019;2019:1389289.
26. Serra S. Precursor neoplastic lesions of the biliary tract. J Clin Pathol. 2014;67(10):875–82.
27. Zen Y, Quaglia A, Heaton N, Rela M, Portmann B. Two distinct pathways of carcinogenesis in primary sclerosing cholangitis. Histopathology. 2011;59(6):1100–10.
28. Zen Y, Sasaki M, Fujii T, Chen TC, Chen MF, Yeh TS, et al. Different expression patterns of mucin core proteins and cytokeratins during intrahepatic cholangiocarcinogenesis from biliary intraepithelial neoplasia and intraductal papillary neoplasm of the bile duct--an immunohistochemical study of 110 cases of hepatolithiasis. J Hepatol. 2006;44(2):350–8.
29. Kim KM, Lee JK, Shin JU, Lee KH, Lee KT, Sung JY, et al. Clinicopathologic features of intraductal papillary neoplasm of the bile duct according to histologic subtype. Am J Gastroenterol. 2012;107(1):118–25.

30. Rocha FG, Lee H, Katabi N, DeMatteo RP, Fong Y, D'Angelica MI, et al. Intraductal papillary neoplasm of the bile duct: a biliary equivalent to intraductal papillary mucinous neoplasm of the pancreas? Hepatology. 2012;56(4):1352–60.
31. Park HJ, Kim SY, Kim HJ, Lee SS, Hong GS, Byun JH, et al. Intraductal papillary neoplasm of the bile duct: clinical, imaging, and pathologic features. AJR Am J Roentgenol. 2018;211(1):67–75.
32. Hachiya H, Kita J, Shiraki T, Iso Y, Shimoda M, Kubota K. Intraductal papillary neoplasm of the bile duct developing in a patient with primary sclerosing cholangitis: a case report. World J Gastroenterol. 2014;20(42):15925–30.
33. Jung G, Park KM, Lee SS, Yu E, Hong SM, Kim J. Long-term clinical outcome of the surgically resected intraductal papillary neoplasm of the bile duct. J Hepatol. 2012;57(4):787–93.
34. Nakanuma Y, Kakuda Y, Uesaka K, Miyata T, Yamamoto Y, Fukumura Y, et al. Characterization of intraductal papillary neoplasm of bile duct with respect to histopathologic similarities to pancreatic intraductal papillary mucinous neoplasm. Hum Pathol. 2016;51:103–13.
35. Wu X, Li B, Zheng C, Chang X, Zhang T, He X, et al. Intraductal papillary neoplasm of the bile duct: a single-center retrospective study. J Int Med Res. 2018;46(10):4258–68.
36. Luvira V, Somsap K, Pugkhem A, Eurboonyanun C, Luvira V, Bhudhisawasdi V, et al. Morphological classification of intraductal papillary neoplasm of the bile duct with survival correlation. Asian Pac J Cancer Prev. 2017;18(1):207–13.
37. Nakanuma Y, Sudo Y. Biliary tumors with pancreatic counterparts. Semin Diagn Pathol. 2017;34(2):167–75.
38. Schlitter AM, Born D, Bettstetter M, Specht K, Kim-Fuchs C, Riener MO, et al. Intraductal papillary neoplasms of the bile duct: stepwise progression to carcinoma involves common molecular pathways. Mod Pathol. 2014;27(1):73–86.
39. Nakanuma Y, Sato Y. Cystic and papillary neoplasm involving peribiliary glands: a biliary counterpart of branch-type intraductal papillary mucinous [corrected] neoplasm? Hepatology. 2012;55(6):2040–1.
40. Lim JH, Zen Y, Jang KT, Kim YK, Nakanuma Y. Cyst-forming intraductal papillary neoplasm of the bile ducts: description of imaging and pathologic aspects. AJR Am J Roentgenol. 2011;197(5):1111–20.
41. Lee SS, Kim MH, Lee SK, Jang SJ, Song MH, Kim KP, et al. Clinicopathologic review of 58 patients with biliary papillomatosis. Cancer. 2004;100(4):783–93.
42. Nakanuma Y, Kakuda Y, Uesaka K. Characterization of intraductal papillary neoplasm of the bile duct with respect to the histopathologic similarities to pancreatic intraductal papillary mucinous neoplasm. Gut Liver. 2019;13(6):617–27.
43. Schlitter AM, Jang KT, Kloppel G, Saka B, Hong SM, Choi H, et al. Intraductal tubulopapillary neoplasms of the bile ducts: clinicopathologic, immunohistochemical, and molecular analysis of 20 cases. Mod Pathol. 2015;28(9):1249–64.
44. Chan KM, Tsai CY, Yeh CN, Yeh TS, Lee WC, Jan YY, et al. Characterization of intrahepatic cholangiocarcinoma after curative resection: outcome, prognostic factor, and recurrence. BMC Gastroenterol. 2018;18(1):180.
45. Cardinale V, Wang Y, Carpino G, Reid LM, Gaudio E, Alvaro D. Mucin-producing cholangiocarcinoma might derive from biliary tree stem/progenitor cells located in peribiliary glands. Hepatology. 2012;55(6):2041–2.
46. Wan XS, Xu YY, Qian JY, Yang XB, Wang AQ, He L, et al. Intraductal papillary neoplasm of the bile duct. World J Gastroenterol. 2013;19(46):8595–604.
47. Kendall T, Verheij J, Gaudio E, Evert M, Guido M, Goeppert B, et al. Anatomical, histomorphological and molecular classification of cholangiocarcinoma. Liver Int. 2019;39(Suppl 1):7–18.
48. Sasaki M, Matsubara T, Yoneda N, Nomoto K, Tsuneyama K, Sato Y, et al. Overexpression of enhancer of zeste homolog 2 and MUC1 may be related to malignant behaviour in intraductal papillary neoplasm of the bile duct. Histopathology. 2013;62(3):446–57.

49. Tsai JH, Yuan RH, Chen YL, Liau JY, Jeng YM. GNAS is frequently mutated in a specific subgroup of intraductal papillary neoplasms of the bile duct. Am J Surg Pathol. 2013;37(12):1862–70.
50. Muraki T, Memis B, Reid MD, Uehara T, Ito T, Hasebe O, et al. Reflux-associated cholecystopathy: analysis of 76 gallbladders from patients with supra-oddi union of the pancreatic duct and common bile duct (pancreatobiliary maljunction) elucidates a specific diagnostic pattern of mucosal hyperplasia as a prelude to carcinoma. Am J Surg Pathol. 2017;41(9):1167–77.
51. Adsay V, Jang KT, Roa JC, Dursun N, Ohike N, Bagci P, et al. Intracholecystic papillary-tubular neoplasms (ICPN) of the gallbladder (neoplastic polyps, adenomas, and papillary neoplasms that are >/=1.0 cm): clinicopathologic and immunohistochemical analysis of 123 cases. Am J Surg Pathol. 2012;36(9):1279–301.
52. Argon A, Barbet FY, Nart D. The relationship between intracholecystic papillary-tubular neoplasms and invasive carcinoma of the gallbladder. Int J Surg Pathol. 2016;24(6):504–11.
53. Warfel KA, Hull MT. Villous papilloma of the gallbladder in association with leukodystrophy. Hum Pathol. 1984;15(12):1192–4.
54. Bennett S, Marginean EC, Paquin-Gobeil M, Wasserman J, Weaver J, Mimeault R, et al. Clinical and pathological features of intraductal papillary neoplasm of the biliary tract and gallbladder. HPB (Oxford). 2015;17(9):811–8.
55. Hashimoto S, Horaguchi J, Fujita N, Noda Y, Kobayashi G, Ito K, et al. Intracholecystic papillary-tubular neoplasm of the gallbladder presenting with jaundice. Intern Med. 2014;53(20):2313–7.
56. Paez Cumpa C, Erimeiku Barahona A, Payeras Capo MA, Amengual Antich I, Garrido Duran C. Hemobilia due to intracholecystic papillary neoplasm. Rev Esp Enferm Dig. 2017;109(1):70–3.
57. Hazarika P, Sharma MK. Intracholecystic papillary-tubular neoplasm of gallbladder: a 5-year retrospective pathological study. Indian J Pathol Microbiol. 2018;61(4):516–9.
58. Muranushi R, Saito H, Matsumoto A, Kato T, Tanaka N, Nakazato K, et al. A case report of intracholecystic papillary neoplasm of the gallbladder resembling a submucosal tumor. Surg Case Rep. 2018;4(1):124.
59. He C, Fukumura Y, Toriyama A, Ogura K, Sasahara N, Mitani K, et al. Pyloric gland adenoma (PGA) of the gallbladder: a unique and distinct tumor from PGAs of the stomach, duodenum, and pancreas. Am J Surg Pathol. 2018;42(9):1237–45.
60. Albores-Saavedra J, Chable-Montero F, Gonzalez-Romo MA, Ramirez Jaramillo M, Henson DE. Adenomas of the gallbladder. Morphologic features, expression of gastric and intestinal mucins, and incidence of high-grade dysplasia/carcinoma in situ and invasive carcinoma. Hum Pathol. 2012;43(9):1506–13.
61. Schaefer IM, Cameron S, Middel P, Homayounfar K, Schworer H, Vieth M, et al. Pyloric gland adenoma of the cystic duct with malignant transformation: report of a case with a review of the literature. BMC Cancer. 2012;12:570.
62. Bray F, Ferlay J, Soerjomataram I, Siegel RL, Torre LA, Jemal A. Global cancer statistics 2018: GLOBOCAN estimates of incidence and mortality worldwide for 36 cancers in 185 countries. CA Cancer J Clin. 2018;68(6):394–424.
63. Stinton LM, Shaffer EA. Epidemiology of gallbladder disease: cholelithiasis and cancer. Gut Liver. 2012;6(2):172–87.
64. Duffy A, Capanu M, Abou-Alfa GK, Huitzil D, Jarnagin W, Fong Y, et al. Gallbladder cancer (GBC): 10-year experience at Memorial Sloan-Kettering Cancer Centre (MSKCC). J Surg Oncol. 2008;98(7):485–9.
65. Henley SJ, Weir HK, Jim MA, Watson M, Richardson LC. Gallbladder cancer incidence and mortality, United States 1999–2011. Cancer Epidemiol Biomark Prev. 2015;24(9):1319–26.
66. Ali AH, Tabibian JH, Nasser-Ghodsi N, Lennon RJ, DeLeon T, Borad MJ, et al. Surveillance for hepatobiliary cancers in patients with primary sclerosing cholangitis. Hepatology. 2018;67(6):2338–51.

67. Chapman R, Fevery J, Kalloo A, Nagorney DM, Boberg KM, Shneider B, et al. Diagnosis and management of primary sclerosing cholangitis. Hepatology. 2010;51(2):660–78.
68. Tabibian JH, Ali AH, Lindor KD. Primary sclerosing cholangitis, part 2: cancer risk, prevention, and surveillance. Gastroenterol Hepatol (N Y). 2018;14(7):427–32.
69. Patel S, Roa JC, Tapia O, Dursun N, Bagci P, Basturk O, et al. Hyalinizing cholecystitis and associated carcinomas: clinicopathologic analysis of a distinctive variant of cholecystitis with porcelain-like features and accompanying diagnostically challenging carcinomas. Am J Surg Pathol. 2011;35(8):1104–13.
70. Roa JC, Tapia O, Manterola C, Villaseca M, Guzman P, Araya JC, et al. Early gallbladder carcinoma has a favorable outcome but Rokitansky-Aschoff sinus involvement is an adverse prognostic factor. Virchows Arch. 2013;463(5):651–61.
71. Nagano T, Ishii G, Nagai K, Ito T, Kawase A, Takahashi K, et al. Structural and biological properties of a papillary component generating a micropapillary component in lung adenocarcinoma. Lung Cancer. 2010;67(3):282–9.
72. Nakanuma Y, Jang KT, Fukushima N, Furukawa T, Hong SM, Kim H, et al. A statement by the Japan-Korea expert pathologists for future clinicopathological and molecular analyses toward consensus building of intraductal papillary neoplasm of the bile duct through several opinions at the present stage. J Hepatobiliary Pancreat Sci. 2018;25(3):181–7.
73. Nassar H, Pansare V, Zhang H, Che M, Sakr W, Ali-Fehmi R, et al. Pathogenesis of invasive micropapillary carcinoma: role of MUC1 glycoprotein. Mod Pathol. 2004;17(9):1045–50.
74. Hara S, Kijima H, Okada K, Igarashi Y. Invasive micropapillary variant of the gallbladder adenocarcinoma and its aggressive potential for lymph node metastasis. Biomed Res. 2010;31(2):89–95.
75. Lei L, Zhang H, Zhang XB, Lonser R, Thompson K, Raza A. Consensus and conflict in invasive micropapillary carcinoma: a case report and review of the literature. J Gastrointest Oncol. 2016;7(Suppl 1):S55–61.
76. Albores-Saavedra J, Nadji M, Henson DE. Intestinal-type adenocarcinoma of the gallbladder. A clinicopathologic study of seven cases. Am J Surg Pathol. 1986;10(1):19–25.
77. Wan X, Shi J, Wang A, Xie Y, Yang X, Zhu C, et al. Gallbladder papillary neoplasms share pathological features with intraductal papillary neoplasm of the bile duct. Oncotarget. 2017;8(19):31532–9.
78. Dursun N, Escalona OT, Roa JC, Basturk O, Bagci P, Cakir A, et al. Mucinous carcinomas of the gallbladder: clinicopathologic analysis of 15 cases identified in 606 carcinomas. Arch Pathol Lab Med. 2012;136(11):1347–58.
79. Ahmad Z, Qureshi A. Primary signet ring cell carcinoma of gall bladder: report of an extremely rare histological type of primary gall bladder carcinoma. BMJ Case Rep. 2010;2010:bcr0420091782.
80. Czyszczon IA, Alatassi H. Signet ring cell carcinoma of the gallbladder in a 22-year-old man: a case report and review of the literature. Int J Surg Pathol. 2010;18(5):358–62.
81. Karabulut Z, Yildirim Y, Abaci I, Ilgici D, Ozyilkan O. Signet-ring cell carcinoma of the gallbladder: a case report. Adv Ther. 2008;25(5):520–3.
82. Pudasainin S, Subedi N, Prasad KB, Rauniyar SK, Bhattacharya SK, Koirala R, et al. Signet ring cell carcinoma of the gallbladder: a case report. Nepal Med Coll J. 2011;13(4):308–10.
83. Saito Y, Okuda H, Yoshida M, Okimasa S, Fukuda T, Yano M, et al. Gallbladder metastasis of renal clear cell carcinoma 15 years after primary cancer excision: a case report. J Med Case Rep. 2018;12(1):162.
84. Eken H, Balci MG, Buyukakincak S, Isik A, Firat D, Cimen O. Rare tumors of the gallbladder: clear cell carcinoma. Int J Surg Case Rep. 2015;9:65–8.
85. Vardaman C, Albores-Saavedra J. Clear cell carcinomas of the gallbladder and extrahepatic bile ducts. Am J Surg Pathol. 1995;19(1):91–9.
86. Gu L, Jiang CH, Xu Q, Liu Q, Luo M, Wu ZY. Primary clear cell carcinoma of hilar bile duct: a case report. J Dig Dis. 2010;11(1):63–5.

87. Roa JC, Tapia O, Cakir A, Basturk O, Dursun N, Akdemir D, et al. Squamous cell and adenosquamous carcinomas of the gallbladder: clinicopathological analysis of 34 cases identified in 606 carcinomas. Mod Pathol. 2011;24(8):1069–78.
88. Song HW, Chen C, Shen HX, Ma L, Zhao YL, Zhang GJ, et al. Squamous/adenosquamous carcinoma of the gallbladder: analysis of 34 cases and comparison of clinicopathologic features and surgical outcomes with adenocarcinoma. J Surg Oncol. 2015;112(6):677–80.
89. Ellouze S, Slim C, Ahmad G, Naourez G, Ali A, Hela M, et al. Hepatoid adenocarcinoma of the gallbladder. World J Surg Oncol. 2011;9:103.
90. Sakamoto K, Monobe Y, Kouno M, Moriya T, Sasano H. Hepatoid adenocarcinoma of the gallbladder: case report and review of the literature. Pathol Int. 2004;54(1):52–6.
91. van den Bos IC, Hussain SM, Dwarkasing RS, Stoop H, Zondervan PE, Krestin GP, et al. Hepatoid adenocarcinoma of the gallbladder: a mimicker of hepatocellular carcinoma. Br J Radiol. 2007;80(960):e317–20.
92. Kim MJ, Yu E, Ro JY. Sarcomatoid carcinoma of the gallbladder with a rhabdoid tumor component. Arch Pathol Lab Med. 2003;127(10):e406–8.
93. Arakawa A, Fujii H, Matsumoto T, Hirai S, Suda K. Loss of heterozygosity in clonal evolution with genetic progression and divergence in spindle cell carcinoma of the gallbladder. Hum Pathol. 2004;35(4):418–23.
94. Furuya Y, Hiroshima K, Wakahara T, Akimoto H, Yanagie H, Harigaya K, et al. Undifferentiated carcinoma of the gallbladder with endothelial differentiation: a case report and literature review. Mol Clin Oncol. 2016;5(6):773–6.
95. Akatsu T, Ueda M, Shimazu M, Wakabayashi G, Aiura K, Tanabe M, et al. Primary undifferentiated spindle-cell carcinoma of the gallbladder presenting as a liver tumor. J Gastroenterol. 2005;40(10):993–8.
96. Guo KJ, Yamaguchi K, Enjoji M. Undifferentiated carcinoma of the gallbladder. A clinicopathologic, histochemical, and immunohistochemical study of 21 patients with a poor prognosis. Cancer. 1988;61(9):1872–9.
97. Javle M, Bekaii-Saab T, Jain A, Wang Y, Kelley RK, Wang K, et al. Biliary cancer: utility of next-generation sequencing for clinical management. Cancer. 2016;122(24):3838–47.
98. Jiao Y, Pawlik TM, Anders RA, Selaru FM, Streppel MM, Lucas DJ, et al. Exome sequencing identifies frequent inactivating mutations in BAP1, ARID1A and PBRM1 in intrahepatic cholangiocarcinomas. Nat Genet. 2013;45(12):1470–3.
99. Shibata T, Arai Y, Totoki Y. Molecular genomic landscapes of hepatobiliary cancer. Cancer Sci. 2018;109(5):1282–91.
100. Roa JC, Roa I, Correa P, Vo Q, Araya JC, Villaseca M, et al. Microsatellite instability in preneoplastic and neoplastic lesions of the gallbladder. J Gastroenterol. 2005;40(1):79–86.
101. Park SK, Andreotti G, Rashid A, Chen J, Rosenberg PS, Yu K, et al. Polymorphisms of estrogen receptors and risk of biliary tract cancers and gallstones: a population-based study in Shanghai, China. Carcinogenesis. 2010;31(5):842–6.
102. Nam AR, Kim JW, Cha Y, Ha H, Park JE, Bang JH, et al. Therapeutic implication of HER2 in advanced biliary tract cancer. Oncotarget. 2016;7(36):58007–21.
103. Iyer P, Shrikhande SV, Ranjan M, Joshi A, Gardi N, Prasad R, et al. ERBB2 and KRAS alterations mediate response to EGFR inhibitors in early stage gallbladder cancer. Int J Cancer. 2019;144(8):2008–19.
104. Silva VW, Askan G, Daniel TD, Lowery M, Klimstra DS, Abou-Alfa GK, et al. Biliary carcinomas: pathology and the role of DNA mismatch repair deficiency. Chin Clin Oncol. 2016;5(5):62.
105. Cha PC, Zembutsu H, Takahashi A, Kubo M, Kamatani N, Nakamura Y. A genome-wide association study identifies SNP in DCC is associated with gallbladder cancer in the Japanese population. J Hum Genet. 2012;57(4):235–7.
106. Khan SA, Emadossadaty S, Ladep NG, Thomas HC, Elliott P, Taylor-Robinson SD, et al. Rising trends in cholangiocarcinoma: is the ICD classification system misleading us? J Hepatol. 2012;56(4):848–54.

107. Raoof M, Singh G. Rising trends in intrahepatic cholangiocarcinoma incidence and mortality: getting at the root cause. Hepatobiliary Surg Nutr. 2019;8(3):301–3.
108. Tyson GL, Ilyas JA, Duan Z, Green LK, Younes M, El-Serag HB, et al. Secular trends in the incidence of cholangiocarcinoma in the USA and the impact of misclassification. Dig Dis Sci. 2014;59(12):3103–10.
109. Welzel TM, McGlynn KA, Hsing AW, O'Brien TR, Pfeiffer RM. Impact of classification of hilar cholangiocarcinomas (Klatskin tumors) on the incidence of intra- and extrahepatic cholangiocarcinoma in the United States. J Natl Cancer Inst. 2006;98(12):873–5.
110. Amin MB; American Joint Committee on Cancer, American Cancer Society. AJCC cancer staging manual. 8th ed. In: Amin MB, Editor-in-chief, Edge SB, et al., Gress DM, RHIT, CTR, Technical editor, Meyer LR, CAPM, Managing editor. Chicago: American Joint Committee on Cancer/Springer; 2017. xvii, 1024 p.
111. DeOliveira ML, Cunningham SC, Cameron JL, Kamangar F, Winter JM, Lillemoe KD, et al. Cholangiocarcinoma: thirty-one-year experience with 564 patients at a single institution. Ann Surg. 2007;245(5):755–62.
112. Nakeeb A, Pitt HA, Sohn TA, Coleman J, Abrams RA, Piantadosi S, et al. Cholangiocarcinoma. A spectrum of intrahepatic, perihilar, and distal tumors. Ann Surg. 1996;224(4):463–73; discussion 73–5.
113. Kloppel G, Adsay V, Konukiewitz B, Kleeff J, Schlitter AM, Esposito I. Precancerous lesions of the biliary tree. Best Pract Res Clin Gastroenterol. 2013;27(2):285–97.
114. Carpino G, Cardinale V, Onori P, Franchitto A, Berloco PB, Rossi M, et al. Biliary tree stem/progenitor cells in glands of extrahepatic and intraheptic bile ducts: an anatomical in situ study yielding evidence of maturational lineages. J Anat. 2012;220(2):186–99.
115. Carpino G, Cardinale V, Renzi A, Hov JR, Berloco PB, Rossi M, et al. Activation of biliary tree stem cells within peribiliary glands in primary sclerosing cholangitis. J Hepatol. 2015;63(5):1220–8.
116. Sato Y, Harada K, Sasaki M, Nakanuma Y. Cystic and micropapillary epithelial changes of peribiliary glands might represent a precursor lesion of biliary epithelial neoplasms. Virchows Arch. 2014;464(2):157–63.
117. Gulamhusein AF, Eaton JE, Tabibian JH, Atkinson EJ, Juran BD, Lazaridis KN. Duration of inflammatory bowel disease is associated with increased risk of cholangiocarcinoma in patients with primary sclerosing cholangitis and IBD. Am J Gastroenterol. 2016;111(5):705–11.
118. Ebata T, Kosuge T, Hirano S, Unno M, Yamamoto M, Miyazaki M, et al. Proposal to modify the International Union Against Cancer staging system for perihilar cholangiocarcinomas. Br J Surg. 2014;101(2):79–88.
119. Hong SM, Pawlik TM, Cho H, Aggarwal B, Goggins M, Hruban RH, et al. Depth of tumor invasion better predicts prognosis than the current American Joint Committee on Cancer T classification for distal bile duct carcinoma. Surgery. 2009;146(2):250–7.
120. Young AL, Igami T, Senda Y, Adair R, Farid S, Toogood GJ, et al. Evolution of the surgical management of perihilar cholangiocarcinoma in a Western Centre demonstrates improved survival with endoscopic biliary drainage and reduced use of blood transfusion. HPB (Oxford). 2011;13(7):483–93.
121. Brunt E, Aishima S, Clavien PA, Fowler K, Goodman Z, Gores G, et al. cHCC-CCA: consensus terminology for primary liver carcinomas with both hepatocytic and cholangiocytic differentation. Hepatology. 2018;68(1):113–26.
122. Albores-Saavedra J, Chable-Montero F, Mendez-Sanchez N, Mercado MA, Vilatoba-Chapa M, Henson DE. Adenocarcinoma with pyloric gland phenotype of the extrahepatic bile ducts: a previously unrecognized and distinctive morphologic variant of extrahepatic bile duct carcinoma. Hum Pathol. 2012;43(12):2292–8.
123. Jarnagin WR, Fong Y, DeMatteo RP, Gonen M, Burke EC, Bodniewicz BJ, et al. Staging, resectability, and outcome in 225 patients with hilar cholangiocarcinoma. Ann Surg. 2001;234(4):507–17; discussion 17–9.

124. Deoliveira ML, Schulick RD, Nimura Y, Rosen C, Gores G, Neuhaus P, et al. New staging system and a registry for perihilar cholangiocarcinoma. Hepatology. 2011;53(4):1363–71.
125. Wardell CP, Fujita M, Yamada T, Simbolo M, Fassan M, Karlic R, et al. Genomic characterization of biliary tract cancers identifies driver genes and predisposing mutations. J Hepatol. 2018;68(5):959–69.
126. Liau JY, Tsai JH, Yuan RH, Chang CN, Lee HJ, Jeng YM. Morphological subclassification of intrahepatic cholangiocarcinoma: etiological, clinicopathological, and molecular features. Mod Pathol. 2014;27(8):1163–73.
127. Kim HJ, Kim JS, Kim BH, Bak YT. Clinicopathologic study of biliary intraepithelial neoplasia in cholangiocarcinoma. Dig Surg. 2018;35(2):116–20.
128. Brooks C, Gausman V, Kokoy-Mondragon C, Munot K, Amin SP, Desai A, et al. Role of fluorescent in situ hybridization, cholangioscopic biopsies, and EUS-FNA in the evaluation of biliary strictures. Dig Dis Sci. 2018;63(3):636–44.
129. Rizvi S, Khan SA, Hallemeier CL, Kelley RK, Gores GJ. Cholangiocarcinoma – evolving concepts and therapeutic strategies. Nat Rev Clin Oncol. 2018;15(2):95–111.
130. Albores-Saavedra J, Cordova-Ramon JC, Chable-Montero F, Dorantes-Heredia R, Henson DE. Cystadenomas of the liver and extrahepatic bile ducts: morphologic and immunohistochemical characterization of the biliary and intestinal variants. Ann Diagn Pathol. 2015;19(3):124–9.
131. Quigley B, Reid MD, Pehlivanoglu B, Squires MH 3rd, Maithel S, Xue Y, et al. Hepatobiliary mucinous cystic neoplasms with ovarian type stroma (so-called "hepatobiliary cystadenoma/cystadenocarcinoma"): clinicopathologic analysis of 36 cases illustrates rarity of carcinomatous change. Am J Surg Pathol. 2018;42(1):95–102.
132. Arnaoutakis DJ, Kim Y, Pulitano C, Zaydfudim V, Squires MH, Kooby D, et al. Management of biliary cystic tumors: a multi-institutional analysis of a rare liver tumor. Ann Surg. 2015;261(2):361–7.
133. Rivero-Soto RJ, Hossein-Zadeh Z, Coleman J, Ahuja V. A mucinous cystic neoplasm originating from the gallbladder: a case report and literature review. Perm J. 2019;23:18–077.
134. Lee CW, Tsai HI, Lin YS, Wu TH, Yu MC, Chen MF. Intrahepatic biliary mucinous cystic neoplasms: clinicoradiological characteristics and surgical results. BMC Gastroenterol. 2015;15:67.
135. Jeong D, Jiang K, Anaya DA. Mucinous cystic neoplasm of the liver masquerading as an echinococcal cyst: radiologic-pathologic differential of complex cystic liver lesions. J Clin Imaging Sci. 2016;6:12.
136. Hsu M, Terris B, Wu TT, Zen Y, Eng HL, Huang WT, et al. Endometrial cysts within the liver: a rare entity and its differential diagnosis with mucinous cystic neoplasms of the liver. Hum Pathol. 2014;45(4):761–7.
137. Nakayama Y, Kato Y, Okubo S, Takahashi D, Okada R, Nishida Y, et al. A case of mucinous cystic neoplasm of the liver: a case report. Surg Case Rep. 2015;1(1):9.
138. Conner JR, Marino-Enriquez A, Mino-Kenudson M, Garcia E, Pitman MB, Sholl LM, et al. Genomic characterization of low- and high-grade pancreatic mucinous cystic neoplasms reveals recurrent KRAS alterations in "high-risk" lesions. Pancreas. 2017;46(5):665–71.
139. Fujikura K, Akita M, Abe-Suzuki S, Itoh T, Zen Y. Mucinous cystic neoplasms of the liver and pancreas: relationship between KRAS driver mutations and disease progression. Histopathology. 2017;71(4):591–600.
140. Gupta A, Dixon E. Epidemiology and risk factors: intrahepatic cholangiocarcinoma. Hepatobiliary Surg Nutr. 2017;6(2):101–4.
141. Saha SK, Zhu AX, Fuchs CS, Brooks GA. Forty-year trends in cholangiocarcinoma incidence in the U.S.: intrahepatic disease on the rise. Oncologist. 2016;21(5):594–9.
142. Shaib Y, El-Serag HB. The epidemiology of cholangiocarcinoma. Semin Liver Dis. 2004;24(2):115–25.
143. Ben-Menachem T. Risk factors for cholangiocarcinoma. Eur J Gastroenterol Hepatol. 2007;19(8):615–7.

144. Kurathong S, Lerdverasirikul P, Wongpaitoon V, Pramoolsinsap C, Kanjanapitak A, Varavithya W, et al. Opisthorchis viverrini infection and cholangiocarcinoma. A prospective, case-controlled study. Gastroenterology. 1985;89(1):151–6.
145. Lowenfels AB. Opisthorchis viverrini infection and cholangiocarcinoma. Gastroenterology. 1985;89(6):1449.
146. Okuda K, Nakanuma Y, Miyazaki M. Cholangiocarcinoma: recent progress. Part 2: molecular pathology and treatment. J Gastroenterol Hepatol. 2002;17(10):1056–63.
147. Okuda K, Nakanuma Y, Miyazaki M. Cholangiocarcinoma: recent progress. Part 1: epidemiology and etiology. J Gastroenterol Hepatol. 2002;17(10):1049–55.
148. Shaib YH, El-Serag HB, Nooka AK, Thomas M, Brown TD, Patt YZ, et al. Risk factors for intrahepatic and extrahepatic cholangiocarcinoma: a hospital-based case-control study. Am J Gastroenterol. 2007;102(5):1016–21.
149. Singal AK, Vauthey JN, Grady JJ, Stroehlein JR. Intra-hepatic cholangiocarcinoma--frequency and demographic patterns: thirty-year data from the M.D. Anderson Cancer Center. J Cancer Res Clin Oncol. 2011;137(7):1071–8.
150. Suzuki Y, Mori T, Yokoyama M, Nakazato T, Abe N, Nakanuma Y, et al. Hepatolithiasis: analysis of Japanese nationwide surveys over a period of 40 years. J Hepatobiliary Pancreat Sci. 2014;21(9):617–22.
151. Welzel TM, Mellemkjaer L, Gloria G, Sakoda LC, Hsing AW, El Ghormli L, et al. Risk factors for intrahepatic cholangiocarcinoma in a low-risk population: a nationwide case-control study. Int J Cancer. 2007;120(3):638–41.
152. Zhang H, Yang T, Wu M, Shen F. Intrahepatic cholangiocarcinoma: epidemiology, risk factors, diagnosis and surgical management. Cancer Lett. 2016;379(2):198–205.
153. Welzel TM, Graubard BI, El-Serag HB, Shaib YH, Hsing AW, Davila JA, et al. Risk factors for intrahepatic and extrahepatic cholangiocarcinoma in the United States: a population-based case-control study. Clin Gastroenterol Hepatol. 2007;5(10):1221–8.
154. Aishima S, Iguchi T, Fujita N, Taketomi A, Maehara Y, Tsuneyoshi M, et al. Histological and immunohistological findings in biliary intraepithelial neoplasia arising from a background of chronic biliary disease compared with liver cirrhosis of non-biliary aetiology. Histopathology. 2011;59(5):867–75.
155. Aishima S, Oda Y. Pathogenesis and classification of intrahepatic cholangiocarcinoma: different characters of perihilar large duct type versus peripheral small duct type. J Hepatobiliary Pancreat Sci. 2015;22(2):94–100.
156. Nakanuma Y, Kakuda Y. Pathologic classification of cholangiocarcinoma: new concepts. Best Pract Res Clin Gastroenterol. 2015;29(2):277–93.
157. Nakanuma Y. Classification of intrahepatic cholangiocarcinoma based on recent progress and new proposal. Nihon Shokakibyo Gakkai Zasshi. 2012;109(11):1865–71.
158. Akita M, Fujikura K, Ajiki T, Fukumoto T, Otani K, Azuma T, et al. Dichotomy in intrahepatic cholangiocarcinomas based on histologic similarities to hilar cholangiocarcinomas. Mod Pathol. 2017;30(7):986–97.
159. Rocken C, Pross M, Brucks U, Ridwelski K, Roessner A. Cholangiocarcinoma occurring in a liver with multiple bile duct hamartomas (von Meyenburg complexes). Arch Pathol Lab Med. 2000;124(11):1704–6.
160. Aishima S, Nishihara Y, Tsujita E, Taguchi K, Soejima Y, Taketomi A, et al. Biliary neoplasia with extensive intraductal spread associated with liver cirrhosis: a hitherto unreported variant of biliary intraepithelial neoplasia. Hum Pathol. 2008;39(6):939–47.
161. Blanc JF, Bernard PH, Carles J, Le Bail B, Balabaud C, Bioulac-Sage P. Cholangiocarcinoma arising in Von Meyenburg complex associated with hepatocellular carcinoma in genetic haemochromatosis. Eur J Gastroenterol Hepatol. 2000;12(2):233–7.
162. Pinho AC, Melo RB, Oliveira M, Almeida M, Lopes J, Graca L, et al. Adenoma-carcinoma sequence in intrahepatic cholangiocarcinoma. Int J Surg Case Rep. 2012;3(4):131–3.

163. Komuta M, Spee B, Vander Borght S, De Vos R, Verslype C, Aerts R, et al. Clinicopathological study on cholangiolocellular carcinoma suggesting hepatic progenitor cell origin. Hepatology. 2008;47(5):1544–56.
164. Nakanuma Y, Sato Y, Ikeda H, Harada K, Kobayashi M, Sano K, et al. Intrahepatic cholangiocarcinoma with predominant "ductal plate malformation" pattern: a new subtype. Am J Surg Pathol. 2012;36(11):1629–35.
165. Sigel CS, Drill E, Zhou Y, Basturk O, Askan G, Pak LM, et al. Intrahepatic cholangiocarcinomas have histologically and immunophenotypically distinct small and large duct patterns. Am J Surg Pathol. 2018;42(10):1334–45.
166. Sia D, Hoshida Y, Villanueva A, Roayaie S, Ferrer J, Tabak B, et al. Integrative molecular analysis of intrahepatic cholangiocarcinoma reveals 2 classes that have different outcomes. Gastroenterology. 2013;144(4):829–40.
167. Sekiya S, Suzuki A. Intrahepatic cholangiocarcinoma can arise from Notch-mediated conversion of hepatocytes. J Clin Invest. 2012;122(11):3914–8.
168. Ishii Y, Sasaki T, Serikawa M, Minami T, Okazaki A, Yukutake M, et al. Elevated expression of cyclooxygenase-2 and microsomal prostaglandin E synthase-1 in primary sclerosing cholangitis: iotamplications for cholangiocarcinogenesis. Int J Oncol. 2013;43(4):1073–9.
169. Chan-On W, Nairismagi ML, Ong CK, Lim WK, Dima S, Pairojkul C, et al. Exome sequencing identifies distinct mutational patterns in liver fluke-related and non-infection-related bile duct cancers. Nat Genet. 2013;45(12):1474–8.
170. Jusakul A, Cutcutache I, Yong CH, Lim JQ, Huang MN, Padmanabhan N, et al. Whole-genome and epigenomic landscapes of etiologically distinct subtypes of cholangiocarcinoma. Cancer Discov. 2017;7(10):1116–35.
171. Andrici J, Goeppert B, Sioson L, Clarkson A, Renner M, Stenzinger A, et al. Loss of BAP1 expression occurs frequently in intrahepatic cholangiocarcinoma. Medicine (Baltimore). 2016;95(2):e2491.
172. Mosbeh A, Halfawy K, Abdel-Mageed WS, Sweed D, Rahman MHA. Nuclear BAP1 loss is common in intrahepatic cholangiocarcinoma and a subtype of hepatocellular carcinoma but rare in pancreatic ductal adenocarcinoma. Cancer Genet. 2018;224–225:21–8.
173. Graham RP, Barr Fritcher EG, Pestova E, Schulz J, Sitailo LA, Vasmatzis G, et al. Fibroblast growth factor receptor 2 translocations in intrahepatic cholangiocarcinoma. Hum Pathol. 2014;45(8):1630–8.
174. Lowery MA, Ptashkin R, Jordan E, Berger MF, Zehir A, Capanu M, et al. Comprehensive molecular profiling of intrahepatic and extrahepatic cholangiocarcinomas: potential targets for intervention. Clin Cancer Res. 2018;24(17):4154–61.
175. Andersen JB, Spee B, Blechacz BR, Avital I, Komuta M, Barbour A, et al. Genomic and genetic characterization of cholangiocarcinoma identifies therapeutic targets for tyrosine kinase inhibitors. Gastroenterology. 2012;142(4):1021–31 e15.
176. Sia D, Villanueva A, Friedman SL, Llovet JM. Liver cancer cell of origin, molecular class, and effects on patient prognosis. Gastroenterology. 2017;152(4):745–61.
177. Goeppert B, Frauenschuh L, Renner M, Roessler S, Stenzinger A, Klauschen F, et al. BRAF V600E-specific immunohistochemistry reveals low mutation rates in biliary tract cancer and restriction to intrahepatic cholangiocarcinoma. Mod Pathol. 2014;27(7):1028–34.
178. Sempoux C, Paradis V, Saxena R. Variant differentiation patterns in primary liver carcinoma. Semin Diagn Pathol. 2017;34(2):176–82.
179. Yoon YI, Hwang S, Lee YJ, Kim KH, Ahn CS, Moon DB, et al. Postresection outcomes of combined hepatocellular carcinoma-cholangiocarcinoma, hepatocellular carcinoma and intrahepatic cholangiocarcinoma. J Gastrointest Surg. 2016;20(2):411–20.
180. Jarnagin WR, Weber S, Tickoo SK, Koea JB, Obiekwe S, Fong Y, et al. Combined hepatocellular and cholangiocarcinoma: demographic, clinical, and prognostic factors. Cancer. 2002;94(7):2040–6.

181. Fowler KJ, Sheybani A, Parker RA 3rd, Doherty S, Brunt EM, Chapman WC, et al. Combined hepatocellular and cholangiocarcinoma (biphenotypic) tumors: imaging features and diagnostic accuracy of contrast-enhanced CT and MRI. AJR Am J Roentgenol. 2013;201(2):332–9.
182. Wells ML, Venkatesh SK, Chandan VS, Fidler JL, Fletcher JG, Johnson GB, et al. Biphenotypic hepatic tumors: imaging findings and review of literature. Abdom Imaging. 2015;40(7):2293–305.
183. Zen C, Zen Y, Mitry RR, Corbeil D, Karbanova J, O'Grady J, et al. Mixed phenotype hepatocellular carcinoma after transarterial chemoembolization and liver transplantation. Liver Transpl. 2011;17(8):943–54.
184. Garancini M, Goffredo P, Pagni F, Romano F, Roman S, Sosa JA, et al. Combined hepatocellular-cholangiocarcinoma: a population-level analysis of an uncommon primary liver tumor. Liver Transpl. 2014;20(8):952–9.
185. Kim KH, Lee SG, Park EH, Hwang S, Ahn CS, Moon DB, et al. Surgical treatments and prognoses of patients with combined hepatocellular carcinoma and cholangiocarcinoma. Ann Surg Oncol. 2009;16(3):623–9.
186. Chu KJ, Lu CD, Dong H, Fu XH, Zhang HW, Yao XP. Hepatitis B virus-related combined hepatocellular-cholangiocarcinoma: clinicopathological and prognostic analysis of 390 cases. Eur J Gastroenterol Hepatol. 2014;26(2):192–9.
187. Park HS, Bae JS, Jang KY, Lee JH, Yu HC, Jung JH, et al. Clinicopathologic study on combined hepatocellular carcinoma and cholangiocarcinoma: with emphasis on the intermediate cell morphology. J Korean Med Sci. 2011;26(8):1023–30.
188. Tickoo SK, Zee SY, Obiekwe S, Xiao H, Koea J, Robiou C, et al. Combined hepatocellular-cholangiocarcinoma: a histopathologic, immunohistochemical, and in situ hybridization study. Am J Surg Pathol. 2002;26(8):989–97.
189. Brunt EM, Paradis V, Sempoux C, Theise ND. Biphenotypic (hepatobiliary) primary liver carcinomas: the work in progress. Hepat Oncol. 2015;2(3):255–73.
190. Theise ND, Yao JL, Harada K, Hytiroglou P, Portmann B, Thung SN, et al. Hepatic 'stem cell' malignancies in adults: four cases. Histopathology. 2003;43(3):263–71.
191. Leung CO, Mak WN, Kai AK, Chan KS, Lee TK, Ng IO, et al. Sox9 confers stemness properties in hepatocellular carcinoma through Frizzled-7 mediated Wnt/beta-catenin signaling. Oncotarget. 2016;7(20):29371–86.
192. Sasaki M, Sato H, Kakuda Y, Sato Y, Choi JH, Nakanuma Y. Clinicopathological significance of 'subtypes with stem-cell feature' in combined hepatocellular-cholangiocarcinoma. Liver Int. 2015;35(3):1024–35.
193. Fujii H, Zhu XG, Matsumoto T, Inagaki M, Tokusashi Y, Miyokawa N, et al. Genetic classification of combined hepatocellular-cholangiocarcinoma. Hum Pathol. 2000;31(9):1011–7.
194. Yano H, Iemura A, Haramaki M, Momosaki S, Ogasawara S, Higaki K, et al. A human combined hepatocellular and cholangiocarcinoma cell line (KMCH-2) that shows the features of hepatocellular carcinoma or cholangiocarcinoma under different growth conditions. J Hepatol. 1996;24(4):413–22.
195. Li L, Qian M, Chen IH, Finkelstein D, Onar-Thomas A, Johnson M, et al. Acquisition of cholangiocarcinoma traits during advanced hepatocellular carcinoma development in mice. Am J Pathol. 2018;188(3):656–71.
196. Moeini A, Sia D, Zhang Z, Camprecios G, Stueck A, Dong H, et al. Mixed hepatocellular cholangiocarcinoma tumors: cholangiolocellular carcinoma is a distinct molecular entity. J Hepatol. 2017;66(5):952–61.
197. Lee JH, Chung GE, Yu SJ, Hwang SY, Kim JS, Kim HY, et al. Long-term prognosis of combined hepatocellular and cholangiocarcinoma after curative resection comparison with hepatocellular carcinoma and cholangiocarcinoma. J Clin Gastroenterol. 2011;45(1):69–75.
198. Zuo HQ, Yan LN, Zeng Y, Yang JY, Luo HZ, Liu JW, et al. Clinicopathological characteristics of 15 patients with combined hepatocellular carcinoma and cholangiocarcinoma. Hepatobiliary Pancreat Dis Int. 2007;6(2):161–5.

199. Desmet VJ. Congenital diseases of intrahepatic bile ducts: variations on the theme "ductal plate malformation". Hepatology. 1992;16(4):1069–83.
200. Jain D, Sarode VR, Abdul-Karim FW, Homer R, Robert ME. Evidence for the neoplastic transformation of Von-Meyenburg complexes. Am J Surg Pathol. 2000;24(8):1131–9.
201. Panda N, Brackett D, Eymard C, Kawai T, Markmann J, Kotton CN, et al. Liver transplantation for recurrent cholangitis from Von Meyenburg complexes. Transplant Direct. 2019;5(3):e428.
202. Jain D, Ahrens W, Finkelstein S. Molecular evidence for the neoplastic potential of hepatic Von-Meyenburg complexes. Appl Immunohistochem Mol Morphol. 2010;18(2):166–71.
203. Desmet VJ. Ludwig symposium on biliary disorders--part I. Pathogenesis of ductal plate abnormalities. Mayo Clin Proc. 1998;73(1):80–9.
204. Parekh V, Peker D. Malignant transformation in Von-Meyenburg complexes: histologic and immunohistochemical clues with illustrative cases. Appl Immunohistochem Mol Morphol. 2015;23(9):607–14.
205. Kaminsky P, Preiss J, Sasatomi E, Gerber DA. Biliary adenofibroma: a rare hepatic lesion with malignant features. Hepatology. 2017;65(1):380–3.
206. Sturm AK, Welsch T, Meissner C, Aust DE, Baretton G. A case of biliary adenofibroma of the liver with malignant transformation: a morphomolecular case report and review of the literature. Surg Case Rep. 2019;5(1):104.
207. Arnason T, Borger DR, Corless C, Hagen C, Iafrate AJ, Makhlouf H, et al. Biliary adenofibroma of liver: morphology, tumor genetics, and outcomes in 6 cases. Am J Surg Pathol. 2017;41(4):499–505.
208. Varnholt H, Vauthey JN, Dal Cin P, Marsh Rde W, Bhathal PS, Hughes NR, et al. Biliary adenofibroma: a rare neoplasm of bile duct origin with an indolent behavior. Am J Surg Pathol. 2003;27(5):693–8.
209. Akin O, Coskun M. Biliary adenofibroma with malignant transformation and pulmonary metastases: CT findings. AJR Am J Roentgenol. 2002;179(1):280–1.
210. Bhathal PS, Hughes NR, Goodman ZD. The so-called bile duct adenoma is a peribiliary gland hamartoma. Am J Surg Pathol. 1996;20(7):858–64.
211. Hasebe T, Sakamoto M, Mukai K, Kawano N, Konishi M, Ryu M, et al. Cholangiocarcinoma arising in bile duct adenoma with focal area of bile duct hamartoma. Virchows Arch. 1995;426(2):209–13.
212. Allaire GS, Rabin L, Ishak KG, Sesterhenn IA. Bile duct adenoma. A study of 152 cases. Am J Surg Pathol. 1988;12(9):708–15.
213. An C, Park S, Choi YJ. Diffusion-weighted MRI in intrahepatic bile duct adenoma arising from the cirrhotic liver. Korean J Radiol. 2013;14(5):769–75.
214. Koga F, Tanaka H, Takamatsu S, Baba S, Takihara H, Hasegawa A, et al. A case of very large intrahepatic bile duct adenoma followed for 7 years. World J Clin Oncol. 2012;3(4):63–6.
215. Albores-Saavedra J, Hoang MP, Murakata LA, Sinkre P, Yaziji H. Atypical bile duct adenoma, clear cell type: a previously undescribed tumor of the liver. Am J Surg Pathol. 2001;25(7):956–60.
216. Arena V, Arena E, Stigliano E, Capelli A. Bile duct adenoma with oncocytic features. Histopathology. 2006;49(3):318–20.
217. Gambarotti M, Medicina D, Baronchelli C, Bercich L, Bonetti F, Facchetti F. Alpha-1-antitrypsin-positive "signet-ring" bile duct adenoma in a patient with M(MALTON) mutation. Int J Surg Pathol. 2008;16(2):218–21.
218. Wei J, Zhang D, Yang J, Xu C. Intrahepatic bile duct adenoma (peribiliary gland hamartoma): a case report and review of literature. Int J Clin Exp Pathol. 2015;8(5):5908–13.
219. Hughes NR, Goodman ZD, Bhathal PS. An immunohistochemical profile of the so-called bile duct adenoma: clues to pathogenesis. Am J Surg Pathol. 2010;34(9):1312–8.
220. Sasaki M, Matsubara T, Kakuda Y, Sato Y, Nakanuma Y. Immunostaining for polycomb group protein EZH2 and senescent marker p16INK4a may be useful to differentiate chol-

angiolocellular carcinoma from ductular reaction and bile duct adenoma. Am J Surg Pathol. 2014;38(3):364–9.
221. Pujals A, Zafrani ES, Calderaro J. Bile duct adenoma should not be designated as a reactive process. Pathol Int. 2015;65(6):338.
222. Klimstra DS, Modlin IR, Coppola D, Lloyd RV, Suster S. The pathologic classification of neuroendocrine tumors: a review of nomenclature, grading, and staging systems. Pancreas. 2010;39(6):707–12.
223. Modlin IM, Shapiro MD, Kidd M. An analysis of rare carcinoid tumors: clarifying these clinical conundrums. World J Surg. 2005;29(1):92–101.
224. Yao JC, Hassan M, Phan A, Dagohoy C, Leary C, Mares JE, et al. One hundred years after "carcinoid": epidemiology of and prognostic factors for neuroendocrine tumors in 35,825 cases in the United States. J Clin Oncol. 2008;26(18):3063–72.
225. Albores-Saavedra J, Batich K, Hossain S, Henson DE, Schwartz AM. Carcinoid tumors and small-cell carcinomas of the gallbladder and extrahepatic bile ducts: a comparative study based on 221 cases from the Surveillance, Epidemiology, and End Results Program. Ann Diagn Pathol. 2009;13(6):378–83.
226. Lee KJ, Cho JH, Lee SH, Lee KH, Park BK, Lee JK, et al. Clinicopathological characteristics of biliary neuroendocrine neoplasms: a multicenter study. Scand J Gastroenterol. 2017;52(4):437–41.
227. Eltawil KM, Gustafsson BI, Kidd M, Modlin IM. Neuroendocrine tumors of the gallbladder: an evaluation and reassessment of management strategy. J Clin Gastroenterol. 2010;44(10):687–95.
228. Matsumoto T, Imai Y, Inokuma T. Neuroendocrine carcinoma of the gallbladder accompanied by pancreaticobiliary maljunction. Clin Gastroenterol Hepatol. 2016;14(3):e29–30.
229. Chen C, Wang L, Liu X, Zhang G, Zhao Y, Geng Z. Gallbladder neuroendocrine carcinoma: report of 10 cases and comparision of clinicopathologic features with gallbladder adenocarcinoma. Int J Clin Exp Pathol. 2015;8(7):8218–26.
230. Tonelli F, Giudici F, Nesi G, Batignani G, Brandi ML. Biliary tree gastrinomas in multiple endocrine neoplasia type 1 syndrome. World J Gastroenterol. 2013;19(45):8312–20.
231. Norton JA, Foster DS, Blumgart LH, Poultsides GA, Visser BC, Fraker DL, et al. Incidence and prognosis of primary gastrinomas in the hepatobiliary tract. JAMA Surg. 2018;153(3):e175083.
232. Maitra A, Tascilar M, Hruban RH, Offerhaus GJ, Albores-Saavedra J. Small cell carcinoma of the gallbladder: a clinicopathologic, immunohistochemical, and molecular pathology study of 12 cases. Am J Surg Pathol. 2001;25(5):595–601.
233. Zhang XY, Gao PT, Yang X, Cai JB, Ding GY, Zhu XD, et al. Reduced selenium-binding protein 1 correlates with a poor prognosis in intrahepatic cholangiocarcinoma and promotes the cell epithelial-mesenchymal transition. Am J Transl Res. 2018;10(11):3567–78.
234. Oshiro H, Matsuo K, Mawatari H, Inayama Y, Yamanaka S, Nagahama K, et al. Mucin-producing gallbladder adenocarcinoma with focal small cell and large cell neuroendocrine differentiation associated with pancreaticobiliary maljunction. Pathol Int. 2008;58(12):780–6.
235. Onishi I, Kitagawa H, Harada K, Maruzen S, Sakai S, Makino I, et al. Intraductal papillary neoplasm of the bile duct accompanying biliary mixed adenoneuroendocrine carcinoma. World J Gastroenterol. 2013;19(20):3161–4.
236. Rugge M, Sonego F, Militello C, Guido M, Ninfo V. Primary carcinoid tumor of the cystic and common bile ducts. Am J Surg Pathol. 1992;16(8):802–7.
237. Noronha YS, Raza AS. Well-differentiated neuroendocrine (carcinoid) tumors of the extrahepatic biliary ducts. Arch Pathol Lab Med. 2010;134(7):1075–9.
238. Ehrlich L, Scrushy M, Meng F, Lairmore TC, Alpini G, Glaser S. Biliary epithelium: a neuroendocrine compartment in cholestatic liver disease. Clin Res Hepatol Gastroenterol. 2018;42(4):296–305.

239. Ligato S, Furmaga W, Cartun RW, Hull D, Tsongalis GJ. Primary carcinoid tumor of the common hepatic duct: a rare case with immunohistochemical and molecular findings. Oncol Rep. 2005;13(3):543–6.
240. Maitra A, Krueger JE, Tascilar M, Offerhaus GJ, Angeles-Angeles A, Klimstra DS, et al. Carcinoid tumors of the extrahepatic bile ducts: a study of seven cases. Am J Surg Pathol. 2000;24(11):1501–10.
241. Parwani AV, Geradts J, Caspers E, Offerhaus GJ, Yeo CJ, Cameron JL, et al. Immunohistochemical and genetic analysis of non-small cell and small cell gallbladder carcinoma and their precursor lesions. Mod Pathol. 2003;16(4):299–308.
242. Li M, Liu F, Zhang Y, Wu X, Wu W, Wang XA, et al. Whole-genome sequencing reveals the mutational landscape of metastatic small-cell gallbladder neuroendocrine carcinoma (GB-SCNEC). Cancer Lett. 2017;391:20–7.

Part II
Diagnosis and Management of Cholangiocarcinoma

Chapter 5
Clinical Epidemiology of Cholangiocarcinoma

Roongruedee Chaiteerakij

Abbreviations

95%CI	95% confidence interval
ABCC2	ATP binding cassette subfamily C member 2
ARPKD	Autosomal recessive polycystic kidney disease
BAP1	BRCA1-associated protein 1
BER	Base excision repair
BiLIN	Biliary intraepithelial neoplasia
CCA	Cholangiocarcinoma
COX-2	Cyclooxygenase-2
CT	Computerized tomography
CUP	Cancers of unknown primary origin
dCCA	Distal CCA
eCCA	Extrahepatic CCA
EGFR	Epidermal growth factor receptor
GSTM1	Glutathione S-transferase Mu 1
GSTO1	Glutathione S-transferase omega-1
GSTT1	Glutathione S-transferase theta 1
HBV	Hepatitis B virus
HCC	Hepatocellular carcinoma
HCV	Hepatitis C virus
hOGG1	Human homolog of the 8-oxoguanine glycosylase 1
IARC	International Agency for Research on Cancer
iCCA	Intrahepatic CCA
ICD	International Classification of Diseases

R. Chaiteerakij (✉)
Division of Gastroenterology, Department of Medicine, Chulalongkorn University, Bangkok, Thailand
e-mail: roon.chaiteerakij@chula.md; roongruedee.c@chula.ac.th

J. H. Tabibian (ed.), *Diagnosis and Management of Cholangiocarcinoma*,
https://doi.org/10.1007/978-3-030-70936-5_5

IL-6	Interleukin-6
iNOS	Inducible nitric oxide synthase
IR	Incidence ratio
MetS	Metabolic syndrome
MRCP	Magnetic resonance cholangiopancreatography
MRI	Magnetic resonance imaging
MRP2	Multidrug resistance-associated protein 2
MTHFR	Methylenetetrahydrofolate reductase
MUTYH, MYH	MutY homolog
NAFLD/NASH	Nonalcoholic fatty liver disease/nonalcoholic steatohepatitis
NAT1	N-acetyltransferase 1
NAT2	N-acetyltransferase 2
NKG2D	Natural killer cell receptor group 2 member D
NOCCA	Nordic Occupational Cancer Study
OR	Odds ratio
pCCA	Hilar/perihilar CCA
PSC	Primary sclerosing cholangitis
SEER	Surveillance, Epidemiology, and End Results
SIRs	Standardized incidence ratios
SNPs	Single nucleotide polymorphisms
STAT3	Signal transducer and activator of transcription 3
TNF	Tumor necrosis factor
TSER	Thymidylate synthase enhancer region
WHO	World Health Organization
XRCC1	X-ray repair cross-complementing protein 1

Introduction

Cholangiocarcinoma (CCA) is the second most common primary liver cancer after hepatocellular carcinoma (HCC). CCA is currently classified into three distinct subtypes based on anatomic location: intrahepatic CCA (iCCA), perihilar CCA (pCCA), and distal CCA (dCCA). Each subtype has its respective risk factors, genetics, clinical characteristics, management, and outcomes [1]. iCCA, also known as peripheral CCA, arises from small intrahepatic bile ducts above the secondary hilar branch of the left and right hepatic ducts. pCCA, the so-called Klatskin tumor, is located between the secondary branches of hepatic duct and the insertion of the cystic duct. dCCA arises in the common bile duct, confined to the area between the cystic duct junction and the ampulla of Vater [2, 3]. pCCA is the most common subtype, accounting for 50–60% of all CCAs, followed by dCCA (20–30%) and iCCA (10–20%) [3, 4]. Sometimes, pCCA and dCCA are grouped together as extrahepatic CCA (eCCA).

Epidemiology

Incidence of CCA

CCA is considered a relatively a rare cancer, with an annual incidence of 0.3–6 per 100,000 people, globally. However, there is substantial variation in its incidence among different geographic regions. The incidence of CCA is much higher in some Asian countries (>6 per 100,000 population in Thailand, South Korea, and China) than in Western countries (0.35–2 per 100,000 persons) (Table 5.1) [5]. This diversity of incidence is explained by variation in host genetic and environmental risk factors.

Table 5.1 Global incidence rates of CCA

Eastern countries	Age-standardized incidence rate per 100,000 people	Western countries	Age-standardized incidence rate per 100,000 people
Thailand – Northeast	85.0	Italy	3.4
Thailand – North	14.5	Germany	3.0
Thailand – Central	14.4	Austria	2.7
South Korea, Gwangju	8.8	United Kingdom	2.2
China, Shanghai	7.6	United States	1.6
China, Qidong	7.5	USA	1.6
South Korea, Daegu	7.3	Denmark	1.3
South Korea, Busan	7.1	France	1.3
Thailand – South	5.7	Finland	1.1
Taiwan	4.7	Poland	0.7
Japan, Osaka	3.5	Spain	0.5
Japan, Hiroshima	3.1	Switzerland	0.5
Hong Kong	2.3	Canada	0.4
Singapore	1.5	Puerto Rico	0.4
Philippines	1.2	Costa Rica	0.3
China, Guangzhou	1	Israel	0.3
Australia	0.4		
New Zealand	0.4		
Vietnam	0.1		

Adapted from Ref. [5]

The incidence of CCA has increased in most countries over the past few decades, with a substantial increase in the incidence of the iCCA subtype in particular [4, 6–8]. For example, the overall incidence of CCA in the United States increased by 65% from 1973 to 2012, with a higher magnitude of increase in the incidence of iCCA than in that of eCCA (350% vs. 20%) [4]. The reasons for the rising trends in CCA, particularly the iCCA subtype, remain unclear, though several have been proposed; namely, the increase in the incidence of some potential risk factors globally (details are discussed below), the better understanding of CCA biology and subtypes, the ability to differentiate iCCA from other cancers found in the liver that were previously diagnosed as cancers of unknown primary origin (CUP) [8], and the changes in World Health Organization (WHO) International Classification of Diseases (ICD) coding system may all have contributed to the increased incidence [3]. However, there are geoepidemiological differences in CCA incidence trends; e.g., the incidence decreased between 1978 and 2002 in Denmark [9] while remaining stable in Burgundy, France, between 1976 and 2005 [10].

Mortality Rate

CCA is a highly lethal cancer. Despite advances in diagnostic methods and treatment modalities, survival remains poor globally [4, 10, 11]. The high mortality rate of CCA is due to (i) its aggressiveness; (ii) late diagnosis, as it is clinically silent in the early stage; and (iii) high recurrence rate after treatment. A population-based study in the United States reported that the mortality rate was stable between 1973 and 2008, with a median overall survival of 7 months, and the median overall survival was 8 and 4 months for eCCA and iCCA patients, respectively [4]. Consistent with these findings, another nationwide study in Thailand reported a high mortality rate, with a 1-year mortality rate of 81.7%, which was stable from 2009 to 2013 [11].

Risk Factors for CCA

Pathogenesis of CCA involves a complex interplay between host genetic susceptibility, host factors, and environmental factors. To date, several diseases/conditions have been identified as risk factors for CCA. These risk factors vary geographically. Some factors are strongly associated with a higher risk of CCA but are less commonly encountered, whereas some factors are associated with a lower risk but are more frequently encountered in the general population. Some emerging factors were reported in recent epidemiologic studies and might in part explain the increasing trend of CCA incidence. Of note, approximately 50–60% of CCA patients in Western populations do not have any identifiable risk factors [12], suggesting that there are other factors yet to be discovered. Risk factors for CCA are summarized in Table 5.2; some of these factors contribute to both iCCA and eCCA subtypes, while others are more specific to either iCCA or eCCA.

Table 5.2 Risk factors for intrahepatic and extrahepatic cholangiocarcinoma [12, 21, 26, 27, 32, 46, 62, 97, 101]

Risk factor	Association with iCCA		Association with eCCA	
	Strength	OR (95%CI)	Strength	OR (95%CI)
Bile duct conditions				
Choledochal cyst	++++	26.71 (15.80–45.16)	++++	34.94 (24.36–50.12)
Caroli's disease	++++	38.13 (14.20–102.38)	++++	96.81 (51.02–183.68)
Primary sclerosing cholangitis	++++	93.4 (27.1–322.2)	++++	453 (104–999) and 34.0 (3.6–323.1)[a]
Hepatolithiasis	++++	50.0 (21.2–117.3) and 6.7 (1.3–33.4)[b]	No association	
Choledocholithiasis	++++	10.08 (5.50–18.49)	++++	18.58 (11.07–31.18)
Cholelithiasis	+++	3.38 (1.93–5.92)	+++	5.92 (3.09–11.32)
Liver fluke infection	+++	4.17 (2.81–6.19)[c]	+++	4.17 (2.81–6.19)[c]
Chronic liver diseases				
Cirrhosis	++++	15.32 (9.33–25.15)	+++	3.82 (2.58–5.65)
Hepatitis B infection	++++	4.57 (3.43–6.09)	++	2.11 (1.64–2.73)
Hepatitis C infection	+++	4.28 (2.98–6.16)	++	1.98 (1.33–2.94)
NAFLD/NASH	++	2.22 (1.52–3.24)	+	1.55 (1.03–2.33)
Metabolic conditions				
Diabetes	++	1.73 (1.47–2.04)	+	1.50 (1.31–1.71)
Obesity	Inconclusive		Inconclusive	
Metabolic syndrome	Inconclusive		Inconclusive	
Toxin and environmental exposure				
Alcohol	+++	3.15 (2.24–4.41)	Inconclusive	
Smoking	+	1.25 (1.05–1.49)	+	1.69 (1.28–2.22)
Thorotrast	++++	300 folds[c]	++++	300 folds[c]
Asbestos	+/++	IR: 1.6–4.35	No association	
Organic solvents[d]	++	IR: 2.34 (1.45–3.57)	No association	
Genetic polymorphisms (see Table 5.3)				

Abbreviations: *IR* incidence ratio, *NAFLD/NASH* nonalcoholic fatty liver disease/nonalcoholic steatohepatitis, *OR (95%CI)* odds ratio (95% confidence interval)

[a]For pCCA and dCCA, respectively

[b]For Asian and Western populations, respectively

[c]Avilable data did not distinguish between iCCA and eCCA

[d]Organic solvents in printing industrial work, e.g., dichloromethane or 1,2-propylene dichloride

Host Factors

Age and Sex

Older age confers risk of CCA development, with a 1.25-fold increased risk of CCA for every 10-year increase in age, analogous to various other malignancies [12]. CCA usually presents in the sixth to seventh decade of life and is more common in males than in females.

Bile Duct Conditions

Most chronic bile duct disorders are established risk factors for CCA. These include choledochal cysts, primary sclerosing cholangitis (PSC), and liver fluke infection. Choledochal cysts and PSC are relatively uncommon in the general population yet are notable in that they can predispose to CCA in young individuals, though older individuals may also be affected by either [13, 14].

Choledochal Cysts and Caroli's Disease

Choledochal cysts, or bile duct cysts, are strongly associated with a long-term risk of both iCCA and eCCA. Choledochal cysts are rare congenital anomalies characterized by dilatation of intrahepatic and/or extrahepatic bile ducts. They are more commonly found in East Asian than Western populations. The prevalence of choledochal cysts is estimated to be 1 in 13,000 in Japan and China and 1 in 150,000 in Western countries [15, 16]. Choledochal cysts are generally categorized into five types based on the anatomical location of bile duct dilatation (Fig. 5.1) [17]. Type I is the most common type, accounting for 60–80%, followed by type IV (15–30%) and type V or Caroli's disease [18, 19] Caroli's disease is characterized by

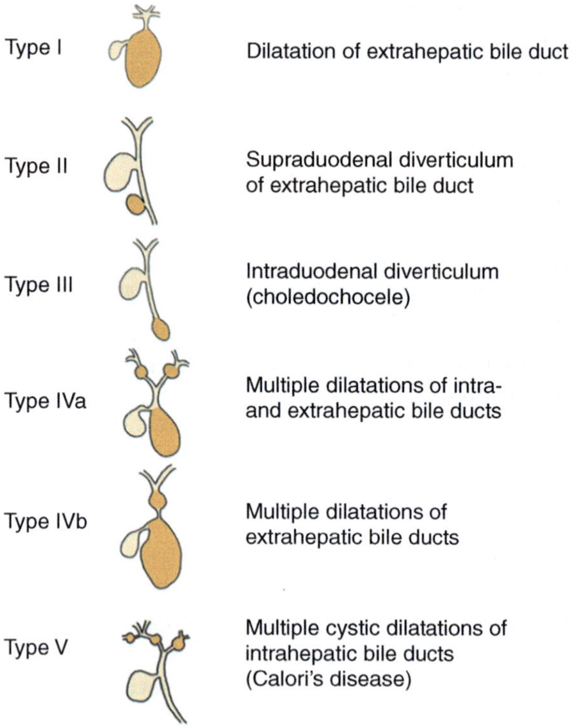

Fig. 5.1 Todani classification of choledochal cyst [17]

multifocal, segmental dilatation of large intrahepatic ducts; when associated with congenital hepatic fibrosis, it is called Caroli's syndrome [20]. Both Caroli's disease and Caroli's syndrome are inherited autosomal recessive diseases and are associated with autosomal recessive polycystic kidney disease (ARPKD).

Approximately 80–90% of patients with choledochal cysts are females [21, 22]. Common presentations are jaundice, abdominal pain, and palpable right upper quadrant mass. An association between choledochal cysts and CCA has long been established. Cholangiocarcinogenesis in choledochal cysts is caused by increased bile acids due to bile stasis and reflux of pancreatic enzymes and chronic cholangitis. These lead to hyperplasia, dysplasia, and subsequent malignant transformation of biliary epithelium of the dilated bile duct wall [23]. Patients with a choledochal cyst have a 20- to 30-fold greater risk for CCA than the general population, though the degree of risk depends on the type of choledochal cyst [24]. The risk increases with age, with a lifetime risk of 10–30% [25]. The odds ratios (95% CI) of choledochal cyst were 26.71 (15.80–45.16) and 34.94 (24.36–50.12) for iCCA and eCCA, respectively [26]. Similarly, Caroli's disease was associated with both iCCA and eCCA with ORs of 38.13 (14.20–102.38) and 96.81 (51.02–183.68), respectively [27]. Individuals with choledochal cyst develop CCA at a much younger age than the general population, with the mean age at the time of developing CCA being only 32 years [25]. Of note, tumors can also arise in undilated parts of the biliary tree.

Surgical excision of choledochal cyst is recommended to prevent development of CCA, except in type III choledochal cyst, where the benefit of surgery does not outweigh the risk. At the time of preventative resection, CCA has been incidentally found in 3–4% of resected specimens [21, 22]. Incomplete cyst excision can lead to recurrent disease and malignant transformation within the cyst remnant [21]. Approximately 3% of patients have been reported to develop CCA after resection, which can occur at 1–32 years post-resection [28, 29]. Lifelong close follow-up is therefore needed [21, 22].

Hepatolithiasis, Cholelithiasis, and Choledocholithiasis

Hepatolithiasis is the presence of a stone in the intrahepatic bile ducts. Similar to a choledochal cyst, it is more prevalent in East Asia (2–25% in Taiwan, China, Hong Kong, South Korea, and Japan) than Western countries (0.6–1.3%) [30]. Hepatolithiasis is an established risk factor for iCCA and has been found to increase the risk of iCCA by 50-fold and seven-fold in Asian and Western populations, respectively [31, 32]. The overall incidence of CCA in patients with hepatolithiasis was reported to be 5–23% [30]. Pathogenesis of CCA in hepatolithiasis includes chronic proliferative cholangitis due to bile stasis, biliary stricture, recurrent cholangitis, and chronic bacterial infection [33, 34].

Cholelithiasis (i.e., gallstones or cholecystolithiasis) and chronic choledocholithiasis (gallstones within the common bile duct) have been shown to increase the risk for CCA in epidemiological studies. A recent meta-analysis of 25 case-control studies from 7 different countries reported associations between both conditions and CCA. Choledocholithiasis was more strongly associated with eCCA than with iCCA, with ORs (95% CI) of 18.58 (11.07–31.18) and 10.08 (5.50–18.49), respectively [26]. The association between cholelithiasis and CCA is less clear; however, cholelithiasis is the most common risk factor of gallbladder cancer [35].

Primary Sclerosing Cholangitis

PSC is an idiopathic biliary disorder characterized by chronic progressive inflammation resulting in fibrosis and stricturing of the intrahepatic and extrahepatic bile ducts. The chronic inflammatory state leads to increased proliferation of biliary epithelial cells. In addition, bile stasis causes increased production of endogenous mutagens in the bile. These and other mechanisms contribute to biliary carcinogenesis [36–38].

PSC is a well-established risk factor for CCA [39]. It is one of the most common causes of CCA in Western populations. An autopsy series reported the presence of CCA in 30–40% of PSC patients [40]. Those with PSC had a 5–36% lifetime risk of CCA, with an annual incidence of 0.6–1.5% [41]. PSC patients develop CCA at a younger age than the general population, typically in their fourth decade of life. The highest incidence of CCA occurs during the first 2 years after PSC is diagnosed [42]. The high rate of CCA development shortly after diagnosis of PSC is likely explained by occult CCA not being detected at the time of PSC diagnosis (and long-standing but undetected history of PSC) rather than de novo CCA occurring after PSC diagnosis [12]. Patients with PSC have a 400-fold to 1500-fold higher risk of CCA than the general population [39]. The relationship of PSC was much stronger in pCCA than iCCA and dCCA, as demonstrated in a large hospital-based case-control study of 2395 CCA cases and 4769 controls, reporting ORs (95% CI) of 453 (104–999), 93.4 (27.1–322.2), and 34.0 (3.57–323.1), for pCCA, iCCA, and dCCA, respectively [12].

Liver Fluke Infection

Liver flukes *Opisthorchis viverrini* and *Clonorchis sinensis* are well-recognized risk factors for CCA. Chronic infection with either fluke is classified as "carcinogenic to human (Group 1)" by the International Agency for Research on Cancer (IARC) [43]. It is a common cause of CCA in East Asia (Korea, China, and Thailand), where liver fluke infection is endemic. It is estimated that 35 million and ten million individuals are infected with *O. viverrini* and *C. sinensis* worldwide, respectively [44, 45]. A meta-analysis of 24 case-control studies showed that individuals with liver fluke infection had a 4.2-fold higher risk for developing CCA than those without the infection [46]. Humans become infected with the liver fluke by ingestion of raw or undercooked fish containing metacercariae, which are the infective stage of liver flukes. Once ingested, the metacercaria excysts in the duodenum, and the young fluke enters the bile duct retrograde through the ampulla of Vater. It takes approximately 1 month for a young fluke to become an adult fluke. The adult fluke resides in the small or medium bile ducts in the liver and can survive for many years therein. The average lifespan of *O. viverrini* is estimated to be approximately 10 years, while *C. sinensis* may live up to 26 years [47, 48].

Liver flukes cause CCA through several mechanisms, including direct mechanical damage by their movements, chronic inflammation, and the effect of their metabolites and antigens secreted into the bile duct. Some of these metabolites are potently immunogenic and induce strong host immune response causing severe inflammation. Some metabolites are directly toxic to the bile duct epithelium, resulting in epithelial desquamation and hyperplasia, followed by periductal fibrosis [49]. Both *O. viverrini* and *C. sinensis* excretory-secretory (ES) antigens can promote cell proliferation [50, 51]. Oxidative DNA damage is another mechanism of liver fluke-induced cholangiocarcinogenesis [52]. Liver fluke infection-related CCA is discussed in further detail in a dedicated chapter in this book (Chap. 11, Waraasawapati et al.).

Chronic Liver Diseases

Chronic liver diseases, including cirrhosis and chronic viral hepatitis B (HBV) and C (HCV) infections, are well-recognized risk factors for HCC. Accumulating epidemiologic evidence has shown that these diseases also confer a risk of CCA, particularly iCCA, suggesting that both HCC and iCCA may share a common pathogenesis [12, 26].

Cirrhosis

A population-based study conducted in Taiwan reported that cirrhosis was significantly associated with CCA, with an OR of 8.0 (6.6–9.8) for iCCA and 3.9 (3.0–5.1) for eCCA [53]. Consistent with these findings, a subsequent study including 2395 CCA patients and 4769 controls conducted in the United States confirmed that non-PSC-related cirrhosis was strongly associated with iCCA and pCCA, with ORs of 13.8 (6.62–28.63) and 14.1 (5.87–33.7), respectively [12]. Nevertheless, the association between cirrhosis and dCCA remains unclear, as does biological plausibility. Cirrhosis could potentially cause CCA via the release of inflammatory cytokines, an increase in cell proliferation, and changes in the liver characterized (e.g., fibrosis) that promote tumor formation [54].

Viral Hepatitis B and C Infections

Similar to cirrhosis, an association of both HBV and HCV infection with CCA has been increasingly suggested. The magnitude of association is more pronounced for iCCA than for eCCA. A recent meta-analysis demonstrated that HBV infection had estimated ORs (95% CI) of 4.57 (3.43–6.09) and 2.11 (1.64–2.73) for iCCA and eCCA, respectively, while HCV infection had ORs (95% CI) of 4.28 (2.98–6.16) and 1.98 (1.33–2.94) for iCCA and eCCA, respectively [26]. It is important to note that these numbers were estimated from mixed populations of those with and without cirrhosis. Thus, the real magnitude of effect of HBV and HCV infection on CCA risk is unrevealed.

Both HBV and HCV infections induce development of biliary intraepithelial neoplasia (BiLIN), a premalignant change of the bile duct. This premalignant condition was found in 16% of explant livers with HBV-related cirrhosis [55]. Likewise, bile duct dysplasia in the intrahepatic ducts was found in 2% of explanted livers of patients with HCV infection [56]. A later study confirmed this finding and reported that BiLIN was found in 82% of cases of HCV cirrhosis [57]. These pathological findings support the plausible biological mechanisms by which these viruses cause iCCA and pCCA. As suggested above, in addition to their associations with cirrhosis, these viruses might have both direct and indirect effects that induce CCA. These viruses encode oncoproteins involved in hepatocarcinogenesis. They also cause a chronic inflammatory state in the liver, which induces oxidative stress and increases levels of reactive oxygen species, causing DNA damage and impairing DNA repair mechanisms, which in turn can cause genetic mutations and cell proliferation followed by malignant transformation [58].

Nonalcoholic Fatty Liver Disease (NAFLD) and Nonalcoholic Steatohepatitis (NASH)

NAFLD is now the most common chronic liver disease in Western countries. The spectrum of NAFLD ranges from simple steatosis, defined as fat accumulation in >5% of hepatocytes, to NASH, which is characterized by steatosis with hepatic inflammation and can progress to liver fibrosis and cirrhosis. NAFLD/NASH has been shown to be associated with HCC and extrahepatic cancers [59–61]. A meta-analysis of seven case-control studies has suggested a possible relationship between NAFLD/NASH and CCA [62]. NAFLD/NASH was more strongly associated with iCCA than eCCA, i.e., ORs were 2.22 (95% CI: 1.52–3.24) and 1.55 (95% CI: 1.03–2.33) for iCCA and eCCA, respectively. A more recent meta-analysis and trial sequential analysis, after removal of confounding factors, confirmed a positive association between NAFLD and iCCA but not with eCCA [63].

It is conceivable that NAFLD contributes to CCA via indirect and direct mechanisms, analogous to chronic viral hepatitis. Indirectly, NAFLD induces chronic hepatic inflammation, leading to progression to NASH and cirrhosis, a recognized independent risk factor for CCA [54]. Directly, NAFLD induces expression of proinflammatory cytokines, particularly interleukin-6 (IL-6) and tumor necrosis factor

(TNF)-alpha, which play a major role in cholangiocarcinogenesis. IL-6 promotes cholangiocyte proliferation [64, 65]. TNF-alpha activated inducible nitric oxide synthase (iNOS) leading to nitric oxide production, which subsequently promoted DNA damage and inhibited DNA repair mechanisms [66]. iNOS activation also upregulated cyclooxygenase-2 (COX-2) expression which is another important mechanism that increases the proliferation of cholangiocytes [67].

Metabolic Conditions

Diabetes, obesity, and metabolic syndrome are pandemic diseases. In recent years, accumulating evidence has suggested that these conditions may confer a significant, although modest, risk of CCA development.

Diabetes

Several meta-analyses have consistently demonstrated the association between type 2 diabetes and CCA [26, 68]. The most recent meta-analysis, including 12 case-control studies of iCCA and 6 case-control studies of eCCA, showed that type 2 diabetes was associated with both iCCA and eCCA with ORs of 1.73 (1.47–2.04) and 1.50 (1.31–1.71), respectively [26]. Mechanisms by which diabetes contributes to CCA are not well understood. One plausible mechanism is related to compensatory hyperinsulinemia due to insulin resistance in diabetes. Insulin binds to insulin receptors on cancer cells and stimulates their growth [69]. Insulin upregulates insulin-like growth factor, which in turn increases proliferation and inhibits apoptosis of cholangiocytes [70]. Another possible mechanism may be linked to indirect effects secondary to other conditions related to diabetes, e.g., obesity, NAFLD, and cirrhosis.

Obesity

Obesity is related to an increased level of leptin, which has been shown to promote tumor growth in a number of cancers [71]. Leptin receptors are mainly expressed in the brain but also in other tissues including normal and malignant cholangiocytes. In vitro data have shown that leptin increases proliferation and migration and decreases apoptosis of CCA cells [72]. Additionally, obesity is related to increased levels of proinflammatory cytokines, particularly IL-6 and TNF [34]. Although obesity has been linked to a number of cancers in the gastrointestinal system, including esophageal, gastric, colorectal, pancreatic, gallbladder, and HCC [73], data on the association between obesity and CCA are controversial. A meta-analysis including 11 cohort studies and 14 case-control studies reported an RR of 1.48 (95% CI, 1.21–1.81) for eCCA [74]. Likewise, data from a meta-analysis of 13 US-based prospective cohort studies and 3 nested case-control studies found that obesity was significantly associated with iCCA with a relative risk of 1.49 (1.32–1.70) [68]. However, a more recent meta-analysis of 7 case-control studies of iCCA and 7 case-control studies of eCCA did not observe such associations with both CCA subtypes, i.e., ORs were 1.14 (0.93–1.39) and 1.20 (0.84–1.70) for iCCA and eCCA, respectively [26]. Whether obesity is associated with an increased risk of CCA needs to be further studied.

Metabolic Syndrome

Metabolic syndrome (MetS) is a group of metabolic disorders that increases the risk of cardiovascular diseases. These disorders include obesity, insulin resistance, hypertension, and dyslipidemia. MetS has been associated with several cancers, including HCC and colorectal cancer; however, the magnitude of association was only fair, with risk estimates ranging from 1.1 to 1.6. Moreover, the risk estimates varied by gender, populations, and definitions of MetS [75]. Regarding CCA, data on an association between MetS and the risk of CCA are limited and inconclusive. The first published evidence came from the Surveillance, Epidemiology, and End Results (SEER)-Medicare database including 743 iCCA cases, which demonstrated a potential relationship between MetS and iCCA with an OR of 1.56 (95% CI 1.32–1.83) [76]. However, this finding was not replicated in a subsequent, large, hospital-based case-control study of 612 iCCA patients [77]. A more recent hospital-based case-control study in China showed that ORs were 2.68 (95% CI: 1.72–4.16) and 1.79 (95% CI: 1.15–2.79) for iCCA and eCCA, respectively [78]. Mechanisms by which MetS is implicated in CCA are not well understood. It may be linked to oxidative stress [79] or simply a surrogate marker for other general cancer risk factors, e.g., physical inactivity, high caloric intake, and low fiber intake [80, 81].

Toxin and Environmental Exposure

Alcohol

Heavy alcohol consumption has been shown to be associated with HCC and various other cancers, including oropharyngeal, esophageal, colorectal, and breast [82]. A relationship between alcohol consumption and iCCA has been observed in most of case-control studies. A meta-analysis including 10 case-control studies reported that alcohol exposure, defined as >80 g per day of alcohol consumption, presence of alcoholic liver disease, or a defined threshold for alcohol exposure, increased the risk of iCCA by 2.8-fold (OR 2.81, 95% CI: 1.52–5.21) [83]. Likewise, a recent meta-analysis of 15 case-control studies demonstrated a strong relationship between alcohol exposure and iCCA, with an OR of 3.15 (95% CI: 2.24–4.41) [26]. Unlike iCCA, the link between alcohol use and eCCA risk remains controversial. A meta-analysis of 6 case-control studies and 1 prospective cohort study did not report a positive association between alcohol consumption and eCCA risk (RR 1.09; 95%

CI: 0.87–1.37) [84], while another meta-analysis including 11 case-control studies found that alcohol exposure, defined as >80 grams per day, any history of exposure, >15 drinks per week, or through ICD9 codes, increased the risk of eCCA, with an OR of 1.75 (95% CI: 1.20–2.55) [26]. Mechanisms of alcohol-associated cancer involve the production of acetaldehyde (the toxic metabolite of alcohol metabolism that affects DNA synthesis and repair) and reactive oxygen species [85].

Tobacco

Tobacco use is known to have a tumorigenic effect in a number of cancers, including CCA [86]. Cigarette smoke contains several compounds that have been shown to be carcinogenetic. One of them is N-nitrosodimethylamine, which has been clearly demonstrated to cause CCA in mice [87]. A large, hospital-based case-control study conducted in the United States reported that ever-smokers had a 1.29-fold greater risk for developing CCA than nonsmokers [12]. When classified by CCA subtypes, smoking was associated with all subtypes, with ORs (95% CI) of 1.21 (1.02–1.43), 1.25 (1.03–1.52), and 1.85 (1.27–2.71) for iCCA, pCCA, and dCCA, respectively [12]. These findings were validated in a meta-analysis consisting of 12 case-control studies reporting an association between smoking and iCCA and eCCA with ORs of 1.25 (95% CI: 1.05–1.49) and 1.69 (95% CI 1.28–2.22), respectively [26].

Thorotrast

Thorotrast, or radioactive thorium dioxide, was widely used as a radiologic intravenous contrast agent between the 1930s and 1950s [88]. It emits alpha particles that have a biologic half-life of 400 years. After injection, Thorotrast accumulates in reticuloendothelial cells. Approximately 60–70% of Thorotrast is deposited in the liver for decades and induces cancer formation with a long latent period after exposure. Cancers induced from Thorotrast include CCA (particularly the iCCA subtype), malignant hemangioendothelioma, and leukemia [89]. Thorotrast exposure increased the risk of CCA by 300 times, with an average time of disease onset 26 years after exposure (range: 3 – over 40 years) [90]. Although Thorotrast has been banned since the 1950s and is no longer used, Thorotrast-induced CCA may still be encountered in those who received this agent decades earlier. The development of CCA by Thorotrast involves multistep carcinogenesis, including microsatellite instability and mutations of the RAS oncogene and the TP53 tumor suppressor gene [91, 92].

Asbestos

Asbestos is a Group 1 human carcinogen classified by the IARC [93]. It is a well-recognized causative agent of mesothelioma and lung cancer (adenocarcinoma, squamous cell carcinoma, and small cell carcinoma) [94]. Mounting epidemiologic evidence has shown a potential association between asbestos exposure and the risk of iCCA (but not of ECC) [95]. Occupational exposure to asbestos for over 30 years conferred a 4.8-fold increased risk of iCCA in one study [96]. Asbestos exposure is believed to be one of the causes of the rising incidence of iCCA in Western populations during recent decades. Standardized incidence ratios of CCA have been found to range from 1.6 to 4.35 among workers who were exposed to asbestos [97].

The presence of asbestos fibers in the liver was reported since the 1980s [98]. Asbestos fibers reach the liver and bile duct via inhalation and ingestion. After inhalation, asbestos fibers can cross the alveolar epithelial barrier to enter the pulmonary lymphatic system, to be further drained into the venous system and spread to other organs, including the liver and bile ducts. If ingested, fibers can penetrate the gastrointestinal mucosa and reach the liver through the portal vein. Once they enter into the tissue, fibers are phagocytosed by macrophages. Activated macrophages release proinflammatory cytokines, leading to a chronic inflammatory state. After a very long latency period (30–40 years) after exposure, malignant transformation of cells may occur through several mechanisms, including chronic inflammation, activation of multiple signaling pathways in cell proliferation, and survival, e.g., the epidermal growth factor receptor (EGFR) pathway, production of reactive oxygen species and reactive nitrogen species, and induction of genetic aberrations [97, 99]. Genetic predisposition also appears to play an important role in asbestos-induced carcinogenesis; individuals who carry the BRCA1-associated protein 1 (BAP1) germline mutations are particularly susceptible to asbestos-induced cancers [97].

Organic Solvents in Printing Industrial Work

The link between chronic exposure to organic solvents used in the printing industry, e.g., dichloromethane or 1,2-propylene dichloride, and CCA has been recently established. A cluster of CCA patients among young proof-printing workers was reported in Japan [100]. The patients were diagnosed with CCA 7–20 years after chemical exposure and developed CCA at young ages (25–45 years). Another report analyzing the Nordic Occupational Cancer Study (NOCCA) database found the increased risk of CCA among workers in the Nordic printing industry; specifically, typographers and printers had an increased risk of iCCA, but not eCCA, with standardized incidence ratios (SIRs) of 2.34 (95% CI: 1.45–3.57) [101].

Genetic Polymorphisms

A number of case-control studies have demonstrated the possible role of genetic predisposition in CCA development. Variants of genes involved in DNA repair mechanisms, metabolizing enzymes, inflammation, and the immune system were shown to contribute to CCA risk.

Table 5.3 summarizes genetic polymorphisms previously identified as factors associated with CCA. Most of these variants have yet to be validated or their

Table 5.3 Studies of the association between genetic variations and risk of cholangiocarcinoma

Risk factor		**Discovery cohort**			Validation cohort	
Genes	Polymorphisms	Country	Number of cases/ controls	OR (95%CI)	Country	Result
Metabolic enzyme-related genes						
GSTO1	GSTO1*A140D	Thailand [115]	30/98	8.5 (2.07–37.85)	United States [116]	Negative
	rs4925	United States [116]	370/740	1.11 (0.92–1.34)	N/A	
GSTM1	Null variant with elevated level of anti-OV antibody	Thailand [117]	129/129	23.53 (4.25–130.31)	N/A	
GSTT1	Null variant in ex-regular drinker	Thailand [117]	129/129	27.93 (1.84–424.60)	N/A	
MTHFR	1298CC	Thailand [118]	219/438	2.0 (1.14–3.48)	N/A	
MTHFR/ TSER	*MTHFR* 677CC with the *TSER* 2R(+) genotype	Korea [119]	47/204	5.38 (1.23–23.56)	N/A	
NAT1	*NAT1*11*	Thailand [120]	216/233	0.10 (0.00–0.58)	N/A	
NAT2	*NAT2*13*	Thailand [120]	216/233	0.35 (0.16–0.77)	N/A	
NAT2	*NAT2*6B*	Thailand [120]	216/233	0.28 (0.12–0.69)	N/A	
NAT2	*NAT2*7A*	Thailand [120]	216/233	0.33 (0.16–0.70)	N/A	
DNA repair-related genes						
MYH	rs3219472	China [121]	59/100	2.82 (0.99–7.99)	N/A	
	rs3219476	China [121]	59/100	0.36 (0.17–0.76)	N/A	
hOGG1/ GSTM1	*hOGG1* codon 326 with *GSTM1* polymorphism	Thailand [122]	25/24	0.06 (0.01–0.53) 0.06 (0.01–0.54) and 0.14 (0.02–1.08)[a]	N/A	
XRCC1	rs1799782	China [123]	127/786	1.9 (1.1–3.5)	N/A	
Others (innate immune system, inflammation, and bile acid)						
NKG2D	rs2617167	Scandinavia [124]	49/368	2.32 (1.47–3.66)	United States [116]	Negative

(continued)

Table 5.3 (continued)

Risk factor		Discovery cohort			Validation cohort	
Genes	Polymorphisms	Country	Number of cases/controls	OR (95%CI)	Country	Result
					England [125]	Negative
NKG2D	rs11053781	Scandinavia [124]	49/368	2.08 (1.31–3.29)	US [116]	Negative
					England [125]	Negative
COX-2	rs689466	United States [116]	370/740	1.36 (1.10–1.69)	United States [116]	Negative
COX-2	rs2143417	United States [116]	370/740	1.52 (1.21–1.91)	United States [116]	Negative
MRP2/ ABCC2	rs3740066	Germany [126]	60/73	1.83 (1.09–3.08)	N/A	

Abbreviations: *ABCC2* ATP binding cassette subfamily C member 2, *COX-2* cyclooxygenase-2, *GSTM1* glutathione S-transferase Mu 1, *GSTO1* glutathione S-transferase omega-1, *GSTT1* glutathione S-transferase theta 1, *hOGG1* human homolog of the 8-oxoguanine glycosylase 1, *MRP2* multidrug resistance-associated protein 2, *MTHFR* methylenetetrahydrofolate reductase, *MYH* MutY homolog, *NAT1* N-acetyltransferase 1, *NAT2* N-acetyltransferase 2, *NKG2D* natural killer cell receptor group 2 member D, *TSER* thymidylate synthase enhancer region, *XRCC1* X-ray repair cross-complementing protein 1

[a]For *hOGG1* Ser/Ser and *GSTM1* null, *hOGG1* Ser/Cys or Cys/Cys and *GSTM1* wild type, and *hOGG1* Ser/Cys or Cys/Cys and *GSTM1* null, respectively

associations with CCA were not replicated. Collectively, these findings imply that genetic susceptibility is complex; it may interact with other host and environmental factor to affect the risk of CCA development at the individual level.

Surveillance and Prevention

Surveillance for CCA

Surveillance for CCA in high-risk populations, e.g., PSC patients and those living in areas endemic for liver fluke infection, has been shown to improve survival of CCA patients. For example, a recent hospital-based study was conducted in a cohort of 830 PSC patients. Of these, 79 patients were diagnosed with hepatobiliary cancer, of whom 68% (54/79) were diagnosed with CCA. Among the 79 PSC patients with hepatobiliary cancer, 51% (40/79) were under hepatobiliary cancer surveillance with annual abdominal imaging (transabdominal ultrasound, computed tomography, or magnetic resonance imaging with magnetic resonance cholangiopancreatopgraphy) and blood tests for serum cancer biomarkers, namely, carbohydrate antigen 19-9 and alpha fetoprotein, every 6–12 months. The other 49% (39/79) of patients who were diagnosed with hepatobiliary cancer were not under surveillance. The study demonstrated that patients in the surveillance group had significantly better survival than those in the no surveillance group, i.e., 5-year survival was 68% vs. 20% ($p < 0.001$) [102].

Another study was conducted in 4225 individuals in Northern Thailand, where *O. viverrini* is highly prevalent. The participants underwent abdominal ultrasound every 6 months for CCA surveillance. After the follow-up period of 5 years, there were 48 patients diagnosed with CCA. When compared to a hospital-based cohort of 192 CCA patients who never underwent ultrasound for surveillance, CCA patients in the surveillance group had a significantly better median survival (31.8 vs. 6.7 months, $p < 0.0001$), and a greater number of CCA patients in the surveillance group were diagnosed at an operable stage (77.1% (37/48) vs. 11.5% (22/192)). CCA surveillance by ultrasound every 6 months improved patient survival by 59% (hazard ratio [HR]: 0.41, 95% CI: 0.20–0.82; $p = 0.012$) [103].

CCA Prevention

Regarding CCA prevention, some medications have been shown to have a possible protective effect against CCA. A large hospital-based case-control study reported the significant inverse association between aspirin use and CCA, with an OR (95% CI) of 0.34 (0.30–0.39). The protective effect of aspirin was consistent for all CCA subtypes, i.e., ORs (95% CI) were 0.35 (0.29–0.42), 0.34 (0.27–0.42), and 0.29 (0.19–0.44) for iCCA, pCCA, and dCCA, respectively [12]. A meta-analysis of 5 observational studies (1 cohort study and 4 case-control study) with 9,200,653 patients, demonstrated that aspirin use was associated with a 44% decreased risk of CCA (OR 0.56, 95% CI: 0.32–0.96) [104]. The mechanisms by which aspirin prevents CCA development include inhibition of COX-2, which is overexpressed in chronic inflammatory states and induces cell proliferation [105], and inhibition of activation of nuclear factor kappa-light-chain-enhancer of activated B cells (NF-κB), a transcription factor that activates genes in inflammation and apoptosis pathways [106].

Another medication shown to have a chemopreventive effect against CCA is metformin, a widely used antidiabetic agent. Data from a case-control study found that diabetic patients who were treated with metformin had a significantly lower risk of iCCA than those not treated with metformin (OR 0.4; 95% CI: 0.2–0.9) [77]. In vitro studies have shown that metformin inhibits proliferation and migration of CCA cells via suppression of NF-κB and signal transducer and activator of transcription 3 (STAT3) pathways [107, 108].

Curcumin is a natural constituent of turmeric (*Curcuma longa*) and has long been used as a traditional anti-inflammatory agent, particularly in South Asia. Increasing evidence from in vitro and in vivo studies have demonstrated the strong antioxidant and anti-inflammatory effects of curcumin for prevention of tumor, including CCA, formation [109]. Curcumin was shown to reduce bile canaliculi alteration and periductal fibrosis in *O. viverrini*-infected hamsters [110, 111]. Curcumin reduced oxidative DNA damage and inhibited of cell proliferation by suppression of the activation of transcription factors NF-kB and JAK2/STAT-3 [112]. Other mechanisms included induction of cell apoptosis, activation of tumor suppressor gene, and inhibition of angiogenesis [109]. Although curcumin has the remarkable anticarcinogenic activities and good safety profile, its clinical use remains currently limited due to its poor solubility, poor absorption, rapid metabolism, and rapid clearance [113]. Development of novel delivery systems to improve solubility and bioavailability, such as nanoparticles, is now underway [114].

Summary

CCA is a highly lethal cancer with geographic variation in its incidence. Some factors confer a strong risk of CCA but are relatively uncommon, whereas other some factors confer a less strong risk but are common in the general population. The high incidence of CCA in some Asian countries is due to the uniquely high prevalence of strong risk factors, in particular liver fluke infection and hepatolithiasis. In Western countries, the incidence of CCA is relatively low, as strong risk factors are comparably less prevalent. The worldwide incidence of CCA has been increasing, partly due to the increasing prevalence of emerging risk factors, e.g., chronic liver diseases and metabolic conditions, as well as due to an improved understanding of CCA biology and classification. Surveillance for CCA in patients with PSC and individuals living in endemic areas of liver fluke infection is associated with improved clinical outcomes.

References

1. Marcano-Bonilla L, Mohamed EA, Mounajjed T, Roberts LR. Biliary tract cancers: epidemiology, molecular pathogenesis and genetic risk associations. Chin Clin Oncol. 2016;5(5):61. https://doi.org/10.21037/cco.2016.10.09.
2. Nakeeb A, Pitt HA, Sohn TA, Coleman J, Abrams RA, Piantadosi S, et al. Cholangiocarcinoma. A spectrum of intrahepatic, perihilar, and distal tumors. Ann Surg. 1996;224(4):463–73; discussion 73–5. https://doi.org/10.1097/00000658-199610000-00005.
3. Khan SA, Tavolari S, Brandi G. Cholangiocarcinoma: epidemiology and risk factors. Liver Int. 2019;39(Suppl 1):19–31. https://doi.org/10.1111/liv.14095.
4. Mukkamalla SKR, Naseri HM, Kim BM, Katz SC, Armenio VA. Trends in incidence and factors affecting survival of patients with cholangiocarcinoma in the United States. J Natl Compr Cancer Netw. 2018;16(4):370–6. https://doi.org/10.6004/jnccn.2017.7056.
5. Banales JM, Cardinale V, Carpino G, Marzioni M, Andersen JB, Invernizzi P, et al. Expert consensus document: cholangiocarcinoma: current knowledge and future perspectives consensus statement from the European Network for the Study of Cholangiocarcinoma

(ENS-CCA). Nat Rev Gastroenterol Hepatol. 2016;13(5):261–80. https://doi.org/10.1038/nrgastro.2016.51.
6. Florio AA, Ferlay J, Znaor A, Ruggieri D, Alvarez CS, Laversanne M, et al. Global trends in intrahepatic and extrahepatic cholangiocarcinoma incidence from 1993 to 2012. Cancer. 2020;126(11):2666–78. https://doi.org/10.1002/cncr.32803.
7. Pinter M, Hucke F, Zielonke N, Waldhor T, Trauner M, Peck-Radosavljevic M, et al. Incidence and mortality trends for biliary tract cancers in Austria. Liver Int. 2014;34(7):1102–8. https://doi.org/10.1111/liv.12325.
8. Saha SK, Zhu AX, Fuchs CS, Brooks GA. Forty-year trends in cholangiocarcinoma incidence in the U.S.: intrahepatic disease on the rise. Oncologist. 2016;21(5):594–9. https://doi.org/10.1634/theoncologist.2015-0446.
9. Jepsen P, Vilstrup H, Tarone RE, Friis S, Sorensen HT. Incidence rates of intra- and extrahepatic cholangiocarcinomas in Denmark from 1978 through 2002. J Natl Cancer Inst. 2007;99(11):895–7. https://doi.org/10.1093/jnci/djk201.
10. Lepage C, Cottet V, Chauvenet M, Phelip JM, Bedenne L, Faivre J, et al. Trends in the incidence and management of biliary tract cancer: a French population-based study. J Hepatol. 2011;54(2):306–10. https://doi.org/10.1016/j.jhep.2010.06.039.
11. Chaiteerakij R, Pan-Ngum W, Poovorawan K, Soonthornworasiri N, Treeprasertsuk S, Phaosawasdi K. Characteristics and outcomes of cholangiocarcinoma by region in Thailand: a nationwide study. World J Gastroenterol. 2017;23(39):7160–7. https://doi.org/10.3748/wjg.v23.i39.7160.
12. Choi JG, Ghoz HM, Peeraphatdit T, Baichoo E, Addissie BD, Harmsen WS, et al. Aspirin use and the risk of cholangiocarcinoma. Hepatology. 2016;64(3):785–96. https://doi.org/10.1002/hep.28529.
13. Tabibian JH, Tabibian N, Aguet JC. Choledochal cyst complications presenting as duodenal obstruction in an 82-year-old patient with gallbladder agenesis. Dig Dis Sci. 2009;54(1):184–7. https://doi.org/10.1007/s10620-008-0317-8.
14. Fung BM, Lindor KD, Tabibian JH. Cancer risk in primary sclerosing cholangitis: epidemiology, prevention, and surveillance strategies. World J Gastroenterol. 2019;25(6):659–71. https://doi.org/10.3748/wjg.v25.i6.659.
15. Wiseman K, Buczkowski AK, Chung SW, Francoeur J, Schaeffer D, Scudamore CH. Epidemiology, presentation, diagnosis, and outcomes of choledochal cysts in adults in an urban environment. Am J Surg. 2005;189(5):527–31; discussion 31. https://doi.org/10.1016/j.amjsurg.2005.01.025.
16. Sato M, Ishida H, Konno K, Naganuma H, Ishida J, Hirata M, et al. Choledochal cyst due to anomalous pancreatobiliary junction in the adult: sonographic findings. Abdom Imaging. 2001;26(4):395–400. https://doi.org/10.1007/s002610000184.
17. Todani T, Watanabe Y, Narusue M, Tabuchi K, Okajima K. Congenital bile duct cysts: classification, operative procedures, and review of thirty-seven cases including cancer arising from choledochal cyst. Am J Surg. 1977;134(2):263–9. https://doi.org/10.1016/0002-9610(77)90359-2.
18. Soares KC, Arnaoutakis DJ, Kamel I, Rastegar N, Anders R, Maithel S, et al. Choledochal cysts: presentation, clinical differentiation, and management. J Am Coll Surg. 2014;219(6):1167–80. https://doi.org/10.1016/j.jamcollsurg.2014.04.023.
19. Ronnekleiv-Kelly SM, Soares KC, Ejaz A, Pawlik TM. Management of choledochal cysts. Curr Opin Gastroenterol. 2016;32(3):225–31. https://doi.org/10.1097/MOG.0000000000000256.
20. Desmet VJ. What is congenital hepatic fibrosis? Histopathology. 1992;20(6):465–77. https://doi.org/10.1111/j.1365-2559.1992.tb01031.x.
21. Soares KC, Kim Y, Spolverato G, Maithel S, Bauer TW, Marques H, et al. Presentation and clinical outcomes of choledochal cysts in children and adults: a multi-institutional analysis. JAMA Surg. 2015;150(6):577–84. https://doi.org/10.1001/jamasurg.2015.0226.

22. Edil BH, Cameron JL, Reddy S, Lum Y, Lipsett PA, Nathan H, et al. Choledochal cyst disease in children and adults: a 30-year single-institution experience. J Am Coll Surg. 2008;206(5):1000–5; discussion 5–8. https://doi.org/10.1016/j.jamcollsurg.2007.12.045.
23. Katabi N, Pillarisetty VG, DeMatteo R, Klimstra DS. Choledochal cysts: a clinicopathologic study of 36 cases with emphasis on the morphologic and the immunohistochemical features of premalignant and malignant alterations. Hum Pathol. 2014;45(10):2107–14. https://doi.org/10.1016/j.humpath.2014.06.016.
24. Madadi-Sanjani O, Wirth TC, Kuebler JF, Petersen C, Ure BM. Choledochal cyst and malignancy: a plea for lifelong follow-up. Eur J Pediatr Surg. 2019;29(2):143–9. https://doi.org/10.1055/s-0037-1615275.
25. Soreide K, Soreide JA. Bile duct cyst as precursor to biliary tract cancer. Ann Surg Oncol. 2007;14(3):1200–11. https://doi.org/10.1245/s10434-006-9294-3.
26. Clements O, Eliahoo J, Kim JU, Taylor-Robinson SD, Khan SA. Risk factors for intrahepatic and extrahepatic cholangiocarcinoma: a systematic review and meta-analysis. J Hepatol. 2020;72(1):95–103. https://doi.org/10.1016/j.jhep.2019.09.007.
27. Petrick JL, Yang B, Altekruse SF, Van Dyke AL, Koshiol J, Graubard BI, et al. Risk factors for intrahepatic and extrahepatic cholangiocarcinoma in the United States: a population-based study in SEER-Medicare. PLoS One. 2017;12(10):e0186643. https://doi.org/10.1371/journal.pone.0186643.
28. Todani T, Tabuchi K, Watanabe Y, Kobayashi T. Carcinoma arising in the wall of congenital bile duct cysts. Cancer. 1979;44(3):1134–41. https://doi.org/10.1002/1097-0142(197909)44:3<1134::aid-cncr2820440350>3.0.co;2-t.
29. Watanabe Y, Toki A, Todani T. Bile duct cancer developed after cyst excision for choledochal cyst. J Hepato-Biliary-Pancreat Surg. 1999;6(3):207–12. https://doi.org/10.1007/s005340050108.
30. Kim HJ, Kim JS, Joo MK, Lee BJ, Kim JH, Yeon JE, et al. Hepatolithiasis and intrahepatic cholangiocarcinoma: a review. World J Gastroenterol. 2015;21(48):13418–31. https://doi.org/10.3748/wjg.v21.i48.13418.
31. Lee TY, Lee SS, Jung SW, Jeon SH, Yun SC, Oh HC, et al. Hepatitis B virus infection and intrahepatic cholangiocarcinoma in Korea: a case-control study. Am J Gastroenterol. 2008;103(7):1716–20. https://doi.org/10.1111/j.1572-0241.2008.01796.x.
32. Donato F, Gelatti U, Tagger A, Favret M, Ribero ML, Callea F, et al. Intrahepatic cholangiocarcinoma and hepatitis C and B virus infection, alcohol intake, and hepatolithiasis: a case-control study in Italy. Cancer Causes Control. 2001;12(10):959–64. https://doi.org/10.1023/a:1013747228572.
33. Nakanuma Y, Terada T, Tanaka Y, Ohta G. Are hepatolithiasis and cholangiocarcinoma aetiologically related? A morphological study of 12 cases of hepatolithiasis associated with cholangiocarcinoma. Virchows Arch A Pathol Anat Histopathol. 1985;406(1):45–58. https://doi.org/10.1007/BF00710556.
34. Rizvi S, Gores GJ. Pathogenesis, diagnosis, and management of cholangiocarcinoma. Gastroenterology. 2013;145(6):1215–29. https://doi.org/10.1053/j.gastro.2013.10.013.
35. Schmidt MA, Marcano-Bonilla L, Roberts LR. Gallbladder cancer: epidemiology and genetic risk associations. Chin Clin Oncol. 2019;8(4):31. https://doi.org/10.21037/cco.2019.08.13.
36. Patel T. Cholangiocarcinoma. Nat Clin Pract Gastroenterol Hepatol. 2006;3(1):33–42. https://doi.org/10.1038/ncpgasthep0389.
37. O'Hara SP, Tabibian JH, Splinter PL, LaRusso NF. The dynamic biliary epithelia: molecules, pathways, and disease. J Hepatol. 2013;58(3):575–82. https://doi.org/10.1016/j.jhep.2012.10.011.
38. O'Hara SP, Gradilone SA, Masyuk TV, Tabibian JH, LaRusso NF. MicroRNAs in cholangiopathies. Curr Pathobiol Rep. 2014;2(3):133–42. https://doi.org/10.1007/s40139-014-0048-9.

39. Fung BM, Tabibian JH. Cholangiocarcinoma in patients with primary sclerosing cholangitis. Curr Opin Gastroenterol. 2020;36(2):77–84. https://doi.org/10.1097/MOG.0000000000000616.
40. Rosen CB, Nagorney DM. Cholangiocarcinoma complicating primary sclerosing cholangitis. Semin Liver Dis. 1991;11(1):26–30. https://doi.org/10.1055/s-2008-1040419.
41. Jesudian AB, Jacobson IM. Screening and diagnosis of cholangiocarcinoma in patients with primary sclerosing cholangitis. Rev Gastroenterol Disord. 2009;9(2):E41–7.
42. Burak K, Angulo P, Pasha TM, Egan K, Petz J, Lindor KD. Incidence and risk factors for cholangiocarcinoma in primary sclerosing cholangitis. Am J Gastroenterol. 2004;99(3):523–6. https://doi.org/10.1111/j.1572-0241.2004.04067.x.
43. IARC Working Group on the Evaluation of Carcinogenic Risks to Humans. Biological agents. Volume 100 B. A review of human carcinogens. IARC Monogr Eval Carcinog Risks Hum. 2012;100(Pt B):1–441.
44. Fang YY, Chen YD, Li XM, Wu J, Zhang QM, Ruan CW. Current prevalence of Clonorchis sinensis infection in endemic areas of China. Zhongguo Ji Sheng Chong Xue Yu Ji Sheng Chong Bing Za Zhi. 2008;26(2):99–103. 9
45. Jongsuksuntigul P, Imsomboon T. Opisthorchiasis control in Thailand. Acta Trop. 2003;88(3):229–32. https://doi.org/10.1016/j.actatropica.2003.01.002.
46. Xia J, Jiang SC, Peng HJ. Association between liver fluke infection and hepatobiliary pathological changes: a systematic review and meta-analysis. PLoS One. 2015;10(7):e0132673. https://doi.org/10.1371/journal.pone.0132673.
47. Sithithaworn P, Haswell-Elkins M. Epidemiology of Opisthorchis viverrini. Acta Trop. 2003;88(3):187–94. https://doi.org/10.1016/j.actatropica.2003.02.001.
48. Attwood HD, Chou ST. The longevity of Clonorchis sinensis. Pathology. 1978;10(2):153–6. https://doi.org/10.3109/00313027809063494.
49. Sripa B, Kaewkes S, Sithithaworn P, Mairiang E, Laha T, Smout M, et al. Liver fluke induces cholangiocarcinoma. PLoS Med. 2007;4(7):e201. https://doi.org/10.1371/journal.pmed.0040201.
50. Thuwajit C, Thuwajit P, Kaewkes S, Sripa B, Uchida K, Miwa M, et al. Increased cell proliferation of mouse fibroblast NIH-3T3 in vitro induced by excretory/secretory product(s) from Opisthorchis viverrini. Parasitology. 2004;129(Pt 4):455–64. https://doi.org/10.1017/s0031182004005815.
51. Kim EM, Kim JS, Choi MH, Hong ST, Bae YM. Effects of excretory/secretory products from Clonorchis sinensis and the carcinogen dimethylnitrosamine on the proliferation and cell cycle modulation of human epithelial HEK293T cells. Korean J Parasitol. 2008;46(3):127–32. https://doi.org/10.3347/kjp.2008.46.3.127.
52. Pinlaor S, Yongvanit P, Hiraku Y, Ma N, Semba R, Oikawa S, et al. 8-nitroguanine formation in the liver of hamsters infected with Opisthorchis viverrini. Biochem Biophys Res Commun. 2003;309(3):567–71. https://doi.org/10.1016/j.bbrc.2003.08.039.
53. Chang JS, Tsai CR, Chen LT. Medical risk factors associated with cholangiocarcinoma in Taiwan: a population-based case-control study. PLoS One. 2013;8(7):e69981. https://doi.org/10.1371/journal.pone.0069981.
54. Razumilava N, Gores GJ. Cholangiocarcinoma. Lancet. 2014;383(9935):2168–79. https://doi.org/10.1016/S0140-6736(13)61903-0.
55. Zarei M, Shasaeefar A, Kazemi K, Dehghani M, Malekhosseini SA, Geramizadeh B. Biliary intraepithelial neoplasia in non-biliary cirrhosis-report from 100 explanted livers: a single center experience. Clin Pathol. 2019;12:2632010X19876934. https://doi.org/10.1177/2632010X19876934.
56. Torbenson M, Yeh MM, Abraham SC. Bile duct dysplasia in the setting of chronic hepatitis C and alcohol cirrhosis. Am J Surg Pathol. 2007;31(9):1410–3. https://doi.org/10.1097/PAS.0b013e318053d122.

57. Wu TT, Levy M, Correa AM, Rosen CB, Abraham SC. Biliary intraepithelial neoplasia in patients without chronic biliary disease: analysis of liver explants with alcoholic cirrhosis, hepatitis C infection, and noncirrhotic liver diseases. Cancer. 2009;115(19):4564–75. https://doi.org/10.1002/cncr.24471.
58. Ralphs S, Khan SA. The role of the hepatitis viruses in cholangiocarcinoma. J Viral Hepat. 2013;20(5):297–305. https://doi.org/10.1111/jvh.12093.
59. Younossi ZM, Otgonsuren M, Henry L, Venkatesan C, Mishra A, Erario M, et al. Association of nonalcoholic fatty liver disease (NAFLD) with hepatocellular carcinoma (HCC) in the United States from 2004 to 2009. Hepatology. 2015;62(6):1723–30. https://doi.org/10.1002/hep.28123.
60. Plaz Torres MC, Bodini G, Furnari M, Marabotto E, Zentilin P, Strazzabosco M, et al. Surveillance for hepatocellular carcinoma in patients with non-alcoholic fatty liver disease: universal or selective? Cancers (Basel). 2020;12(6). https://doi.org/10.3390/cancers12061422.
61. Liu SS, Ma XF, Zhao J, Du SX, Zhang J, Dong MZ, et al. Association between nonalcoholic fatty liver disease and extrahepatic cancers: a systematic review and meta-analysis. Lipids Health Dis. 2020;19(1):118. https://doi.org/10.1186/s12944-020-01288-6.
62. Wongjarupong N, Assavapongpaiboon B, Susantitaphong P, Cheungpasitporn W, Treeprasertsuk S, Rerknimitr R, et al. Non-alcoholic fatty liver disease as a risk factor for cholangiocarcinoma: a systematic review and meta-analysis. BMC Gastroenterol. 2017;17:149. https://doi.org/10.1186/s12876-017-0696-4.
63. Corrao S, Natoli G, Argano C. Nonalcoholic fatty liver disease is associated with intrahepatic cholangiocarcinoma and not with extrahepatic form: definitive evidence from meta-analysis and trial sequential analysis. Eur J Gastroenterol Hepatol. 2020. https://doi.org/10.1097/meg.0000000000001684.
64. Wehbe H, Henson R, Meng F, Mize-Berge J, Patel T. Interleukin-6 contributes to growth in cholangiocarcinoma cells by aberrant promoter methylation and gene expression. Cancer Res. 2006;66(21):10517–24. https://doi.org/10.1158/0008-5472.CAN-06-2130.
65. Trussoni CE, Tabibian JH, Splinter PL, O'Hara SP. Lipopolysaccharide (LPS)-induced biliary epithelial cell NRas activation requires epidermal growth factor receptor (EGFR). PLoS One. 2015;10(4):e0125793. https://doi.org/10.1371/journal.pone.0125793.
66. Jaiswal M, LaRusso NF, Shapiro RA, Billiar TR, Gores GJ. Nitric oxide-mediated inhibition of DNA repair potentiates oxidative DNA damage in cholangiocytes. Gastroenterology. 2001;120(1):190–9. https://doi.org/10.1053/gast.2001.20875.
67. Ishimura N, Bronk SF, Gores GJ. Inducible nitric oxide synthase upregulates cyclooxygenase-2 in mouse cholangiocytes promoting cell growth. Am J Physiol Gastrointest Liver Physiol. 2004;287(1):G88–95. https://doi.org/10.1152/ajpgi.00539.2003.
68. Petrick JL, Thistle JE, Zeleniuch-Jacquotte A, Zhang X, Wactawski-Wende J, Van Dyke AL, et al. Body mass index, diabetes and intrahepatic cholangiocarcinoma risk: the liver cancer pooling project and meta-analysis. Am J Gastroenterol. 2018;113(10):1494–505. https://doi.org/10.1038/s41395-018-0207-4.
69. Vigneri R, Goldfine ID, Frittitta L. Insulin, insulin receptors, and cancer. J Endocrinol Investig. 2016;39(12):1365–76. https://doi.org/10.1007/s40618-016-0508-7.
70. Cai HH, Sun YM, Bai JF, Shi Y, Zhao HL, Miao Y. Relationship between the GH-IGFs axis and the proliferation of bile duct cancer cell line QBC939 in vitro. Hepatob Pancreat Dis Int. 2008;7(1):76–81.
71. Dutta D, Ghosh S, Pandit K, Mukhopadhyay P, Chowdhury S. Leptin and cancer: pathogenesis and modulation. Indian J Endocrinol Metab. 2012;16(Suppl 3):S596–600. https://doi.org/10.4103/2230-8210.105577.
72. Fava G, Alpini G, Rychlicki C, Saccomanno S, DeMorrow S, Trozzi L, et al. Leptin enhances cholangiocarcinoma cell growth. Cancer Res. 2008;68(16):6752–61. https://doi.org/10.1158/0008-5472.CAN-07-6682.

73. Lauby-Secretan B, Scoccianti C, Loomis D, Grosse Y, Bianchini F, Straif K, et al. Body fatness and cancer – viewpoint of the IARC Working Group. N Engl J Med. 2016;375(8):794–8. https://doi.org/10.1056/NEJMsr1606602.
74. Li LQ, Gan Y, Li WZ, Wu CM, Lu ZX. Overweight, obesity and the risk of gallbladder and extrahepatic bile duct cancers: a meta-analysis of observational studies. Obesity. 2016;24(8):1786–802. https://doi.org/10.1002/oby.21505.
75. Esposito K, Chiodini P, Colao A, Lenzi A, Giugliano D. Metabolic syndrome and risk of cancer: a systematic review and meta-analysis. Diabetes Care. 2012;35(11):2402–11. https://doi.org/10.2337/dc12-0336.
76. Welzel TM, Graubard BI, Zeuzem S, El-Serag HB, Davila JA, McGlynn KA. Metabolic syndrome increases the risk of primary liver cancer in the United States: a study in the SEER-Medicare Database. Hepatology. 2011;54(2):463–71. https://doi.org/10.1002/hep.24397.
77. Chaiteerakij R, Yang JD, Harmsen WS, Slettedahl SW, Mettler TA, Fredericksen ZS, et al. Risk factors for intrahepatic cholangiocarcinoma: association between metformin use and reduced cancer risk. Hepatology. 2013;57(2):648–55. https://doi.org/10.1002/hep.26092.
78. Xiong JP, Lu X, Xu WY, Bai Y, Huang HC, Bian J, et al. Metabolic syndrome and the risk of cholangiocarcinoma: a hospital-based case-control study in China. Cancer Manag Res. 2018;10:3849–55. https://doi.org/10.2147/Cmar.S175628.
79. Roberts CK, Sindhu KK. Oxidative stress and metabolic syndrome. Life Sci. 2009;84(21–22):705–12. https://doi.org/10.1016/j.lfs.2009.02.026.
80. Kim J, Tanabe K, Yokoyama N, Zempo H, Kuno S. Association between physical activity and metabolic syndrome in middle-aged Japanese: a cross-sectional study. BMC Public Health. 2011;11:624. https://doi.org/10.1186/1471-2458-11-624.
81. Kunzmann AT, Coleman HG, Huang WY, Kitahara CM, Cantwell MM, Berndt SI. Dietary fiber intake and risk of colorectal cancer and incident and recurrent adenoma in the Prostate, Lung, Colorectal, and Ovarian Cancer Screening Trial. Am J Clin Nutr. 2015;102(4):881–90. https://doi.org/10.3945/ajcn.115.113282.
82. LoConte NK, Brewster AM, Kaur JS, Merrill JK, Alberg AJ. Alcohol and cancer: a statement of the American Society of Clinical Oncology. J Clin Oncol. 2018;36(1):83–93. https://doi.org/10.1200/Jco.2017.76.1155.
83. Palmer WC, Patel T. Are common factors involved in the pathogenesis of primary liver cancers? A meta-analysis of risk factors for intrahepatic cholangiocarcinoma. J Hepatol. 2012;57(1):69–76. https://doi.org/10.1016/j.jhep.2012.02.022.
84. Ye XH, Huai JP, Ding J, Chen YP, Sun XC. Smoking, alcohol consumption, and the risk of extrahepatic cholangiocarcinoma: a meta-analysis. World J Gastroenterol. 2013;19(46):8780–8. https://doi.org/10.3748/wjg.v19.i46.8780.
85. Seitz HK, Becker P. Alcohol metabolism and cancer risk. Alcohol Res Health. 2007;30(1):38–41, 4–7.
86. Jacob L, Freyn M, Kalder M, Dinas K, Kostev K. Impact of tobacco smoking on the risk of developing 25 different cancers in the UK: a retrospective study of 422,010 patients followed for up to 30 years. Oncotarget. 2018;9(25):17420–9. https://doi.org/10.18632/oncotarget.24724.
87. Flavell DJ, Lucas SB. Promotion of N-nitrosodimethylamine-initiated bile duct carcinogenesis in the hamster by the human liver fluke, Opisthorchis viverrini. Carcinogenesis. 1983;4(7):927–30. https://doi.org/10.1093/carcin/4.7.927.
88. Abbatt JD. History of the use and toxicity of thorotrast. Environ Res. 1979;18(1):6–12.
89. Mori T, Kido C, Fukutomi K, Kato Y, Hatakeyama S, Machinami R, et al. Summary of entire Japanese thorotrast follow-up study: updated 1998. Radiat Res. 1999;152(6 Suppl):S84–7.
90. Levy DW, Rindsberg S, Friedman AC, Fishman EK, Ros PR, Radecki PD, et al. Thorotrast-induced hepatosplenic neoplasia: CT identification. AJR Am J Roentgenol. 1986;146(5):997–1004. https://doi.org/10.2214/ajr.146.5.997.

91. Liu D, Momoi H, Li L, Ishikawa Y, Fukumoto M. Microsatellite instability in thorotrast-induced human intrahepatic cholangiocarcinoma. Int J Cancer. 2002;102(4):366–71. https://doi.org/10.1002/ijc.10726.
92. Kamikawa T, Amenomori M, Itoh T, Momoi H, Hiai H, Machinami R, et al. Analysis of genetic changes in intrahepatic cholangiocarcinoma induced by thorotrast. Radiat Res. 1999;152(6 Suppl):S118–24.
93. IARC Working Group on the Evaluation of Carcinogenic Risks to Humans. Arsenic, metals, fibres, and dusts. IARC Monogr Eval Carcinog Risks Hum. 2012;100(Pt C):11–465.
94. Uguen M, Dewitte JD, Marcorelles P, Lodde B, Pougnet R, Saliou P, et al. Asbestos-related lung cancers: a retrospective clinical and pathological study. Mol Clin Oncol. 2017;7(1):135–9. https://doi.org/10.3892/mco.2017.1277.
95. Farioli A, Straif K, Brandi G, Curti S, Kjaerheim K, Martinsen JI, et al. Occupational exposure to asbestos and risk of cholangiocarcinoma: a population-based case-control study in four Nordic countries. Occup Environ Med. 2018;75(3):191–8. https://doi.org/10.1136/oemed-2017-104603.
96. Brandi G, Di Girolamo S, Farioli A, de Rosa F, Curti S, Pinna AD, et al. Asbestos: a hidden player behind the cholangiocarcinoma increase? Findings from a case-control analysis. Cancer Causes Control. 2013;24(5):911–8. https://doi.org/10.1007/s10552-013-0167-3.
97. Brandi G, Tavolari S. Asbestos and intrahepatic cholangiocarcinoma. Cells. 2020;9(2). https://doi.org/10.3390/cells9020421.
98. Szendroi M, Nemeth L, Vajta G. Asbestos bodies in a bile duct cancer after occupational exposure. Environ Res. 1983;30(2):270–80. https://doi.org/10.1016/0013-9351(83)90213-x.
99. Ospina D, Villegas VE, Rodriguez-Leguizamon G, Rondon-Lagos M. Analyzing biological and molecular characteristics and genomic damage induced by exposure to asbestos. Cancer Manag Res. 2019;11:4997–5012. https://doi.org/10.2147/CMAR.S205723.
100. Kumagai S, Kurumatani N, Arimoto A, Ichihara G. Cholangiocarcinoma among offset colour proof-printing workers exposed to 1,2-dichloropropane and/or dichloromethane. Occup Environ Med. 2013;70(7):508–10. https://doi.org/10.1136/oemed-2012-101246.
101. Vlaanderen J, Straif K, Martinsen JI, Kauppinen T, Pukkala E, Sparen P, et al. Cholangiocarcinoma among workers in the printing industry: using the NOCCA database to elucidate the generalisability of a cluster report from Japan. Occup Environ Med. 2013;70(12):828–30. https://doi.org/10.1136/oemed-2013-101500.
102. Ali AH, Tabibian JH, Nasser-Ghodsi N, Lennon RJ, DeLeon T, Borad MJ, et al. Surveillance for hepatobiliary cancers in patients with primary sclerosing cholangitis. Hepatology. 2018;67(6):2338–51. https://doi.org/10.1002/hep.29730.
103. Siripongsakun S, Vidhyarkorn S, Charuswattanakul S, Mekraksakit P, Sungkasubun P, Yodkhunnathum N, et al. Ultrasound surveillance for cholangiocarcinoma in an endemic area: a prove of survival benefits. J Gastroenterol Hepatol. 2018;33(7):1383–8. https://doi.org/10.1111/jgh.14074.
104. Lapumnuaypol K, Tiu A, Thongprayoon C, Wijarnpreecha K, Ungprasert P, Mao MA, et al. Effects of aspirin and non-steroidal anti-inflammatory drugs on the risk of cholangiocarcinoma: a meta-analysis. QJM. 2019;112(6):421–7. https://doi.org/10.1093/qjmed/hcz039.
105. Boonmasawai S, Akarasereenont P, Techatraisak K, Thaworn A, Chotewuttakorn S, Palo T. Effects of selective COX-inhibitors and classical NSAIDs on endothelial cell proliferation and migration induced by human cholangiocarcinoma cell culture. J Med Assoc Thail. 2009;92(11):1508–15.
106. Elwood PC, Gallagher AM, Duthie GG, Mur LA, Morgan G. Aspirin, salicylates, and cancer. Lancet. 2009;373(9671):1301–9. https://doi.org/10.1016/S0140-6736(09)60243-9.
107. Wandee J, Prawan A, Senggunprai L, Kongpetch S, Kukongviriyapan V. Metformin sensitizes cholangiocarcinoma cell to cisplatin-induced cytotoxicity through oxidative stress mediated mitochondrial pathway. Life Sci. 2019;217:155–63. https://doi.org/10.1016/j.lfs.2018.12.007.

108. Saengboonmee C, Seubwai W, Cha'on U, Sawanyawisuth K, Wongkham S, Wongkham C. Metformin exerts antiproliferative and anti-metastatic effects against cholangiocarcinoma cells by targeting STAT3 and NF-kB. Anticancer Res. 2017;37(1):115–23. https://doi.org/10.21873/anticanres.11296.
109. Hu RW, Carey EJ, Lindor KD, Tabibian JH. Curcumin in hepatobiliary disease: pharmacotherapeutic properties and emerging potential clinical applications. Ann Hepatol. 2017;16(6):835–41. https://doi.org/10.5604/01.3001.0010.5273.
110. Jattujan P, Pinlaor S, Charoensuk L, Arunyanart C, Welbat JU, Chaijaroonkhanarak W. Curcumin prevents bile canalicular alterations in the liver of hamsters infected with Opisthorchis viverrini. Korean J Parasitol. 2013;51(6):695–701. https://doi.org/10.3347/kjp.2013.51.6.695.
111. Pinlaor S, Prakobwong S, Hiraku Y, Pinlaor P, Laothong U, Yongvanit P. Reduction of periductal fibrosis in liver fluke-infected hamsters after long-term curcumin treatment. Eur J Pharmacol. 2010;638(1–3):134–41. https://doi.org/10.1016/j.ejphar.2010.04.018.
112. Prakobwong S, Khoontawad J, Yongvanit P, Pairojkul C, Hiraku Y, Sithithaworn P, et al. Curcumin decreases cholangiocarcinogenesis in hamsters by suppressing inflammation-mediated molecular events related to multistep carcinogenesis. Int J Cancer. 2011;129(1):88–100. https://doi.org/10.1002/ijc.25656.
113. Wahlstrom B, Blennow G. A study on the fate of curcumin in the rat. Acta Pharmacol Toxicol (Copenh). 1978;43(2):86–92. https://doi.org/10.1111/j.1600-0773.1978.tb02240.x.
114. Liu W, Zhai Y, Heng X, Che FY, Chen W, Sun D, et al. Oral bioavailability of curcumin: problems and advancements. J Drug Target. 2016;24(8):694–702. https://doi.org/10.3109/1061186X.2016.1157883.
115. Marahatta SB, Punyarit P, Bhudisawasdi V, Paupairoj A, Wongkham S, Petmitr S. Polymorphism of glutathione S-transferase omega gene and risk of cancer. Cancer Lett. 2006;236(2):276–81. https://doi.org/10.1016/j.canlet.2005.05.020.
116. Chaiteerakij R, Juran BD, Aboelsoud MM, Harmsen WS, Moser CD, Giama NH, et al. Association between variants in inflammation and cancer-associated genes and risk and survival of cholangiocarcinoma. Cancer Med. 2015;4(10):1599–602. https://doi.org/10.1002/cam4.501.
117. Honjo S, Srivatanakul P, Sriplung H, Kikukawa H, Hanai S, Uchida K, et al. Genetic and environmental determinants of risk for cholangiocarcinoma via Opisthorchis viverrini in a densely infested area in Nakhon Phanom, northeast Thailand. Int J Cancer. 2005;117(5):854–60. https://doi.org/10.1002/ijc.21146.
118. Songserm N, Promthet S, Sithithaworn P, Pientong C, Ekalaksananan T, Chopjitt P, et al. MTHFR polymorphisms and Opisthorchis viverrini infection: a relationship with increased susceptibility to cholangiocarcinoma in Thailand. Asian Pac J Cancer Prev. 2011;12(5):1341–5.
119. Ko KH, Kim NK, Yim DJ, Hong SP, Park PW, Rim KS, et al. Polymorphisms of 5,10-methylenetetrahydrofolate reductase (MTHFR C677T) and thymidylate synthase enhancer region (TSER) as a risk factor of cholangiocarcinoma in a Korean population. Anticancer Res. 2006;26(6B):4229–33.
120. Prawan A, Kukongviriyapan V, Tassaneeyakul W, Pairojkul C, Bhudhisawasdi V. Association between genetic polymorphisms of CYP1A2, arylamine N-acetyltransferase 1 and 2 and susceptibility to cholangiocarcinoma. Eur J Cancer Prev. 2005;14(3):245–50.
121. You SH, Wang X, Huang S, Wang M, Ji GZ, Xia JR, et al. MYH rs3219476 and rs3219472 polymorphisms and risk of cholangiocarcinoma. Mol Med Rep. 2013;7(1):347–51. https://doi.org/10.3892/mmr.2012.1175.
122. Zeng L, You G, Tanaka H, Srivatanakul P, Ohta E, Viwatthanasittiphong C, et al. Combined effects of polymorphisms of DNA-repair protein genes and metabolic enzyme genes on the risk of cholangiocarcinoma. Jpn J Clin Oncol. 2013;43(12):1190–4. https://doi.org/10.1093/jjco/hyt138.

123. Huang WY, Gao YT, Rashid A, Sakoda LC, Deng J, Shen MC, et al. Selected base excision repair gene polymorphisms and susceptibility to biliary tract cancer and biliary stones: a population-based case-control study in China. Carcinogenesis. 2008;29(1):100–5. https://doi.org/10.1093/carcin/bgm247.
124. Melum E, Karlsen TH, Schrumpf E, Bergquist A, Thorsby E, Boberg KM, et al. Cholangiocarcinoma in primary sclerosing cholangitis is associated with NKG2D polymorphisms. Hepatology. 2008;47(1):90–6. https://doi.org/10.1002/hep.21964.
125. Wadsworth CA, Dixon PH, Taylor-Robinson S, Kim JU, Zabron AA, Wong JH, et al. Polymorphisms in natural killer cell receptor protein 2D (NKG2D) as a risk factor for cholangiocarcinoma. J Clin Exp Hepatol. 2019;9(2):171–5. https://doi.org/10.1016/j.jceh.2018.06.521.
126. Hoblinger A, Grunhage F, Sauerbruch T, Lammert F. Association of the c.3972C>T variant of the multidrug resistance-associated protein 2 Gene (MRP2/ABCC2) with susceptibility to bile duct cancer. Digestion. 2009;80(1):36–9. https://doi.org/10.1159/000212990.

Chapter 6
Biochemical Indicators of Cholangiocarcinoma

Sukanya Luang, Masahiko Minamiya, and Nobuo Sakaguchi

Abbreviations

AFP	Alpha-fetoprotein
AID	Activation-induced cytidine deaminase
AMPN	Aminopeptidase N
APC	Adenomatous polyposis coli
APOBEC	Apolipoprotein B mRNA editing enzyme
ARID1A	AT-rich interactive domain-containing protein 1A
AUC	Area under the curve
BAP1	BRCA1-associated protein 1
BAR	Beta-catenin/armadillo-related protein
B-CADHERIN	Brain cadherin (catenin cell-cell adhesion complex)
BCL2	B-cell lymphoma 2
BCLX5	B-cell lymphoma-extra large 5
BCLXL	B-cell lymphoma-extra large
BRAF	v-Raf murine sarcoma viral oncogene homolog

S. Luang
Department of Biochemistry, Faculty of Medicine, Khon Kaen University, Khon Kaen, Thailand
e-mail: sukany@kku.ac.th

M. Minamiya
Gene Osaka Clinic Inc., Osaka, Japan
e-mail: info@osa.g-cg.jp

N. Sakaguchi (✉)
Department of Immunology, Graduate School of Medical Sciences, Kumamoto University, Kumamoto, Japan

Department of Microbiology and Cell Biology, Tokyo Metropolitan Institute of Medical Science, Kamikitazawa, Setagaya-ku, Tokyo, Japan
e-mail: nobusaka@kumamoto-u.ac.jp

J. H. Tabibian (ed.), *Diagnosis and Management of Cholangiocarcinoma*,
https://doi.org/10.1007/978-3-030-70936-5_6

BRCA1	Breast cancer susceptibility gene I
BRCA2	Breast cancer susceptibility gene II
BSEP	Bile salt export pump
CA 19-9	Carbohydrate antigen 19-9
CCA	Cholangiocarcinoma
CCND1	Cyclin D1
CDC6	Cell division cycle 6
CDK6	Cyclin-dependent kinase 6
CDKN2A	Cyclin-dependent kinase inhibitor 2
CEA	Carcinoembryonic antigen
cfDNA	Cell-free DNA
COX-2	Cyclooxygenase 2
CTC	Circulating tumor cell
CYP1A2	Cytochrome P450 family 1 subfamily A member 2
dCCA	Distal cholangiocarcinoma
EGFR	Epidermal growth factor receptor
EpCAM	Epithelial cell adhesion molecule
ERB-2	Erb-B2 receptor tyrosine kinase 2
EVs	Extracellular vesicles
FBXW7	F-box and WD repeat domain containing 7
FGF19	Fibroblast growth factor 19
FGFR2	Fibroblast growth factor receptor 2
FIC1	Familial intrahepatic cholestasis type 1
FXR	Farnesoid X receptor
GANP	Germinal center-associated nuclear protein
GSTO1	Glutathione S-transferase omega 1
HBV	Hepatitis B virus
HCC	Hepatocellular carcinoma
HCV	Hepatitis C virus
HOXD9	Homeobox protein Hox-D9
iCCA	Intrahepatic cholangiocarcinoma
IDH1	Isocitrate dehydrogenase [ADP(+) 1]
IDH2	Isocitrate dehydrogenase [ADP(+) 2]
KEAP1	Kelch-like ECH-associated protein 1
K-RAS	Ki-ras2 Kirsten rat sarcoma viral oncogene homolog
LTO1	LTO1 maturation factor of ABCE1
mAb	Monoclonal antibody
MCL1	Induced myeloid leukemia cell differentiation protein
MDM2	Mouse double minute 2 homolog
MDR3	Multidrug resistance gene 3
miR	MicroRNA
MRP2	Multidrug resistance-associated protein 2
MTHFR	Methylenetetrahydrofolate reductase
MVs	Microvesicles
MYC	v-Myc myelocytomatosis viral oncogene homolog

NAT2	Arylamine N-acetyltransferase 2
ncRNA	Noncoding RNA
NF1	Neurofibromin 1
NKG2D	Natural killer cell lectin-like receptor subfamily 2D
OPCML	Opioid binding protein/cell adhesion molecule-like
p14arf	An alternative reading frame product of the CDKN2A locus
p16	Cyclin-dependent kinase inhibitor protein p16 (INK4a)
PBRM1	Protein polybromo-1
pCCA	Perihilar cholangiocarcinoma
PD-1/PD-L2	Programmed cell death 1/programmed death ligand 2
PI3KCA	Phosphoinositide 3-kinase p110
PIGR	Polymeric immunoglobulin receptor
PTEN	Phosphatase and tensin homolog
RAD51AP1	RAD51 associating protein-1
RASSF1A	Ras association domain family 1 isoform A
ROS1	ROS proto-oncogene 1
shRNA	Short hairpin RNA
SIN1	Stress-activated map kinase-interacting protein 1
Axin-1	Axis inhibition protein 1
SMAD4	Small body mothers against decapentaplegic 4
SOCS3	Suppressor of cytokine signaling 3
TGF-β	Transforming growth factor-β
TP53	Tumor protein p53
TYMS	Thymidylate synthetase
UNG	Uracil nucleotide glycosidase
VNN1	Vanin1
XRCC1	X-ray repair cross-complementing protein 1

Introduction

Cholangiocarcinoma (CCA) is the second most common liver malignancy worldwide and is particularly common in Southeast Asian countries such as Thailand, Cambodia, and Laos. A major feature of CCA is its heterogeneity, including of its risk factors and causes. For example, many cases of CCA in Northeastern Thailand are related to liver fluke infection and presumably originate over time as a result of inflammatory damage by the stenosis in the bile duct(s) [1–3]. In contrast, CCAs in the other countries are accompanied with sporadic genetic abnormalities commonly detected in various malignancies (oncogenic genetic alteration) [4, 5]. This heterogeneity of CCA complicates many aspects of its clinical management, including diagnosis, prognosis, and surveillance.

Early biomarker analysis of patient sera led to the finding that carbohydrate antigen 19-9 (CA19-9) and other carcinoembryonic markers are valid for the diagnosis and follow-up of CCA patients [6]. Genome-wide next-generation gene sequencing (NGS) of CCA tumor cells has facilitated the accumulation of further information and formulation of a more comprehensive classification of CCAs as compared to earlier compendia of genetic data. Here, we show currently available standard biomarkers in sections "Classification of CCA", "Classical Serum Markers", and "Earlier Analyses of Gene Mutation and Amplification in CCA" and propose the advanced biomarker/gene marker strategy by combination with the data of the genome alterations of the individual CCAs in sections "Challenges of Highly Specific Biomarkers", and "Recent Classification of CCAs with Large-Scale Analysis of Multi-omics".

Classification of CCA

The clinical diagnosis of CCA involves tumor classification depending on tumor location: intrahepatic (iCCA), perihilar (pCCA), and distal (dCCA). (i) Primary sclerosing cholangitis (PSC) is one of the primary causes of CCA development in the western world. It is a chronic disease of the intrahepatic and extrahepatic bile ducts due to inflammation and scarring. (ii) Parasitic infestation with *Opisthorchis viverrini* and *Clonorchis sinensis* is the significant risk factors of CCA in Asia, particularly in Southeast Asia. Due to the food-consumption behavior of humans to eat raw or undercooked fish, worms can infect humans via ingestion and inhabit in the bile ducts, gallbladder, and pancreatic duct [7]. (iii) Hepatolithiasis is one type of the gallstone disease with the stones in the intrahepatic bile ducts proximal to either the left or right hepatic duct. Hepatolithiasis-associated CCA with a high incidence in East Asian countries, such as Taiwan, China, Hong Kong, South Korea, and Japan [8–11], may arise after the prolonged inflammation (recurrent or chronic inflammatory) of bile duct epithelium [12, 13]. (iv) Hepatitis virus infections, especially with hepatitis B and C viruses (HBV and HCV), are the causes of hepatocellular carcinoma (HCC). The epidemiologic evidence suggests chronic HBV and HCV infection may be involved in an increased incidence of iCCA [14–16].

Classical Serum Markers

CCA is a "silent killer" in part due to the difficulty of being diagnosed before the advanced or metastatic stage. The CCA diagnosis depends on various components, including clinical findings, imaging techniques, biochemical data, and histological information. Standard serum liver tests occasionally find initial changes in CCA (e.g., ALP, ALT, and total bilirubin). The current serum biomarkers for CCA are CA 19-9, carcinoembryonic antigen (CEA), mucins, and alpha-fetoprotein (AFP) and are reviewed herein (Table 6.1).

Carbohydrate antigen 19-9 (CA 19-9) is an epitope on the sialyl-Lewis antigens (Lew^a and Lew^b, etc.) which are produced by biliary, pancreatic, gastric, colonic, endometrial, and salivary epithelial cells [17]. It is a routine diagnostic marker for

Table 6.1 The diagnostic value of serum markers for CCA

Marker	Cutoff value	Sensitivity (%)	Specificity (%)	PPV (%)	NPV (%)	Accuracy (%)	Ref.	Application
CA 19-9	129 U/mL	79.0	98.0	78.6	99.4	96.2	[19]	Useful for cancer diagnosis, especially pancreatobiliary
	125.1 U/mL	76.7	80.0	79.3	77.4	–	[32]	
	>37 KU/L	77.1	84.8	65.9	90.7	82.7	[20]	
CEA	12.1 μg/L	53.3	86.7	80.0	65.0	70.0	[23]	A broad-spectrum tumor marker, useful especially in colorectal carcinoma
	22 μg/L	68.6	81.5	58.5	87.2	78.0	[20]	
CA 19-9 + CEA	–	76.7	83.3	81.1	78.1	80.0	[23]	Combination of two markers provides better sensitivity and specificity
CA 19-9 + AFP	–	86.7	83.3	83.9	86.2	85.0	[32]	
CEA + AFP	–	83.0	87.0	86.2	83.9	85.0	[31, 32]	
MUC4	–	27.0	93.0	82.0	51.0	–	[26]	Low sensitivity for CCA but useful for diagnosing primary sclerosing cholangitis
cfDNA								Useful for differential diagnosis of CCA from other biliary diseases
OPCML	–	80.0	90.0	88.9	81.9	85.0	[55]	
HOXD9	–	67.5	90.0	87.1	73.5	78.8	[55]	
OPCML + HOXD9	–	62.5	100.0	100.0	71.7	81.3	[55]	
MicroRNA								
Bile miR-191 + miR-486-3p + miR-1274b + miR-16 + miR-484	–	67.0	96.0	94.4	74.4	–	[44]	Useful for differential diagnosis of CCA from other biliary diseases

PPV positive predictive value, *NPV* negative predictive value hepatobiliary and pancreatic malignancies, while it is not applicable for the tumors in the Lew^{a-} Lew^{b-} patients [18]. CA19-9 is a CCA marker with relatively high sensitivity (approx 79%) and specificity (approx 98%) when using a cutoff value of 129 U/mL [19]. Other cutoff values have been studied (e.g., in the context of PSC), and performance characteristics may depend on the presence of other underlying disease(s). Indeed, CA19-9 level may also increase in patients with cholangitis or pancreatobiliary ductal obstruction; therefore, CCA prediction by serum CA 19-9 is only reliable if combined with and interpreted in the context of other clinical data [20].

Carcinoembryonic antigen (CEA) is a cell membrane-associated glycoprotein and shows the different expression patterns between healthy tissues and cancer cells. While it is a marker for colorectal and other adenocarcinomas [21, 22], CEA indicates approximately 53% sensitivity and 87% specificity for CCA diagnosis [23]. If combined with CA19-9, CEA gives valuable information on CCA prediction with 63% sensitivity and 87% specificity [4]. Besides, CEA is useful to predict the long-term survival after resection of CCA [24], and the higher expression levels of CEA and CA19-9 are related to the reduced overall survival of CCA patients [23].

Mucins are the glycoproteins secreted into the extracellular space from the epithelial cells. Various human malignancies show the changes in the expression levels of transmembrane mucins of MUC1, MUC2, MUC4, MUC5AC, MUC13, and MUC16 [25]. MUC4 expression increased highly and significantly in the advanced CCA patients of the poor prognosis group. MUC4 has a sensitivity (approx 27%) and specificity (approx 93%) for CCA [26]. Another biomarker, MUC5AC, is expressed in the bronchial, gastric, and endocervix epithelium, but not in the normal intrahepatic biliary tree. Serum MUC5AC is positive in CCA patients with a 2.5-fold higher risk of death [27]. The ratio of MUC5AC expression between serum and bile is useful for the differential diagnosis of CCAs from cholangitis and biliary stones [28].

Serum alpha-fetoprotein (AFP) is a useful marker for hepatocellular carcinoma (HCC) and can be also for other cancers (gastrointestinal, pancreatic, biliary, nonseminomatous germ cell testicular, and germ cell ovarian cancers) [29]. Approximately 20% of CCA patients show a high AFP level (>20 ng/mL) [30]. AFP shows a high specificity for HCC diagnosis but low specificity (and sensitivity) for CCA diagnosis. However, AFP can be useful in combination with either one of the other markers such as CA19-9 (86.67% sensitivity and 83.33% specificity), CA125 (80.00% sensitivity and 86.67% specificity), CEA (83.33% sensitivity and 86.67% specificity), and CA242 (88.90% sensitivity and 89.7% specificity) [31, 32].

Earlier Analyses of Gene Mutation and Amplification in CCA

Analysis of gene expression and SNP microarray of CCAs demonstrated various alterations in oncogenic signaling pathways of CCND1 and FGF19 genes (amplification), KRAS and BRAF genes (mutation), and activation of inflammatory signaling pathways. The genetic alterations also classified CCAs into congenital

Table 6.2 Molecular abnormalities associated with CCA

Origin/normal function	Gene (and/or protein)
I. *Congenital abnormality*	
Transport	MDR3, BSEP, MRP2, FIC1
Metabolism	CYP1A2, GST01, ARY2, BAR (FXR)
DNA repair and modification	MTHFR, TYMS, XRCC1
Tumor surveillance	NKG2D, COX-2
II. *Acquired mutation*	
Tumor suppressor	APC, BRCA1, E-CADHERIN, p16, p14arf, PTEN, RASSSF1A, **SMAD4**[a], **TP53**[a]
Transcription regulation	**ARID1A**[a], KEAP1
Apoptosis	AXIN1, BCL2, BCLXL, BCLX5, MCL1
Cell growth	**BAP1**[a], CCND1, CDK6, FGFR2, ROS1, **CDKN2A**[a]
Oncogene	BRAF, B-CADHERIN, EGFR (ERB1), **ERB2**[a] (HER2), **K-RAS**[a], MDM2, MYC
DNA damage and repair	BRCA2, RAD51AP1
Regulation of bile production	FGF19
Proteasomal protein degradation	**FBXW7**[a]
Glucose metabolism	**IDH1**[a], **IDH2**[a]
Ribosome biosynthesis	LTO1
Signal transduction	NF1, **PBRM1**[a], **PI3KCA**, SOCS3

Ref: Peter et al. [65]
[a]Boldface indicates genes of high mutation frequency

abnormality group and acquired mutation group (Table 6.2) [33]. The current biomarker study may not be directly applicable as a diagnostic tool to predict the prognosis and the future severity of the disease, but may be useful when used in combination with the genetic study such as the number of affected genes and the critically impaired genes in CCAs. The five reports of clinical cases calculated higher-frequency gene alterations [34–38]; these included molecules of tumor suppressors (SMAD4, TP53, RASSF1A), transcription regulation (ARID1A), cell growth (BAP1, CDKN2A), oncogene [ERB-2 (HER2), K-RAS, B-RAF], protease protein degradation (FBXW7), glucose metabolism (IDH1, IDH2), and signal transduction (PBRM1, PI3KCA). A study of circulating tumor cell (CTC) DNA confirmed the high degree correlation of mutational frequencies with published datasets of CCA in TP53 (38-8%), ARID1A (36-4%), KRAS (28-5%), IDH1 (32-4%), BAP1 (29-1%), PBRM1 (21-1%), SMAD4 (9-4%), PIK3CA (9-3%), and CDKN2A (7-0%) [39].

Previous studies with smaller numbers of CCA cases attempted to identify the critical differences in gene alterations to account for the geographic differences in CCA development and prognosis. As mentioned earlier, CCAs are highly heterogeneous, in large part due to the etiological, environmental, anatomical, cellular, and genetic factors. CCAs with liver fluke infection, for example, are different than those of non-liver fluke-infected patients. Therefore, it has been difficult to discover the most appropriate biomarker among the conventional ones (or a novel one). Researchers have probably studied CCAs as different category tumors originating with different genetic alterations; though this may have offered some advantages, it may have also somewhat impeded understanding and generalization of genetic changes and clinical treatment of CCA.

Challenges of Highly Specific Biomarkers

Many technologies have been applied to improve diagnostic accuracy, particularly at an early stage of disease, and in order to best target therapeutic options. These are reviewed in the forthcoming paragraphs. Extracellular vesicles (EVs) are classified into microvesicles (MVs) and exosomes according to their size and biogenesis. MVs directly bud from the plasma membrane, and their size ranges between 100 and 1000 nm. Exosomes originate from multivesicular bodies; their size is smaller than 100 nm, and they float at a density of 1.13–1.19 g ml^{-1} in sucrose gradients [40–42]. EVs are found in blood, urine, saliva, bile, and ascites. They carry the disease biomarkers as specific proteins, lipids, RNA species, DNA, and metabolite [42, 43]. Proteomics analysis evaluated the abundance of oncogenic proteins in CCA cell-derived EVs and found aminopeptidase N (AMPN), vanin1 (VNN1), and polymeric immunoglobulin receptor (PIGR) in early-stage CCA to have an area under the curve (AUC) of 0.88, 0.88, and 0.84, respectively. The miR profiles from extracellular vesicles from human bile revealed miR-based panels of miR-191, miR-486-3p, miR-1274b, miR-16, and miR-484 to be valuable for CCA diagnosis, with 67% sensitivity and 96% specificity, which gives similar diagnostic potential compared to CA19-9 with the specified cutoff value [44].

Circulating nucleic acid as cell-free DNA (cfDNA) is released in plasma and other body fluids from tumor cells. Investigation of cfDNA can assess the genetic and epigenetic alterations of individual patients, particularly those who are diagnosed in advanced stages of the disease and with limited therapeutic options. It can determine single-nucleotide mutations [45–48], aberrations in DNA methylation [49, 50], copy number aberrations [45, 50, 51], and gene expression alterations [52, 53]. For example, molecular analysis of cfDNA can help screen for FGFR2 mutations both in the primary tumor and metastatic lesions to examine the gain of drug resistance against the BFJ398 inhibitor in patients with ICC. Multiple mutations of the FGFR2 gene affect the FGFR2 kinase domain and create a significant oncogenic alteration in cancer cells that should be critically monitored for decision-making in clinical treatment [54]. Other epigenetic changes, including DNA methylation, also provide useful information, such as cfDNA hypermethylation of opioid binding protein/cell adhesion molecule-like (OPCML: AUC, 0.85; sensitivity, 80%; specificity, 90%; accuracy, 85%) and homeobox protein Hox-D9 (HOXD9: AUC, 0.789;

sensitivity, 67.5%; specificity, 90%; accuracy, 78.75%), to differentially diagnose CCA with a higher percentage compared to other biliary diseases [55].

Circulating noncoding RNA (ncRNA) may regulate gene transcription, transcript stability, and translation of protein-coding transcripts [56]. Altered expressions of serum and plasma miR-21 and miR-26a in patients are useful for diagnosis and the prediction of patient survival [57, 58]. CCA patient serum also shows the downregulation of miR-150-5p expression [59, 60]. MicroRNA is aberrantly expressed in CCAs as well as in all types of human tumors [61].

Circulating tumor cells (CTCs) overexpress epithelial cell adhesion molecule (EpCAM), an indicator of having lost cell-to-cell adhesion capacity and a propensity for metastasis. CCA has high-level expression of EpCAM, with a sensitivity of 93.7%, as shown by enrichment-immunofluorescence in situ hybridization (SE-iFISH) [62].

Recent Classification of CCAs with Large-Scale Analysis of Multi-omics

Application of NGS and omics examination for larger-scale clinical samples has provided a comprehensive concept in the classification of CCAs. A world cooperative study of the combined datasets of a large whole-genome sequencing, whole-exome sequencing, copy number alterations, transcriptomes, and epigenomes proposed the classification of CCAs of 489 cases from 10 countries. It classified four types of CCA clusters based on tumor etiologies, anatomical locations, and the cellular origin, the tumor characteristics, and clinical features, as summarized below [63].

The first factor for clustering is history of liver fluke infection, and the second factor is genomic modification caused by increased DNA hypermethylation of CpG island shores and high levels of mutations in H3K27me3-associated promoters. Cluster 1, liver fluke (+)/genomic modification (-), and Cluster 2, liver fluke (+)/genomic modification (+), show recurrent mutations of TP53, ARID1A and BRCA1/2, and ERBB2 amplification. These clusters show a poor prognosis. Cluster 3, liver fluke (-)/genomic modification (-), and Cluster 4, liver fluke (-)/genomic modification (+), show recurrent mutations in epigenetic-related genes, i.e., BAP1 and IDH1/2, as well as FGFR rearrangements, and have high PD-1/PD-L2 expression. Clusters 3 and 4 show better prognosis. The higher-rate alterations of various genes in CCAs during clinical treatment are one of the causes of the worse prognosis.

Development of CCA is associated with metabolic syndrome, hepatolithiasis, congenital biliary tract malformations, bile duct cysts with the risk factors of chronic inflammation involving the biliary tract, several toxic and environmental factors such as nitrosamine-contaminated food, asbestos, dioxins, vinyl chlorides and thorotrast, smoking, and alcohol intake [32, 64]. Exposure to various long-term risk factors results in the proliferation and genetic and epigenetic alterations of cholangiocytes and their malignant transformation [64, 65].

Additionally, any stimulus that causes oxidative stress can be oncogenic. Several CCA cell lines induce aberrant expression of activation-induced cytidine deaminase (AID) as an initiator of gene alteration [66]. AID initiates somatic hypermutation at the immunoglobulin V-region gene and class switch regions in B lymphocytes [67]. The cytidine deamination potentially causes the DNA injuries, resulting in mutation of the promoter regions and coding regions of various critical genes by the assist of the associated protein complex of RNA polymerase II, transcription elongation factor Spt5, UNG, and GANP [68, 69].

Current studies suggested that aberrant expression of cytidine deaminase molecules resulted in altering the genome. TGF-β stimulation causes the aberrant AID expression in multiple cancer cells of the digestive system [70–72]. Virus infection may evoke the APOBEC family cytidine deaminase proteins as the endogenous defense molecules [68]. Typically, human APOBEC3B is involved in the development of breast cancers [73]. These cytidine deaminase molecules enter into the nucleus together with the RNA exportation component GANP [69]. Aberrant expression of the APOBEC family cytidine deaminase protein associated with GANP might alter the genome randomly at the transcription-competent nucleosome, resulting in chromosome translocation, gene deletion, and mutations [72–74]. Therefore, it is difficult to predict and determine the genome alteration in individual CCA cells. Nevertheless, identification of novel biomarkers is an essential issue to monitor the gene mutations and chromosome modifications.

Future Perspective

Combination of Standard Cancer Biomarker Plus CCA-Selective Biomarkers

Diagnosis and treatment of patients with CCA needs to be guided and advanced by incorporation of comprehensive tools, including with conventional biomarkers as well as patient-specific genetic and cellular abnormalities. As an initial tool, CA19-9 can be useful but still provides only a small piece of the overall picture and future clinical course. Preoperative or postoperative genetic information of tumor cells provides a vital avenue for better treatment. Surgical specimens provide the most information on genetic abnormalities of primary CCA foci. One approach to optimize nonsurgical specimens is to enrich CTCs in peripheral blood or ascites fluid by the antibody trap method using high-affinity monoclonal antibodies against a standard biomarker that appears commonly in CCA tumors (e.g., CA19-9, Muc5a). Antibody trapping of CTCs from CCA patients with magnetic beads enhances the tumor cells that are actively mutating and metastasizing in the cancer patient. Direct capturing of tumor cells under the microscope also provides insight regarding genetic alterations of the individual primary CCA lesion. Such tumor cells demonstrate the genetic alterations and the critical causes of a highly malignant trait of cell proliferation, drug resistance, mutation, and anti-apoptotic properties. The genetic information includes the alterations in tumor suppressor genes such as p53, PTEN, p16, and CDC6 and the methylation status of CpG islands at the promoter regions of selected target genes; changes for CTNNB1, WNT5B, and AKT gene expression; somatic gene copy numbers of immune cells; mutations of BAP1 and IDH1/2; and the upregulation of FGFRs and PI3K signaling.

Cancer Therapy with an Infusion of Tumor Suppressor Genes and shRNA Vectors

Gene transfection therapy is one of the promising procedures for targeting of specific tumors. To develop next-generation cancer treatment, we need to solve two kinds of complicated issues. First, authentic and precise targeting depends on the identification of abnormalities of individual cancer cells. This is a cost-consuming and probably the most challenging issue for advanced clinical treatment. Practically, the procedure needs to target the most common genetic alterations associated with oncogenesis and cell proliferation. Gene alterations of CCAs include congenital molecular abnormalities of various functions such as molecular transport, cell metabolism, DNA repair and modification, and tumor surveillance as well as acquired mutations of multiple genes. The target genes for this procedure are diverse; therefore, rapid and convenient screening of individual patients is necessary. At present, however, we need to select several active target genes for the practical use.

The second issue is vector selection for gene therapy. The choices for vectors are many and will develop more in the future. One candidate vector is the lentivirus vector, which is highly effective in introducing genes into tumor cells [75]. The gene knockdown procedure into cancer cells is capable of targeting a cancer-specific abnormality with short hairpin RNA. Also, the human telomerase gene promoter can facilitate targeting of cancer cells [76]. One of the challenges of vector selection is as follows: the regular protocol of gene therapy is with drip infusion of five genes to the cancer patients in The Gene Osaka Clinic Inc. (http://www.g-cg.jp/) (Osaka, Japan). Drip infusion of five constructs (ten million virus titers/each gene at one time in a week) is undertaken five or six times as a single course under the informed consent. The patient receives the course at least twice. The clinical outcome of CCA patients often shows marked decrease of cancer biomarkers with p53, PTEN, p16, CDC6-shRNA, and Gankirin-shRNA in combination with standard cancer therapy [77]. In principle, gene therapy causes the adverse side effect of virus particle infusion-associated inflammation and possibly allergic response; this includes fever (~38 °C), nausea, diarrhea, vomiting, and hypotension. In some cases, transient increases of ALT, AST, CRP, and white blood cell count occur.

The promise held by gene therapy against CCA will growingly contribute to the improvement of patient outcomes. The exchange of information, knowledge, and technical skills are necessary for this and other advancements in CCA treatment.

Conclusion

A hopeful approach for better cancer treatment depends on rapid and accurate diagnosis and targeted therapy based on individual cancer genetic information. Strategic biomarkers play an important role in this regard and are a subject of continued research.

Acknowledgments The authors thank Drs. Sopit Wongkham and Atit Silsirivanit (Khon Kaen University, Thailand) for continuous support and encouragement.

References

1. Chalnuvati T, Paosawadhi A, Sripranoth M, Manasatith S, Viranuvatti V. Carcinoma of the cystic duct associated with opisthorchiasis. Southeast Asian J Trop Med Public Health. 1976;7:482–6.
2. Bridgewater J, Galle P, Khan S, Llovet J, Park J, Patel T, et al. Guidelines for the diagnosis and management of intrahepatic cholangiocarcinoma. J Hepatol. 2014;13:1268–89.
3. Yothiasong S, Thanee M, Namwat N, Yongvanit P, Boonmars T, Puapairol A, et al. Opisthorchis viverrini infection activates the PI3K/AKT/PTRN and Wnt/β-catenin signaling pathways in a cholangiocarcinogenesis model. Asian Pac J Cancer Prev. 2014;15:10463–8.
4. Patel T. Increasing incidence and mortality of primary intrahepatic cholangiocarcinoma in the United States. Hepatology. 2001;33:1353–7.
5. Montomli J, Erichsen R, Norgaard M, Hoye M, Hansen JB, Jacobsen JB. Survival of patients with primary liver cancer in central and northeastern Denmark, 1998–2009. Clin Epidemiol. 2011;3(Suppl 1):3–10.
6. Qin XL, Wang ZR, Shi JS, Lu M, Wang L, He QR. Utility of serum CA19-9 in diagnosis of cholangiocarcinoma: in comparison with CEA. World J Gastroenterol. 2004;10:427–32.
7. Smout MJ, Laha T, Mulvenna J, Sripa B, Suttiprapa S, Jones A, et al. A granulin-like growth factor secreted by the carcinogenic liver fluke, *Opisthorchis viverrini*, promotes proliferation of host cells. PLoS Pathog. 2009;5(10):e1000611.
8. Su CH, Lui WY, P'eng FK. Relative prevalence of gallstone diseases in Taiwan. A nationwide cooperative study. Dig Dis Sci. 1992;37:764–8.
9. Kim MH, Lim BC, Myung SJ, Lee SK, Ohrr HC, Kim YT, et al. Epidemiological study on Korean gallstone disease: a nationwide cooperative study. Dig Dis Sci. 1999;44:1674–83.
10. Kim YH, Park SJ, Jang JY, Ahn YJ, Park YC, Yoon YB, et al. Changing patterns of gallstone disease in Korea. World J Surg. 2004;28:206–10.
11. Tazuma S. Gallstone disease: epidemiology, pathogenesis, and classification of biliary stones (common bile duct and intrahepatic). Best Pract Res Clin Gastroenterol. 2006;20:1075–83.
12. Nakanuma Y, Terada T, Tanaka Y, Ohta G. Are hepatolithiasis and cholangiocarcinoma aetiologically related? A morphological study of 12 cases of hepatolithiasis associated with cholangiocarcinoma. Virchows Arch A Pathol Anat Histopathol. 1985;406:45–58.

13. Rizvi S, Gores GJ. Pathogenesis, diagnosis, and management of cholangiocarcinoma. Gastroenterology. 2013;145:1215–29.
14. Alvaro D, Crocetti E, Ferretti S, Bragazzi MC, Capocaccia R, AISF Cholangiocarcinoma Committee. Descriptive epidemiology of cholangiocarcinoma in Italy. Dig Liver Dis. 2010;42(7):490–5.
15. Fwu CW, Chien YC, You SL, Nelson KE, Kirk GD, Kuo HS, et al. Hepatitis B virus infection and risk of intrahepatic cholangiocarcinoma and non-Hodgkin lymphoma: a cohort study of parous women in Taiwan. Hepatology. 2011;53(4):1217–25.
16. Shin HR, Lee CU, Park HJ, Seol SY, Chung JM, Choi HC, et al. Hepatitis B and C virus, Clonorchis sinensis for the risk of liver cancer: a case–control study in Pusan, Korea. Int J Epidemiol. 1996;25:933–40.
17. Laulu S, Roberts W. Performance characteristics of five automated ca19.9 assays. Am J Clin Pathol. 2007;127(3):436–40.
18. Tempero MA, Uchida E, Takasaki H, Burnett DA, Steplewski Z, Pour PM. Relationship of carbohydrate antigen 19-9 and Lewis antigens in pancreatic cancer. Cancer Res. 1987;47:5501–3.
19. Levy C, Lymp J, Angulo P, Gores GJ, Larusso N, Lindor KD. The value of serum CA 19-9 in predicting cholangiocarcinomas in patients with primary sclerosing cholangitis. Dig Dis Sci. 2005;50(9):1734–40.
20. Charatcharoenwitthaya P, Enders FB, Halling KC, Lindor KD. Utility of serum tumor markers, imaging, and biliary cytology for detecting cholangiocarcinoma in primary sclerosing cholangitis. Hepatology. 2008;48(4):1106–17.
21. Sørensen CG, Karlsson WK, Pommergaard H-C, Burcharth J, Rosenberg J. The diagnostic accuracy of carcinoembryonic antigen to detect colorectal cancer recurrence – a systematic review. Int J Surg. 2016;25:134–44.
22. Das V, Kalita J, Pal M. Predictive and prognostic biomarkers in colorectal cancer: a systematic review of recent advances and challenges. Biomed Pharmacother. 2017;87:8–19.
23. Li Y, Li DJ, Chen J, Liu W, Li JW, Jiang P, et al. Application of joint detection of AFP, CA19-9, CA125 and CEA in identification and diagnosis of cholangiocarcinoma. Asian Pac J Cancer Prev. 2015;16(8):3451–5.
24. Loosen SH, Roderburg C, Kauertz KL, Koch A, Vucur M, Schneider AT, et al. CEA but not CA19-9 is an independent prognostic factor in patients undergoing resection of cholangiocarcinoma. Sci Rep. 2017;7:16975–85.
25. Kufe DW. Mucins in cancer: function, prognosis and therapy. Nat Rev Cancer. 2009;9(12):874–85.
26. Matull WR, Andreola F, Loh A, Adiguzel Z, Deheragoda M, Qureshi U, et al. MUC4 and MUC5AC are highly specific tumour-associated mucins in biliary tract cancer. Br J Cancer. 2008;98:1675–81.
27. Boonla C, Wongkham S, Sheehan JK, Wongkham C, Bhudhisawasdi V, Tepsiri N, et al. Prognostic value of serum MUC5AC mucin in patients with cholangiocarcinoma. Cancer. 2003;98:1438–43.
28. Danese E, Ruzzenente O, Ruzzenente A, Iacono C, Bertuzzo F, Gelati M, et al. Assessment of bile and serum mucin5AC in cholangiocarcinoma: diagnostic performance and biologic significance. Surgery. 2014;156(5):1218–24.
29. Zhang BH, Yang BH, Tang ZY. Randomized controlled trial of screening for hepatocellular carcinoma. J Cancer Res Clin Oncol. 2004;130:417–22.
30. Liver Cancer Study Group of Japan. Primary liver cancer in Japan. Clinicopathologic features and results of surgical treatment. Ann Surg. 1990;211(3):277–87.
31. Tao LY, Cai L, He XD, Liu W, Qu Q. Comparison of serum tumor markers for intrahepatic cholangiocarcinoma and hepatocellular carcinoma. Am Surg. 2010;76(11):1210–3.
32. Gahlot G, Joshi G. Evaluation of the importance of the serum levels of CA-125, CA19-9, CA-19-9, carcinoembryonic antigen and alpha fetoprotein for diagnosis of cholangiocarcinoma. Int J Adv Sci Eng Technol. 2018;6(1):2321–8991.

33. Shiao MS, Chiablaem K, Charoensawan V, Ngamphaiboon N, Jinawath N. Emergence of intrahepatic cholangiocarcinoma: how high-throughput technologies expedite the solutions for a rare cancer type. Front Genet. 2018;9:309–25.
34. Nakamura H, Arai Y, Totoki Y, Shirota T, Elzawahry A, Kato M, et al. Genomic spectra of biliary tract cancer. Nat Genet. 2015;47(9):1003–10.
35. Zou S, Li J, Zhou H, Frech C, Jiang X, Chu JS, et al. Mutational landscape of intrahepatic cholangiocarcinoma. Nat Commun. 2014;5:5696–707.
36. Churi CR, Shroff R, Wang Y, Rashid A, Kang HC, Weatherly J, et al. Mutation profiling in cholangiocarcinoma: prognostic and therapeutic implications. PLoS One. 2014;9(12):e115383–406.
37. Farshidfar F, Zheng S, Gingras MC, Newton Y, Shih J, Robertson AG, et al. Integrative genomic analysis of cholangiocarcinoma identifies distinct IDH-mutant molecular profiles. Cell Rep. 2017;18:2780–94.
38. Ross JS, Wang K, Gay L, Al-Rohil R, Rand JV, Jones DM, et al. New routes to targeted therapy of intrahepatic cholangiocarcinomas revealed by next-generation sequencing. Oncologist. 2014;19:235–42.
39. Ettrich TJ, Schwerdel S, Dolnik A, Beuter F, Blatte TJ, Schmidt SA, et al. Genotyping of circulating tumor DNA in cholangiocarcinoma reveals diagnostic and prognostic information. Sci Rep. 2019;9:13261–72.
40. Théry C, Zitvogel L, Amigorena S. Exosomes: composition, biogenesis and function. Nat Rev Immunol. 2002;2:569–79.
41. Théry C, Witwer KW, Aikawa E, Alcaraz MJ, Anderson JD, Andriantsitohaina R. Minimal information for studies of extracellular vesicles 2018 (MISEV2018): a position statement of the international society for extracellular vesicles and update of the misev2014 guidelines. J Extracell Vesicles. 2018;7(1):1535750.
42. Raposo G, Stoorvogel W. Extracellular vesicles: exosomes, microvesicles, and friends. J Cell Biol. 2013;200(4):373–83.
43. Yáñez-Mó M, Siljander PR, Andreu Z, Zavec AB, Borràs FE, Buzas EI, et al. Biological properties of extracellular vesicles and their physiological functions. J Extracell Vesicles. 2015;4:27066.
44. Li L, Masica D, Ishida M, Tomuleasa C, Umegaki S, Kalloo AN, Georgiades C, et al. Human bile contains microRNA-laden extracellular vesicles that can be used for cholangiocarcinoma diagnosis. Hepatology. 2014;60(3):896–907.
45. Chan KCA, Jiang P, Zheng YWL, Liao GJWW, Sun H, Wong J, et al. Cancer genome scanning in plasma: detection of tumor-associated copy number aberrations, single-nucleotide variants, and tumoral heterogeneity by massively parallel sequencing. Clin Chem. 2013;59:211–24.
46. Dawson S-JJ, Tsui DWY, Murtaza M, Biggs H, Rueda OM, Chin S-FF, et al. Analysis of circulating tumor DNA to monitor metastatic breast cancer. N Engl J Med. 2013;368:1199–209.
47. Cohen JD, Li L, Wang Y, Thoburn C, Afsari B, Danilova L, et al. Detection and localization of surgically resectable cancers with a multi-analyte blood test. Science. 2018;359:926–30.
48. Murtaza M, Dawson SJ, Tsui DWY, Gale D, Forshew T, Piskorz AM, et al. Non-invasive analysis of acquired resistance to cancer therapy by sequencing of plasma DNA. Nature. 2013;497:108–12.
49. Chan KCA, Jiang P, Chan CWM, Sun K, Wong J, Hui EP, et al. Noninvasive detection of cancer-associated genome-wide hypomethylation and copy number aberrations by plasma DNA bisulfite sequencing. Proc Natl Acad Sci U S A. 2013;110:18761–8.
50. Wen L, Li J, Guo H, Liu X, Zheng S, Zhang D, et al. Genome-scale detection of hypermethylated CpG islands in circulating cell-free DNA of hepatocellular carcinoma patients. Cell Res. 2015;25:1250–64.
51. Heitzer E, Ulz P, Geigl JB, Speicher MR. Non-invasive detection of genome-wide somatic copy number alterations by liquid biopsies. Mol Oncol. 2016;10:494–502.
52. Tsui NBY, Jiang P, Wong YF, Leung TY, Chan KCA, Chiu RWK, et al. Maternal plasma RNA sequencing for genome-wide transcriptomic profiling and identification of pregnancy-associated transcripts. Clin Chem. 2014;60:954–62.

53. Koh W, Pan W, Gawad C, Fan HC, Kerchner GA, Wyss-Coray T, et al. Noninvasive in vivo monitoring of tissue-specific global gene expression in humans. Proc Natl Acad Sci U S A. 2014;111:7361–6.
54. Goyal L, Saha SK, Liu LY, Siravegna G, Leshchiner I, Ahronian LG, et al. Polyclonal secondary FGFR2 mutations drive acquired resistance to FGFR inhibition in patients with FGFR2 fusion-positive cholangiocarcinoma. Cancer Discov. 2017;7(3):252–63.
55. Wasenang W, Chaiyarit P, Proungvitaya S, Limpaiboon T. Serum cell-free DNA methylation of OPCML and HOXD9 as a biomarker that may aid in differential diagnosis between cholangiocarcinoma and other biliary diseases. Clin Epigenetics. 2019;11(1):39–49.
56. Salati M, Braconi C. Noncoding RNA in cholangiocarcinoma. Semin Liver Dis. 2019;39(1):13–25.
57. Sun C, Zhu J, Wu B, Chen J, Zhu Z, Cai P, et al. Diagnostic and prognostic value of microRNAs in cholangiocarcinoma: a systematic review and meta-analysis. Cancer Manag Res. 2018;10:2125–39.
58. Wu X, Xia M, Chen D, Wu F, Lv Z, Zhan Q, et al. Profiling of downregulated blood-circulating miR-150-5p as a novel tumor marker for cholangiocarcinoma. Tumour Biol. 2016;37(11):15019–29.
59. Wang LJ, Zhang KL, Zhang N, Ma XW, Yan SW, Cao DH, et al. Serum miR-26a as a diagnostic and prognostic biomarker in cholangiocarcinoma. Oncotarget. 2015;6(21):18631–40.
60. Wang LJ, He CC, Sui X, Cai MJ, Zhou CY, Ma JL, et al. MiR-21 promotes intrahepatic cholangiocarcinoma proliferation and growth in vitro and in vivo by targeting PTPN14 and PTEN. Oncotarget. 2015;6(8):5932–46.
61. Volinia S, Calin GA, Liu CG, Ambs S, Cimmino A, Petrocca F, et al. A microRNA expression signature of human solid tumors defines cancer gene targets. Proc Natl Acad Sci U S A. 2006;103(7):2257–61.
62. Wang L, Li Y, Xu J, Zhang A, Wang X, Tang R, et al. Quantified postsurgical small cell size CTCs and EpCAM+ circulating tumor stem cells with cytogenetic abnormalities in hepatocellular carcinoma patients determine cancer relapse. Cancer Lett. 2018;412:99–107.
63. Jusakul A, Cutcutache I, Yong CH, Lim JQ, Huang MN, Padmanabhan N, et al. Whole-genome and epigenetic landscapes of etiologically distinct subtypes of cholangiocarcinoma. Cancer Discov. 2017;7:1116–35.
64. Banales J, Cardinale V, Carpino G, Marzioni M, Anderson J, Inernizzi P, et al. Expert consensus document: cholangiocarcinoma: current knowledge and future perspectives consensus statement from the European Network for the study of Cholangiocarcinoma (ENS-CCA). Nat Rev Gastroenterol Hepatol. 2016;13:261–89.
65. Labib PL, Goodchild G, Pereira SP. Molecular pathogenesis of cholangiocarcinoma. BMC Cancer. 2019;19:185–201.
66. Chan-On W, Kuwahara K, Kobayashi N, Ohta K, Shimasaki T, Sripa B, et al. Cholangiocarcinomas associated with long-term inflammation express the activation-induced cytidine deaminase and germinal center–associated nuclear protein involved in immunoglobulin V-region diversification. Int J Oncol. 2009;35:287–95.
67. Muramatsu M, Kinoshita K, Fagarasan S, Yamada S, Shinkai Y, Honjo T. Class switch recombination and hypermutation require activation-induced cytidine deaminase (AID), a potential RNA editing enzyme. Cell. 2000;102:553–63.
68. Maeda K, Singh SK, Eda K, Kitabatake M, Pham P, Goodman MF, et al. GANP-mediated recruitment of activation-induced cytidine deaminase to cell nuclei and to immunoglobulin variable region DNA. J Biol Chem. 2010;285:23945–53.
69. Singh SK, Maeda K, Eid MMA, Almofty AM, Ono M, Pham P, et al. GANP regulates targeting of AID to the immunoglobulin variable region by regulating transcription and nucleosome occupancy. Nat Commun. 2013;4:1830.
70. Endo Y, Marusawa H, Chiba T. Involvement of activation-induced cytidine deaminase in the development of colitis-associated colorectal cancers. J Gastroenterol. 2011;1:6–10.

71. Marusawa H, Takai A, Chiba T. Role of activation-induced cytidine deaminase in inflammation-associated cancer development. Adv Immunol. 2011;111:109–41.
72. Matsumoto Y, Marusawa H, Kinoshita K, Endo Y, Kou T, Morisawa T, et al. Helicobacter pylori infection triggers aberrant expression of activation-induced cytidine deaminase in gastric epithelium. Nat Med. 2007;13:470–6.
73. Burns MB, Lackey L, Carpenter MA, Rathore A, Land AM, Leonard B, et al. APOBEC3B is an enzymatic source of mutation in breast cancer. Nature. 2013;494:366–70.
74. Eid MM, Maeda K, Almofty SA, Singh SK, Shimoda M, Sakaguchi N. GANP regulates the choice of DNA repair pathway by DNA-PKcs interaction in AID-dependent IgV region diversification. J Immunol. 2014;192:5529–39.
75. Milone MC, O'Doherty U. Clinical use of lentiviral vectors. Leukemia. 2018;32:1529–41.
76. Fukazawa T, Maeda Y, Sladek FM, Owen-Schaub LB. Development of a cancer-targeted tissue-specific promoter system. Cancer Res. 2004;64:363–9.
77. Higashitsuji H, Itoh K, Nagao T, Dawson S, Nonoguchi K, Kido T, et al. Reduced stability of retinoblastoma protein by gankyrin, an oncogenic ankyrin-repeat protein overexpressed in hepatomas. Nat Med. 2000;6(1):96–9.

Chapter 7
Imaging of Cholangiocarcinoma

Karoly Viragh, Maitraya Patel, Shaden Mohammad, Monica Deshmukh, and Anokh Pahwa

Abbreviations

US	Ultrasound
CT	Computed tomography
MRI	Magnetic resonance imaging
PET	Positron emission tomography
CCA	Cholangiocarcinoma
iCCA	Intrahepatic CCA
pCCA	Perihilar CCA
dCCA	Distal CCA

Introduction

The *objective* of this chapter is to provide a comprehensive overview of the non-invasive imaging techniques employed in the diagnosis and management of *cholangiocarcinoma* (CCA).

As discussed extensively in other chapters, CCA is a malignancy arising from the biliary ductal epithelium. It is the most common type of biliary ductal cancer and the second most common liver cancer after hepatocellular carcinoma, although with

K. Viragh (✉) · S. Mohammad · M. Deshmukh · A. Pahwa
Department of Radiology, Olive View-UCLA Medical Center, Sylmar, CA, USA
e-mail: KVIRAGH@DHS.LACOUNTY.GOV; SMOHAMMAD@DHS.LACOUNTY.GOV; MDESHMUKH@DHS.LACOUNTY.GOV; APAHWA@DHS.LACOUNTY.GOV

M. Patel
Department of Radiology, Ronald Reagan UCLA Medical Center, Los Angeles, CA, USA
e-mail: MPATEL@MEDNET.UCLA.EDU

J. H. Tabibian (ed.), *Diagnosis and Management of Cholangiocarcinoma*,
https://doi.org/10.1007/978-3-030-70936-5_7

Table 7.1 Major non-invasive imaging modalities for cholangiocarcinoma management and their advantages/disadvantages with respect to technique and clinical indication

Major non-invasive imaging modalities for cholangiocarcinoma management				
Technique	US	CT	MR	FDG PET/CT
Mechanism	Sound-wave reflection	X-ray attenuation	Magnetic relaxation	Glucose metabolism
Availability	+++	++	+	+
Cost	+	++	+++	+++
Ionizing radiation	None	+++	None	+++
Artifact/operator dependence	+++	+	++	+
Bile ducts/stones	++	++	+++	++
Inflammation	+	+++	+++	+++
Local neoplasm	+	+++	+++	+++
Lymph node/metastatic disease	+	+++	+++	+++
Vascular involvement	+	+++	+++	++

overall relatively low prevalence. Prompt and accurate imaging diagnosis of CCA is challenging due to the heterogeneous nature of this malignancy, which is reflected by the variability and nonspecific nature of imaging findings.

Similar to the clinicopathologic classification, the traditional *imaging classification* of CCA is based on anatomic location and divides tumors into intrahepatic (iCCA), perihilar (pCCA), and distal (dCCA) types [1]. Regardless of location, CCAs are subdivided into three specific growth patterns, each with characteristic imaging findings: mass-forming subtype, periductal-infiltrating subtype, and intraductal growth subtype [1]. In general, iCCA most commonly presents as a mass-forming lesion, while pCCA and dCCA more commonly present with a periductal-infiltrating growth pattern [2]. The classification and corresponding imaging features of CCA reflect the heterogeneity in genetics, pathology, and prognosis of the underlying tissue (Table 7.1).

Imaging Modalities

In general, imaging modalities can be grouped as *non-invasive* and *invasive techniques*. The non-invasive techniques require, at most, the placement of an intravenous (IV) line and contrast administration. On the other hand, invasive techniques include the placement of advanced catheters, endoscopes, needle puncture of organs, and sedation/anesthesia. The major *non-invasive techniques* include ultrasound (US), computed tomography (CT), magnetic resonance imaging (MRI), nuclear imaging such as positron emission tomography (PET), and hybrid imaging (such as PET/CT). These modalities are discussed in detail below (Table 7.2). Radiography and fluoroscopy are not specifically used for non-invasive imaging but

Table 7.2 Most common imaging characteristics of the different types of cholangiocarcinoma

Typical imaging characteristics of cholangiocarcinoma		
Anatomic location	Typical growth pattern	Typical imaging appearance
iCCA	Mass-forming	*Primary characteristics* US: hypoechoic/targetoid (but variable) CT/MR: irregular, peripheral arterial hyperenhancement with gradual centripetal delayed enhancement FDG PET: intense FDG uptake *Secondary characteristics* Biliary ductal dilation with abrupt cutoff at stricture or mass with normal-caliber distal duct Hepatic lobar atrophy Hepatic capsular retraction Satellite nodules Vascular encasement without invasion
pCCA	Periductal infiltrating	Biliary ductal dilation with abrupt cutoff at stricture or mass with normal-caliber distal duct
dCCA	Periductal infiltrating	Biliary ductal dilation with abrupt cutoff at stricture or mass with normal-caliber distal duct

only insofar as they are needed in general patient management and as guidance for invasive evaluations. Invasive imaging techniques such as transhepatic cholangiography (THC), endoscopic retrograde cholangiopancreatography (ERCP), endoscopic ultrasound (EUS), intraductal ultrasound, choledochoscopy/cholangioscopy, and similar techniques will not be discussed in the present chapter.

Role of Non-invasive Imaging

Non-invasive imaging plays three major roles in the diagnosis and management of CCA:

1. *Diagnosis*: Imaging helps localize suspicious lesions and can suggest CCA as a differential diagnosis based on appearance. Nevertheless, tissue sampling and pathological analysis remain the gold standard for diagnosis.
2. *Staging*: Imaging is used to evaluate the extent of malignancy at different time points in the course of the disease such as initial staging, restaging after therapy, and surveillance after complete response to therapy. While the exact local extent of disease (T staging) is often difficult to accurately evaluate, lymph node status (N staging) and distal metastases (M staging) are best detected by imaging.
3. *Surgical planning*: Surgery is the only potentially curative therapy currently available. Imaging provides comprehensive preoperative planning information, including vascular and biliary involvement with anatomic variants as well as measurement of liver volume. Imaging is also used to evaluate potential postoperative complications.

Approach to Imaging

Patients with CCA present with nonspecific clinical symptoms. When suspected, imaging workup usually begins with transabdominal US, which is closely followed usually by a contrast-enhanced CT of the abdomen and/or MRI with magnetic resonance cholangiopancreatography (MRCP) for more comprehensive evaluation. In general, a contrast-enhanced MRI/MRCP examination of the abdomen provides the most comprehensive evaluation of the biliary tract. A complete staging examination may then be performed with CT of the chest, abdomen, and pelvis, or a PET/CT from skull base to thighs. Tissue sampling is usually obtained for diagnostic confirmation.

Transabdominal Ultrasound (US) (Figs. 7.1, 7.2, and 7.3)

Introduction

While some centers have described success in identification and staging of CCA with US, this technique is *most commonly utilized as an initial examination* in light of its low cost and broad availability, to assess for biliary ductal dilation in patients with jaundice or elevated bilirubin and alkaline phosphatase. Alternatively, it may be used in patients with known CCA to assess for progressive biliary dilation, hepatic metastasis, or abscess, and as guidance for image-guided biopsy or drainage. The ability of US to identify, stage, and plan for resectability is surpassed by MRI and CT [3].

A meta-analysis in 2012 described the *performance of US* in the assessment of ductal extent of tumor to have an accuracy of 59–82% [4]. Sensitivity and specificity for identifying portal vein involvement ranged from 75% to 83% and 93% to 100%, respectively [4]. No data were provided regarding hepatic artery involvement, lymph node status, or distant metastasis. This meta-analysis was limited in that US was performed in only three studies included in the analysis, and these studies were quite old (1992–1995) [4]. In general, given its limitations, US can identify, characterize, and in some cases provide relevant staging information in CCA.

Technique

Transabdominal US evaluation of the bile ducts should be performed after fasting for 6 hours to minimize bowel gas and allow for gallbladder distention. Using a curvilinear 5–7 mHz transducer, evaluation should include grayscale images of the confluence of the bile ducts at the porta hepatis, longitudinal and transverse images

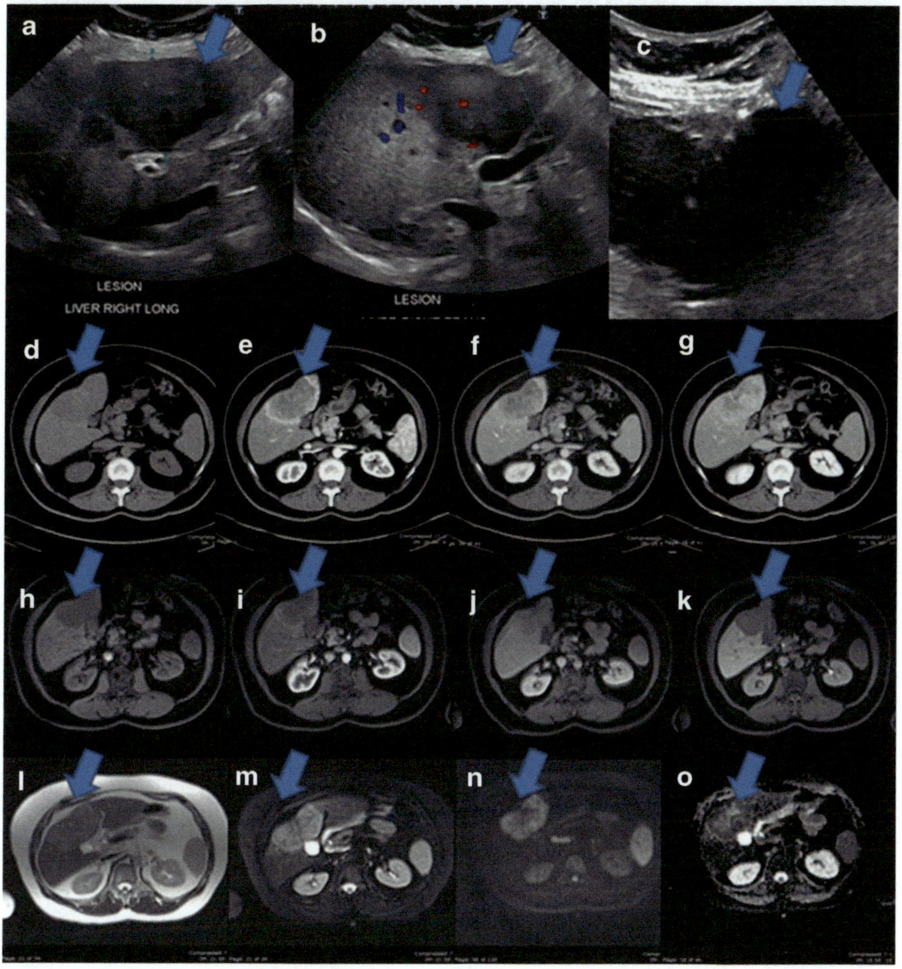

Fig. 7.1 Intrahepatic cholangiocarcinoma (iCCA) with mass-forming growth pattern (blue arrows), which is the most common subtype of iCCA. Grayscale (**a**) and color Doppler (**b**) US images obtained as initial screening, demonstrating a hypoechoic mass with hypovascularity. US was also used as guidance (**c**) for percutaneous biopsy later in the management. The echogenic linear foci correspond to the biopsy needle within the lesion. Multiphasic CT images with iodinated contrast in the non-contrast (**d**), arterial (**e**), portal venous (**f**), and 3-minute delayed (**g**) phases confirmed the large hepatic mass with typical findings of peripheral arterial hyperenhancement and delayed progressive central enhancement. The mass is associated with capsular retraction and regional hepatic atrophy. Multiphasic MR images with a hepatobiliary contrast agent in the non-contrast (**h**), arterial (**i**), portal venous (**j**), and 20-minute delayed hepatobiliary phase (**k**) demonstrated the hepatic mass similarly to CT. Of note, no contrast uptake is seen on the hepatobiliary phase in the lesion, confirming non-hepatic cellular content. The mass shows mild T2 hyperintensity on the nonfat-saturated (**l**) and fat-saturated (**m**) T2 sequences, as well as marked restricted diffusion with DWI hyperintensity (**n**) and ADC hypointensity (**o**)

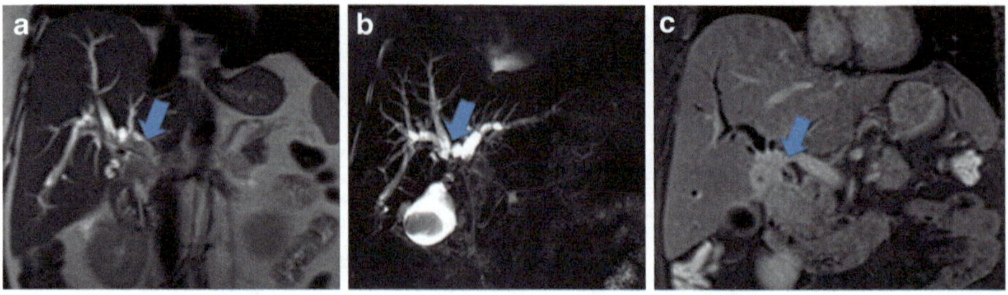

Fig. 7.2 Perihilar cholangiocarcinoma ("Klatskin tumor") with mass-forming growth pattern. Coronal T2 (**a**), MRCP (**b**), and contrast-enhanced T1 FS (**c**) images demonstrate an indistinct T2 mildly hyperintense lesion with delayed enhancement at the confluence of the hepatic ducts (blue arrows) causing marked intrahepatic biliary ductal dilation

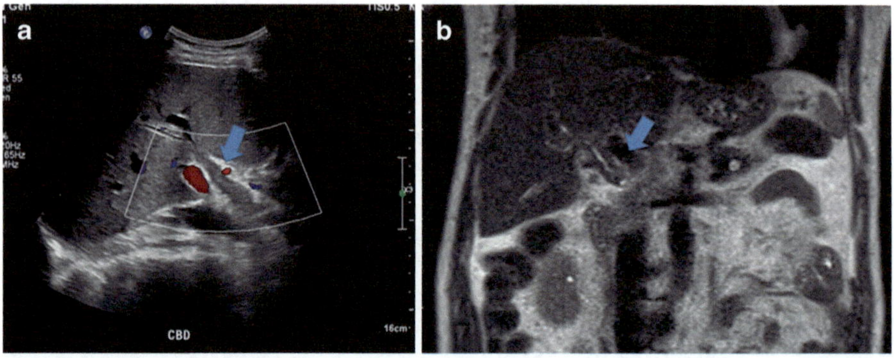

Fig. 7.3 Extrahepatic combined perihilar/distal cholangiocarcinoma (combined pCCA/dCCA) with periductal infiltrating growth pattern. Color Doppler abdominal ultrasound (**a**) demonstrates thickened common bile duct with tumor(blue arrow). Coronal T2-weighted MR (**b**) demonstrates long segment thickening of the common bile duct in a periductal infiltrating pattern (blue arrow)

of the right- and left-sided ducts, images of the hepatoduodenal ligament to visualize the extrahepatic common bile duct, and images of the pancreatic head to assess the distal common bile duct [5]. In addition, Doppler ultrasound images are used to distinguish between bile ducts and blood vessels as well as to evaluate for blood flow.

Contrast-enhanced ultrasound (*CEUS*) is a newer technique approved by the FDA in 2016 to augment assessment of liver lesions in addition to the traditional grayscale and Doppler evaluation. Sonographic contrast agents are gas-filled microbubbles stabilized by an albumin-, surfactant-, and phospholipid-containing shell. The microbubbles are smaller than 7 μm and circulate freely into capillary beds. They are purely microvascular agents and do not demonstrate an interstitial or equilibrium phase, unlike conventional CT and MRI contrast agents. They are eliminated by the lungs and liver within 10–15 minutes of injection and have no nephrotoxic effects. The only sonographic contrast agent currently FDA-approved in the USA for liver imaging consists of sulfur hexafluoride lipid-type A microspheres. This agent is well tolerated by most patients, with only rare adverse events. There is an FDA warning for rare cardiopulmonary events after administration of the agent. The *role of CEUS is to assess dynamic phases of contrast enhancement in order to differentiate between different types of focal lesions*. The arterial phase starts within 10–20 seconds of injection and lasts for 35–40 seconds after injection. The portal venous phase occurs after arrival of the contrast into the portal system and lasts for 2 minutes after injection. The late phase (4–6 minutes after injection) is characterized by clearing of the microbubbles from the system [6, 7].

Imaging

Mass-forming subtype The mass-forming subtype of CCA usually demonstrates a homogenous mass with an irregular but well-defined margin [5]. A hypoechoic halo around the tumor is present approximately 35% of the time, which may represent proliferating tumor [8]. Tumors <3 cm are generally hypoechoic or isoechoic, while those >3 cm tend to be hyperechoic for unclear reasons but potentially secondary to stromal properties. Four enhancement patterns of the mass-forming subtype of CCA have been described with CEUS on the arterial phase: peripheral irregular rim-like enhancement, heterogeneous hyperenhancement, homogenous hyperenhancement, and heterogeneous hypoenhancement, in descending frequency. On the portal venous and late phases, mass-forming CCA tends to be hypoechoic. Smaller lesions tend to be more homogenous in enhancement in the arterial phase than larger lesions, likely due to their higher component of tumor cells to fibrous tissue and necrosis. Delayed enhancement described on CT and MRI is not seen on CEUS, as these agents are strictly intravascular. The iCCA with mass-forming growth pattern is often associated with biliary ductal dilation peripheral to the lesion and subsequent lobar atrophy. Frequently, biliary ductal crowding secondary to mass effect may be the only indicator for the presence of a mass.

Periductal-infiltrating subtype The periductal-infiltrating subtype of CCA may present on ultrasound as a small, mass-like lesion or as diffuse bile duct thickening [5]. Obliteration of the bile duct lumen depends on the extent of tumor. On CEUS, these tumors tend to appear heterogeneously enhancing in the arterial phase, with hypoenhancement in portal and late phases. Dilation of intrahepatic bile ducts with a normal-caliber common bile duct or disconnected bile ducts at the porta hepatis is a nonspecific finding, but one that is commonly seen with pCCA.

Intraductal growth subtype The intraductal growth subtype of CCA may manifest on ultrasound as localized or diffuse bile duct dilation with or without an echogenic intraductal polypoid lesion. Marked biliary dilation without a visible polypoid lesion can be explained by anechoic mucin production by this tumor. With CEUS, the polypoid component, if visible, will show arterial phase homogenous hyperenhancement and hypoenhancement in the portal and late phases [6, 9].

Additional Considerations

Staging Vascular involvement can be evaluated by color Doppler assessment of the portal vein, hepatic veins, and hepatic artery, but as described above, its role is limited in accurate staging of CCA. Similarly, when identified, porta hepatic lymphadenopathy, common bile duct involvement, or metastatic disease can provide relevant information regarding the tumor; however, ultrasound is limited in reliably assessing for these.

HCC vs. iCCA Patients with chronic fibroinflammatory liver disease are at risk for both HCC and iCCA. Differentiating between the two has significant implications for transplantation. Intrahepatic biliary dilation peripheral to a mass is seen 31% of the time in iCCA, compared to 2% in patients with HCC, which can be a clue in distinguishing between the two [5]. With CEUS, both iCCA and HCC demonstrate hyperenhancement in the arterial phase. iCCA tends to demonstrate earlier (<60 seconds after contrast injection) and a greater degree of washout compared to HCC, which has later (>60 seconds after injection) and milder degrees of washout. When combined, early onset and marked degree of washout as a diagnostic criterion for iCCA has been reported to have a 78.8% sensitivity, 88% specificity, and an 84.3% diagnostic accuracy [7].

Mimickers of CCA Other entities that may mimic CCA on sonography, some of which coexist with CCA, include primary sclerosing cholangitis (PSC), AIDS cholangiopathy, recurrent pyogenic cholangitis, and Mirizzi syndrome. Finally, gallbladder cancer when it infiltrates into the liver may mimic an iCCA.

Computed Tomography (CT) (Fig. 7.1)

Introduction

Contrast-enhanced CT is a major workhorse in the imaging evaluation of CCA, commonly used in diagnosis, staging, and surgical planning. The *advantages* of CT include fast and robust data acquisition with relative operator independence, wide access and low cost compared to MRI and hybrid imaging, excellent depiction of vasculature, and good depiction of the hepatobiliary system with better spatial resolution than MRI. The major *disadvantages* include ionizing radiation, less powerful soft tissue resolution compared to MRI, and the usage of iodinated contrast, which may affect renal function ("contrast-induced nephropathy").

Technique

CT scans are diagnostic imaging procedures that use X-rays to create cross-sectional images of the body based on X-ray attenuation through different tissues. Tissue densities are measured in Hounsfield units (HU), with water by definition having a density of 0 HU. Consequently, other structures have relative densities compared to water, including air (−1000 HU), fat (−50 to −120 HU), soft tissues (0–80 HU), and bone (+1000 HU). Modern CT imaging of the abdomen uses multidetector CT scanners with helical volumetric acquisitions for improved speed and processing [10].

Intravenous contrast is routinely used to improve lesion detection and characterization. The purpose of a contrast-enhanced CT is to determine if pathology is present in a lesion (site of anatomic abnormality) by highlighting the contrast accumulation in the lesion compared to normal surrounding structures. Lesions can be hypoenhancing or hyperenhancing compared to surrounding tissues. Lesion vascularity can change depending on the timing of CT. Multiphase CT is performed to determine the behavior of a lesion compared to normal surrounding structures over time. Contrast dosage is standardized based on patient weight. *Positive oral contrast* (denser than tissue) is not routinely utilized in the imaging of CCA. If there is concern for alimentary tract obstruction or other relevant pathology, a combination of positive oral contrast in the form of water-soluble agents (most commonly meglumine/diatrizoate sodium [Gastrografin]) or negative oral contrast (less dense than tissue) can be useful. At our institution, we routinely administer negative oral contrast (500 cc of water given to patient immediately prior to scanning) to better distinguish the extrahepatic bile ducts from the duodenum and pancreatic head.

The routine *imaging protocol* of a multiphasic contrast-enhanced CT in the evaluation of suspected CCA is the routine "liver protocol," which consists of a (1) pre-contrast phase, (2) late arterial phase, (3) portal venous phase, and (4) delayed phase. Pre-contrast (non-contrast) imaging is useful to detect intraductal stones and casts and distinguish between subsequent enhancement versus intrinsic density or calcification. Late arterial phase imaging is performed 30–40 seconds after contrast injection. The late arterial phase can determine arterial anatomy for pre-surgical planning and assess for peripheral tumoral enhancement. Portal venous phase imaging occurs 70–80 seconds after contrast injection and is best for assessment of the liver parenchyma as well as the rest of the abdomen/pelvis for metastases and other disease processes. The delayed post-contrast imaging occurs from 180 to 240 seconds and up to 15 minutes after contrast injection, and it is used to evaluate for washout or persistent enhancement in the suspicious liver lesion [9].

Of note, the utilization of solely non-contrast CT for cholangiocarcinoma evaluation is not routinely recommended and is usually not appropriate by the American College of Radiology Appropriateness Criteria [11]. While a non-contrast CT may reveal biliary ductal dilation or an indistinct mass, the diagnostic performance is thought to be suboptimal for complete staging. This has not been specifically studied for cholangiocarcinoma but has been documented in similar clinical scenarios [12]. In patients with kidney disease, an MRI/MRCP may be more appropriate (see section "MRI/MRCP"), but consultation with the radiologist is suggested.

Imaging

Mass-forming subtype The mass-forming subtype of CCA is typically homogenous and hypoattenuating on non-contrast images. Hepatolithiasis may be seen on the pre-contrast images as calcifications, heterogeneous hyperdense material, or less commonly hypodense foci indicating cholesterol/fat. Irregular peripheral rim-like hyperenhancement is common on the late arterial phase, followed by gradual centripetal enhancement on delay phase. Additional CT findings include hepatic capsular retraction, satellite nodules, vascular encasement without tumor thrombus, atrophy of the involved liver segment, and portal vein obliteration. Vascular encasement without thrombus is a hallmark CT feature and can help distinguish CCA from hepatocellular carcinoma [9]. Another typical feature is delayed phase gradual centripetal enhancement, the degree of which is related to the volume of viable tumor in the periphery relative to central fibrosis and/or necrosis [13, 14].

Periductal-infiltrating subtype Periductal-infiltrating CCA is characterized by growth along a dilated or narrowed bile duct without mass formation. It manifests as an elongated, spiculated, or branch-like abnormality. Late arterial and portal venous phase CT imaging findings include diffuse periductal thickening and hyperenhancement without obliteration of the bile duct. The bile ducts involved may be narrowed or dilated depending on the degree of longitudinal tumor extent (e.g., the distal margin), with the bile ducts peripheral to the lesion usually being dilated. If intrahepatic-only, the lesions tend to be localized to one liver segment or lobe. Early periductal-infiltrating CCA can be difficult to differentiate from benign biliary strictures. CT secondary signs such as irregular thickening of the bile ducts, asymmetric bile duct narrowing, regional lymph node enlargement, and an adjacent soft tissue lesion can help distinguish early periductal-infiltrating tumor from a benign biliary stricture [15]. The periductal-infiltrating subtype can be seen in combination with mass-forming subtype in the periphery of the liver. Of note, CT may underestimate the proximal longitudinal tumor extent in perihilar CCA [3].

Intraductal growth subtype Intraductal CCA can have variable imaging presentation. Typical appearances include ductal dilation with or without skip lesions, a papillary mass, ductal ectasia without a mass, cast-like lesions, and focal stricture with or without biliary tumors. On pre-contrast CT, the intraductal subtype typically presents as a hypo- or isoattenuating mass compared with the surrounding liver. On post-contrast imaging intraductal tumors exhibit enhancement but show less robust enhancement compared to other intrahepatic subtypes and show progressive enhancement during the arterial and hepatic venous phase. In some cases, only intrahepatic bile duct dilatation, without an intraductal mass or stricture, may be seen. Alternatively, focal ductal dilation with intraductal mass can be seen [2]. This tumor frequently demonstrates extensive superficial spreading, resulting in diffuse involvement. The true extent of the tumor is difficult to determine on CT; therefore ERCP and biopsy are often utilized to determine true extent of tumor [16].

Additional Considerations

Dual-energy CT (DECT) is a new technique that acquires dual-energy datasets with two different X-ray energy spectra using two tubes operating at high and low voltages with corresponding detectors mounted orthogonally. DECT generates color-coded iodine overlay images from a single contrast-enhanced CT acquisition. DECT creates more quantitatively accurate attenuation measurement. The iodine-specific images improve detection and characterization of lesions with slight differences in attenuation and of small lesions. Currently, DECT is being studied in differentiating intrahepatic mass-forming CCAs from small liver abscesses. Early studies are finding increased accuracy of DECT for differentiating small intrahepatic mass-forming CCAs and liver abscesses compared to conventional CT. This has potential for future imaging implications for CCA [17].

CT cholangiography is a rarely used examination of the biliary system with either oral or intravenous administration of special iodinated contrast agents, which opacify the bile ducts through hepatobiliary excretion [18–20]. This technique has been practically replaced by MRI/MRCP in clinical practice (discussed below) due to its potential contrast-related adverse effects and dependence on normal hepatic function and lack of high-grade biliary obstruction, which is a hallmark of CCA [21–24]. Nevertheless, studies have shown acceptable performance in depicting biliary anatomy, stones, PSC, and CCA [21], and CT cholangiography is still used in research and rare perioperative settings [20].

MRI/MRCP (Figs. 7.1, 7.2, 7.3, 7.4, and 7.5)

Introduction

The *advantages* of MRI include lack of ionizing radiation and superior soft tissue contrast resolution which aids in tumor detection, surgical planning, and potentially prognosis. MRI, with appropriate protocols, can be a highly useful problem-solving adjunct in cases of equivocal imaging on other modalities. Specifically, contrast-enhanced MRI with MRCP (i.e., MRI/MRCP) has been shown to be as accurate as contrast-enhanced CT with conventional ERCP for detecting CCA [25]. When combined with MRA, MRI/MRCP is a valuable preoperative tool to aid with lesion characterization to assess surgical resectability, tumor extent, vascular involvement, and vascular mapping [26]. Furthermore, given the lack of ionizing radiation, MRI can safely be used for surveillance for CCA in appropriate high-risk populations, including those with a background of primary sclerosing cholangitis [27–30].

The main *disadvantages* of MRI are its relatively high cost, potential limitations to its access in some clinical settings, and potential patient safety considerations. Non-MRI-compatible devices, including certain pacemakers, may be disrupted in

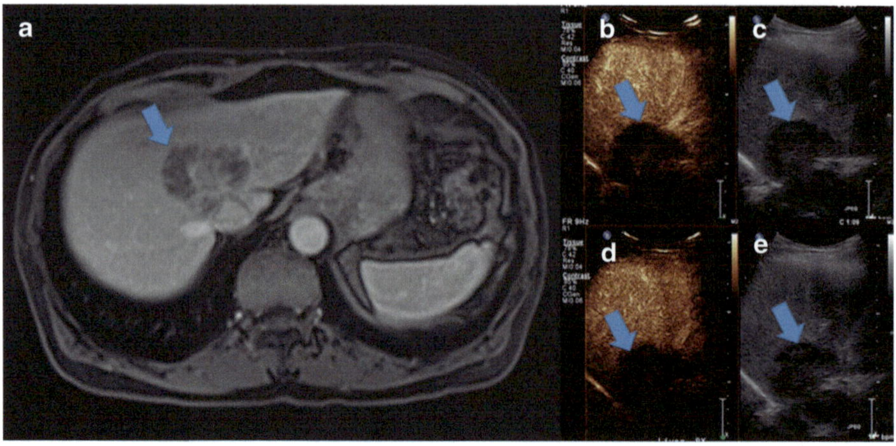

Fig. 7.4 A 76-year-old man presented with diverticulitis and a liver lesion that was initially thought to represent abscess (blue arrows). Axial T1 FS contrastenhanced MRI (**a**) demonstrated mass-like growth concerning for cholangiocarcinoma. Contrast-enhanced ultrasound at 33 seconds (**b** and **c**) and 69 seconds (**d** and **e**) post-injection demonstrated a persistently hypovascular mass. Pathology confirmed cholangiocarcinoma

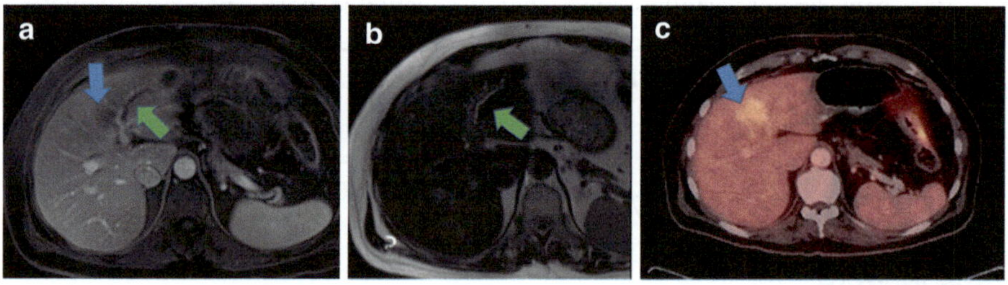

Fig. 7.5 Intrahepatic cholangiocarcinoma with mass-forming growth pattern demonstrates the common finding of suspicious segmental biliary ductal dilation (green arrow) with associated indistinct mass (blue arrow) that demonstrates hypoenhancement on the T1 FS image (**a**), indistinct mild T2 hyperintensity (**b**), and moderate-to-intense FDG uptake on the fused PET/CT image (**c**)

strong electromagnetic fields. Additionally, the presence of ferromagnetic implants or foreign bodies is relative contraindication to MRI in most settings. Appropriate patient screening is necessary prior to any MR imaging. In some cases, even the presence of MRI-safe foreign bodies or implants may result in significant susceptibility artifact that renders the evaluation of adjacent organ systems impossible. Patient tolerance for closed-bore MRI may also be a limiting factor in some cases, particularly given the length of an MR exam compared to CT, although the introduction of more wide-bore (open) systems and the use of anxiolytic premedication may mitigate these concerns. Another disadvantage is the potential side effects and complications of contrast use. Historically, the development of a scleroderma-likely fibrotic condition called nephrogenic systemic fibrosis (NSF) was a rare, but feared, complication of MRI contrast. NSF is most frequently associated with older contrast agents that weakly bind gadolinium to their chelate; however, unconfounded cases of NSF have not been observed with newer, more stable, macrocyclic chelates [31]. Gadolinium deposition in the brain has been recently documented, but the clinical significance is currently unknown [32].

The signal characteristics on T1- and T2-weighted images and dynamic contrast enhancement (DCE) roughly correlate with pathologic findings of CCA, and, in particular, the degree of tumoral fibrosis, which may be beneficial as a prognostic indicator. For instance, the expected central fibrosis typical of CCA correlates with lower central T2 signal and homogenous delayed enhancement, whereas depending on the degree of increased T2 signal intensity, findings may be indicative of desmoplastic changes with coagulative necrosis or mucinous CCA [33].

Technique

MR imaging should encompass the entire liver, biliary tract, and pancreas, and protocols should include at least axial T1- and T2-weighted imaging with MRCP and dynamic contrast enhancement (DCE) [34]. MRCP techniques rely on heavily T2-weighted, and therefore fluid-sensitive, sequences that highlight fluid-filled bile ducts and effectively suppress background soft tissue. MRCP is an ideal non-invasive technique for visualizing bile ducts and for localizing biliary abnormalities, which is frequently performed prior to conventional ERCP. Imaging can be performed on both 1.5 and 3T MR systems. Although higher field strength 3T imaging provides improved spatial resolution and a better signal-to-noise ratio over 1.5T, it may also magnify artifacts. The low field strength of most open MRI systems may limit their use in abdominal imaging, although robust performance data is not available.

Additional sequences that can provide useful information for lesion characterization include in- and opposed-phase imaging, diffusion-weighted imaging (DWI), the use of hepatobiliary-specific contrast agents, subtraction imaging, and MR angiography. In- and opposed-phase imaging allows for the identification of intracellular fat, which can aid in differential diagnosis. For example, the presence of intracellular fat in a tumor with an atypical enhancement pattern in a cirrhotic liver would still suggest a diagnosis of hepatocellular carcinoma rather than CCA. Malignant lesions typically have a lower apparent diffusion coefficient and would therefore appear brighter on DWI. Additionally, the increased signal of malignant lesions and relative suppression of signal in adjacent structures on DWI can increase the conspicuity of small lesions adjacent to blood vessels. Using hepatobiliary contrast agents can also potentially increase lesion-to-liver contrast. Subtraction imaging can sometimes help when there is minimal or subtle contrast enhancement, particularly if there is concurrent tumor hemorrhage or other cause of intrinsic T1 hyperintensity. There may be a future role for placing MR receiver coils directly in bile ducts, which would allow for extremely high resolution, high contrast, and high signal-to-noise ratio imaging, albeit at a cost of a restricted field of view [35].

Imaging

Mass-forming subtype Satellite nodules are seen around the main tumor in 10–20% of cases and commonly result from portal vein involvement [2, 35]. Classically, the masses are irregularly contoured, T1 hypointense, and mildly T2 hyperintense and demonstrate an early and prominent continuous rim of peripheral enhancement that fills centripetally and gradually over time. The early peripheral enhancement is more prominent on MRI than on CT. Increasing enhancement on delayed phase imaging (6 minutes or later) is often seen in more densely fibrotic areas of tumor. There may be associated capsular retraction and distal biliary radical dilation, the latter of which can help distinguish primary CCA from metastatic adenocarcinoma to the liver [33]. Vascular encasement is common, while intravascular tumor thrombus is rare [9]. On DWI, there is a typical "target" pattern of signal intensity, with centrally low signal that corresponds to areas of fibrosis and peripheral diffusion restriction (bright signal on DWI) in areas of highly cellular tumor involvement [2]. Hepatobiliary-specific contrast agents demonstrate gradually increasing enhancement of normal liver parenchyma secondary to the active transport of the contrast from the extracellular sinusoidal space into the hepatocytes via organic anion transporting polypeptides (OATP) transporters [36]. Malignant cells lack the appropriate receptor for transport of contrast into the intracellular space, and therefore do not enhance in the more delayed phases. This results in "pseudo-washout" of tumoral contrast in the transitional phase (beyond 3–4 minutes) relative to the enhancing background liver, in contradistinction to the described delayed enhancement seen with more traditional extracellular contrast agents. The hepatobiliary phase (20 minutes) is characterized by relatively homogenous enhancement of the liver parenchyma and lack of enhancement in malignant tissue. Occasionally, there may be intermingled hyperintensity on a background of signal hypointensity in CCA during the hepatobiliary phase, which is thought to reflect pooling of contrast material in fibrous stroma. Further, the degree of enhancement in the hepatobiliary phase may relate to the degree of tumoral fibrosis, which in turn may be a negative prognostic indicator. A peripheral hypointense rim in the hepatobiliary phase corresponds to the more vascular peripheral tumor [2].

Periductal-infiltrating subtype Infiltrating tumor grows along a usually abnormal (either dilated or narrowed) bile duct without associated mass formation. Eventually, diffuse periductal thickening will result in obliteration of the bile duct lumen. While distinguishing a benign from malignant stricture can be difficult by imaging, features that suggest malignancy include a long segment of ductal involvement (>2 cm), asymmetric narrowing of the duct with more significant thickening (>2 mm), abnormal ring-like ductal enhancement, or an associated soft tissue mass or adenopathy [9, 37]. Gradual tapering of the duct does not help distinguish benign from malignant strictures. Differential considerations for a malignant biliary stricture include primary periductal-infiltrating CCA or periportal lymphangitic metastases.

However, metastatic disease is more likely to involve the biliary system diffusely (as opposed to segmental involvement more commonly seen with CCA) and is less likely to result in significant biliary dilation [9].

Intraductal growth subtype Intraductal growth pattern CCA, while rare, is typically mucinous CCA and demonstrates low T1 and high T2 signal [33]. Commonly, biliary dilation above and below the tumor may relate to the excessive mucin production with partial ductal obstruction. This pattern of involvement is analogous to pancreatic intraductal papillary mucinous neoplasm. On imaging, intraductal-growing tumors may present as marked duct ectasia with or without a visible papillary mass, an intraductal polypoid mass with localized duct dilation, intraductal cast-like lesions that can be mistaken for intraductal stones, or focal stricture-like lesions with proximal biliary dilation [9].

Additional Considerations

Limitations As with CT, imaging of the cirrhotic liver may present a diagnostic dilemma, particularly for smaller tumors which present with less typical imaging features, and commonly demonstrate more homogenous arterial enhancement, an enhancement pattern that can overlap greatly with hepatocellular carcinoma [2]. While MRCP is an ideal non-invasive technique for localizing biliary abnormalities, there is a limited ability to distinguish benign from malignant strictures on imaging alone, and subsequent ERCP is often still needed for diagnosis and intervention. Moreover, reactive inflammation related to biliary intervention (tissue sampling) and decompression (stenting) can be difficult to distinguish from tumor-associated fibrosis rendering tumor identification unreliable and images obtained after intervention of the biliary tree oftentimes nondiagnostic [38].

Magnetic resonance spectroscopy (*MRS*) allows for the assessment of specific metabolites and their relative concentration in a given sample of tissue based on slight differences in their respective resonant frequencies. Historically, MRS has been used in brain imaging, although attempts have been made to apply it to increase the specificity of imaging in other organ systems. In liver imaging, and specifically when trying to assess focal hepatic lesions, its use has been limited by significant respiratory, cardiac, and peristalsis-related motion artifact. Elevated choline peaks are generally associated with malignant lesions, although the ability to distinguish benign from malignant hepatic tumors based on choline peaks has not been well established [39]. Additionally, MRS has been used to evaluate the chemical composition of bile as a potential marker for benign versus malignant biliary disease, although, again, its role in clinical practice remains unclear [40].

Hybrid/Molecular (PET/CT, PET/MR, New Molecular Agents) (Figs. 7.5 and 7.6)

Introduction

There is a growing armament of diagnostic and therapeutic tools that rely on hybrid and molecular imaging. While these are increasingly used in the imaging of biliary tumors, they remain usually second-line in clinical practice next to conventional MR and CT imaging.

Hybrid imaging refers to the fusion of an anatomy-oriented imaging examination (most commonly CT and MR) with a physiology-oriented imaging examination (most commonly PET), which results in a PET/CT or PET/MR. In practice, the two different imaging examinations are usually still acquired separately, although nearly simultaneously. The fusion of the images is accomplished at the time of post-acquisition data processing, when imaging data from the two studies is combined and displayed as a fused image. Because of the complementary nature of anatomic and physiologic imaging, hybrid imaging is thought to improve disease detection and characterization. Physiology-oriented imaging is sometimes referred to as *molecular imaging* because the injected labeled material selectively binds to molecules within the living organism (such as cellular receptors). It is important to note, however, that even a traditionally anatomy-oriented imaging modality such as MR may provide functional/physiologic imaging (MR spectroscopy) and, vice versa, a primarily physiology-oriented imaging study may provide anatomic/morphologic information (such as spatial location).

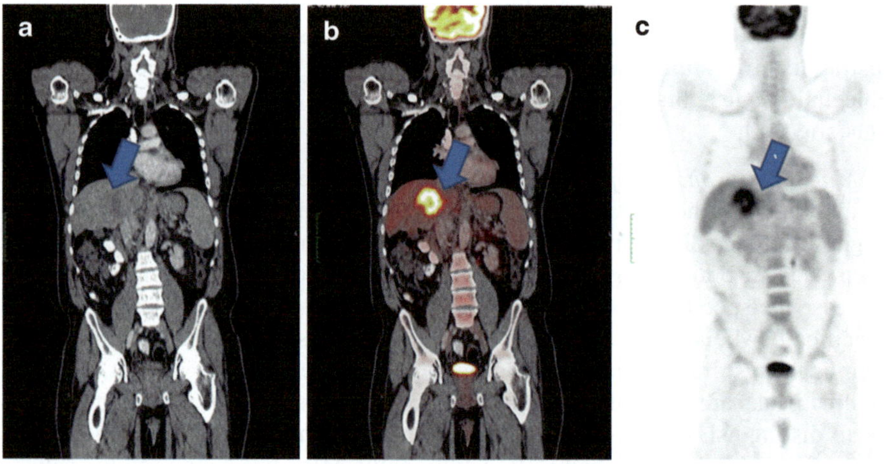

Fig. 7.6 Intrahepatic cholangiocarcinoma with mass-forming growth pattern on a PET/CT staging study (blue arrows). The non-contrast CT image (**a**) shows the hypodense mass that has intense FDG uptake (SUVmax 9.2) on PET (**c**), compatible with aggressive malignancy, which is nicely illustrated on the fused PET/CT image (**b**). No suspicious lymph nodes or distal metastases are seen. (Courtesy of Dr. Martin Auerbach, MD)

Diagnostic anatomic imaging (CT, MR) was discussed above in detail. Diagnostic physiologic imaging of neoplasms in clinical practice employs radiotracers (radioisotope-labeled contrast agents) that target features of increased metabolism characteristic of neoplastic growth. These include increased glucose metabolism, increased DNA, amino acid, or lipid synthesis, as well as the overexpression of certain molecular markers, receptors, and antigens.

Technique

The best studied and most useful radiotracer in clinical practice is *18-fluorodeoxyglucose* (*FDG*), which targets cells with increased glucose metabolism. FDG is a glucose-analog molecule labeled with fluorine-18 radionuclide, which decays through positron emission with a half-life of 110 minutes and provides the basis for imaging. FDG gets taken up by the cells along with regular glucose through the insulin-independent GLUT-1/3 transporters and is trapped in the intracellular space by hexokinase. Unlike glucose, FDG cannot undergo glycolysis and thus remains in the cell. Its normal biodistribution includes uptake in the tissues with significant metabolic activity (such as the brain, heart, liver, tonsils), the urinary system (since it is renally excreted), and variably other organs (such as the bowel). Since glucose competes with FDG in cellular uptake, normal glucose levels are important for imaging examinations. Proper diabetic management and overnight fasting are recommended for most examinations. Avoidance of exercise for 1–2 days is also critical to avoid increased radiotracer into the muscles.

FDG uptake and distribution in the body is imaged with *PET scanners*, which is commonly performed concomitantly with CT and occasionally with MR. The injected FDG radiotracer material emits positrons which almost immediately interact with nearby electrons resulting in particle annihilation and two photons of 511 keV energy, which travel approximately 180 degrees away from the point of annihilation and are detected by the PET camera (coincidence detection). The PET images can be acquired over the whole body or occasionally over a certain region of interest. The images are fused with the near-simultaneously obtained CT or MR to obtain PET/CT and PET/MR images. The CT or MR data is also used in the processing of PET data for attenuation correction, that is, to correct for the absorption and scattering related to the different organs.

Interpretation of PET is qualitative and semiquantitative. Qualitatively, the distribution and intensity of radiotracer activity is described visually in comparison to the liver and/or blood pool activity. Thus, radiotracer activity that appears less than, equal to, and greater than liver corresponds to low, moderate, and intense activity levels. Semiquantitatively, a standardized uptake value (SUV) can be calculated as a measure of FDG uptake and metabolic activity [41]. The SUV represents the amount of radiotracer concentration within a region of interest (tumor) relative to the average radiotracer concentration in the body. The SUV is often presented as a unitless number assuming that tissue density is 1 g/mL. Typically, the highest measured SUV level (SUVmax) is reported for best reproducibility. While SUVmax is often considered an "objective" measure, since it is normalized to the amount of contrast injected and the body size, it is still technique-dependent (hence referred to as semiquantitative). Therefore, absolute SUVs are not used, and comparisons between different studies and patients should be interpreted with caution. In general, an SUVmax above liver level (i.e., SUVmax > 2.5) is considered suspicious for malignancy in the appropriate setting (the differential consideration being inflammation/infection or other hypermetabolic state). This may also be quantified as the tumor-to-liver ratio (TLR = SUVmax of tumor/SUVmax of liver).

Imaging

Regarding biliary tract imaging, the use of PET/CT has been studied more extensively than PET/MR, but nevertheless, the overall data are much more limited than for CT and MR alone. In general, the different CCA subtypes are mostly distinguished based on their CT or MR features (described in detail above), whereas the PET portion provides physiologic information about metabolism to increase the accuracy of the examination and provide ancillary staging information.

PET/CT In PET/CT, PET imaging is fused with CT. While PET/CT is a clinical workhorse for the diagnosis, staging, treatment planning, and response monitoring of a variety of malignancies, its role in the management of biliary tract cancers remains debated [42, 43]. Though traditionally considered second-line to CT/MR in general, there is growing evidence that PET/CT can make a difference in management in up to 20% of cases [43].

A number of small studies assessed the diagnostic performance of PET/CT in the evaluation of CCA and locoregional/distant metastatic disease [44–49]. The available data was pooled by a meta-analysis from 2019, which reanalyzed 47 studies with a pooled total 2125 patients [43]. For *primary tumor detection*, the meta-analysis reported a pooled PET/CT sensitivity and specificity of 95.7% and 38.1% [43]. Subgroup analysis revealed a sensitivity and specificity of 94.2% and 68.3% for iCCA, 91.9% and 21.9% for pCCA, and 95.3% and 27.7% for dCCA [43]. The high sensitivity likely reflects the aggressive nature of CCAs, with associated increased glucose metabolism. The low specificity is mostly seen in extrahepatic CCA types (pCCA and dCCA) likely as a result of false positives from concomitant cholangitis, post-procedural inflammation, and the presence of biliary stents.

For the diagnosis of *metastatic disease*, the sensitivity and specificity were 88.4% and 69.1% for lymph node involvement, as well as 85.4% and 89.7% for other distant metastases [43]. For the diagnosis *of relapsed disease* after a disease-free period, the sensitivity and specificity of 90.1% and 83.5% were reported [43]. Furthermore, PET/CT changed management in 15% of the cases, of which the majority was disease upstaging [43].

With regard to the usage of a SUV, the meta-analysis suggested a "cutoff SUVmax" >3.5 [43]. The study also found that higher SUVmax at baseline was associated with worse prognosis [43]. In general, iCCA has more avid FDG uptake than eCCA (dCCA and dCCA), which is thought to be secondary to its more common mass-forming morphology and different genetics [50]. On the other hand, periductal-infiltrating and hilar lesions tend to have smaller tumor volume with increased fibrosis and decreased cellularity; hence FDG avidity is less.

Limitations include overlap between benign and malignant neoplasms, low uptake in indolent/low-grade tumors/mucinous tumors, insensitivity to microscopic disease (generally, lesions <8 mm), and false positive results secondary to inflammation in the setting of biliary stenting and cholangitis.

PET/MR In PET/MR, PET imaging is fused with MRI in order to take advantage of the higher intrinsic soft tissue resolution provided by MR over CT [51]. Most of the other advantages to PET/MR are also related to the nature of MR imaging, including multiplanar image acquisition capability (CT can only acquire data axially), a larger variety of multiparametric MR sequences providing more extensive evaluation, and less radiation dose (only the PET part has ionizing radiation) [52]. Two available scanner designs include the sequential PET and MR scanners (near-simultaneous data acquisition) and the single integrated PET/MR scanners (simultaneous data acquisition) [52]. Needless to say, these are very expensive units and of limited availability.

Very few studies are available with respect to PET/MR imaging of biliary tract neoplasms. Of note is a retrospective multicenter study of 37 patients with newly diagnosed iCCA which found that PET/MR changed significantly the surgical management in 11 (30%) patients despite having other imaging with a combination of CT, MR, and/or PET/CT [53]. Another small retrospective study of six patients with CCA who underwent baseline PET/MR imaging suggested inverse correlation between the SUVmax measured on PET with the ADC measured on MRI [54]. However, robust diagnostic performance data are not available.

Thus, given cost-effectiveness concerns and the relatively widespread availability of regular CT, MR, and PET/CT scanners, PET/MR is currently almost never used in clinical management outside of a few very highly specialized centers.

Additional Considerations

Other biliary tract cancers Combined HCC/CCA is a rare primary liver tumor which, due to its very low prevalence, is even less well studied. In a retrospective cohort of 46 patients with cHCC/CCA, higher FDG uptake was associated with higher tumor stage, lymph node metastasis, and poorer tumor differentiation of the CCA component, as well as decreased overall survival [55]. Other CCA-related malignancies (such as gallbladder and ampullary carcinoma) will not be discussed in the current chapter.

Other radiotracers Although there are a growing number of other PET radiotracers in addition to FDG, most are still within the realm of research or rarely useful. For example, gallium-68 FAPI, a marker of cancer-associated fibroblasts, was shown to have intense uptake in a group of 12 patients with CCA, suggesting correlation with the characteristic desmoplastic/fibrotic reaction produced by many CCAs, which is promising for future use [56]. On the other hand, gallium-68 pentixafor, which binds to a marker of poorly differentiated cells, and carbon-11 choline, a marker of lipid metabolism, were not found to be helpful [57]. CCAs that have neuroendocrine features may show uptake of somatostatin receptor analogs (gallium-68 DOTA agents on PET or indium-111 pentetreotide/octreotide on scintigraphy); however, these agents are not routinely used in the imaging of biliary cancers, unless a neuroendocrine tumor is suspected [58].

Older non-PET oncologic radiotracers such as gallium-67 citrate may show uptake in CCAs but are almost never used in current practice. Other nuclear imaging studies may be performed as accessory studies in the management of biliary tract tumors. For example, a hepatobiliary scintigraphic scan may be obtained with a technetium-99m-labeled hepatobiliary agent (e.g., Tc-99m HIDA) to evaluate for biliary obstruction or postoperative bile leaks. On a technetium-99m sulfur colloid scan, iCCA is a "cold spot" secondary to the lack of macrophages within the tumor.

Therapeutics For patients with locally advanced unresectable iCCA, local therapy with yttrium-90 microsphere transarterial radioembolization (Y-90 TARE) may be an option [59]. In this procedure, a percutaneously introduced microcatheter is selectively advanced into the hepatic arterial branch feeding the iCCA, and radioactive Yttrium-90 microspheres are then administered. The therapeutic effect is from the emission of beta radiation. These patients may undergo a technetium-99m macroaggregated albumin (MAA) scan prior to the radioembolization to assess for significant hepato-pulmonary shunts to avoid unnecessary radiation to the lungs.

Molecular imaging also relates to the emerging field of *radiogenomics*, in which imaging appearance (imaging phenotype) is correlated with underlying specific genes and mutations (genotype) that can be targeted by specific therapies. A small study of 22 cases of iCCA found positive correlation between genes associated with glucose metabolism and intense FDG activity with SUVmax > 9 and corresponding negative correlation with the expression of tumor suppressor genes [60]. Based on the analysis, the study also suggested that iCCA with intense FDG activity may not respond well to gemcitabine or cisplatin [60].

Conclusion

In conclusion, non-invasive imaging plays a powerful role in the diagnosis and management of CCA. Currently, US is mainly used for initial screening, while CT and MR/MRCP are the major primary tools for imaging evaluation. While hybrid and molecular imaging is an active area of research with growing importance, its current clinical use in the evaluation of biliary malignancies is not first-line and mostly limited to PET/CT.

References

1. Lim JH. Cholangiocarcinoma: morphologic classification according to growth pattern and imaging findings. AJR Am J Roentgenol. 2003;181(3):819–27.
2. Seo N, Kim DY, Choi JY. Cross-sectional imaging of intrahepatic cholangiocarcinoma: development, growth, spread, and prognosis. AJR Am J Roentgenol. 2017;209(2):W64–w75.
3. Joo I, Lee JM, Yoon JH. Imaging diagnosis of intrahepatic and perihilar cholangiocarcinoma: recent advances and challenges. Radiology. 2018;288(1):7–13.
4. Ruys AT, van Beem BE, Engelbrecht MR, Bipat S, Stoker J, Van Gulik TM. Radiological staging in patients with hilar cholangiocarcinoma: a systematic review and meta-analysis. Br J Radiol. 2012;85(1017):1255–62.
5. Bloom CM, Langer B, Wilson SR. Role of US in the detection, characterization, and staging of cholangiocarcinoma. Radiographics. 1999;19(5):1199–218.
6. D'Onofrio M, Crosara S, De Robertis R, Canestrini S, Mucelli RP. Contrast-enhanced ultrasound of focal liver lesions. AJR Am J Roentgenol. 2015;205(1):W56–66.
7. Lyshchik A, Kono Y, Dietrich CF, Jang HJ, Kim TK, Piscaglia F, et al. Contrast-enhanced ultrasound of the liver: technical and lexicon recommendations from the ACR CEUS LI-RADS Working Group. Abdom Radiol (NY). 2018;43(4):861–79.
8. Wernecke K, Henke L, Vassallo P, von Bassewitz DB, Diederich S, Peters PE, et al. Pathologic explanation for hypoechoic halo seen on sonograms of malignant liver tumors: an in vitro correlative study. AJR Am J Roentgenol. 1992;159(5):1011–6.
9. Chung YE, Kim MJ, Park YN, Choi JY, Pyo JY, Kim YC, et al. Varying appearances of cholangiocarcinoma: radiologic-pathologic correlation. Radiographics. 2009;29(3):683–700.
10. Rubin GD. Computed tomography: revolutionizing the practice of medicine for 40 years. Radiology. 2014;273(2 Suppl):S45–74.
11. American College of Radiology Appropriateness Criteria [Internet]. 2020 [Cited 6/16/2020].
12. Jee HB, Park MJ, Lee HS, Park M-S, Kim M-J, Chung YE. Is non-contrast CT adequate for the evaluation of hepatic metastasis in patients who cannot receive iodinated contrast media? PLoS One. 2015;10(7):e0134133.
13. Lacomis JM, Baron RL, Oliver JH 3rd, Nalesnik MA, Federle MP. Cholangiocarcinoma: delayed CT contrast enhancement patterns. Radiology. 1997;203(1):98–104.
14. Valls C, Guma A, Puig I, Sanchez A, Andia E, Serrano T, et al. Intrahepatic peripheral cholangiocarcinoma: CT evaluation. Abdom Imaging. 2000;25(5):490–6.
15. Han JK, Lee JM. Intrahepatic intraductal cholangiocarcinoma. Abdom Imaging. 2004;29(5):558–64.
16. Han JK, Choi BI, Kim AY, An SK, Lee JW, Kim TK, et al. Cholangiocarcinoma: pictorial essay of CT and cholangiographic findings. Radiographics. 2002;22(1):173–87.
17. Kim JE, Kim HO, Bae K, Cho JM, Choi HC, Choi DS. Differentiation of small intrahepatic mass-forming cholangiocarcinoma from small liver abscess by dual source dual-energy CT quantitative parameters. Eur J Radiol. 2017;92:145–52.
18. Hyodo T, Kumano S, Kushihata F, Okada M, Hirata M, Tsuda T, et al. CT and MR cholangiography: advantages and pitfalls in perioperative evaluation of biliary tree. Br J Radiol. 2012;85(1015):887–96.
19. Caoili EM, Paulson EK, Heyneman LE, Branch MS, Eubanks WS, Nelson RC. Helical CT cholangiography with three-dimensional volume rendering using an oral biliary contrast agent: feasibility of a novel technique. AJR Am J Roentgenol. 2000;174(2):487–92.
20. Tabibian JH, Macura SI, O'Hara SP, Fidler JL, Glockner JF, Takahashi N, et al. Micro-computed tomography and nuclear magnetic resonance imaging for noninvasive, live-mouse cholangiography. Lab Invest. 2013;93(6):733–43.
21. Saad WE, Ginat D. Computed tomography and magnetic resonance cholangiography. Tech Vasc Interv Radiol. 2008;11(2):74–89.
22. Okuda Y, Taura K, Seo S, Yasuchika K, Nitta T, Ogawa K, et al. Usefulness of operative planning based on 3-dimensional CT cholangiography for biliary malignancies. Surgery. 2015;158(5):1261–71.

23. Ogawa M, Ozawa Y, Ohta K, Sekiguchi T, Omata S, Urano M, et al. Usefulness of 3D balanced turbo-field-echo MR sequence evaluating the branching pattern of the intrahepatic bile ducts: comparison with drip infusion CT cholangiography. Abdom Radiol (NY). 2017;42(7):1888–95.
24. Dilger SKN, Nelson N, Venkatesh SK, Ehman EC, Fidler JL, Fletcher JG, et al. Computed tomography cholangiography using the magnetic resonance contrast agent gadoxetate disodium: a phantom study. Investig Radiol. 2019;54(9):572–9.
25. Park HS, Lee JM, Choi JY, Lee MW, Kim HJ, Han JK, et al. Preoperative evaluation of bile duct cancer: MRI combined with MR cholangiopancreatography versus MDCT with direct cholangiography. AJR Am J Roentgenol. 2008;190(2):396–405.
26. Sahani D, Mehta A, Blake M, Prasad S, Harris G, Saini S. Preoperative hepatic vascular evaluation with CT and MR angiography: implications for surgery. Radiographics. 2004;24(5):1367–80.
27. Razumilava N, Gores GJ, Lindor KD. Cancer surveillance in patients with primary sclerosing cholangitis. Hepatology. 2011;54(5):1842–52.
28. Ali AH, Tabibian JH, Nasser-Ghodsi N, Lennon RJ, DeLeon T, Borad MJ, et al. Surveillance for hepatobiliary cancers in patients with primary sclerosing cholangitis. Hepatology. 2018;67(6):2338–51.
29. Fung BM, Lindor KD, Tabibian JH. Cancer risk in primary sclerosing cholangitis: epidemiology, prevention, and surveillance strategies. World J Gastroenterol. 2019;25(6):659–71.
30. Fung BM, Tabibian JH. Cholangiocarcinoma in patients with primary sclerosing cholangitis. Curr Opin Gastroenterol. 2020;36(2):77–84.
31. Shah AH, Olivero JJ. Gadolinium-induced nephrogenic systemic fibrosis. Methodist Debakey Cardiovasc J. 2017;13(3):172–3.
32. Gulani V, Calamante F, Shellock FG, Kanal E, Reeder SB. Gadolinium deposition in the brain: summary of evidence and recommendations. Lancet Neurol. 2017;16(7):564–70.
33. Maetani Y, Itoh K, Watanabe C, Shibata T, Ametani F, Yamabe H, et al. MR imaging of intrahepatic cholangiocarcinoma with pathologic correlation. AJR Am J Roentgenol. 2001;176(6):1499–507.
34. Olthof SC, Othman A, Clasen S, Schraml C, Nikolaou K, Bongers M. Imaging of cholangiocarcinoma. Visc Med. 2016;32(6):402–10.
35. Sainani NI, Catalano OA, Holalkere NS, Zhu AX, Hahn PF, Sahani DV. Cholangiocarcinoma: current and novel imaging techniques. Radiographics. 2008;28(5):1263–87.
36. Campos JT, Sirlin CB, Choi JY. Focal hepatic lesions in Gd-EOB-DTPA enhanced MRI: the atlas. Insights Imaging. 2012;3(5):451–74.
37. Engelbrecht MR, Katz SS, van Gulik TM, Lameris JS, van Delden OM. Imaging of perihilar cholangiocarcinoma. AJR Am J Roentgenol. 2015;204(4):782–91.
38. Caserta MP, Sakala M, Shen P, Gorden L, Wile G. Presurgical planning for hepatobiliary malignancies: clinical and imaging considerations. Magn Reson Imaging Clin N Am. 2014;22(3):447–65.
39. Qayyum A. MR spectroscopy of the liver: principles and clinical applications. Radiographics. 2009;29(6):1653–64.
40. Sharif AW, Williams HR, Lampejo T, Khan SA, Bansi DS, Westaby D, et al. Metabolic profiling of bile in cholangiocarcinoma using in vitro magnetic resonance spectroscopy. HPB (Oxford). 2010;12(6):396–402.
41. Kinahan PE, Fletcher JW. Positron emission tomography-computed tomography standardized uptake values in clinical practice and assessing response to therapy. Semin Ultrasound CT MR. 2010;31(6):496–505.
42. Donswijk ML, Hess S, Mulders T, Lam MG. [18F]Fluorodeoxyglucose PET/computed tomography in gastrointestinal malignancies. PET Clin. 2014;9(4):421–41, v–vi.
43. Lamarca A, Barriuso J, Chander A, McNamara MG, Hubner RA, ÓReilly D, et al. (18) F-fluorodeoxyglucose positron emission tomography ((18)FDG-PET) for patients with biliary tract cancer: systematic review and meta-analysis. J Hepatol. 2019;71(1):115–29.

44. Ma KW, Cheung TT, She WH, Chok KSH, Chan ACY, Dai WC, et al. Diagnostic and prognostic role of 18-FDG PET/CT in the management of resectable biliary tract cancer. World J Surg. 2018;42(3):823–34.
45. Annunziata S, Caldarella C, Pizzuto DA, Galiandro F, Sadeghi R, Giovanella L, et al. Diagnostic accuracy of fluorine-18-fluorodeoxyglucose positron emission tomography in the evaluation of the primary tumor in patients with cholangiocarcinoma: a meta-analysis. Biomed Res Int. 2014;2014:247693.
46. Moon CM, Bang S, Chung JB, Park SW, Song SY, Yun M, et al. Usefulness of 18F-fluorodeoxyglucose positron emission tomography in differential diagnosis and staging of cholangiocarcinomas. J Gastroenterol Hepatol. 2008;23(5):759–65.
47. Lee Y, Yoo IR, Boo SH, Kim H, Park HL, Hyun OJ. The role of F-18 FDG PET/CT in intrahepatic cholangiocarcinoma. Nucl Med Mol Imaging. 2017;51(1):69–78.
48. Petrowsky H, Wildbrett P, Husarik DB, Hany TF, Tam S, Jochum W, et al. Impact of integrated positron emission tomography and computed tomography on staging and management of gallbladder cancer and cholangiocarcinoma. J Hepatol. 2006;45(1):43–50.
49. Kim JY, Kim MH, Lee TY, Hwang CY, Kim JS, Yun SC, et al. Clinical role of 18F-FDG PET-CT in suspected and potentially operable cholangiocarcinoma: a prospective study compared with conventional imaging. Am J Gastroenterol. 2008;103(5):1145–51.
50. Sabate-Llobera A, Gracia-Sanchez L, Reynes-Llompart G, Ramos E, Llado L, Robles J, et al. Differences on metabolic behavior between intra and extrahepatic cholangiocarcinomas at (18)F-FDG-PET/CT: prognostic implication of metabolic parameters and tumor markers. Clin Transl Oncol. 2019;21(3):324–33.
51. Gaertner FC, Furst S, Schwaiger M. PET/MR: a paradigm shift. Cancer Imaging. 2013;13:36–52.
52. Paspulati RM, Gupta A. PET/MR imaging in cancers of the gastrointestinal tract. PET Clin. 2016;11(4):403–23.
53. Ferrone C, Goyal L, Qadan M, Gervais D, Sahani DV, Zhu AX, et al. Management implications of fluorodeoxyglucose positron emission tomography/magnetic resonance in untreated intrahepatic cholangiocarcinoma. Eur J Nucl Med Mol Imaging. 2020;47(8):1871–84.
54. Kong E, Chun KA, Cho IH. Quantitative assessment of simultaneous F-18 FDG PET/MRI in patients with various types of hepatic tumors: correlation between glucose metabolism and apparent diffusion coefficient. PLoS One. 2017;12(7):e0180184.
55. Lim CH, Moon SH, Cho YS, Choi JY, Lee KH, Hyun SH. Prognostic value of (18) F-fluorodeoxyglucose positron emission tomography/computed tomography in patients with combined hepatocellular-cholangiocarcinoma. Eur J Nucl Med Mol Imaging. 2019;46(8):1705–12.
56. Kratochwil C, Flechsig P, Lindner T, Abderrahim L, Altmann A, Mier W, et al. (68)Ga-FAPI PET/CT: tracer uptake in 28 different kinds of cancer. J Nucl Med. 2019;60(6):801–5.
57. Chotipanich C, Promteangtrong C, Kunawudhi A, Chanwat R, Sricharunrat T, Suratako S, et al. (11)C-Choline and FDG PET/CT imaging of primary cholangiocarcinoma: a comparative analysis. Asia Ocean J Nucl Med Biol. 2015;3(1):18–25.
58. Pauwels E, Cleeren F, Bormans G, Deroose CM. Somatostatin receptor PET ligands – the next generation for clinical practice. Am J Nucl Med Mol Imaging. 2018;8(5):311–31.
59. Lee EJ, Chung HW, Jo JH, So Y. Radioembolization for the treatment of primary and metastatic liver cancers. Nucl Med Mol Imaging. 2019;53(6):367–73.
60. Ahn KS, Kang KJ, Kim YH, Kim TS, Song BI, Kim HW, et al. Genetic features associated with (18)F-FDG uptake in intrahepatic cholangiocarcinoma. Ann Surg Treat Res. 2019;96(4):153–61.

Chapter 8
Pathological Diagnosis of Cholangiocarcinoma

Carlie Sigel and Tao Wang

Abbreviations

AFP	Alpha-fetoprotein
BilIN	Biliary intraepithelial neoplasia
CEA	Carcinoembryonic antigen
CT	Computed tomography
DIA	Digital image analysis
ERCP	Endoscopic retrograde cholangiopancreatography
EUS	Endoscopic ultrasound
FISH	Fluorescent *in situ* hybridization
FNA	Fine needle aspiration
HCC	Hepatocellular carcinoma
IMP3	Insulin-like growth factor-I mRNA binding protein-3
IPNB	Intraductal papillary neoplasms of bile ducts
KRAS	Kristen rat sarcoma
MCN	Mucinous cystic neoplasm
NGS	Next-generation sequencing
PSC	Primary sclerosing cholangitis
pVHL	von Hippel-Lindau protein
TFF1	Trefoil factor 1

C. Sigel (✉)
Department of Pathology, Memorial Sloan Kettering Cancer Center, New York, NY, USA
e-mail: sigelc@mskcc.org

T. Wang
Department of Pathology and Molecular Medicine, Queen's University, Kingston, ON, Canada
e-mail: tao.wang@kingstonhsc.ca

J. H. Tabibian (ed.), *Diagnosis and Management of Cholangiocarcinoma*,
https://doi.org/10.1007/978-3-030-70936-5_8

Cholangiocarcinoma Diagnosis

Definitive histologic classification and staging of cholangiocarcinoma can be achieved by evaluation of surgically resected material. Given the advanced presentation of many patients with cholangiocarcinoma, radiologic guidance is commonly used to obtain small tissue samples for histologic or cytologic evaluation so that pathologists can reach a definitive diagnosis to guide therapy. There are many challenges to cholangiocarcinoma diagnosis on small biopsies. Noninvasive biopsy techniques require significant operator skill, and tumor cell yields can be low due to due to infiltrative tumor growth patterns, necrosis, and a relatively low tumor concentration compared to tumor-associated stroma. Furthermore, markedly reactive changes due to bile duct strictures or stenting can be difficult to distinguish from cancer. Nonetheless, the diagnosis can be established using morphologic criteria and, when indicated, immunohistochemistry, ancillary cytogenetics, and molecular-based techniques.

Tissue Acquisition Techniques

The tissue acquisition technique for diagnosis of cholangiocarcinoma (CCA) depends on the site of disease and the clinical features of individual patients. Tissue acquisition for intrahepatic CCA is typically obtained by percutaneous approach with radiologic guidance by computed tomography or ultrasound to obtain cores of tissue (FNB) and/or fine needle aspirate (FNA). Rapid onsite adequacy can be used to improve diagnostic yield.

Extrahepatic CCA can be sampled using several methods [1]. Intraductal forceps biopsy or fine needle biopsy can obtained by endoscopic retrograde cholangiopancreatography (ERCP) utilizing standard or mini-forceps with fluoroscopic guidance and/or specialized forceps under cholangioscopic; when retrograde access is not feasible due to anatomical or other factors, the same may be performed by percutaneous transhepatic cholangiography (PTC). The sensitivity and specificity of biopsy is 62–78% and 100%, respectively [2–4]. Cells in biliary fluid can be obtained for cytologic examination by direct aspiration during ERCP or via percutaneous drainage, and cytology techniques generally have near 100% specificity. Biliary fluid cytology has a low sensitivity (6–32%) for detecting malignancy and is commonly performed in conjunction with cytologic evaluation of bile duct brushings, which have a higher pooled sensitivity of 45% [1, 5]. Bile duct brushing obtained by ERCP or PTC involves scraping cells from the superficial biliary mucosa at the level of the bile duct lesion. The brush, charged with cellular material, is carefully smeared directly on a glass slide. The slide is reserved for air drying or fixed by very rapidly placing it in an alcohol-based fixative; any delay between the smearing and fixation creates artifactual distortion that hinders diagnosis. Alternatively, the cells can be dislodged from the brush using agitation into a container with a fixative appropriate for liquid-based cytology preparation [6]. Liquid-based media is a flexible collection technique because the cells can be applied to slide using various proprietary techniques such as CytoSpin™ (Thermo Fisher Scientific, Waltham, MA), ThinPrep^{R} (Hologic, Inc., Marlborough, MA), or BD SurePath™ prep (Becton, Dickinson and Company, Franklin Lakes, NJ). Also, tissue fragments can be centrifuged into a cell pellet and fixed with formalin into a cell block. Cytology diagnosis, DNA-based testing, fluorescence *in situ* hybridization (FISH), and immunocytochemistry, as indicated, can be performed on material placed in liquid-based fixative. As an alternative or compliment to ERCP, bile duct masses may also be sampled using endoscopic ultrasound (EUS)-guided FNA/FNB. Like bile duct brushings, FNAs can be prepared as direct smears, liquid-based preparations, and cell blocks. FNA has a high sensitivity and specificity for extrahepatic CCA (82% and 87.5%) [7, 8]. Because of the transduodenal approach of EUS, distal bile duct lesions are technically easier and safer to access compared to peri-hilar lesions, although overall complication rates are low in experienced hands [7].

Precursor Neoplastic Lesions

Three main precursor lesions exist: biliary intraepithelial neoplasia (BilIN), intraductal papillary neoplasm of the bile ducts (IPNB), and mucinous cystic neoplasm (MCN) These are each discussed in the forthcoming subsections (see also Chap. 3, Nakanuma et al., for complementary information).

Biliary Intraepithelial Neoplasia

Non-mass-forming dysplasia of the bile duct epithelium, termed "biliary intraepithelial neoplasia," is an incidental microscopic finding and putative precursor of CCA. The atypical epithelium is flat or micropapillary and confined to the lumen. There are two tiers in grade (low and high), and lesions are graded based on the highest degree of atypia [9]. Diagnosis of low grade reflects pseudostratification of nuclei, increased nuclear-cytoplasmic ratio, and nuclear hyperchromasia. High-grade BilIN lesions have increasing architectural complexity such as micropapillae, loss of cellular polarity, and marked nuclear atypia.

Due to the non-mass-forming nature of BilIN, it is rarely discovered prior to the development of carcinoma, and thus little is known about its natural history. However, patients with primary sclerosing cholangitis (PSC) are at markedly increased risk of CCA, with lifetime risk approaching 10% [10]. Retrospective studies in patients with PSC have shown strong associations between the presence of intestinal metaplasia, low- and high-grade BilIN, and CCA [11–13]. The inflammation-metaplasia-dysplasia-carcinoma model of progression in PSC is supported by the finding of increasing cytogenetic abnormalities as lesions progress

[14]. This model of progression in PSC is similar to that of inflammatory bowel disease, and there is also evidence it may be applicable to other clinical contexts, such as liver fluke-associated CCA [15].

Intraductal Papillary Neoplasm of the Bile Ducts

Single or multifocal grossly exophytic proliferations of neoplastic biliary epithelium within the bile ducts are termed intraductal papillary neoplasms of bile ducts (Fig. 8.1a). These premalignant neoplasms are seen in association with an invasive carcinoma in 74% of resected cases [16]. In East Asian populations, there is evidence of association between IPNB and hepatolithiasis, but many IPNB also arise in the absence of a predisposing condition [17, 18]. The histology comprises villous or finger-like branching fibrovascular cores lined by dysplastic cuboidal to columnar epithelium of biliary, intestinal, oncocytic, or gastric differentiation [19] (Fig. 8.1b). The mucin expression profiles are similar to those of their pancreatic counterparts; the pancreatobiliary type expresses MUC1, the intestinal type expresses MUC2, and while gastric and oncocytic types express MUC5AC and MUC6 [16].

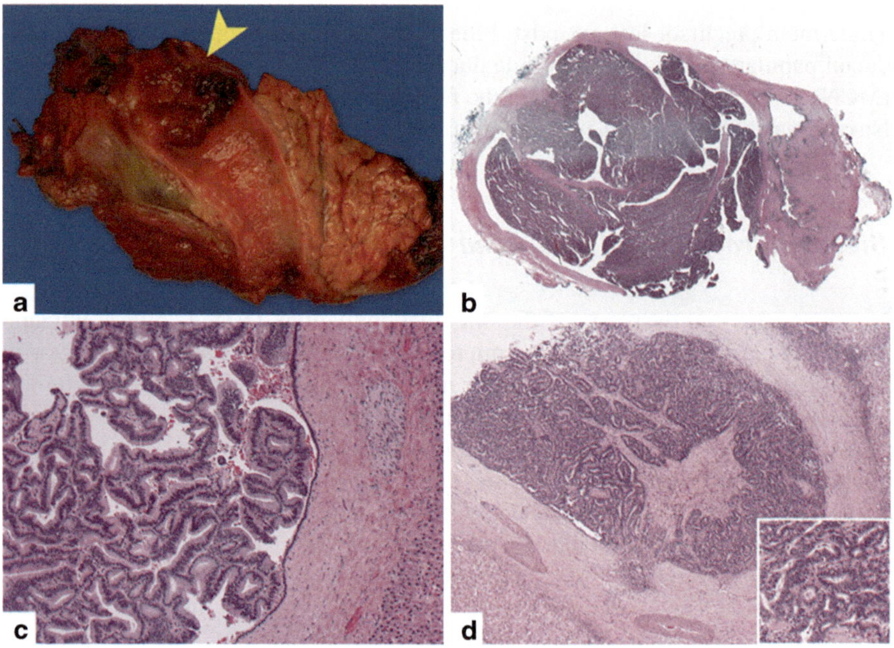

Fig. 8.1 (**a–d**) Grossly, an intraductal papillary neoplasm of the bile ducts (IPNB) is an exophytic and papillary lesion within the lumen of the bile duct (**a**). IPNB of the common bile duct fills and expands the duct lumen on low power histology (**b**). Branching and tubular architecture is typical of low-grade IPNB (**c**), while marked cytologic atypia and complex architecture are present in IPNB with high-grade dysplasia (**d**)

IPNB are graded in two tiers: low- and high-grade based on the highest level of cytological atypia and cellular organization in a given lesion (Fig. 8.1c, d). Recently, dividing IPNB into two types has been proposed due to clinical, pathologic, and genetic differences [20, 21]. Type 1 is similar to pancreatic intraductal papillary mucinous neoplasm and mainly in the intrahepatic bile duct, whereas type 2 is more architecturally complex with solid and tubular components, is more often associated with invasive adenocarcinoma at resection, and mainly involves the extrahepatic bile ducts [20].

A rarer and morphologically distinct mass-forming neoplasm exists that lacks the mucinous characteristics of IPNB. These lesions typically show predominantly compact tubular-glandular architecture with minimal papillae and are usually associated with high-grade dysplasia and invasive carcinoma (up to 80%) [22]. These lesions are designated "intraductal tubulopapillary neoplasm of the bile duct" and are also morphologically similar to their pancreatic analog [22].

Mucinous Cystic Neoplasm of the Liver and Biliary System

CCAs may arise, albeit rarely (approximately 6%), in association with mucinous cystic neoplasm of the liver and biliary system, placing it in the category of precursor neoplastic lesion [23]. MCN is a cystic neoplasm arising without clear communication with the bile duct. These neoplasms are well-demarcated grossly and contain fluid. The defining histologic feature is the combination of cystic glands and ovarian-type stroma. The neoplastic glands are lined by epithelial cells that are columnar (often mucinous), cuboidal (non-mucinous), or attenuated [23]. Invasive cholangiocarcinoma may be present in radiologically/grossly solid components of MCNs. Although typically flat, some neoplasms have papillary projections. The ovarian-type stroma must be identified for diagnosis but may only be focal and is highlighted by immunohistochemical stains for ER or PR. Rarely, MCN has high-grade dysplasia; the lining is typically low-grade.

Peri-hilar and Distal Extrahepatic Bile Duct Adenocarcinomas

Gross Evaluation

Peri-hilar CCA arises from the common hepatic duct, whereas distal CCA arises from the common bile duct. Resection specimens are evaluated by gross assessment of tumor size, appearance, location, relationship to adjacent structures, distance to margins, and the presence of lymph nodes. Most tumors have a firm white or tan appearance with poorly defined infiltrative margins. For peri-hilar tumors, the macroscopic involvement of the common hepatic duct and its branches is important to document. Extension of these neoplasms along bile ducts leading to strictures is common. Peri-hilar resections usually include partial hepatectomy, and thus extension into liver parenchyma, branches of the portal vein, hepatic artery, or second-order biliary radicals can occasionally be seen grossly, and the documentation of tumor involvement is an element of tumor staging. The resection margins, proximal/distal bile ducts and soft tissue margins, are examined for the distance to tumor, with samples taken for microscopy.

For distal extrahepatic CCA, the resection is often a Whipple specimen. Likewise, the tumor is described in relation to the adjacent structures such as the pancreas, duodenum, and ampulla. The depth of invasion from the bile duct wall is key for pathologic T staging of distal CCA, which is assessed by gross measurement and confirmed with microscopy of the tumor at its widest invasive span. For distal CCA, the most important margin is often the proximal bile duct margin, but all other margins (uncinate, pancreatic neck, luminal gastrointestinal) are sampled, typically in a shave section, for microscopy.

Histology

The majority of extrahepatic CCAs have a histologic appearance similar to conventional pancreatic ductal adenocarcinoma. The infiltrating and irregularly angulated glands may appear scattered among residual biliary structures or occur within an obliterative desmoplastic stroma (Fig. 8.2). The cells are usually columnar and often contain intracellular mucin. Among the varied histologic subtypes described are intestinal, foveolar, mucinous, signet ring cell, clear cell, hepatoid, and micropapillary [24]. Rare CCA subtypes with a distinctive appearance include adenosquamous, sarcomatoid, and undifferentiated carcinomas. Lymphovascular invasion is common, which is reflected in the high proportion of resections with positive lymph nodes (39% to 76%) [25–27]. Perineural invasion is also common and, coupled with the tumors' tendency to extend along the existing ducts, results in high rates of positive resection margins (13–37%) [28–31]. Frozen section analysis with further resection on intraoperatively positive margins can result in improved survival [28, 29].

Differential Diagnosis of Extrahepatic Cholangiocarcinoma and Distal Bile Duct Carcinoma

The differential diagnosis of extrahepatic CCAs includes reactive peri-ductal glands in the setting of inflammation, metastatic lesions, and direct extension from primary pancreatic, ampullary, or duodenal tumors. Malignant glands are

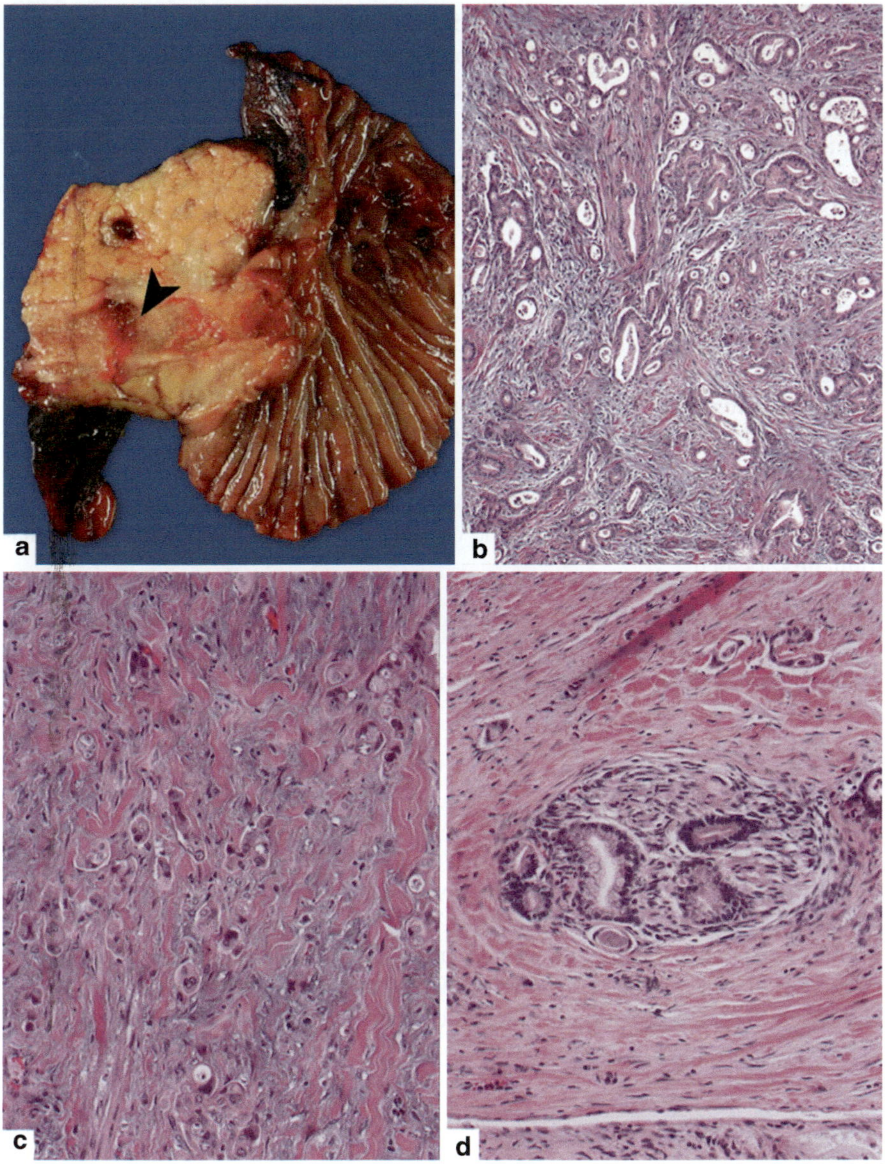

Fig. 8.2 Irregularly infiltrating glands and intra-tumoral desmoplastic stroma typify well-differentiated distal (**a**) and peri-hilar (**b**) CCAs. Poorly differentiated CCAs of the distal (**c**) and peri-hilar (**d**) bile ducts have poorly formed glands and single cell infiltration

distinguished from reactive glands by the irregular infiltration and degree of cytomorphologic atypia. This can be difficult in the setting of severe inflammation. Immunohistochemistry for p53 (abnormal overexpression or loss of expression) and/or SMAD4 (loss of expression) may be of value in distinguishing between reactive versus neoplastic, but these stains are aberrant in only approximately half of extrahepatic CCAs [32, 33]. Therefore, non-aberrant staining does not exclude neoplasia. Another nonneoplastic mimicker is IgG4-related cholangitis, which can appear similar on cholangiography to PSC or cholangiocarcinoma [34]. Serum IgG4 is a useful ancillary test, but its sensitivity and specificity vary depending on the thresholds used [35]. Biopsies of IgG4 cholangitis may show lymphoplasmacytic inflammation and fibrosis, with significantly increased IgG4 plasma cells by immunohistochemistry [36].

With respect to neoplastic differential diagnoses, the extrahepatic bile ducts are uncommon locations for distant metastasis, but attention to the history of other prior malignancies is still important, particularly if the histomorphology is unusual. Far more commonly, the extrahepatic bile ducts may be involved by direct extension of adenocarcinoma from an adjacent organ. Extension of primary pancreatic ductal adenocarcinoma or ampullary adenocarcinoma into the bile duct may be morphologically and immunohistochemically indistinguishable from extrahepatic CCA. Therefore, the distinction is usually made based on gross and microscopic assessment of where the epicenter and/or bulk of the tumor is anatomically located.

Intrahepatic Cholangiocarcinoma

Gross Evaluation

Intrahepatic CCA is an adenocarcinoma arising from the second-order bile ducts and smaller branches. Resections for intrahepatic CCAs are typically partial hepatectomies. The macroscopic configuration can be mass forming (Fig. 8.3a), periductal infiltrating (Fig. 8.3b), or mixed. The gross appearance is firm, white, and fibrous. Gross assessment of tumor size, presence of multifocality, vascular involvement, capsular involvement, and extrahepatic extension are all important factors for pathologic T staging. There is a hepatic parenchymal margin, but distal biliary branches at the margin are important to evaluate due to the propensity for periductal tumoral extension.

Histology

There are two major histologic subtypes of intrahepatic CCA: small duct and large duct. Other rare subtypes include adenosquamous carcinoma, mucinous carcinoma, signet ring cell carcinoma, mucoepidermoid carcinoma, lymphoepithelioma-like carcinoma, and sarcomatous carcinoma [37].

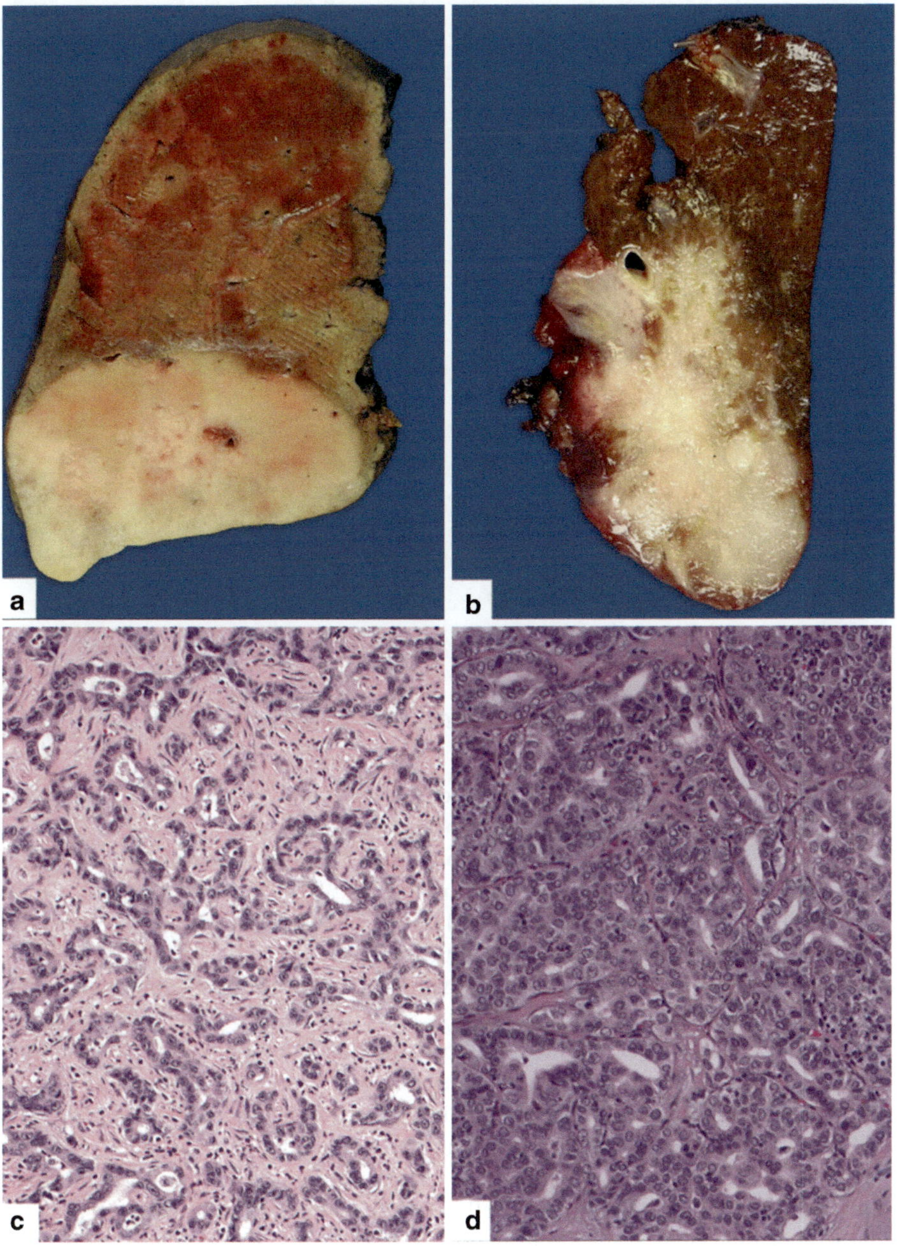

Fig. 8.3 (**a**–**f**) Mass-forming intrahepatic cholangiocarcinoma is well-circumscribed, firm, and fibrous in texture (**a**). A poorly circumscribed gross margin reflects peri-ductal infiltration of intrahepatic cholangiocarcinoma (**b**). Well-differentiated small duct type intrahepatic cholangiocarcinoma has distinct tubular or anastomosing glands, such as this cholangiolar pattern (**c**). Marked glandular complexity and sheets of cells are seen in moderately differentiated (**d**) and poorly differentiated (**e**) small duct type cholangiocarcinomas. The ductal malformation subtype of cholangiocarcinoma (**f**)

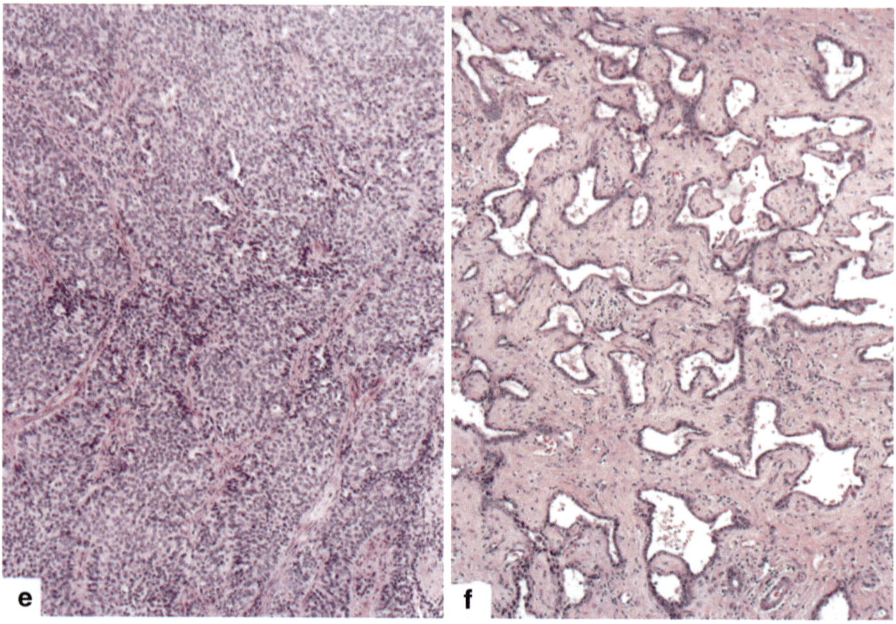

Fig. 8.3 (continued)

Intrahepatic Cholangiocarcinoma: Small Duct Subtype

Small duct subtype has also been called "peripheral," "cholangiolar," and "bile ductular," since they are more likely to present away from the liver hilum and resemble to reactive biliary proliferations. The prevalence of this phenotype is regionally dependent, comprising approximately 40–90% of intrahepatic CCAs [38, 39]. The predominantly tubuloglandular architecture shows remarkable inter-tumoral and intra-tumoral heterogeneity [38]. The patterns of the infiltrating glands include simple tubules, anastomosing tubules, confluent tubules with slit-like lumens, and dilated and solid sheets of cells (Fig. 8.3c–e). Micropapillary arrangements can be seen. The cells are cuboidal, polygonal, or low columnar with cytoplasm that can range from pale and amphophilic to plump and eosinophilic. The neoplastic cells may appear hepatoid but they do not express hepatocellular markers. Small collections of luminal mucin and intracellular mucin can be present in a minority of cases [38]. Many tumors have densely hyalinized intra-tumoral stroma. The tumor cells infiltrate and entrap hepatocytes at the tumor-liver interface. Some small duct type intrahepatic CCAs have architecture resembling ductal plate malformation or biliary adenofibroma (Fig. 8.3f) [40]. Very well-differentiated tumors with a uniformly anastomosing tubular pattern resembling the ductular reaction have been referred to as cholangiolocellular carcinoma, but they lack a unique genotype and may not be a distinct entity (Fig. 8.3c) [41].

Intrahepatic Cholangiocarcinoma: Large Duct Subtype

Large duct subtype intrahepatic CCAs have had prior descriptive labels including "hilar type," "peri-hilar type," and "bile duct type," which reflect the resemblance of this subtype to extrahepatic and peri-hilar CCAs. The histology consists of irregularly infiltrating glands with large-caliber lumens frequently containing mucin (Fig. 8.4a). Cells lining the glands are cuboidal to columnar and often contain intracytoplasmic mucin. The intra-tumoral stroma is characteristically desmoplastic and abundant. Higher-grade carcinomas have increasing architectural complexity and loss of glandular differentiation (Fig. 8.4b). Smaller infiltrating glands resembling the small duct subtype can be seen in variable proportion, and, in some instances, there is infiltration of single cells with signet ring cell appearance. The large duct subtype of intrahepatic CCA frequently exhibits perineural invasion [38].

Differential Diagnosis of Intrahepatic Cholangiocarcinoma

The diagnosis of intrahepatic CCA requires distinction from reactive biliary glands and benign biliary proliferations. Similar to extrahepatic bile ducts, IgG4-related cholangitis can also involve the intrahepatic ducts. Other malignancies such as hepatocellular carcinoma and metastasis from the lung, breast, and upper gastrointestinal tracts and extrahepatic pancreaticobiliary system also enter the differential. The *Immunohistochemistry of Cholangiocarcinoma* section in this chapter provides information on the use of stains in resolving the site of tumor origin.

Small biopsies containing well-differentiated CCA may present a challenge in diagnosis. Carcinoma is distinguished from bile duct adenomas and reactive biliary proliferations based on larger nucleus size, atypical cytological

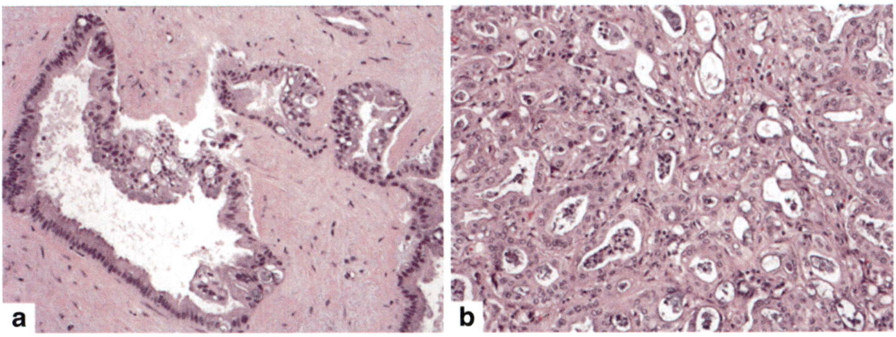

Fig. 8.4 (**a**, **b**) Large duct type intrahepatic cholangiocarcinoma resembles extrahepatic cholangiocarcinoma with widely spaced large-caliber infiltrating glands (**a**). Higher-grade tumors have a higher density of infiltrating glands with more complexity (**b**)

features, and irregular distribution of infiltrating glands. The Ki-67 proliferation index of adenomas is low compared to cholangiocarcinoma (average = 2% versus 23%) [42]. The immunohistochemical marker for p16 (*CDKN2A*) is expressed in most adenomas and bile ductular proliferations but less so in carcinoma [43].

Morphologic features are often sufficient for distinguishing CCA from hepatocellular carcinoma because CCA has tubuloglandular differentiation, mucin production, and intra-tumoral stroma. These features are absent in hepatocellular carcinoma (HCC), excepting the rare scirrhous or sclerosing variant of HCC [44, 45]. Poorly differentiated primary liver carcinomas require immunohistochemistry to exclude hepatocellular differentiation.

The histology of intrahepatic CCA overlaps with several extrahepatic adenocarcinomas. Fortunately, most well-differentiated intrahepatic CCAs have anastomosing glands and sclerotic stroma; this "cholangiolar pattern" of the small duct subtype has been shown to be specific for intrahepatic cholangiocarcinoma, particularly when combined with positive albumin RNA *in situ* hybridization [46]. Unfortunately, the large duct subtype of intrahepatic CCA resembles extrahepatic bile duct and pancreas adenocarcinomas both histologically and immunophenotypically. In the event of large tumors involving the liver hilum with a large duct phenotype, it can be impossible on a histologic basis to distinguish the large duct subtype of intrahepatic CCA from a peri-hilar CCA. Clinical and radiologic correlation plays a key role in these scenarios.

Combined Hepatocellular-Cholangiocarcinoma

Carcinomas containing areas with both hepatocellular and cholangiocytic differentiation are classified as combined hepatocellular-cholangiocarcinoma. Genomic studies have revealed that most cases of primary liver carcinoma with this bi-phenotypic morphology represent proliferations derived from the same clone [47, 48]. Tumors that show two distinct genomic profiles between the phenotypes may represent "collision tumors" which arose as separate primaries [48]. Collision tumors are currently excluded from the WHO classification of combined hepatocellular-cholangiocarcinoma, although there is still debate on this matter [37]. The two phenotypic components in combined hepatocellular-cholangiocarcinoma may be regionally distinct or intermixed. There is no defining proportion required for either component, but diagnosis is based on recognition of the two morphologies on routine hematoxylin and eosin (H&E)-stained slides (Fig. 8.5). Immunohistochemistry to demonstrate both hepatocellular (Arginase-1, HepPar1) and biliary (CK7, CK19) phenotype may be useful to support the diagnosis, but this technique is ancillary to the H&E morphology [37].

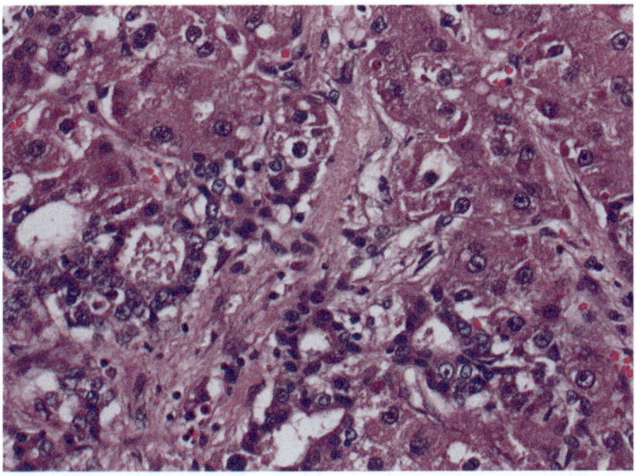

Fig. 8.5 Combined hepatocellular-cholangiocarcinoma has distinct histologic components

Table 8.1 Staining patterns in cholangiocarcinoma

Staining pattern	Intrahepatic cholangiocarcinoma, small duct type	Intrahepatic cholangiocarcinoma, large duct type	Extrahepatic cholangiocarcinoma
Positive	CK7 CK19 CK20 (−/focal positive) Albumin mRNA *in situ* Mucicarmine (focal) CD56 MUC1	CK7 CK19 CK20 (−/focal positive) Mucicarmine CA19–9 S100P TFF1 MUC5AC MUC6 MUC1	CK7 CK19 CA19–9 S100P IMP3 Maspin Methionyl-tRNA synthetase 1 Claudin-18 Mucicarmine
Negative	HepPar1 Arginase-1 Alpha-fetoprotein Polyclonal CEA (canalicular pattern) CD10 (canalicular pattern)	Albumin mRNA *in situ*	Albumin mRNA *in situ* Smad-4 pVHL

Abbreviations: *CEA* Carcinoembryonic antigen, *TFF1* trefoil factor 1, *IMP3* insulin-like growth factor-I mRNA binding protein-3, *pVHL* von Hippel-Lindau protein

Immunohistochemistry of Cholangiocarcinoma

Immunohistochemistry plays a larger role in assessing intrahepatic CCAs compared to their extrahepatic counterparts because of the differential diagnosis with hepatocellular carcinoma (HCC) and the propensity of a wide variety of other adenocarcinomas to metastasize to the liver. A summary of immunohistochemical labeling patterns is shown in Table 8.1. The distinction of CCA from non-hepatic adenocarcinomas relies on the integration of morphology, ancillary tests, as well as clinical context and radiological findings. When a patient has a known prior extra-biliary adenocarcinoma, for instance, comparison should be made with prior histology to exclude metastasis.

CCAs of all types are positive for CK7 and CK19 while negative or only focally positive for CK20. This keratin labeling pattern is by no means specific for CCA over adenocarcinoma from another site but is supportive evidence that an established primary liver carcinoma is CCA (as opposed to HCC). Typical HCCs only rarely or weakly label with CK7, which is a marker of poor prognosis, while strong CK7 labeling is supportive of CCA [49]. The fibrolamellar variant of HCC is a clinically and genetically distinct variant which is strongly CK7 positive, but its morphology is so distinctive that it is unlikely to be mistaken for CCA. Mucicarmine is a histochemical stain that can be used to highlight intracellular mucin, which also supports glandular differentiation. Most CCAs are negative for hepatocytic lineage markers HepPar1, Arginase-1, and alpha-fetoprotein (AFP) [50–52].

Immunohistochemical approaches to evaluating intrahepatic tumors commonly involve excluding metastasis using a panel of markers given the keratin profile alone is nonspecific. In brief, these are generally useful ancillary tests for clarifying tumor origin, but interpretation requires an understanding of the sensitivity and specificity of these markers for their target sites. For example, TTF-1 and Napsin A are positive in the vast majority of lung adenocarcinomas and are generally negative in intrahepatic CCAs, but these stains have been reported positive in anywhere from 5–47% of extrahepatic CCAs [53–55]. This wide range may be related to the use of different antibody clones between different institutions. CDX2 is often positive in luminal gastrointestinal tract tumors, but it can stain CCA in roughly 30% of cases, albeit patchy or with weaker intensity [55–57]. Estrogen receptor (ER) and progesterone receptor (PR) have high specificity for breast and gynecologic origin but modest sensitivity [58, 59]. Other markers for mammary origin such as GATA-3, mammaglobin, and GCDFP-15 also show modest sensitivity and specificity [55, 60]. Some popular or emerging markers, such as PAX8 (renal, gynecologic, thyroid), NKX3.1 (prostate), and SATB2 (colon), have lower rates of cross-reactivity with CCA, in the range of 5–10% [55]. In summary, most popular immunohistochemical lineage markers are not entirely specific and may show staining in at least a subset of CCAs. Prudence dictates caution in drawing conclusions about site of origin based on immunohistochemistry without knowledge of the clinical and radiological setting.

Many markers have been evaluated for the differential expression in small versus large duct intrahepatic CCA. These stains are generally not employed in routine diagnosis. The large duct type is more likely to stain with CA19-9, S100P, and TFF1, while the small duct type labels with CD56. There is also differential mucin expression since MUC5AC and MUC6 label large duct while MUC1 labels both small and large duct types [38, 61, 62].

Albumin In Situ *Hybridization*

Until recently, there were no lineage-specific markers for CCA. While this remains the case for extrahepatic CCA, albumin mRNA expression has emerged as a relatively specific marker for primary liver cancers of both hepatocellular and cholangiocellular origin. Improvements in automated *in situ* hybridization staining methods have increased the availability of this marker for clinical use, but at the time of this writing, although commercial availability has improved, it is still not widely in use. Interpretation of albumin labeling requires familiarity with the possible range of staining patterns. The stain is often patchy and a positive result requires at least 5% of tumor cells to label [63]. Labeling of entrapped hepatocytes must be excluded. Albumin mRNA ISH has an 89% sensitivity for intrahepatic CCA [46]. It is also positive in almost all hepatocellular carcinomas. Albumin does not stain pancreatic adenocarcinomas, extrahepatic CCA, and gastric adenocarcinomas. The specificity is imperfect since it has been reported to occasionally label non-hepatic neoplasms such as acinar cell carcinoma of the pancreas, ductal breast carcinoma, gallbladder carcinoma, gastroesophageal junction carcinoma, lung carcinoma, and yolk sac tumors [46, 63–65]. The percentages of intrahepatic CCAs labeling for albumin in a given study are affected by the proportion of tumors of the large duct phenotype, which do not tend to express albumin [38, 66].

Cytology

Biliary brushings and drainage fluid are used to diagnose extrahepatic biliary lesions. For the diagnosis of malignant strictures, biliary brushings have variable sensitivity that ranges from 18% to 67%, with a pooled sensitivity of 45% by meta-analysis [5, 67]. The specificity is consistently high, with most studies approaching 99% [5]. Since the sampling utilizes an exfoliative technique, it is not possible to distinguish between a noninvasive intraductal carcinoma and an invasive carcinoma (Fig. 8.6). Fine needle aspiration may be performed for the diagnosis of both extra- and intrahepatic neoplasms. For extrahepatic cholangiocarcinoma, a direct comparison of FNA with brushing showed that FNA has a much higher sensitivity (73% vs 44%) [4].

The cytologic criteria for the diagnosis of cholangiocarcinoma are similar for both exfoliative and aspiration techniques [Table 8.2]. The diagnosis requires the identification of multiple atypical cytological features such as two distinct cell populations, cellular disorganization, cellular crowding and three-dimensionality, increased nuclear-cytoplasmic ratio, nuclear molding, nuclear size variation of >4:1 ratio in cellular clusters, coarse/clumped chromatin, irregular thickening and indentations of the nuclear membrane, and poor cellular cohesion leading to a background

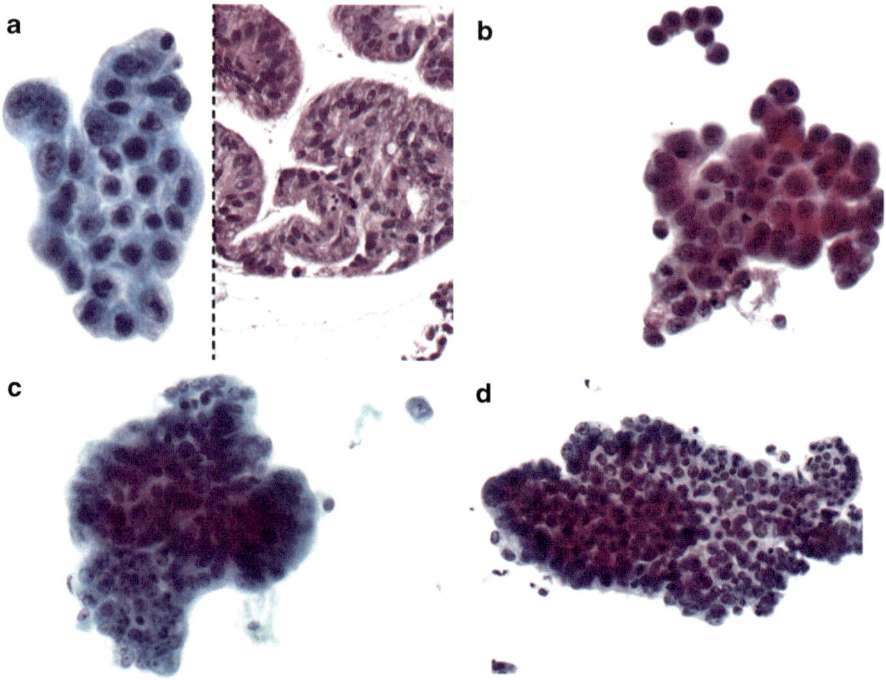

Fig. 8.6 (**a**–**d**) Clusters of ductal epithelium with reactive atypia in the setting of a stent (**a**, ThinPrep, 400× (left) cell block (right)) or primary sclerosing cholangitis (**b**, ThinPrep, 400×) is cohesive and lacks three-dimensional architecture. Intraductal papillary neoplasms with high-grade atypia demonstrate three-dimensional architecture and anisonucleosis, but cannot be distinguished from invasive adenocarcinoma (**c**, ThinPrep, 400×). Adenocarcinoma has crowded epithelial clusters with marked anisonucleosis and chromatin alterations (**d**, ThinPrep, 400×)

Table 8.2 Cytological features of reactive biliary mucosa and cholangiocarcinoma in bile duct brushing

Reactive biliary mucosa	Cholangiocarcinoma
Admixed inflammatory cells	Two distinct populations
Prominent nucleoli	Three-dimensional clusters
Lower nucleus-cytoplasmic ratio	Poor cellular cohesion and single atypical cells
Anisonucleosis up to 1:3 ratio	Increased nucleus-cytoplasmic ratio
Absent coarse chromatin	Nucleus molding
Smooth nucleus membranes	Anisonucleosis >4:1 ratio in clusters
Absent to rare single atypical cells	Coarse chromatin
	Irregularities of the nuclear membrane
	Marked cellular disorganization
	Marked cellular crowding

with single atypical cells [68–71]. The presence of inflammation due to primary sclerosing cholangitis or biliary stenting prior to endoscopic brush sampling of biliary disease creates significant diagnostic difficulties, yet specificity remains high even in this context (97%) [72]. A comparison of stent-associated changes with confirmed malignant cytology indicates that three-dimensional architecture, anisonucleosis (≥1:6), coarse chromatin, and single atypical cells are features significantly associated with malignancy (Fig. 8.6) [73].

The Papanicolaou Society classification system for the reporting of pancreaticobiliary cytology was published in 2015 [74] and provides useful terminology and criteria for the diagnosis of biliary cytology specimens. The system utilizes six diagnostic categories that include nondiagnostic, negative for malignancy, atypical, benign neoplastic, other neoplastic, suspicious for malignancy, and malignant.

Ancillary Techniques for Enhancing Biopsy Diagnosis

FISH, molecular analysis, digital image analysis, and immunohistochemistry have been investigated to improve the suboptimal sensitivity for extrahepatic CCA in biliary brushing specimens [Table 8.3]. Apart from FISH, few are widely used in practice [75]. FISH for CCA is available as a commercial kit that evaluates pericentromeric regions of chromosomes 3, 7, 17, and band 9p21 in biliary brushing cytology [76]. Cells are evenly spread onto a slide which is then incubated with hybridization probes that correspond to the areas of interest. Each probe has a different fluorescent marker and the stained cells are analyzed under a fluorescence

Table 8.3 Performance characteristics of biliary brushing and ancillary techniques for the diagnosis of cholangiocarcinoma

Test	Sensitivity (%)	Specificity (%)
Routine cytology [81, 101–103]	20.1–56	89–100
Biopsy [2–4]	62–78	100
FISH [83, 103]	41–45	95–100
KRAS mutation testing [83, 102]	29–38	96–100
TP53 mutation testing [102]	42	100
Digital image analysis for aneuploidy [67, 101]	39–45	77–89
Routine cytology + FISH [103]	57	89
Routine cytology + *KRAS* [102]	83	91
Routine cytology + DIA [67]	42.9	77
FISH + KRAS mutation testing [83]	54	96
Cytology + next-generation sequencing [81, 104]	56	97
Cytology + next-generation sequencing + FISH [81, 104]	66–73	97–100

Abbreviations: *DIA* Digital image analysis, *FISH* fluorescence *in situ* hybridization, *KRAS* Kirsten rat sarcoma microscope. Aneuploidy or polysomy, which is defined as >2 copies in 2 or more probes, is considered a positive result if seen in more than 5 cells. FISH has a sensitivity of 34–52% for detecting malignancy in pancreatobiliary brushings [77]. The specificity of FISH is more variable and generally lower than cytology, reported at 89–100% [77, 78]. Combining FISH and cytology, particularly in equivocal cases, increases the sensitivity by roughly 20–30% in several studies without reducing specificity [79–81]. Digital image analysis for the detection of aneuploidy performs with a similar sensitivity to cytology and has high specificity [75].

Molecular techniques can enhance small biopsy diagnosis and potentially predict response to targeted therapy. For aiding diagnosis, testing is used in the context of the more prevalent genotypes of CCA at various anatomic sites. For extrahepatic CCA, the most common genetic alterations include *TP53* (47%), *KRAS* (37%), and *SMAD4* (30%) [82]. Options for molecular analysis on biliary brushings include single mutation testing or next-generation sequencing (NGS). *KRAS* testing is the most widely studied and reportedly increases the sensitivity of biliary brushing diagnostics to a degree roughly equivalent to the effect of combining cytology and FISH [83]. Limitations to *KRAS* testing include the lower prevalence of *KRAS* mutations in CCAs compared to pancreatic carcinomas and the fact that *KRAS* is an early genetic event in pancreatobiliary neoplasia and, therefore, the mutation can be detected in the absence of high-grade dysplasia or carcinoma [83–86].

There is less published experience with next-generation sequencing (NGS), but it seems to have similar sensitivity to FISH and equal specificity to cytology. NGS improves testing accuracy when used in combination with other methods [81]. An advantage of NGS is the possibility of testing cell-free DNA in exfoliative specimens [81]. One study showed combined NGS and cytology results achieved a sensitivity of 76%, elevated from 67% sensitivity of cytology alone, but it should be noted both suspicious and positive diagnoses were considered positive [81, 87]. An emerging technique is to perform NGS on the residual supernatant fluid after centrifugation of a liquid-based specimen [88].

For intrahepatic CCA, the most common mutations and prevalence estimates are *IDH1/2* (12–30%), *BAP1* (20–32%), *ARID1A* (20%), *TP53* (20%), PBRM1 (20%), and *FGFR2* rearrangements (14%) [89–91]. The hotspot mutation for IDH1 p.R132X is rarely seen in other epithelial neoplasms in the differential diagnosis, including extrahepatic CCA. A caveat is that rare HCCs have been reported with this mutation [90]. Histological features such as plump eosinophilic cells may suggest the genotype [92]. Currently there is no surrogate immunohistochemical testing available for the *IDH1* mutations found in CCA. Because intrahepatic CCAs are often amenable to core biopsies, sequencing of cytology aspirates is not commonly performed.

Several immunohistochemical markers have been reported to improve the sensitivity of biopsy and/or cytology for the diagnosis of extrahepatic CCA, such as S100 (expression), IMP3 (expression), pVHL (loss), CD10 (loss), SMAD4 (loss), Claudin-18 (expression), Maspin (expression), methionyl-tRNA synthetase 1 (expression), and p53 (expression), but published experience is limited, and these markers are not widely used in practice [93–99].

In summary, routine cytology and the ancillary techniques are all highly specific tests for CCA, but they are limited by low sensitivity such that negative results are of limited value. FISH is the most widely studied and utilized adjunct to cytology, while NGS is emerging to provide a similar improvement in test sensitivity and use in identification of patients eligible for targeted therapy.

Pathologic Grading and Staging

There is no specific grading system for CCA; most tumors are graded on a semiquantitative assessment of the proportion of tumor with gland formation. A tumor with ≥95% gland formation is well differentiated, between 50 and 95% gland formation is moderately differentiated, and less than 50% is poorly differentiated [100]. This system is similar to that of other gastrointestinal tumors. Pathologic staging of CCA is specific for tumors arising intrahepatic, extrahepatic, and distal bile duct as detailed by the Union for International Cancer Control eighth edition AJCC staging manual [100].

Conclusion

Routine histopathology and cytology remain the most definitive methods for diagnosing and classifying CCA. In resection specimens, histopathology provides not only the diagnosis but also crucial staging and prognostic parameters. In biopsies and aspirates, the technique and adequacy of tissue acquisition can have a significant impact on the sensitivity and specificity of the diagnosis. Well-established laboratory methods such as immunohistochemistry and *in situ* hybridization can provide valuable ancillary information to aid diagnosis, but pathologists and clinicians should be aware of existing caveats and limitations. Newer advances in molecular pathology and digital image analysis may become increasingly utilized in the near future and enhance clinical management.

References

1. Brugge W, Dewitt J, Klapman JB, Ashfaq R, Shidham V, Chhieng D, et al. Techniques for cytologic sampling of pancreatic and bile duct lesions. Diagn Cytopathol. 2014;42(4):333–7. https://doi.org/10.1002/dc.23096.
2. Kitajima Y, Ohara H, Nakazawa T, Ando T, Hayashi K, Takada H, et al. Usefulness of transpapillary bile duct brushing cytology and forceps biopsy for improved diagnosis in patients with biliary strictures. J Gastroenterol Hepatol. 2007;22(10):1615–20. https://doi.org/10.1111/j.1440-1746.2007.05037.x.

3. Jung GS, Huh JD, Lee SU, Han BH, Chang HK, Cho YD. Bile duct: analysis of percutaneous transluminal forceps biopsy in 130 patients suspected of having malignant biliary obstruction. Radiology. 2002;224(3):725–30. https://doi.org/10.1148/radiol.2242011501.
4. Gonzalez-Aguirre A, Covey AM, Brown KT, Brody LA, Boas FE, Sofocleous CT, et al. Comparison of biliary brush biopsy and fine needle biopsy in the diagnosis of biliary strictures. Minim Invasive Ther Allied Technol. 2018;27(5):278–83. https://doi.org/10.1080/13645706.2018.1427597.
5. Navaneethan U, Njei B, Lourdusamy V, Konjeti R, Vargo JJ, Parsi MA. Comparative effectiveness of biliary brush cytology and intraductal biopsy for detection of malignant biliary strictures: a systematic review and meta-analysis. Gastrointest Endosc. 2015;81(1):168–76. https://doi.org/10.1016/j.gie.2014.09.017.
6. Vadmal MS, Byrne-Semmelmeier S, Smilari TF, Hajdu SI. Biliary tract brush cytology. Acta Cytol. 2000;44(4):533–8. https://doi.org/10.1159/000328525.
7. Onoyama T, Matsumoto K, Takeda Y, Kawata S, Kurumi H, Koda H, et al. Endoscopic ultrasonography-guided fine needle aspiration for extrahepatic cholangiocarcinoma: a safe tissue sampling modality. J Clin Med. 2019;8(4):417. https://doi.org/10.3390/jcm8040417.
8. Jo JH, Cho CM, Jun JH, Chung MJ, Kim TH, Seo DW, et al. Same-session endoscopic ultrasound-guided fine needle aspiration and endoscopic retrograde cholangiopancreatography-based tissue sampling in suspected malignant biliary obstruction: a multicenter experience. J Gastroenterol Hepatol. 2019;34(4):799–805. https://doi.org/10.1111/jgh.14528.
9. Basturk O, Hong SM, Wood LD, Adsay NV, Albores-Saavedra J, Biankin AV, et al. A revised classification system and recommendations from the baltimore consensus meeting for neoplastic precursor lesions in the pancreas. Am J Surg Pathol. 2015;39(12):1730–41. https://doi.org/10.1097/PAS.0000000000000533.
10. Martins EB, Fleming KA, Garrido MC, Hine KR, Chapman RW. Superficial thrombophlebitis, dysplasia, and cholangiocarcinoma in primary sclerosing cholangitis. Gastroenterology. 1994;107(2):537–42. https://doi.org/10.1016/0016-5085(94)90182-1.
11. Lewis JT, Talwalkar JA, Rosen CB, Smyrk TC, Abraham SC. Precancerous bile duct pathology in end-stage primary sclerosing cholangitis, with and without cholangiocarcinoma. Am J Surg Pathol. 2010;34(1):27–34. https://doi.org/10.1097/PAS.0b013e3181bc96f9.
12. Bergquist A, Glaumann H, Stal P, Wang GS, Broome U. Biliary dysplasia, cell proliferation and nuclear DNA-fragmentation in primary sclerosing cholangitis with and without cholangiocarcinoma. J Intern Med. 2001;249(1):69–75. https://doi.org/10.1046/j.1365-2796.2001.00775.x.
13. Fleming KA, Boberg KM, Glaumann H, Bergquist A, Smith D, Clausen OP. Biliary dysplasia as a marker of cholangiocarcinoma in primary sclerosing cholangitis. J Hepatol. 2001;34(3):360–5. https://doi.org/10.1016/s0168-8278(00)00034-9.
14. Kerr SE, Barr Fritcher EG, Campion MB, Voss JS, Kipp BR, Halling KC, et al. Biliary dysplasia in primary sclerosing cholangitis harbors cytogenetic abnormalities similar to cholangiocarcinoma. Hum Pathol. 2014;45(9):1797–804. https://doi.org/10.1016/j.humpath.2014.05.008.
15. Hughes NR, Pairojkul C, Royce SG, Clouston A, Bhathal PS. Liver fluke-associated and sporadic cholangiocarcinoma: an immunohistochemical study of bile duct, peribiliary gland and tumour cell phenotypes. J Clin Pathol. 2006;59(10):1073–8. https://doi.org/10.1136/jcp.2005.033712.
16. Rocha FG, Lee H, Katabi N, RP DM, Fong Y, D'Angelica MI, et al. Intraductal papillary neoplasm of the bile duct: a biliary equivalent to intraductal papillary mucinous neoplasm of the pancreas? Hepatology. 2012;56(4):1352–60. https://doi.org/10.1002/hep.25786.
17. Yeh TS, Tseng JH, Chen TC, Liu NJ, Chiu CT, Jan YY, et al. Characterization of intrahepatic cholangiocarcinoma of the intraductal growth-type and its precursor lesions. Hepatology. 2005;42(3):657–64. https://doi.org/10.1002/hep.20837.

18. Nakanuma Y, Sato Y, Ojima H, Kanai Y, Aishima S, Yamamoto M, et al. Clinicopathological characterization of so-called "cholangiocarcinoma with intraductal papillary growth" with respect to "intraductal papillary neoplasm of bile duct (IPNB)". Int J Clin Exp Pathol. 2014;7(6):3112–22.
19. Fukumura Y, Nakanuma Y, Kakuda Y, Takase M, Yao T. Clinicopathological features of intraductal papillary neoplasms of the bile duct: a comparison with intraductal papillary mucinous neoplasm of the pancreas with reference to subtypes. Virchows Arch. 2017;471(1):65–76. https://doi.org/10.1007/s00428-017-2144-9.
20. Nakanuma Y, Jang KT, Fukushima N, Furukawa T, Hong SM, Kim H, et al. A statement by the Japan-Korea expert pathologists for future clinicopathological and molecular analyses toward consensus building of intraductal papillary neoplasm of the bile duct through several opinions at the present stage. J Hepatobiliary Pancreat Sci. 2018;25(3):181–7. https://doi.org/10.1002/jhbp.532.
21. Yang CY, Huang WJ, Tsai JH, Cheng A, Chen CC, Hsu HP, et al. Targeted next-generation sequencing identifies distinct clinicopathologic and molecular entities of intraductal papillary neoplasms of the bile duct. Mod Pathol. 2019;32(11):1637–45. https://doi.org/10.1038/s41379-019-0306-9.
22. Schlitter AM, Jang KT, Kloppel G, Saka B, Hong SM, Choi H, et al. Intraductal tubulopapillary neoplasms of the bile ducts: clinicopathologic, immunohistochemical, and molecular analysis of 20 cases. Mod Pathol. 2015;28(9):1249–64. https://doi.org/10.1038/modpathol.2015.61.
23. Quigley B, Reid MD, Pehlivanoglu B, Squires MH 3rd, Maithel S, Xue Y, et al. Hepatobiliary mucinous cystic neoplasms with ovarian type stroma (so-called "hepatobiliary cystadenoma/cystadenocarcinoma"): clinicopathologic analysis of 36 cases illustrates rarity of carcinomatous change. Am J Surg Pathol. 2018;42(1):95–102. https://doi.org/10.1097/PAS.0000000000000963.
24. Tumours of the gallbladder and extrahepatic bile ducts. In: Klimstra DS LA, Paradis V, Shirmacher P, editors. WHO classification of tumours: digestive system tumours. 5th ed: IARC; 2019. p. 265–94.
25. Komaya K, Ebata T, Shirai K, Ohira S, Morofuji N, Akutagawa A, et al. Recurrence after resection with curative intent for distal cholangiocarcinoma. Br J Surg. 2017;104(4):426–33. https://doi.org/10.1002/bjs.10452.
26. Mao K, Liu J, Sun J, Zhang J, Chen J, Pawlik TM, et al. Patterns and prognostic value of lymph node dissection for resected perihilar cholangiocarcinoma. J Gastroenterol Hepatol. 2016;31(2):417–26. https://doi.org/10.1111/jgh.13072.
27. Andrianello S, Paiella S, Allegrini V, Ramera M, Pulvirenti A, Malleo G, et al. Pancreaticoduodenectomy for distal cholangiocarcinoma: surgical results, prognostic factors, and long-term follow-up. Langenbeck's Arch Surg. 2015;400(5):623–8. https://doi.org/10.1007/s00423-015-1320-0.
28. Zhang XF, Squires MH 3rd, Bagante F, Ethun CG, Salem A, Weber SM, et al. The impact of intraoperative re-resection of a positive bile duct margin on clinical outcomes for hilar cholangiocarcinoma. Ann Surg Oncol. 2018;25(5):1140–9. https://doi.org/10.1245/s10434-018-6382-0.
29. Otsuka S, Ebata T, Yokoyama Y, Mizuno T, Tsukahara T, Shimoyama Y, et al. Clinical value of additional resection of a margin-positive distal bile duct in perihilar cholangiocarcinoma. Br J Surg. 2019;106(6):774–82. https://doi.org/10.1002/bjs.11125.
30. Shinohara K, Ebata T, Shimoyama Y, Mizuno T, Yokoyama Y, Yamaguchi J, et al. A study on radial margin status in resected perihilar cholangiocarcinoma. Ann Surg. 2019; https://doi.org/10.1097/SLA.0000000000003305.
31. Wellner UF, Shen Y, Keck T, Jin W, Xu Z. The survival outcome and prognostic factors for distal cholangiocarcinoma following surgical resection: a meta-analysis for the 5-year survival. Surg Today. 2017;47(3):271–9. https://doi.org/10.1007/s00595-016-1362-0.

32. Chuang SC, Lee KT, Tsai KB, Sheen PC, Nagai E, Mizumoto K, et al. Immunohistochemical study of DPC4 and p53 proteins in gallbladder and bile duct cancers. World J Surg. 2004;28(10):995–1000. https://doi.org/10.1007/s00268-004-7447-8.
33. Argani P, Shaukat A, Kaushal M, Wilentz RE, Su GH, Sohn TA, et al. Differing rates of loss of DPC4 expression and of p53 overexpression among carcinomas of the proximal and distal bile ducts. Cancer. 2001;91(7):1332–41.
34. Nakazawa T, Naitoh I, Hayashi K, Okumura F, Miyabe K, Yoshida M, et al. Diagnostic criteria for IgG4-related sclerosing cholangitis based on cholangiographic classification. J Gastroenterol. 2012;47(1):79–87. https://doi.org/10.1007/s00535-011-0465-z.
35. Nakazawa T, Naitoh I, Hayashi K, Miyabe K, Simizu S, Joh T. Diagnosis of IgG4-related sclerosing cholangitis. World J Gastroenterol. 2013;19(43):7661–70. https://doi.org/10.3748/wjg.v19.i43.7661.
36. Deshpande V, Sainani NI, Chung RT, Pratt DS, Mentha G, Rubbia-Brandt L, et al. IgG4-associated cholangitis: a comparative histological and immunophenotypic study with primary sclerosing cholangitis on liver biopsy material. Mod Pathol. 2009;22(10):1287–95. https://doi.org/10.1038/modpathol.2009.94.
37. Tumours of the liver and intrahepatic bile ducts. In: Paradis V FM, Park YN, Schirmacher P, editors. WHO classification of tumours: digestive system tumours. 5th ed: IARC; 2019. p. 217–64.
38. Sigel CS, Drill E, Zhou Y, Basturk O, Askan G, Pak LM, et al. Intrahepatic cholangiocarcinomas have histologically and immunophenotypically distinct small and large duct patterns. Am J Surg Pathol. 2018;42(10):1334–45. https://doi.org/10.1097/PAS.0000000000001118.
39. Komuta M, Govaere O, Vandecaveye V, Akiba J, Van Steenbergen W, Verslype C, et al. Histological diversity in cholangiocellular carcinoma reflects the different cholangiocyte phenotypes. Hepatology. 2012;55(6):1876–88. https://doi.org/10.1002/hep.25595.
40. Nakanuma Y, Sato Y, Ikeda H, Harada K, Kobayashi M, Sano K, et al. Intrahepatic cholangiocarcinoma with predominant "ductal plate malformation" pattern: a new subtype. Am J Surg Pathol. 2012;36(11):1629–35. https://doi.org/10.1097/PAS.0b013e31826e0249.
41. Balitzer D, Joseph NM, Ferrell L, Shafizadeh N, Jain D, Zhang X, et al. Immunohistochemical and molecular features of cholangiolocellular carcinoma are similar to well-differentiated intrahepatic cholangiocarcinoma. Mod Pathol. 2019;32(10):1486–94. https://doi.org/10.1038/s41379-019-0290-0.
42. Tsokos CG, Krings G, Yilmaz F, Ferrell LD, Gill RM. Proliferative index facilitates distinction between benign biliary lesions and intrahepatic cholangiocarcinoma. Hum Pathol. 2016;57:61–7. https://doi.org/10.1016/j.humpath.2016.06.019.
43. Sasaki M, Matsubara T, Kakuda Y, Sato Y, Nakanuma Y. Immunostaining for polycomb group protein EZH2 and senescent marker p16INK4a may be useful to differentiate cholangiolocellular carcinoma from ductular reaction and bile duct adenoma. Am J Surg Pathol. 2014;38(3):364–9. https://doi.org/10.1097/PAS.0000000000000125.
44. Hatano M, Ojima H, Masugi Y, Tsujikawa H, Hiraoka N, Kanai Y, et al. Steatotic and nonsteatotic scirrhous hepatocellular carcinomas reveal distinct clinicopathological features. Hum Pathol. 2019;86:222–32. https://doi.org/10.1016/j.humpath.2018.11.024.
45. Okamura N, Yoshida M, Shibuya A, Sugiura H, Okayasu I, Ohbu M. Cellular and stromal characteristics in the scirrhous hepatocellular carcinoma: comparison with hepatocellular carcinomas and intrahepatic cholangiocarcinomas. Pathol Int. 2005;55(11):724–31. https://doi.org/10.1111/j.1440-1827.2005.01891.x.
46. Brackett DG, Neyaz A, Arora K, Masia R, Mattia A, Zukerberg L, et al. Cholangiolar pattern and albumin in situ hybridisation enable a diagnosis of intrahepatic cholangiocarcinoma. J Clin Pathol. 2020;73(1):23–9. https://doi.org/10.1136/jclinpath-2019-206055.
47. Brunt EM, Paradis V, Sempoux C, Theise ND. Biphenotypic (hepatobiliary) primary liver carcinomas: the work in progress. Hepat Oncol. 2015;2(3):255–73. https://doi.org/10.2217/hep.15.8.

48. Brunt E, Aishima S, Clavien PA, Fowler K, Goodman Z, Gores G, et al. cHCC-CCA: consensus terminology for primary liver carcinomas with both hepatocytic and cholangiocytic differentiation. Hepatology. 2018;68(1):113–26. https://doi.org/10.1002/hep.29789.
49. Lee SH, Lee JS, Na GH, You YK, Kim DG. Immunohistochemical markers for hepatocellular carcinoma prognosis after liver resection and liver transplantation. Clin Transpl. 2017;31(1):e12852. https://doi.org/10.1111/ctr.12852.
50. Geramizadeh B, Seirfar N. Diagnostic value of arginase-1 and glypican-3 in differential diagnosis of hepatocellular carcinoma, cholangiocarcinoma and metastatic carcinoma of liver. Hepat Mon. 2015;15(7):e30336. https://doi.org/10.5812/hepatmon30336v2.
51. Radwan NA, Ahmed NS. The diagnostic value of arginase-1 immunostaining in differentiating hepatocellular carcinoma from metastatic carcinoma and cholangiocarcinoma as compared to HepPar-1. Diagn Pathol. 2012;7:149. https://doi.org/10.1186/1746-1596-7-149.
52. Lau SK, Prakash S, Geller SA, Alsabeh R. Comparative immunohistochemical profile of hepatocellular carcinoma, cholangiocarcinoma, and metastatic adenocarcinoma. Hum Pathol. 2002;33(12):1175–81. https://doi.org/10.1053/hupa.2002.130104.
53. Surrey LF, Frank R, Zhang PJ, Furth EE. TTF-1 and Napsin-A are expressed in a subset of cholangiocarcinomas arising from the gallbladder and hepatic ducts: continued caveats for utilization of immunohistochemistry panels. Am J Surg Pathol. 2014;38(2):224–7. https://doi.org/10.1097/PAS.0000000000000138.
54. Lino-Silva LS, Salcedo-Hernandez RA, Garcia-Gomez MA, Ruiz-Garcia EB, Aguilar-Romero JM, Dominguez-Rodriguez JA, et al. Thyroid transcription factor-1 expression in adenocarcinomas of the bile duct. Int J Surg Pathol. 2016;24(1):24–8. https://doi.org/10.1177/1066896915603121.
55. Conner JR, Hornick JL. Metastatic carcinoma of unknown primary: diagnostic approach using immunohistochemistry. Adv Anat Pathol. 2015;22(3):149–67. https://doi.org/10.1097/PAP.0000000000000069.
56. Tang H, Wang Z, Lv W, Meng X. The expression and clinicopathological role of CDX2 in intrahepatic cholangiocarcinoma. Intractable Rare Dis Res. 2018;7(2):106–11. https://doi.org/10.5582/irdr.2018.01047.
57. Liu F, Gao Z, Shen D, Zhao H, Wang C, Ye Y, et al. Significance of SATB2 expression in colon cancer and its differential diagnosis in digestive tract adenocarcinoma and ovarian primary and metastatic carcinoma. Pathol Res Pract. 2019;215(7):152430. https://doi.org/10.1016/j.prp.2019.04.022.
58. Nash JW, Morrison C, Frankel WL. The utility of estrogen receptor and progesterone receptor immunohistochemistry in the distinction of metastatic breast carcinoma from other tumors in the liver. Arch Pathol Lab Med. 2003;127(12):1591–5. https://doi.org/10.1043/1543-2165(2003)127<1591:TUOERA>2.0.CO;2.
59. Wei S, Said-Al-Naief N, Hameed O. Estrogen and progesterone receptor expression is not always specific for mammary and gynecologic carcinomas: a tissue microarray and pooled literature review study. Appl Immunohistochem Mol Morphol. 2009;17(5):393–402. https://doi.org/10.1097/PAI.0b013e31819faa07.
60. Agostini-Vulaj D, Bratton LE, Dunne RF, JMM C, Zhou Z, Findeis-Hosey JJ, et al. Incidence and significance of GATA3 positivity in pancreatic ductal adenocarcinoma and cholangiocarcinoma. Appl Immunohistochem Mol Morphol. 2019; https://doi.org/10.1097/PAI.0000000000000764.
61. Rhee H, Ko JE, Chung T, Jee BA, Kwon SM, Nahm JH, et al. Transcriptomic and histopathological analysis of cholangiolocellular differentiation trait in intrahepatic cholangiocarcinoma. Liver Int. 2018;38(1):113–24. https://doi.org/10.1111/liv.13492.
62. Akita M, Fujikura K, Ajiki T, Fukumoto T, Otani K, Azuma T, et al. Dichotomy in intrahepatic cholangiocarcinomas based on histologic similarities to hilar cholangiocarcinomas. Mod Pathol. 2017;30(7):986–97. https://doi.org/10.1038/modpathol.2017.22.

63. Nasir A, Lehrke HD, Mounajjed T, Said S, Zhang L, Yasir S, et al. Albumin in situ hybridization can be positive in adenocarcinomas and other tumors from diverse sites. Am J Clin Pathol. 2019;152(2):190–9. https://doi.org/10.1093/ajcp/aqz032.
64. Askan G, Deshpande V, Klimstra DS, Adsay V, Sigel C, Shia J, et al. Expression of markers of hepatocellular differentiation in pancreatic acinar cell neoplasms: a potential diagnostic pitfall. Am J Clin Pathol. 2016;146(2):163–9. https://doi.org/10.1093/ajcp/aqw096.
65. Lin F, Shi J, Wang HL, Ma XJ, Monroe R, Luo Y, et al. Detection of albumin expression by RNA in situ hybridization is a sensitive and specific method for identification of hepatocellular carcinomas and intrahepatic cholangiocarcinomas. Am J Clin Pathol. 2018;150(1):58–64. https://doi.org/10.1093/ajcp/aqy030.
66. Retracted. Histopathology. 2019; https://doi.org/10.1111/his.14046.
67. Baron TH, Harewood GC, Rumalla A, Pochron NL, Stadheim LM, Gores GJ, et al. A prospective comparison of digital image analysis and routine cytology for the identification of malignancy in biliary tract strictures. Clin Gastroenterol Hepatol. 2004;2(3):214–9. https://doi.org/10.1016/s1542-3565(04)00006-0.
68. Cohen MB, Wittchow RJ, Johlin FC, Bottles K, Raab SS. Brush cytology of the extrahepatic biliary tract: comparison of cytologic features of adenocarcinoma and benign biliary strictures. Mod Pathol. 1995;8(5):498–502.
69. Renshaw AA, Madge R, Jiroutek M, Granter SR. Bile duct brushing cytology: statistical analysis of proposed diagnostic criteria. Am J Clin Pathol. 1998;110(5):635–40. https://doi.org/10.1093/ajcp/110.5.635.
70. Avadhani V, Hacihasanoglu E, Memis B, Pehlivanoglu B, Hanley KZ, Krishnamurti U, et al. Cytologic predictors of malignancy in bile duct brushings: a multi-reviewer analysis of 60 cases. Mod Pathol. 2017;30(9):1273–86. https://doi.org/10.1038/modpathol.2017.51.
71. Heath JE, Goicochea LB, Staats PN. Biliary stent-related alterations can be distinguished from adenocarcinoma on bile duct brushings using a limited number of cytologic features. J Am Soc Cytopathol. 2015;4(5):282–9. https://doi.org/10.1016/j.jasc.2015.06.006.
72. Trikudanathan G, Navaneethan U, Njei B, Vargo JJ, Parsi MA. Diagnostic yield of bile duct brushings for cholangiocarcinoma in primary sclerosing cholangitis: a systematic review and meta-analysis. Gastrointest Endosc. 2014;79(5):783–9. https://doi.org/10.1016/j.gie.2013.09.015.
73. Goyal A, Sharaiha RZ, Alperstein SA, Siddiqui MT. Cytologic diagnosis of adenocarcinoma on bile duct brushings in the presence of stent associated changes: a retrospective analysis. Diagn Cytopathol. 2018;46(10):826–32. https://doi.org/10.1002/dc.24052.
74. Pitman MB, Layfield LJ. The papanicolaou society of cytopathology system for reporting pancreaticobiliary cytology. Cham: Springer; 2015.
75. Layfield L. Role of ancillary techniques in biliary cytopathology specimens. Acta Cytol. 2020;64(1–2):175–81. https://doi.org/10.1159/000498976.
76. Gonda TA, Glick MP, Sethi A, Poneros JM, Palmas W, Iqbal S, et al. Polysomy and p16 deletion by fluorescence in situ hybridization in the diagnosis of indeterminate biliary strictures. Gastrointest Endosc. 2012;75(1):74–9. https://doi.org/10.1016/j.gie.2011.08.022.
77. Barr Fritcher EG, Kipp BR, Halling KC, Clayton AC. FISHing for pancreatobiliary tract malignancy in endoscopic brushings enhances the sensitivity of routine cytology. Cytopathology. 2014;25(5):288–301. https://doi.org/10.1111/cyt.12170.
78. Kipp BR, Stadheim LM, Halling SA, Pochron NL, Harmsen S, Nagorney DM, et al. A comparison of routine cytology and fluorescence in situ hybridization for the detection of malignant bile duct strictures. Am J Gastroenterol. 2004;99(9):1675–81. https://doi.org/10.1111/j.1572-0241.2004.30281.x.
79. Brooks C, Gausman V, Kokoy-Mondragon C, Munot K, Amin SP, Desai A, et al. Role of fluorescent in situ hybridization, cholangioscopic biopsies, and EUS-FNA in the evaluation of biliary strictures. Dig Dis Sci. 2018;63(3):636–44. https://doi.org/10.1007/s10620-018-4906-x.
80. von Seth E, Ouchterlony H, Dobra K, Hjerpe A, Arnelo U, Haas S, et al. Diagnostic performance of a stepwise cytological algorithm for biliary malignancy in primary sclerosing cholangitis. Liver Int. 2019;39(2):382–8. https://doi.org/10.1111/liv.14007.

81. Kushnir VM, Mullady DK, Das K, Lang G, Hollander TG, Murad FM, et al. The diagnostic yield of malignancy comparing cytology, fish, and molecular analysis of cell free cytology brush supernatant in patients with biliary strictures undergoing endoscopic retrograde cholangiography (ERC): a prospective study. J Clin Gastroenterol. 2019;53(9):686–92. https://doi.org/10.1097/MCG.0000000000001118.
82. Lowery MA, Ptashkin R, Jordan E, Berger MF, Zehir A, Capanu M, et al. Comprehensive molecular profiling of intrahepatic and extrahepatic cholangiocarcinomas: potential targets for intervention. Clin Cancer Res. 2018;24(17):4154–61. https://doi.org/10.1158/1078-0432.CCR-18-0078.
83. Kipp BR, Fritcher EG, Clayton AC, Gores GJ, Roberts LR, Zhang J, et al. Comparison of KRAS mutation analysis and FISH for detecting pancreatobiliary tract cancer in cytology specimens collected during endoscopic retrograde cholangiopancreatography. J Mol Diagn. 2010;12(6):780–6. https://doi.org/10.2353/jmoldx.2010.100016.
84. Sturm PD, Rauws EA, Hruban RH, Caspers E, Ramsoekh TB, Huibregtse K, et al. Clinical value of K-ras codon 12 analysis and endobiliary brush cytology for the diagnosis of malignant extrahepatic bile duct stenosis. Clin Cancer Res. 1999;5(3):629–35.
85. Schlitter AM, Born D, Bettstetter M, Specht K, Kim-Fuchs C, Riener MO, et al. Intraductal papillary neoplasms of the bile duct: stepwise progression to carcinoma involves common molecular pathways. Mod Pathol. 2014;27(1):73–86. https://doi.org/10.1038/modpathol.2013.112.
86. Abraham SC, Lee JH, Hruban RH, Argani P, Furth EE, Wu TT. Molecular and immunohistochemical analysis of intraductal papillary neoplasms of the biliary tract. Hum Pathol. 2003;34(9):902–10. https://doi.org/10.1016/s0046-8177(03)00337-x.
87. Dudley JC, Zheng Z, McDonald T, Le LP D-SD, Borger D, et al. Next-generation sequencing and fluorescence in situ hybridization have comparable performance characteristics in the analysis of pancreaticobiliary brushings for malignancy. J Mol Diagn. 2016;18(1):124–30. https://doi.org/10.1016/j.jmoldx.2015.08.002.
88. Harbhajanka A, Michael CW, Janaki N, Gokozan HN, Wasman J, Bomeisl P, et al. Tiny but mighty: use of next generation sequencing on discarded cytocentrifuged bile duct brushing specimens to increase sensitivity of cytological diagnosis. Modern Pathol Off J U S Can Acad Pathol Inc. 2020; https://doi.org/10.1038/s41379-020-0577-1.
89. Jiao Y, Pawlik TM, Anders RA, Selaru FM, Streppel MM, Lucas DJ, et al. Exome sequencing identifies frequent inactivating mutations in BAP1, ARID1A and PBRM1 in intrahepatic cholangiocarcinomas. Nat Genet. 2013;45(12):1470–3. https://doi.org/10.1038/ng.2813.
90. Farshidfar F, Zheng S, Gingras MC, Newton Y, Shih J, Robertson AG, et al. Integrative genomic analysis of cholangiocarcinoma identifies distinct IDH-mutant molecular profiles. Cell Rep. 2017;18(11):2780–94. https://doi.org/10.1016/j.celrep.2017.02.033.
91. Boscoe AN, Rolland C, Kelley RK. Frequency and prognostic significance of isocitrate dehydrogenase 1 mutations in cholangiocarcinoma: a systematic literature review. J Gastrointest Oncol. 2019;10(4):751–65. https://doi.org/10.21037/jgo.2019.03.10.
92. Wang T, Drill E, Vakiani E, Pak LM, Boerner T, Askan G, et al. Distinct histomorphological features are associated with IDH1 mutation in intrahepatic cholangiocarcinoma. Hum Pathol. 2019;91:19–25. https://doi.org/10.1016/j.humpath.2019.05.002.
93. Levy M, Lin F, Xu H, Dhall D, Spaulding BO, Wang HL. S100P, von Hippel-Lindau gene product, and IMP3 serve as a useful immunohistochemical panel in the diagnosis of adenocarcinoma on endoscopic bile duct biopsy. Hum Pathol. 2010;41(9):1210–9. https://doi.org/10.1016/j.humpath.2010.01.014.
94. Tokumitsu T, Sato Y, Yamashita A, Moriguchi-Goto S, Kondo K, Nanashima A, et al. Immunocytochemistry for Claudin-18 and Maspin in biliary brushing cytology increases the accuracy of diagnosing pancreatobiliary malignancies. Cytopathology. 2017;28(2):116–21. https://doi.org/10.1111/cyt.12368.
95. Chen L, Huang K, Himmelfarb EA, Zhai J, Lai JP, Lin F, et al. Diagnostic value of maspin in distinguishing adenocarcinoma from benign biliary epithelium on endoscopic bile duct biopsy. Hum Pathol. 2015;46(11):1647–54. https://doi.org/10.1016/j.humpath.2015.07.005.

96. Kanzawa M, Sanuki T, Onodera M, Fujikura K, Itoh T, Zen Y. Double immunostaining for maspin and p53 on cell blocks increases the diagnostic value of biliary brushing cytology. Pathol Int. 2017;67(2):91–8. https://doi.org/10.1111/pin.12505.
97. Ieni A, Todaro P, Crino SF, Barresi V, Tuccari G. Endoscopic ultrasound-guided fine-needle aspiration cytology in pancreaticobiliary carcinomas: diagnostic efficacy of cell-block immunocytochemistry. Hepatobiliary Pancreat Dis Int. 2015;14(3):305–12. https://doi.org/10.1016/s1499-3872(15)60367-8.
98. Tretiakova M, Antic T, Westerhoff M, Mueller J, Himmelfarb EA, Wang HL, et al. Diagnostic utility of CD10 in benign and malignant extrahepatic bile duct lesions. Am J Surg Pathol. 2012;36(1):101–8. https://doi.org/10.1097/PAS.0b013e31822fbc95.
99. Jang SI, Kwon NH, Lim BJ, Nahm JH, Park JS, Kang CM, et al. New staining method using methionyl-tRNA synthetase 1 antibody for brushing cytology of bile duct cancer. Gastrointest Endosc. 2019; https://doi.org/10.1016/j.gie.2019.12.017.
100. Edge SB, American Joint Committee on Cancer. AJCC cancer staging manual. 8th ed. New York: Springer; 2017.
101. Fritcher EG, Kipp BR, Halling KC, Oberg TN, Bryant SC, Tarrell RF, et al. A multivariable model using advanced cytologic methods for the evaluation of indeterminate pancreatobiliary strictures. Gastroenterology. 2009;136(7):2180–6. https://doi.org/10.1053/j.gastro.2009.02.040.
102. Huang P, Zhang H, Zhang XF, Zhang X, Lyu W, Fan Z. Evaluation of intraductal ultrasonography, endoscopic brush cytology and K-ras, P53 gene mutation in the early diagnosis of malignant bile duct stricture. Chin Med J. 2015;128(14):1887–92. https://doi.org/10.4103/0366-6999.160508.
103. Kaura K, Sawas T, Bazerbachi F, Storm AC, Martin JA, Gores GJ, et al. Cholangioscopy biopsies improve detection of cholangiocarcinoma when combined with cytology and FISH, but not in patients with PSC. Dig Dis Sci. 2019; https://doi.org/10.1007/s10620-019-05866-2.
104. Gonda TA, Viterbo D, Gausman V, Kipp C, Sethi A, Poneros JM, et al. Mutation profile and fluorescence in situ hybridization analyses increase detection of malignancies in biliary strictures. Clin Gastroenterol Hepatol. 2017;15(6):913–9 e1. https://doi.org/10.1016/j.cgh.2016.12.013.

Chapter 9
Challenges in Diagnosing Cholangiocarcinoma: Pulling Together Biochemical, Radiological, and Cytopathological Data

S. Franssen, D. M. de Jong, L. M. J. W. van Driel, and B. Groot Koerkamp

Abbreviations

ACUP	Adenocarcinoma of unknown primary
AFP	Alpha-fetoprotein
AJCC	American Joint Committee on Cancer
ALP	Alkaline phosphatase
ALT	Alanine transaminase
AST	Aspartate aminotransferase
BAP	Biofilm-associated protein
CA19.9	Carbohydrate antigen 19.9
CCA	Cholangiocarcinoma
CD10	Cluster of differentiation 10
CEA	Carcinoembryonic antigen
CT	Computed tomography
dCCA	Distal cholangiocarcinoma
ELISA	Enzyme-linked immunosorbent assay
ER	Estrogen receptor
ERCP	Endoscopic retrograde cholangiopancreatography
EUS	Endoscopic ultrasound
FISH	Fluorescence in situ hybridization
FNA	Fine needle aspiration

S. Franssen and D. M. de Jong contributed equally with all other contributors.

S. Franssen · B. Groot Koerkamp (✉)
Department of Surgery, Erasmus MC Cancer Institute, Rotterdam, The Netherlands
e-mail: s.franssen@erasmusmc.nl; b.grootkoerkamp@erasmusmc.nl

D. M. de Jong · L. M. J. W. van Driel
Department of Gastroenterology and Hepatology, Erasmus MC, Rotterdam, The Netherlands
e-mail: d.m.dejong@erasmusmc.nl; l.m.j.w.vandriel@erasmusmc.nl

J. H. Tabibian (ed.), *Diagnosis and Management of Cholangiocarcinoma*,
https://doi.org/10.1007/978-3-030-70936-5_9

GATA-3	GATA binding protein 3
GGT	Gamma-glutamyl transferase
HCC	Hepatocellular carcinoma
HepPar-1	Hepatocyte-specific antigen
HES	Hypereosinophilic syndrome
iCCA	Intrahepatic cholangiocarcinoma
IgG4	Immunoglobulin G4
LI-RADS	Liver Imaging Reporting and Data System
MRCP	Magnetic resonance cholangiopancreatography
MRI	Magnetic resonance imaging
NGS	Next-generation sequencing
PAX-8	Paired box gene 8
pCCA	Perihilar cholangiocarcinoma
PDAC	Pancreatic ductal adenocarcinoma
PET	Positron emission tomography
SUV	Standardized uptake value
TTF-1	Thyroid transcription factor 1

Introduction

The previous chapters in this book have focused on one of the three main diagnostic modalities for CCA: biochemical (Chap. 6), imaging (Chap. 7), and pathological (Chap. 8). In the present chapter, we discuss how these three modalities come together in the diagnostic work-up of patients with a suspicion of CCA, with a focus on important pitfalls.

The aim of the diagnostic work-up of CCA is efficient diagnosis and staging of the disease to guide subsequent management. This work-up presents several challenges. The first diagnostic challenge is that CCA involves three disease entities that differ in genomic alterations, signs, and symptoms; intrahepatic (iCCA), perihilar (pCCA), and distal cholangiocarcinoma (dCCA). Therefore, they each have their own diagnostic approaches and AJCC staging system (Chap. 8). Moreover, distinguishing these different entities is important to guide proper management. The main aspect they share is that they all arise from the epithelial lining of the biliary tree, albeit in different anatomical locations: iCCA arises upstream from the second-order biliary ducts, then pCCA until the origin of the cystic duct, and then dCCA until the ampulla. These boundaries are ambiguous, and at the interface the diagnoses cannot be discerned with certainty.

The second challenge is that a definitive diagnosis can only be made with pathological evaluation. This, in itself, comprises two challenges. Firstly, for most other cancers, it is straightforward to obtain tissue, because they are mostly large and have easy access for tissue acquisition. pCCA and dCCA, however, are mostly small lesions with periductal growth (rather than mass-forming) and are difficult to visualize and biopsy. Despite the effort to obtain enough tissue by means of brushing, intraductal biopsies, and/or endoscopic ultrasound (EUS)-guided fine needle aspiration (FNA), sensitivity does not exceed 74% (Chap. 8). Secondly, even when enough tissue has been obtained, the pathological evaluation can be challenging. For example, iCCA is the only CCA that is typically large and mass-forming, but at pathological evaluation, iCCA may be difficult to distinguish from hepatocellular carcinoma (HCC) or metastatic disease (e.g., pancreatic cancer).

The third challenge is that several nonmalignant diseases can masquerade as CCA. For example, a dominant stricture in primary sclerosing cholangitis (PSC) can be benign or due to pCCA (or dCCA) [1–6]. After repeated failed attempts of pathological confirmation, the suspicion of CCA can remain high enough to justify resection. Therefore, approximately 5–10% of patients undergo a major hepatic or pancreatic resection for a disease that may turn out to be benign at pathological assessment of the resected specimen [7].

In this chapter we first discuss the current standard diagnostic work-up of iCCA, pCCA, and dCCA. The focus of the chapter is thereafter on the challenges of the diagnostic work-up. These challenges are illustrated with case presentations.

Standard Diagnostic Work-Up

The aim of the diagnostic work-up is to confidently diagnose and stage the disease in order to guide subsequent treatment. Staging should distinguish patients with (borderline) resectable, locally advanced (i.e., unresectable), and metastatic disease. Patients with (borderline) resectable CCA are considered for curative-intent resection, patients with locally advanced disease for systemic treatment (palliative and sometimes for induction) or locoregional treatments, and patients with metastatic disease for palliative systemic treatment.

iCCA

Patients with iCCA mostly present with nonspecific abdominal complaints and weight loss. Approximately 15% of iCCA patients present with jaundice, because the tumor is growing toward the liver hilum. Carbohydrate antigen (CA) 19.9 is elevated in most patients, and about 5% of patients have elevated alpha-fetoprotein (AFP) above 200 ng/mL [8]. At imaging, one or multiple lesions are seen in the liver. Multiple lesions can involve a single large lesion with smaller nearby satellites or several lesions spread across the liver. Computed tomography (CT) imaging demonstrates peripheral enhancement of the lesions with subsequent central filling (Chap. 7). CT of the abdomen and chest can detect nodal and distant metastases (e.g., lung and peritoneum). Enlarged locoregional lymph nodes can be present in the hepatoduodenal and gastrohepatic ligament. More distant lymph nodes (e.g., aortocaval) represent metastatic disease (stage IV) [9]. Magnetic resonance imaging (MRI) is unlikely to change management based on CT. A positron emission tomography (PET) scan is not part of the standard work-up but may detect metastatic disease in some patients [10]. Imaging can generally distinguish iCCA from HCC. The other differential diagnosis of iCCA is metastatic disease with primary tumors in the colon, esophagus, stomach, pancreas, and breast. Upper and lower endoscopy and mammography are recommended if imaging is not consistent with iCCA [11, 12].

A solitary lesion of iCCA is resectable if a margin-negative resection is anticipated with an adequate liver remnant volume (Chap. 14). Selected patients with two or three lesions can also be considered for resection. A biopsy is unlikely to change management if presentation and imaging are consistent with iCCA. Most patients have locally advanced or metastatic disease. These patients should undergo biopsy if they are eligible for locoregional or systemic treatment. Pathological examination of iCCA is difficult, as no pathognomonic immunohistochemistry markers are available (Chap. 8). The diagnosis is mainly made by ruling out HCC and metastatic disease. Historically, iCCA has often been mislabeled as adenocarcinoma of unknown primary (ACUP). Sometime iCCA is detected incidentally in patients with liver cirrhosis who undergo surveillance for early detection of HCC. These lesions tend to be small and can be difficult to distinguish from HCC.

pCCA

Patients with pCCA mostly present with painless jaundice and often weight loss. Blood tests generally show elevated bilirubin, except in the earliest of stages. Ultrasound shows dilated intrahepatic bile ducts, and sometimes a mass can be visualized in the liver hilum. The extrahepatic bile duct and gallbladder are not distended, contrary to distal bile duct obstruction in dCCA and pancreatic cancer. CT of the abdomen may show a small mass (typically less than 3 cm) at the confluence of the left and right bile duct, with proximal biliary dilatation. Masses larger than 3 cm mostly represent iCCA or metastases that have grown toward the liver hilum. CT of the chest is performed to rule out metastatic disease. Patients with metastatic disease may have metastases in the liver, lung, peritoneum, or lymph nodes beyond the hepatoduodenal ligament (e.g., aortocaval). PET scans may detect otherwise occult metastatic disease in a small percentage of patients but are not routinely recommended.

Analogous to iCCA, pCCA is resectable if a complete resection with adequate future liver remnant appears feasible. Resectability of pCCA depends on biliary extension of the tumor, as defined by the Bismuth classification [13]. Resectability also depends on vascular involvement; portal vein reconstruction may be required for a margin-negative resection. Hepatic artery reconstruction is less commonly performed as it increases surgical risk and has worse long-term survival. While CT appears more reliable to assess vascular involvement, magnetic resonance cholangiopancreatography (MRCP) provides superior delineation of the extent of biliary involvement.

Most patients require biliary drainage prior to resection or systemic treatment. An intraductal brushing or biopsy should be performed at the time of drainage but has a sensitivity below 74%, even when adding FISH or NGS (Chap. 8). Percutaneous biliary drainage should be avoided in patients eligible for liver transplantation, because it may cause seeding along the biopsy tract [14]. The differential diagnosis includes several nonmalignant diseases such as IgG4-mediated cholangitis and stone disease [7]. Presentation and imaging may provide clues for the likelihood of benign disease.

It is important to complete all imaging prior to biliary drainage, as stents distort imaging [15]. Surgical resection is sometimes performed in the absence of pathological confirmation of cancer, [7] in particular when presentation and imaging are highly suspicious for pCCA. Metastatic disease (e.g., intrahepatic metastases) should be confirmed by biopsy to avoid withholding surgery for distant lesions that may appear malignant but are in fact benign.

dCCA

Patients with dCCA typically present with painless jaundice and weight loss. Serum bilirubin level is elevated. Ultrasound and CT demonstrate dilated intra- and extrahepatic bile ducts and a distended gallbladder, without an obvious mass in the head of the pancreas. CT may also demonstrate an intraductal mass, stricture, or enhancing wall thickening. CT of the abdomen and chest can detect distant metastatic disease (i.e., in the liver, lungs, or peritoneum). Most patients, however, do not have metastatic disease at presentation, because a small dCCA quickly causes jaundice, thereby prompting clinical evaluation. MRI and PET have no substantial impact on diagnosis and staging of dCCA.

An intraductal brushing or biopsy to confirm malignancy can be performed with endoscopic retrograde cholangiopancreatography (ERCP) (or percutaneously when ERCP is not feasible). However, sensitivity of a brushing is below 50% and of an intraductal biopsy no more than 75% (Chap. 8). Results of such specimens may repeatedly come back as negative or inconclusive. Moreover, ERCP is an invasive procedure with a 3–8% risk of pancreatitis, in addition to other potential adverse events [16]. EUS with FNA is a good alternative for pathological confirmation in dCCA, with a comparably high sensitivity and specificity (82% and 88%) reported in some studies [17, 18]. Importantly, if cancer is highly likely based on presentation and imaging, it will remain (highly) likely even after an inconclusive brush or biopsy; therefore, an ERCP with brush or biopsy is only justified if biliary drainage is needed or if the multidisciplinary team agrees to withhold surgical resection if the pathology result comes back negative or inconclusive. With regard to the need for biliary drainage, most but not all dCCA patients will undergo ERCP and stent placement to relieve biliary obstruction, in particular if bilirubin is too high for immediate surgery (e.g., >15 mg/dL) or if surgery is infeasible within 1 or 2 weeks. However, fit patients with a very high suspicion of resectable dCCA have fewer complications if they undergo resection without prior biliary drainage [19]. For patients who are nonoperative candidates, pathological confirmation is generally considered a prerequisite prior to palliative systemic treatment.

The differential diagnosis of dCCA includes several nonmalignant diseases such as IgG4-mediated cholangitis and stone disease. Presentation and imaging may provide clues for the likelihood of benign disease. The distal bile duct is surrounded by the pancreas; pancreatic ductal adenocarcinoma arising close to the distal bile duct may thus be indistinguishable from dCCA. Even pathological examination cannot distinguish dCCA from pancreatic ductal adenocarcinoma (PDAC) with certainty. Both cancers, however, require the same surgical procedure (i.e., pancreatoduodenectomy). Preoperative certainty about the diagnosis is only relevant for patients with (borderline) resectable PDAC who may benefit from neoadjuvant chemotherapy.

EUS may play a role in lymph node staging [20]. EUS-guided biopsy of enlarged aortocaval lymph nodes, for example, may confirm distant metastatic disease. This will be further discussed in Chap. 13.

Case Presentations

Case 1: IgG4-Related Sclerosing Cholangitis

A 72-year-old male patient presented with pain, itching, and jaundice for 2 weeks. Blood tests revealed fluctuating but generally abnormal liver enzyme tests and a high bilirubin level (Table 9.1). CT and MRCP showed a mass at the biliary confluence and an enlarged hilar lymph node (Fig. 9.1a). The diagnosis of pCCA was

Table 9.1 Lab results at initial presentation, upon referral, and after start of treatment in a 72-year-old male presenting with pain, itching, and jaundice (case 1)

Lab results	Initial presentation	Referral	2 weeks after treatment	Normal value
AST	74	58	20	<35 U/L
ALT	126	85	35	<45 U/L
Total bilirubin	7.1	1.2	0.7	<1.0 mg/dL
ALP	339	227	93	<115 U/L
GGT	319	228	153	<55 U/L
CA19.9	30	18	20	<35 kU/L
Creatinine	139	161	126	65–115 μmol/L
IgG4	x	12	6.0	0.08–1.4 g/L

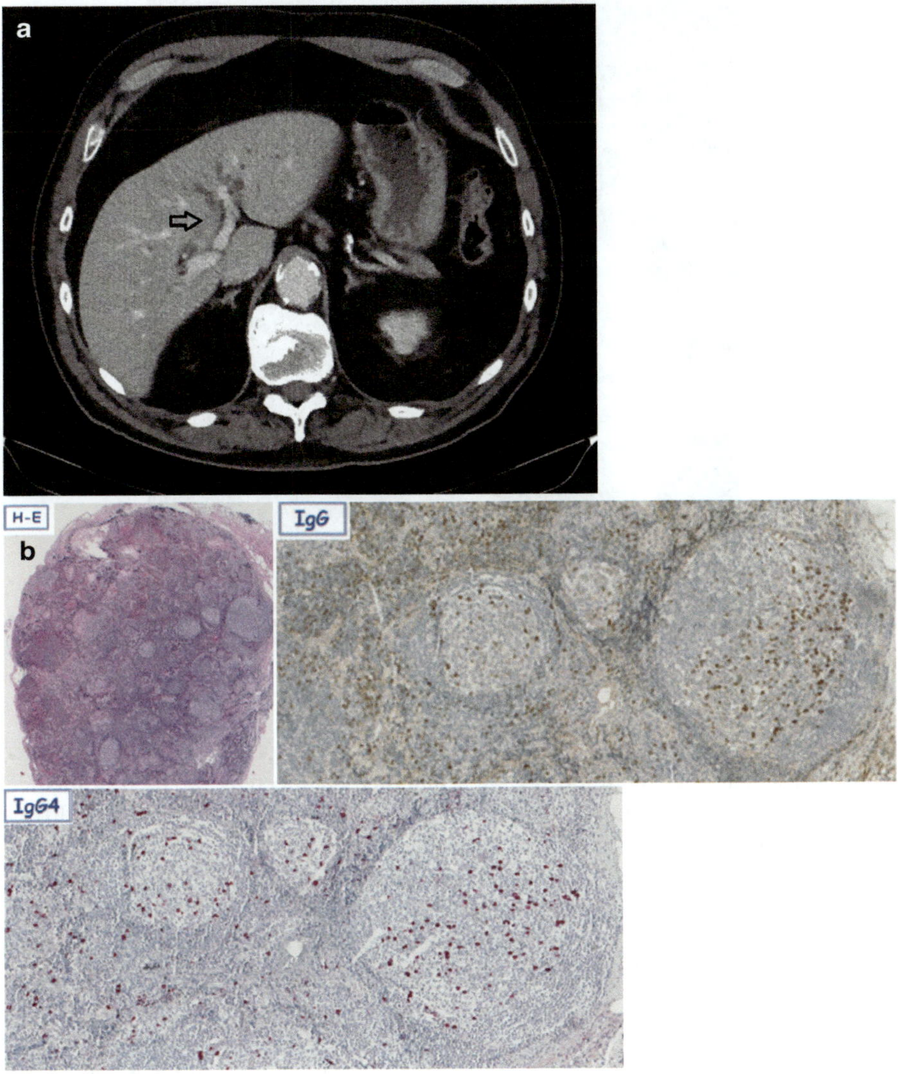

Fig. 9.1 Case 1: IgG4-related sclerosing cholangitis. (**a**) CT at first presentation: centrally obstructing tumor with dilatation of the intrahepatic bile ducts. (**b**) Pathology: lymph node biopsy with normal architecture (follicle formation) and sinus histiocytosis. Immunohistochemistry shows IgG- and IgG4-positive plasma cells. (**c**) CT after prednisone treatment: decrease in both size of tumor and dilatation of the intrahepatic bile ducts

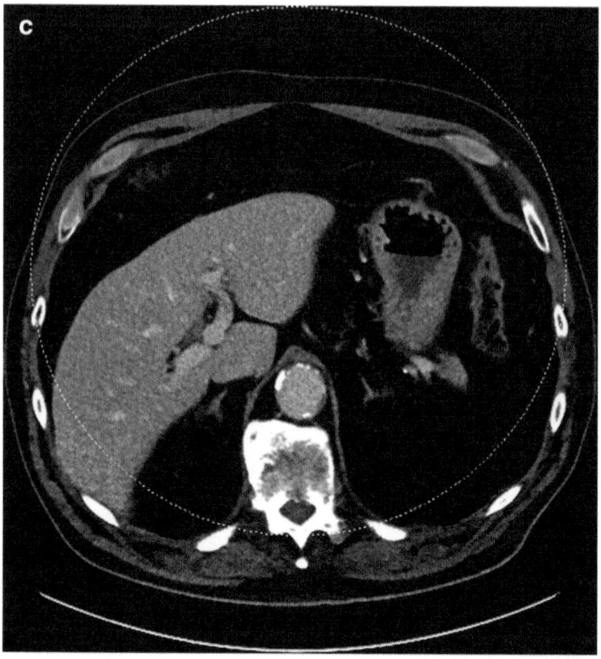

Fig. 9.1 (continued)

discussed with the patient. The patient was referred to a tertiary referral center. Upon presentation to the referral center, jaundice had decreased. His past medical history included a skin rash, lymphadenopathy, infections of the feet, and diffuse skeletal hyperostosis. No clear diagnosis had been found for all these conditions. The patient was discussed in a multidisciplinary meeting. MRI and CT scan reassessment were suspicious for pCCA showing a perihilar mass with bilateral involvement of the second-order bile ducts (i.e., Bismuth IV) without vascular involvement (Fig. 9.1a). An extended right hemihepatectomy to remove the mass was technically feasible.

No ERCP had been performed given serum bilirubin had normalized without treatment (Table 9.1). Moreover, CA19.9 was normal, and serum IgG4 was 12 g/L (i.e., five times the upper limit of normal). Thus, IgG4-related sclerosing cholangitis appeared more likely than pCCA, because of highly elevated IgG4, spontaneous normalization of bilirubin, and previously unexplained systemic symptoms. A few years prior, a biopsy of mediastinal lymph nodes had been performed; this biopsy was reassessed, and IgG4 staining was positive (Fig. 9.1b). Treatment with 40 mg prednisone daily was commenced. Within a few days, the patient experienced improvement of his symptoms. Not only did his jaundice disappear, but he also described improvement of all other symptoms. Repeat imaging (Fig. 9.1c) showed near normalization of the bile duct dilatation and disappearance of the mass. Repeat blood tests (Table 9.1) showed normalization of cholestasis. Treatment response confirmed the diagnosis of IgG4-related sclerosing cholangitis, and surgical intervention was appropriately averted.

This case illustrates how cross-sectional imaging that is very suspicious for pCCA may mimic IgG4-related sclerosing cholangitis (and vice versa). In particular, if IgG4 is highly elevated (i.e., at least twice the upper limit of normal), the possibility of IgG4-related sclerosing cholangitis should be carefully considered. Other clues of IgG4 disease in this case were the spontaneous improvement of symptoms, fluctuating or normalizing serum bilirubin without biliary drainage, and (previously) unexplained symptoms involving other organ systems, highlighting the importance of a thorough patient review. Of note is that although the presence of compatible histology and immunohistochemistry is essential, it is not considered sufficient because appropriate clinical findings and laboratory tests are required [15].

Case 2: IgG4-Related Sclerosing Cholangitis II

A 65-year-old female patient presented with jaundice, nausea, and malaise. Her past medical history included hypertension and mild asthma for which she used inhalation medication. Her family history revealed a brother with autoimmune pancreatitis and no family members with cancer. On physical examination no abnormalities were seen besides jaundice and mild abdominal tenderness. Lab results showed elevated bilirubin, AST, and ALT (Table 9.2). Abdominal ultrasound, CT, and MRI showed dilated intrahepatic bile ducts (Fig. 9.2a, b). On MRI a small mass was seen at the biliary confluence. The patient was referred to a tertiary center.

Upon presentation to the referral center, the patient reported spontaneous improvement of symptoms. Lab results showed that serum bilirubin had decreased without biliary drainage and serum IgG4 level was normal. Imaging was reviewed at the multidisciplinary meeting and showed thickening of the tail of the pancreas suggestive of autoimmune pancreatitis. A treatment trial of prednisone 40 mg daily was started. On repeat CT 2 weeks later, the small mass, dilated intrahepatic bile ducts, and pancreatic tail enlargement largely resolved (Fig. 9.2c, d).

Table 9.2 Lab results at initial presentation, upon referral, and after start of treatment in a 65-year-old female presenting with jaundice, nausea, and malaise (case 2)

Lab results	Initial presentation	Referral	2 weeks after treatment	Normal value
AST	221	110	28	<35 U/L
ALT	565	294	79	<45 U/L
Total bilirubin	8.7	3.3	1.5	<1.0 mg/dL
ALP	445	657	213	<115 U/L
GGT	236	521	174	<55 U/L
CA19.9	x	38	15	<35 kU/L
Creatinine	72	70	80	65–115 μmol/L

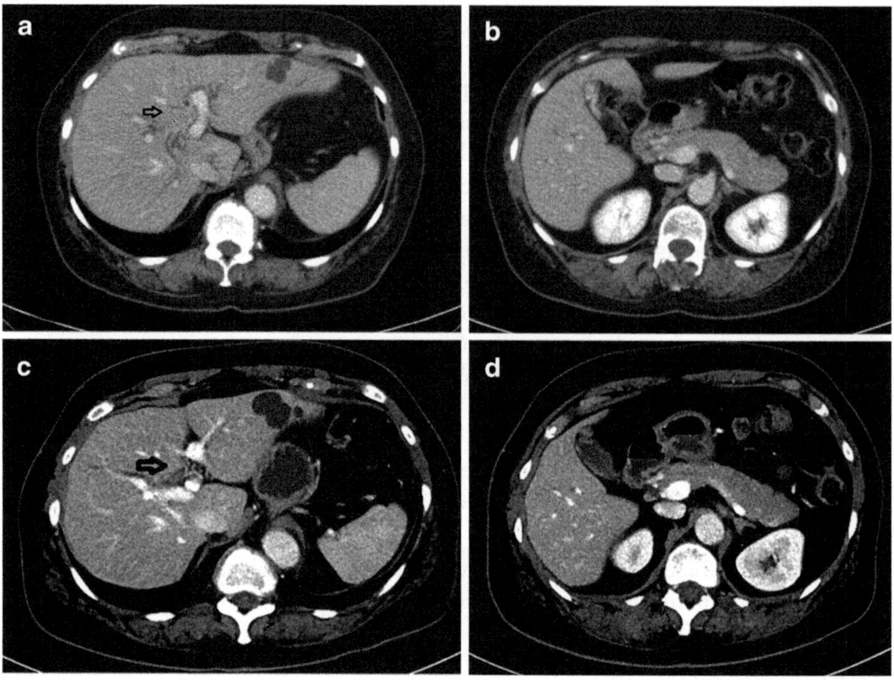

Fig. 9.2 Case 2: IgG4-related sclerosing cholangitis. (**a**) CT at first presentation: centrally obstructing liver tumor with dilatation of the intrahepatic bile ducts. (**b**) CT at first presentation: pancreas showing mild swelling ("sausage"-like appearance), compatible with autoimmune pancreatitis. (**c**) CT after prednisone treatment: decrease in both size of liver tumor and dilatation of the intrahepatic bile ducts. (**d**) CT after prednisone treatment: pancreas showing less swelling

This case illustrates that not all patients with IgG4-related sclerosing cholangitis have elevated serum IgG4 levels. In a large retrospective study by Tanaka et al., 84% of the patients with IgG4-related sclerosing cholangitis had elevated IgG4 levels at first presentation [21]. Fluctuating symptoms and spontaneous improving cholestasis require consideration of IgG4-related sclerosing cholangitis [21]. Moreover, patients with IgG4-related sclerosing cholangitis may have concomitant autoimmune pancreatitis, as illustrated herein [22–25].

Case 3: Stone Disease

A 58-year-old female patient presented with sudden onset abdominal pain and lab results consistent with cholestasis. On MRCP she had gallstones and isolated left intrahepatic bile duct dilatation (Fig. 9.3a) suggestive of Mirizzi syndrome. She underwent an ERCP, at which time a stenosis was seen in the left hepatic duct, and a plastic stent was placed. She subsequently underwent a laparoscopic subtotal

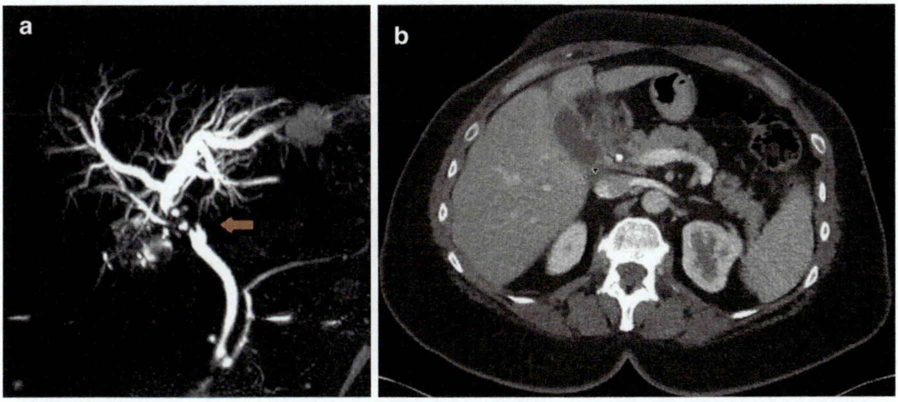

Fig. 9.3 Case 3: Stone disease. (**a**) MRI/MRCP: dilatation of the perihilar and intrahepatic bile ducts with obstructing cystic duct stone suspicious for Mirizzi syndrome (**b**) CT scan: thickening of the hepatic duct suspicious for cholangiocarcinoma

cholecystectomy for acute cholecystitis. A necrotic gallbladder with multiple stones and pus was removed. A postoperative type "A" bile leak was treated with an ERCP to replace the migrated plastic stent. There was a persistent stenosis in the common hepatic and left intrahepatic duct. Brush cytology of this stenosis was diagnosed as adenocarcinoma. The patient was referred to a tertiary referral center.

Upon presentation to the referral center, the patient endorsed improvement in appetite and resolution of abdominal pain. On physical examination no abnormalities were found. Lab results showed improved AST/ALT but persistently elevated ALP (Table 9.3). CT and MRCP showed persistent dilatation of the intrahepatic bile ducts with thickening of the hepatic duct (Fig. 9.3a, b) suspicious for pCCA. However, reassessment of the brush cytology at the referral center did not confirm the diagnosis of adenocarcinoma but showed only atypical cells [26]. ERCP in combination with cholangioscopy was then performed for better evaluation of the stricture. Surprisingly, it showed that the left hepatic duct was obstructed by a large uncalcified stone, which was not seen on previous cross-sectional imaging and mistaken for Mirizzi syndrome. With lithotripsy the stone was fragmented and then removed with balloon sweeping. Bilateral stents were placed to optimize bile flow. She underwent progressive stenting to treat the associated benign ductal stenosis. Twelve months later, she was asymptomatic with no signs of cholestasis.

This case illustrates the difficulty for pathologists to differentiate severe inflammation from adenocarcinoma (see also Chap. 8). Brushings and biopsies should be reviewed independently by an expert pathologist. Moreover, inflammation (and consequent benign stricturing) due to stone disease can mimic pCCA on imaging. In addition, chronic hepaticolithiasis is in itself a risk factor for CCA, which further complicates the differential diagnosis and work-up. Finally, both CT and MRI may not show uncalcified intrahepatic stones (i.e., false negative findings) that are found upon cholangioscopy.

Table 9.3 Lab results on first presentation, at referral, and 2 weeks after treatment in a 58-year-old female presenting with sudden onset abdominal pain (case 3)

Lab results	Initial presentation	Referral	2 weeks after treatment	Normal value
AST	59	32	50	<35 U/L
ALT	64	34	77	<45 U/L
Total bilirubin	0.4	0.2	0.3	<1.0 mg/dL
ALP	207	190	249	<115 U/L
GGT	198	177	299	<55 U/L
CA19.9	x	12	24	<35 kU/L
Creatinine	52	63	66	65–115 μmol/L

Case 4: Infectious Disease

A 20-year-old Caucasian male patient presented with acute abdominal pain in the right upper quadrant and jaundice. The symptoms started nearly 3 weeks prior to presentation, and he had noticed jaundice for about a week. Two weeks later his symptoms spontaneously improved. He had traveled to Croatia and France in the past 5 years. On physical examination of the abdomen, only slight tenderness in the right upper quadrant was noted. Lab results showed mildly elevated ALP and GGT, and serology was negative for hepatitis A, B, C, and E (Table 9.4). Serology for *Echinococcus granulosus* was positive (titer 1:160). An MRI showed cystic dilatation of the intrahepatic bile ducts, predominantly in the left liver, with possible stone formation (Fig. 9.4a). No masses or lymphadenopathy were seen. Since these findings were atypical for echinococcal infection and the differential diagnosis included iCCA, the patient was referred to a tertiary center.

At a multidisciplinary meeting, a differential diagnosis was established including focal Caroli syndrome, iCCA, HCC, and infectious diseases like echinococcal cysts. However, imaging was atypical for each of the differential diagnoses. A repeat CT scan showed several new hypodensities with eggshell calcifications in liver segments 2, 3, 4, and 8 (Fig. 9.4b). Serology came back highly positive for both *Echinococcus granulosus* (ELISA 58.4 U/mL) and *Echinococcus multilocularis* (ELISA IgG: 6400). All things considered, *Echinococcus multilocularis* infection was considered most likely. A PET scan was performed, which did not show extrahepatic manifestation of the disease. The patient was started on albendazole treatment 400 mg twice daily, and periodic repeat imaging will be performed to monitor the treatment effect. Surgery is the only curative option but is reserved for after albendazole has decreased the extent of disease in order to preserve as much liver tissue as possible.

This case illustrates how infection in the liver, in this instance *Echinococcus multilocularis,* can mimic iCCA. Echinococcosis is a zoonotic infection caused by tapeworms of the *Echinococcus* genus. It is a rare condition, though it has shown progressive spread to non-endemic areas in Northern Europe. Imaging features are variable, and initial misdiagnosis is common. Imaging findings include infiltrating lesions with irregular non-enhancing margins, small cystic

Table 9.4 Lab results at initial presentation, upon referral, and after start of treatment in a 20-year-old Caucasian male presenting with acute abdominal pain in the right upper quadrant and jaundice (case 4)

Lab results	Initial presentation	Referral	After treatment	Normal value
AST	28	25	31	<35 U/L
ALT	86	19	18	<45 U/L
Total bilirubin	0.6	0.4	0.2	<1.0 mg/dL
ALP	160	97	74	<115 U/L
GGT	191	74	27	<55 U/L
CA19.9	x	7	x	<35 kU/L
IgG4	x	0.5	x	0.08–1.4 g/L

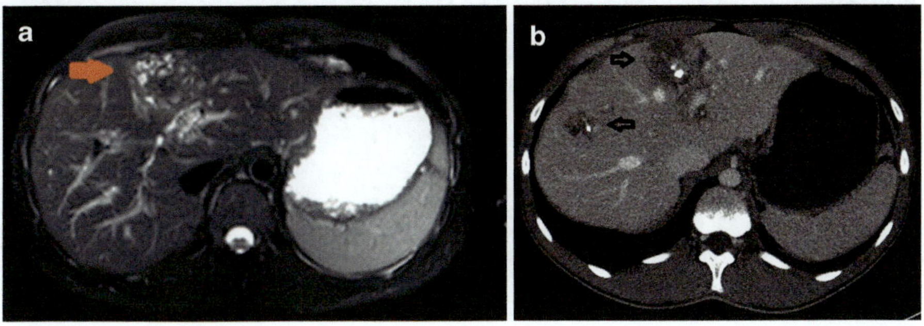

Fig. 9.4 Case 4: Infectious diseases. (**a**) MRI at first presentation: predominantly cystic-appearing liver lesion. (**b**) CT scan: clear calcifications within the lesions, raising suspicion for echinococcosis

components, scattered calcifications, and irregular septa within necrotic cavities [27]. Serology is often positive, and cross-reaction with *Echinococcus granulosus* is possible [28].

Case 5: Infectious Disease II

A 44-year-old healthy female patient presented with complaints of itching. No abnormalities were detected on physical examination. Lab results showed no abnormalities besides elevated total bilirubin of 1.75 mg/dL (Table 9.5). An abdominal CT scan showed a 5-centimeter hypodense liver mass with multiple satellites (Fig. 9.5). Subsequently, a PET scan was performed that showed uptake in the liver lesion (SUV of 7). The patient was diagnosed with unresectable iCCA and scheduled for palliative chemotherapy. She then came to a tertiary referral center for a second opinion.

Detailed patient history at referral found that she had traveled to Thailand 3 months prior. An MRI was performed which showed an irregular lesion, atypical for iCCA (Fig. 9.5a). A new CT showed that one lesion had a major decrease in size

Table 9.5 Lab results at initial presentation, upon referral, and after start of treatment in a 44-year-old female patient presenting with complaints of itching (case 5)

Lab results	Initial presentation	Referral	After treatment	Normal value
AST	15	20	16	<35 U/L
ALT	13	26	14	<45 U/L
Total bilirubin	1.8	1.6	1.4	<1.0 mg/dL
ALP	38	89	51	<115 U/L
GGT	10	18	12	<55 U/L
CA19.9	X	2	x	<35 kU/L

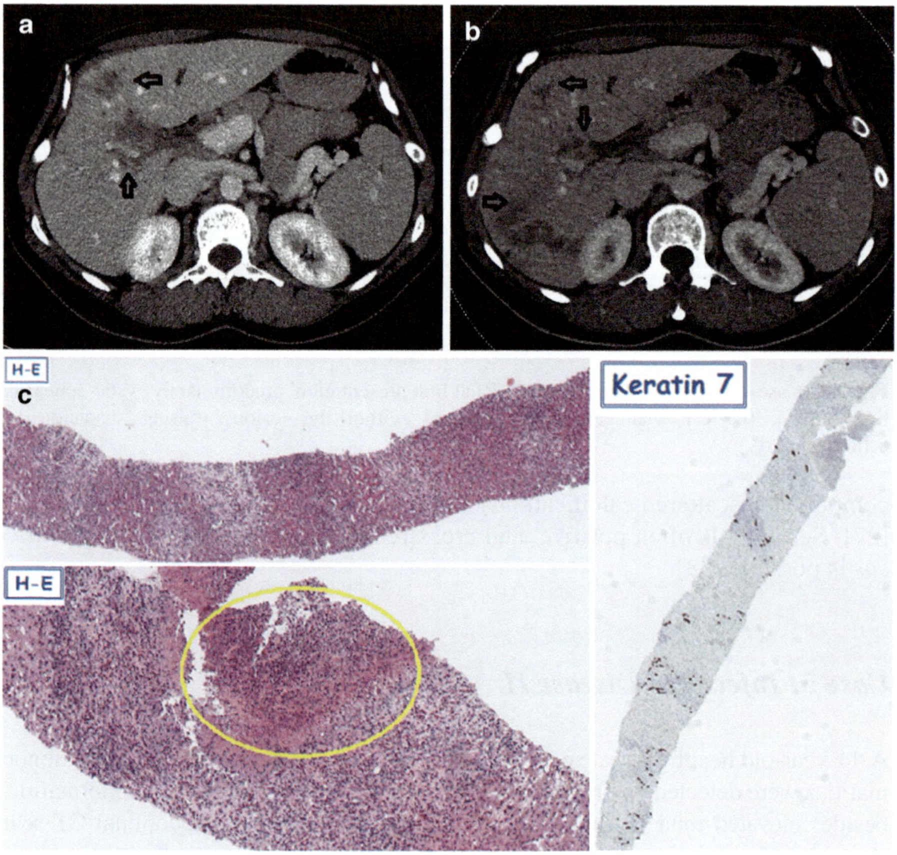

Fig. 9.5 Case 5: Infectious diseases II (**a**) CT at first presentation: irregular central hypodense liver lesion. (**b**) CT after a month: multiple irregular peripheral hypodense masses, resolution of central lesions. (**c**) Pathology: HE liver biopsy with preserved architecture, necrosis (yellow circle), and prominent eosinophilic infiltration. Immunohistochemistry: Keratin 7 highlights the original bile ducts along with some ductular reaction

and change in shape without treatment, and new lesions had developed in segments 6 and 7 (Fig. 9.5b). Blood tests showed that she had severe eosinophilia. A percutaneous liver biopsy showed necrosis and a histiocytic reaction without malignancy (Fig. 9.5c). An eosinophilic infiltrate and a slight increase in IgG4-positive cells were seen. The blood tests and biopsy were consistent with hypereosinophilic syndrome (HES).

The work-up continued with excluding autoimmune diseases and parasitic infections. Autoimmune serology was negative. However, *Fasciola hepatica* serology was positive on indirect immunofluorescent-antibody test and ELISA. The patient was treated with triclabendazole, her symptoms resolved, and imaging showed marked improvement of the liver lesions.

This case, similar to the previous one, illustrates how infectious diseases can mimic CCA. In this case, the patient had infiltrative liver lesions resembling iCCA, but the liver lesions were caused by a liver fluke (*Fasciola hepatica*) that she most likely contracted during her travels in Thailand. Detailed information regarding liver flukes can be found in Chap. 11.

Case 6: Adenocarcinoma of Unknown Primary

A 45-year-old female patient with a past medical history of stage III Hodgkin lymphoma, stage II papillary thyroid carcinoma, and stage I breast carcinoma presented with fatigue. On physical examination of the abdomen, tenderness in the upper abdomen was noted. Lab results showed abnormal liver tests (Table 9.6). A CT was performed and showed multiple bilobar liver lesions suspicious for liver metastases. A PET scan found no extrahepatic disease. A liver biopsy was performed, and pathological examination showed a poorly differentiated adenocarcinoma. Immunohistochemical analyses ruled out her previous malignancies as well as colorectal cancer. Upper endoscopy ruled out esophageal and gastric cancer. She was diagnosed with ACUP and started systemic chemotherapy with carboplatin and paclitaxel. She came to a tertiary referral center for a second opinion.

A new CT was performed that showed a large liver tumor with peripheral enhancement and capsular retraction (Fig. 9.6a, b). Outside pathology was reviewed and showed that the tumor cells were of epithelial origin, and therefore a lymphoma was excluded. Immunohistochemical profile (negative staining for thyroglobulin, TTF-1, and PAX-8) ruled out a thyroid (papillary) carcinoma. Moreover, negative staining for GATA-3, ER, and BAP loss (which were all positive in her breast carcinoma) together with the inconsistent histomorphology excluded metastasis from her breast carcinoma. Both histomorphology and immunohistochemical profile were consistent with iCCA (Fig. 9.6c). Based on imaging and pathology, she was diagnosed with iCCA. She is currently undergoing treatment with systemic chemotherapy (gemcitabine and cisplatin) and concomitant hepatic arterial infusion pump chemotherapy with floxuridine. Several studies have found 5-year OS of about 20% with combined systemic and intra-arterial chemotherapy for unresectable iCCA [29].

Table 9.6 Lab results on initial presentation in a 45-year-old female presenting with abdominal tenderness in the upper abdomen (case 6)

Lab results	Initial presentation	Normal value
AST	124	<35 U/L
ALT	147	<45 U/L
Total bilirubin	0.5	<1.0 mg/dL
ALP	518	<115 U/L
CEA	1	<5 μg/L
CA19.9	16	<35 kU/L

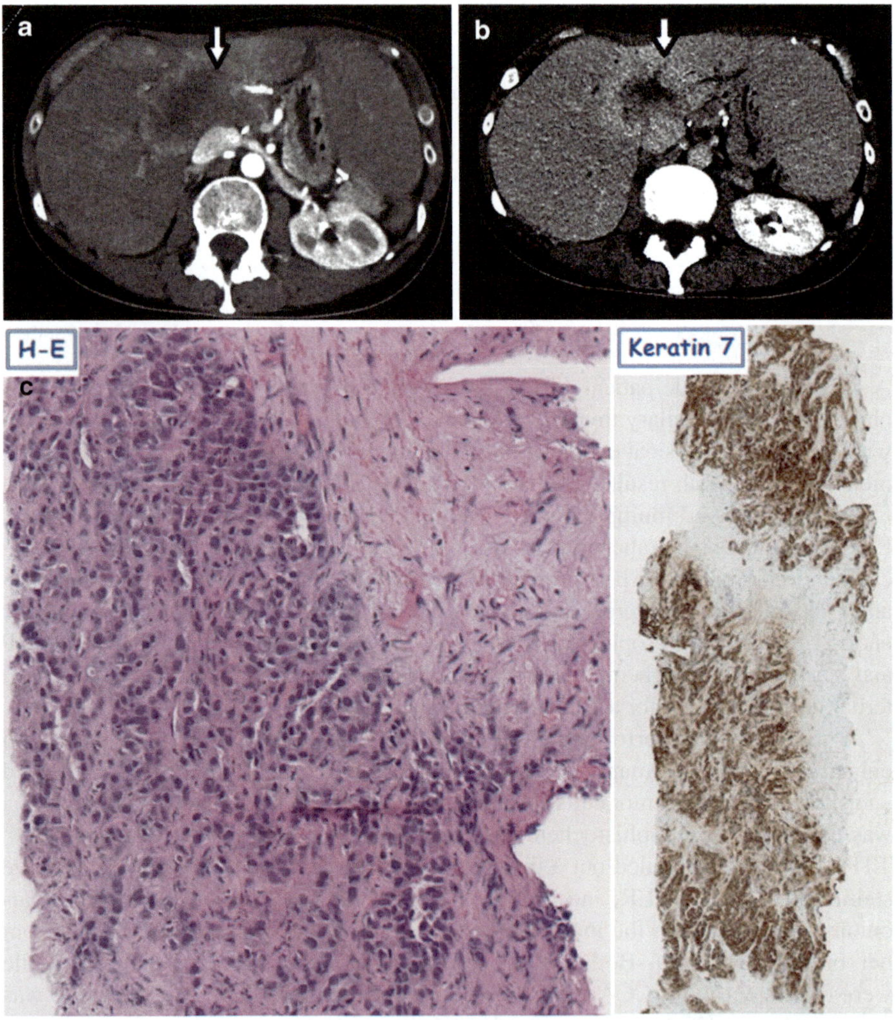

Fig. 9.6 Case 6: Adenocarcinoma of unknown primary origin. (**a**) Arterial phase CT scan demonstrating peripheral enhancement and capsular retraction. (**b**) Venous phase CT scan. (**c**) Pathology: HE liver biopsy with small gland formation. Immunohistochemistry: cytokeratin 7 positivity in tumor cells

This case illustrates that radiologists and pathologists are sometimes unfamiliar with the imaging and immunohistochemical profile of iCCA, thus resulting in an incorrect diagnosis of ACUP by medical oncologists. ACUP in the liver should only be diagnosed after ruling out iCCA by a multidisciplinary team experienced with iCCA.

Case 7: Cirrhotic Liver

A 62-year-old male patient with a past medical history of sarcoidosis treated with steroids, obesity, and alcohol abuse disorder was diagnosed with a Child-Pugh B7 liver cirrhosis. Due to continued alcohol use, a liver transplantation was contraindicated. Biannual abdominal ultrasound was performed for HCC surveillance.

After 3 years of follow-up, a hypodense lesion was seen on ultrasound. Lab results showed normal liver tests and tumor markers (Table 9.7). An MRI scan showed a lesion with a diameter of 14 mm in segment 7 (Fig. 9.7a). The lesion showed rim hyperenhancement, without decrease in intensity from earlier to later phase (i.e., non-peripheral washout). The lesion was classified as LI-RADS M (i.e., malignant but not HCC) (Fig. 9.7b).

A CT scan of the chest and a PET scan were performed to rule out metastatic disease. A liver biopsy was performed, and pathology reported adenocarcinoma with an immunohistochemical profile inconsistent with hepatocellular differentiation (no HepPar-1 or AFP expression and no canalicular pattern of expression with CD10 and polyclonal CEA). The tumor cells, however, did stain positive for markers of biliary differentiation (such as keratin 7 and keratin 19), and together with BerEp-4 expression and histomorphology, this was consistent with iCCA (Fig. 9.7c). Radiofrequency ablation was performed without complications.

This case demonstrates that cirrhosis is a risk factor for iCCA [30]. Indeed, iCCA is more common in cirrhosis than previously recognized. Most new hepatic lesions represent HCC, but small lesions may be difficult to distinguish from iCCA. Treatment of the new liver lesion in this patient would have been ablation regardless of a diagnosis of HCC or iCCA. However, distinguishing iCCA from HCC is relevant in patients that may be eligible for liver transplantation, because survival outcomes are worse for iCCA after transplantation (Chap. 15). Moreover, systemic and locoregional treatments differ between iCCA and HCC (discussed further in Chaps 17 and 18).

Table 9.7 Lab results on initial presentation in a 62-year-old male with a past medical history of alcohol abuse disorder and Child-Pugh B7 liver cirrhosis (case 7)

Lab results	Initial presentation	Normal value
AST	33	<35 U/L
ALT	30	<45 U/L
Total bilirubin	0.8	<1.0 mg/dL
ALP	108	<115 U/L
CEA	2.0	<5 μg/L
AFP	9	<10 μg/L
Ca 19.9	18	<35 kU/L

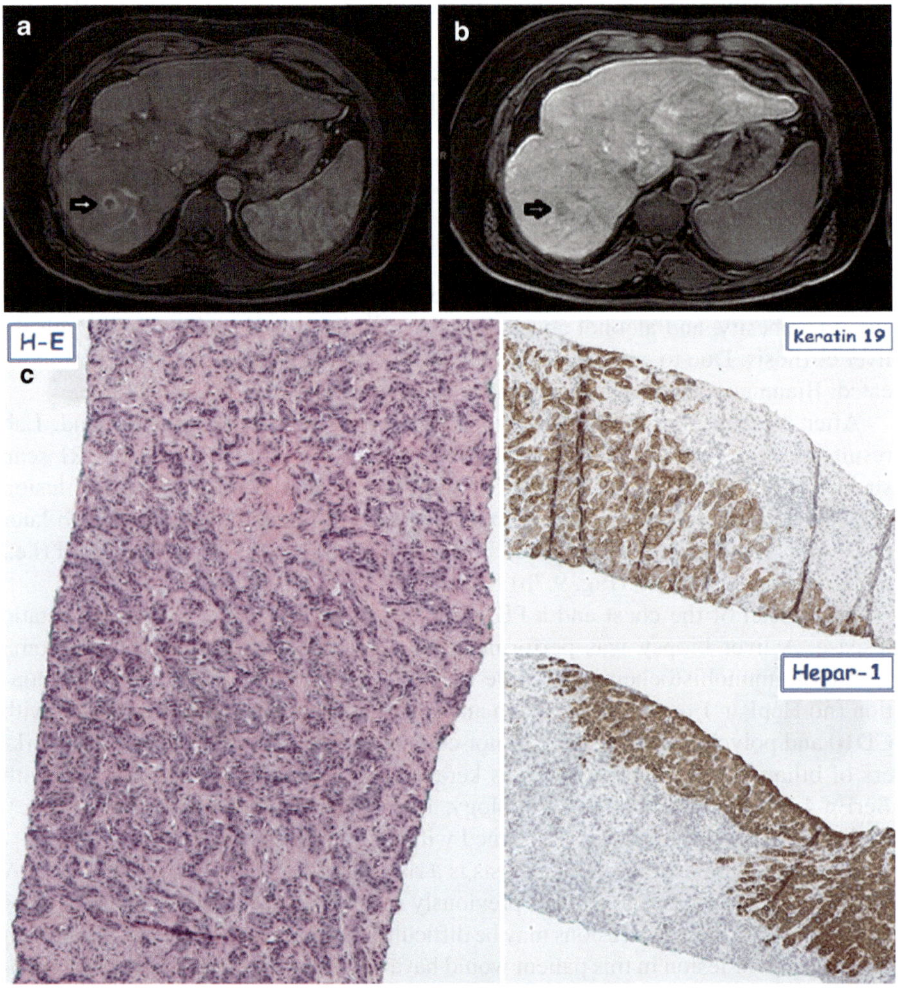

Fig. 9.7 Case 7: Cirrhotic liver. (**a**) MRI (portal venous phase, Primovist contrast): cirrhotic liver, with a peripherally enhancing spheroid lesion in segment 7. (**b**) MRI (late phase, Primovist contrast): in this phase, after contrast injection, the lesion can still be seen. (**c**) Pathology: HE liver biopsy with adenocarcinoma, with relatively small gland formation. Immunohistochemistry: cytokeratin 19 positivity in tumor cells. HepPar-1 highlights the preexistent hepatocytes (tumor cells are negative)

Case 8: Primary Sclerosing Cholangitis

A 54-year-old male patient presented with jaundice, itching, and malaise. His past medical history included mild ulcerative proctitis and PSC. Blood tests revealed elevated liver enzyme tests and bilirubin level (Table 9.8). An abdominal CT scan showed a liver with irregular surface contour with minimal dilatation of the intrahepatic bile ducts, discontinuous narrowing of the bile ducts, and slight arterial enhancement of the common hepatic duct and the cystic duct junction (Fig. 9.8a). A well-defined mass was not identifiable.

ERCP was performed, and the fluoroscopic images showed a significant stenosis of the common hepatic duct and cystic duct conjunction extending proximally to the confluence of the left and right main ducts (Bismuth-Corlette type II classification). Intraductal brushing and biopsy was performed, and a plastic stent was placed across the stenosis (Fig. 9.8b). Malignancy was not found in the obtained specimens.

Irregular wall thickening at the level of the dominant stenosis was seen at MRCP, and combined with high signal on diffusion-weighted imaging, the diagnosis CCA was deemed more likely than a benign stricture. Based on the clinical presentation and imaging, CCA was sufficiently likely to proceed with surgical resection. Because of the extent of the stenosis on fluoroscopy, a right hemihepatectomy with extrahepatic bile duct resection was performed, and pathological examination showed a well-differentiated perihilar adenocarcinoma.

This case illustrates the difficulty of diagnosing CCA in patients with PSC. Interpreting imaging is often challenging due to pre-existing biliary strictures and intraductal tumor growth without clear extra-ductal mass forming. Moreover, pathology is often inconclusive.

Table 9.8 Lab results at initial presentation in a 54-year-old male presenting with jaundice, itching, and malaise (case 8)

Lab results	Initial presentation	Normal value
AST	182	<35 U/L
ALT	230	<45 U/L
Total bilirubin	101	<1.0 mg/dL
ALP	350	<115 U/L
CEA	3.55	<5 μg/L
AFP	3	<10 μg/L
Ca 19.9	56	<35 kU/L

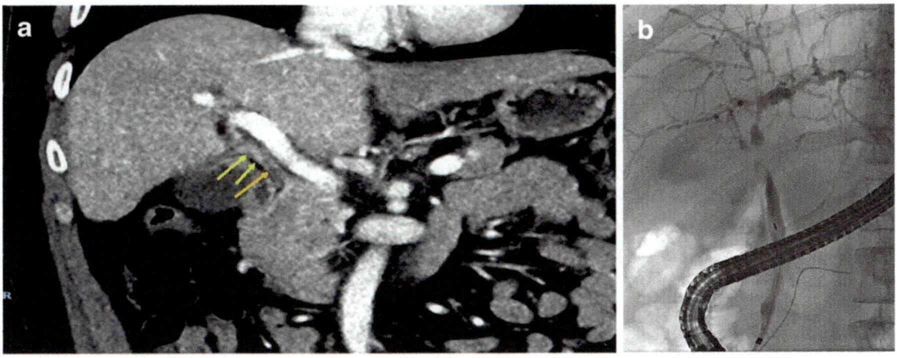

Fig. 9.8 Case 8: Primary sclerosing cholangitis. (**a**) CT at first presentation (coronal view): thickening and slight enhancement of the common hepatic duct (two yellow arrows). No wall thickening is seen at the common bile duct (orange arrow). (**b**) ERCP: significant stenosis of the common hepatic duct and cystic duct conjunction extending to the confluence of the left and right main ducts

Conclusion

In this chapter, and by way of these eight illustrative cases, we have demonstrated that the diagnostic work-up of patients with (suspected) CCA is a challenging multidisciplinary effort including gastroenterologists, surgeons, medical oncologists, radiologists, and pathologists, among others. The differential diagnosis should include IgG4-related sclerosing cholangitis, stone disease, parasitic disease, and metastatic disease from extrahepatic primary cancers, and in some cases even more esoteric disorders may be included. A meticulous patient history, physical examination, and evaluation of imaging and laboratory tests by multidisciplinary experts are required to determine the correct diagnosis and identify the best course of management.

In addition, for the subset of cases which evade definitive diagnosis despite these measures, continued developments in diagnostic tools, including but not limited to molecular biological (e.g., "omics"-based approaches) and other advanced techniques, are clinically needed and anticipated.

Acknowledgments The authors thank Dr. Michael Doukas for providing and reassessing the pathology slides and Dr. Roy Dwarkasing for providing and reassessing the radiological images.

References

1. Fung BM, Tabibian JH. Cholangiocarcinoma in patients with primary sclerosing cholangitis. Curr Opin Gastroenterol. 2020;36(2):77–84.
2. Hilscher MB, Tabibian JH, Carey EJ, Gostout CJ, Lindor KD. Dominant strictures in primary sclerosing cholangitis: a multicenter survey of clinical definitions and practices. Hepatol Commun. 2018;2(7):836–44.
3. Fung BM, Lindor KD, Tabibian JH. Cancer risk in primary sclerosing cholangitis: epidemiology, prevention, and surveillance strategies. World J Gastroenterol. 2019;25(6):659–71.
4. Ali AH, Tabibian JH, Nasser-Ghodsi N, Lennon RJ, DeLeon T, Borad MJ, et al. Surveillance for hepatobiliary cancers in patients with primary sclerosing cholangitis. Hepatology. 2018;67(6):2338–51.
5. Tabibian JH, Lindor KD. Challenges of cholangiocarcinoma detection in patients with primary sclerosing cholangitis. J Anal Oncol. 2012;1(1):50–5.
6. Fung BM, Fejleh MP, Tejaswi S, Tabibian JH. Cholangioscopy and its role in primary sclerosing cholangitis. Eur Med J Hepatol. 2020;8(1):42–53.
7. Corvera CU, Blumgart LH, Darvishian F, Klimstra DS, DeMatteo R, Fong Y, et al. Clinical and pathologic features of proximal biliary strictures masquerading as hilar cholangiocarcinoma. J Am Coll Surg. 2005;201(6):862–9.
8. Liver Cancer Study Group of J. Primary liver cancer in Japan. Clinicopathologic features and results of surgical treatment. Ann Surg. 1990;211(3):277–87.
9. Amin MB, Greene FL, Edge SB, Compton CC, Gershenwald JE, Brookland RK, et al. The Eighth Edition AJCC Cancer Staging Manual: Continuing to build a bridge from a population-based to a more "personalized" approach to cancer staging. CA Cancer J Clin. 2017;67(2):93–9.
10. Corvera CU, Blumgart LH, Akhurst T, RP DM, D'Angelica M, Fong Y, et al. 18F-fluorodeoxyglucose positron emission tomography influences management decisions in patients with biliary cancer. J Am Coll Surg. 2008;206(1):57–65.
11. Bridgewater J, Galle PR, Khan SA, Llovet JM, Park JW, Patel T, et al. Guidelines for the diagnosis and management of intrahepatic cholangiocarcinoma. J Hepatol. 2014;60(6):1268–89.

12. Weber SM, Ribero D, O'Reilly EM, Kokudo N, Miyazaki M, Pawlik TM. Intrahepatic cholangiocarcinoma: expert consensus statement. HPB (Oxford). 2015;17(8):669–80.
13. Bismuth H, Corlette MB. Intrahepatic cholangioenteric anastomosis in carcinoma of the hilus of the liver. Surg Gynecol Obstet. 1975;140(2):170–8.
14. Darwish Murad S, Kim WR, Harnois DM, Douglas DD, Burton J, Kulik LM, et al. Efficacy of neoadjuvant chemoradiation, followed by liver transplantation, for perihilar cholangiocarcinoma at 12 US centers. Gastroenterology. 2012;143(1):88–98 e3. quiz e14.
15. Benson AB, D'Angelica MI, Abbott DE, Abrams TA, Alberts SR, Anaya DA, et al. Guidelines insights: hepatobiliary cancers, version 2.2019. J Natl Compr Cancer Netw. 2019;17(4):302–10.
16. Kochar B, Akshintala VS, Afghani E, Elmunzer BJ, Kim KJ, Lennon AM, et al. Incidence, severity, and mortality of post-ERCP pancreatitis: a systematic review by using randomized, controlled trials. Gastrointest Endosc. 2015;81(1):143–9 e9.
17. Onoyama T, Matsumoto K, Takeda Y, Kawata S, Kurumi H, Koda H, et al. Endoscopic ultrasonography-guided fine needle aspiration for extrahepatic cholangiocarcinoma: a safe tissue sampling modality. J Clin Med. 2019;8(4):417.
18. Jo JH, Cho CM, Jun JH, Chung MJ, Kim TH, Seo DW, et al. Same-session endoscopic ultrasound-guided fine needle aspiration and endoscopic retrograde cholangiopancreatography-based tissue sampling in suspected malignant biliary obstruction: a multicenter experience. J Gastroenterol Hepatol. 2019;34(4):799–805.
19. van der Gaag NA, de Castro SM, Rauws EA, Bruno MJ, van Eijck CH, Kuipers EJ, et al. Preoperative biliary drainage for periampullary tumors causing obstructive jaundice; DRainage vs. (direct) OPeration (DROP-trial). BMC Surg. 2007;7:3.
20. Malikowski T, Levy MJ, Gleeson FC, Storm AC, Vargas Valls EJ, Topazian MD, et al. EUS-FNA is effective for lymph node staging in patients with cholangiocarcinoma. Hepatology. 2019;72(3)940–48.
21. Tanaka A, Tazuma S, Okazaki K, Nakazawa T, Inui K, Chiba T, et al. Clinical features, response to treatment, and outcomes of igg4-related sclerosing cholangitis. Clin Gastroenterol Hepatol. 2017;15(6):920–6 e3.
22. Ohara H, Okazaki K, Tsubouchi H, Inui K, Kawa S, Kamisawa T, et al. Clinical diagnostic criteria of IgG4-related sclerosing cholangitis 2012. J Hepatobiliary Pancreat Sci. 2012;19(5):536–42.
23. Okazaki K, Uchida K, Miyoshi H, Ikeura T, Takaoka M, Nishio A. Recent concepts of autoimmune pancreatitis and IgG4-related disease. Clin Rev Allergy Immunol. 2011;41(2):126–38.
24. Montano-Loza AJ, Lalor E, Mason AL. Recognizing immunoglobulin G4 related overlap syndromes in patients with pancreatic and hepatobiliary diseases. Can J Gastroenterol. 2008;22(10):840–6.
25. Kamisawa T, Nakazawa T, Tazuma S, Zen Y, Tanaka A, Ohara H, et al. Clinical practice guidelines for IgG4-related sclerosing cholangitis. J Hepatobiliary Pancreat Sci. 2019;26(1):9–42.
26. Layfield LJ, Pitman MB, DeMay RM, Shidham VB. Pancreaticobiliary tract cytology: journey toward "bethesda" style guidelines from the papanicolaou society of cytopathology. Cytojournal. 2014;11:18.
27. Chouhan MD, Wiley E, Chiodini PL, Amin Z. Hepatic alveolar hydatid disease (*Echinococcus multilocularis*), a mimic of liver malignancy: a review for the radiologist in non-endemic areas. Clin Radiol. 2019;74(4):247–56.
28. Ito A, Ma L, Schantz PM, Gottstein B, Liu YH, Chai JJ, et al. Differential serodiagnosis for cystic and alveolar echinococcosis using fractions of *Echinococcus granulosus* cyst fluid (antigen B) and *E. multilocularis* protoscolex (EM18). Am J Trop Med Hyg. 1999;60(2):188–92.
29. Cercek A, Boerner T, Tan BR, Chou JF, Gonen M, Boucher TM, et al. Assessment of hepatic arterial infusion of floxuridine in combination with systemic gemcitabine and oxaliplatin in patients with unresectable intrahepatic cholangiocarcinoma: a phase 2 clinical trial. JAMA Oncol. 2019;6(1):60–7.
30. Shaib YH, El-Serag HB, Davila JA, Morgan R, McGlynn KA. Risk factors of intrahepatic cholangiocarcinoma in the United States: a case-control study. Gastroenterology. 2005;128(3):620–6.

Chapter 10
PSC-Associated Cholangiocarcinoma: Diagnostic and Therapeutic Considerations

Silvia Cagnin, James H. Tabibian, and Luca Fabris

Abbreviations

AIH	Autoimmune hepatitis
ALP	Alkaline phosphatase
CA	Carbohydrate antigen
CCA	Cholangiocarcinoma
CD	Crohn's disease
COX	Cyclooxygenase
CT	Computer tomography
DWI	Diffusion-weighted imaging
ECM	Extracellular matrix
ERCP	Endoscopic retrograde cholangiopancreatography
EUS	Endoscopic ultrasound
EV	Extracellular vesicle
F-FDG	F-Fluoro-deoxyglucose
FISH	Fluorescence in situ hybridization
FNA	Fine needle aspiration
FUT	Fucosyltransferase

S. Cagnin
Department of Molecular Medicine, University of Padua School of Medicine, Padua, Italy

J. H. Tabibian
Division of Gastroenterology, Department of Medicine, Olive View-UCLA Medical Center, Sylmar, CA, USA

David Geffen School of Medicine at UCLA, Los Angeles, CA, USA

L. Fabris (✉)
Department of Molecular Medicine, University of Padua School of Medicine, Padua, Italy

Digestive Disease Section, Liver Center, Yale University, New Haven, CT, USA
e-mail: luca.fabris@unipd.it; luca.fabris@yale.edu

J. H. Tabibian (ed.), *Diagnosis and Management of Cholangiocarcinoma*,
https://doi.org/10.1007/978-3-030-70936-5_10

GP2	Glycoprotein 2
HCC	Hepatocellular carcinoma
IBD	Inflammatory bowel disease
lncRNA	Long noncoding RNA
LT	Liver transplantation
miRNA	Micro-ribonucleic acid
MRCP	Magnetic resonance cholangiopancreatography
MRI	Magnetic resonance imaging
NO	Nitric oxide
pCCA	Perihilar cholangiocarcinoma
PET	Positron emission tomography
PSC	Primary sclerosing cholangitis
TRAIL	Tumor necrosis factor-related apoptosis-inducing ligand
UC	Ulcerative colitis
US	Ultrasonography

Primary Sclerosing Cholangitis: Background and Risk of Malignancies

Primary sclerosing cholangitis (PSC) is a chronic liver disease of unknown etiology but likely sustained by immune-mediated mechanisms, featuring ductopenic bile duct injury, cholestasis, peribiliary fibrosis, and associated multifocal strictures alternating with segmental ductal ectasia [1, 2]. Since PSC can target any segment of the biliary tree, including either the intrahepatic or the extrahepatic portions, PSC is currently divided into three main variants (or subtypes) according to the level and extent of biliary involvement (Table 10.1): classic PSC, small-duct PSC, and autoimmune hepatitis (AIH)-associated PSC.

A unique feature of PSC is its strong association with inflammatory bowel disease (IBD), with chronic ulcerative colitis (UC) comprising nearly 75–80% of these cases, while Crohn's disease (CD) and indeterminate colitis comprise approximately 10–15% and 5–10%, respectively [3]. Although the clinical course of the disease is

Table 10.1 Different subtypes of primary sclerosing cholangitis [1, 2, 56]

Subtype	Biliary involvement	Clinical features and risk of malignancy
Classic (90%)	Small and large bile ducts	70–80% of patients have IBD; increased risk of colon cancer and gallbladder cancer, cholangiocarcinoma, and hepatocellular carcinoma
Small-duct (5%)	Only small bile ducts	May progress to classic subtype; associated with longer survival and lower risk of cholangiocarcinoma than the classic subtype
AIH-associated (5%)	Small and large bile ducts	Associated with interface hepatitis. Higher than expected levels of aminotransferases and IgG; patients usually younger than 25 years at diagnosis (35% of children with PSC); better prognosis than the classic subtype but worse than autoimmune hepatitis alone

quite heterogeneous, most patients progress to end-stage liver disease and require liver transplantation (LT) [4]. Currently, PSC is still regarded as an "orphan" disease, given the lack of effective therapies in hindering disease progression. Though LT has significantly improved long-term survival of PSC patients with end-stage liver disease, up to 40–50% of deaths remain cancer-related and make PSC a bona fide premalignant condition [5]. Among cancers associated with PSC, cholangiocarcinoma (CCA) is the most diagnosed and lethal tumor, but PSC patients can also develop colorectal (especially when PSC is associated with UC) and gallbladder cancer [6]. Unlike other chronic liver diseases, the risk of hepatocellular carcinoma (HCC) is quite low, and it seems to be related to the progression to cirrhosis [7, 8].

Among the three anatomical subtypes of CCA, the one most commonly diagnosed in PSC patients is the perihilar form (pCCA), as generally observed in CCA patients even in the absence of a PSC background. Morphologically, CCA frequently presents as an obstructive biliary stricture without evidence of a mass on cross-sectional imaging [9]. There are some important distinctive features of PSC-associated CCA. In PSC patients, the lifetime risk of CCA development is 7–14% (corresponding to a 400- to 1500-fold increase in respect to the general population), with a 10-year cumulative incidence of 7–9% according to multiple studies [10–12]. Interestingly, CCA development is not related to the duration of the disease, in contrast with what is generally observed with other primary liver malignancies, HCC in particular, commonly arising in a cirrhotic setting [6]. Of note, one third of the CCAs detected in PSC is diagnosed within the first year from the PSC diagnosis, thus suggesting that a long-standing disease becomes symptomatic because of the tumor [13]. Moreover, since PSC strikes young individuals, in their third to fifth decade, PSC-associated CCA develops about 20 years earlier than in CCA patients without PSC [8].

PSC-related factors predisposing to CCA are still largely unknown. A recent study indicates duration and severity of PSC, age at diagnosis, smoking, alcohol consumption, or a history of colorectal dysplasia as factors bearing an increased CCA risk [5]. On the other hand, small-duct PSC and pediatric patients have a low risk of CCA development [6, 14]. As aforementioned, PSC patients also have a lifetime risk of gallbladder cancer ranging from 3 to 14%, whereas patients with PSC and UC have a fourfold increased risk of colorectal cancer when compared to patients with UC alone. Among other epithelial cancers, the risk of developing HCC is also slightly increased, ranging from 0.3 to 2.8% [5].

Pathogenesis of PSC-Associated CCA: The Archetype of a Premalignant Condition Sustained by Fibroinflammatory Lesions

The pathogenesis of PSC involves both environmental and inherited factors, with a yet unidentified environmental trigger probably activating a persistent cholangiocyte injury in genetically predisposed individuals. This injury is associated with a pronounced accumulation of fibrotic tissue, which prevails on the inflammatory infiltrate, with the development of the typical "onion skin-like" lesions, the hallmark of the disease [1, 4]. These lesions are made up of activated fibroblasts and macrophages and by a concentric peribiliary deposition of new extracellular matrix (ECM) components, in particular collagen type I and fibronectin, which induce progressive narrowing of the damaged bile ducts, eventually resulting in ductopenia [4, 15]. Moreover, ECM components, by binding soluble mediators (growth factors, chemokines, cytokines) via low-affinity non-covalent interactions, create gradients that further stimulate recruitment of fibroblasts and inflammatory cells to the damaged ducts leading to cholangiocyte proliferation and neoangiogenesis [16].

Remarkably, in CCA, neoplastic bile ducts are embedded in a dense desmoplastic tissue populated by myofibroblasts (cancer-associated fibroblasts) and macrophages (tumor-associated macrophages), together with a variety of innate and adaptive immune cells, encompassing T lymphocytes, macrophages, and neutrophils, which reproduces the prominent fibroinflammatory reaction featuring PSC [17–19] (Fig. 10.1). This observation lends support to the concept that PSC is paradigmatic of the pathogenetic sequence from fibroinflammation to cancer, driven by a proficient microenvironment characterized by qualitative and quantitative changes in ECM components associated with a dense myofibroblast gathering (Fig. 10.2). Moreover, either pro-inflammatory mediators released in the periductal milieu or

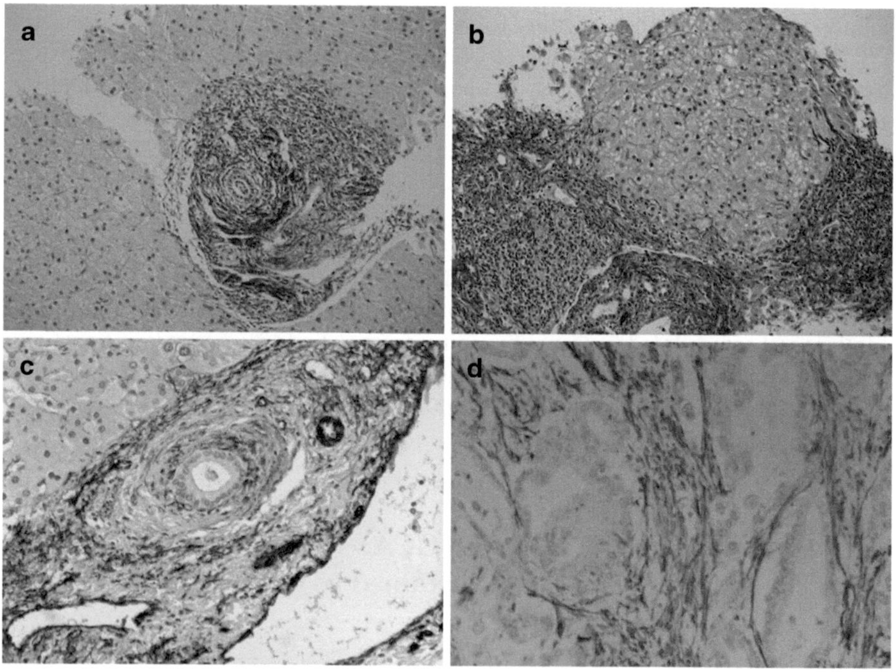

Fig. 10.1 Primary sclerosing cholangitis (**a**, **c**) and cholangiocarcinoma (**b**, **d**) share an exuberant fibrotic reaction embedding the bile ducts (**a**, **b**, Masson's trichrome), densely populated by activated myofibroblasts laying closely adjacent to cholangiocytes (**c**, **d**, immunohistochemistry for alpha-smooth muscle actin). Magnification **a**, **b**, 100×; **c**, 200×; **d**, 400×

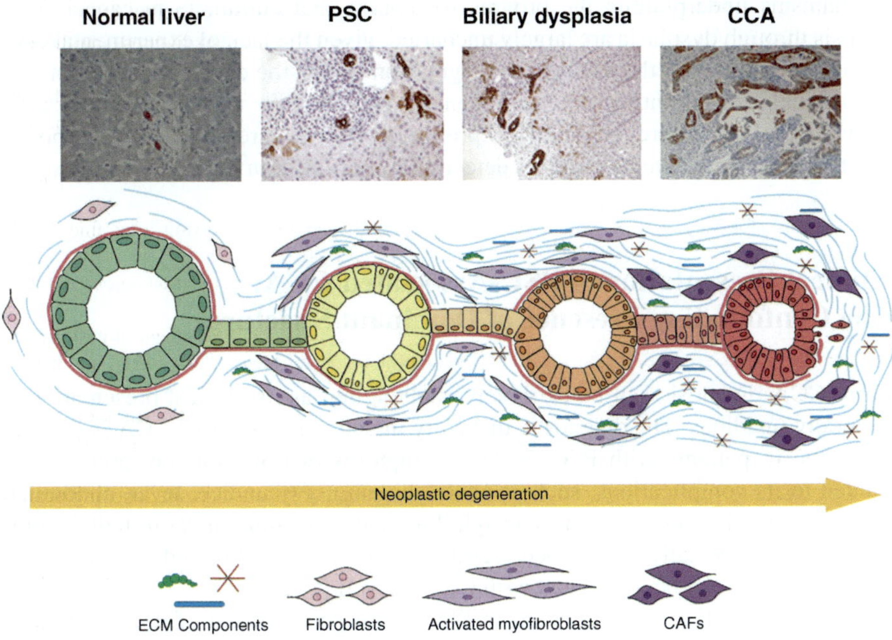

Fig. 10.2 In primary sclerosing cholangitis (PSC), the histopathological sequence from fibroinflammation to biliary dysplasia and cancer (cholangiocarcinoma, CCA) is faithfully reproduced. The peribiliary microenvironment behaves as the main director of this sequence, sustained by ECM changes and prominent myofibroblast accumulation. Up-sided micrographs are derived from human liver biopsies immunostained by the biliary marker keratin-7. Magnification, 100×

cholestasis cooperates with the inciting effects of the fibrotic stroma. IL-6, nitric oxide (NO), and reactive nitrogen and oxygen species induce DNA damage and promote epithelial cell proliferation while inhibiting apoptosis. TNF-α is also involved in the upregulation of inducible NO synthase.

Once cholangiocytes have gained a malignant phenotype, they release further growth factors, cytokines and chemokines acting as a feed-forward loop that potentiate CCA invasiveness [6]. The tumor necrosis factor-related apoptosis-inducing ligand (TRAIL), a pro-apoptotic death receptor agonist, might also be involved in the sequence PSC-CCA by activating a sublethal pro-apoptotic signaling that induces chromosomal instability [20]. Furthermore, cholestasis that may exert several effects on malignant transformation of the biliary epithelium has been shown, as related to the activation of receptor tyrosine kinases, such as the epidermal growth factor receptor leading to cell proliferation, and of cyclooxygenase-2 (COX-2), which, beyond promoting proliferation, stimulates angiogenesis and inhibits apoptosis [21, 22]. Of note, development of an abundant stromal reaction nearby the tumoral ducts (so-called tumor reactive stroma) is a common trait in many epithelial malignancies with pronounced invasive properties, including, beyond CCA, pancreatic ductal adenocarcinoma and invasive ductal breast carcinoma among others, where it provides a scaffold sustaining tumor cell dissemination [23]. However, the mechanisms underpinning the progressive course that culminate in cancer from fibrosis through dysplasia are largely uncharted, given the lack of experimental conditions able to model the PSC-CCA progression. Thus, the development of an animal model recapitulating this pathogenetic sequence is eagerly awaited, as a valuable tool to capture the pathways promoting biliary carcinogenesis and, possibly, to identify putative biomarkers detecting tumor onset in the earliest stages.

Clinical Presentation of PSC-Associated CCA: The Confounding Presence of Dominant Strictures

Early CCA diagnosis can be extremely challenging, as its clinical presentation is generally insidious. The diagnostic difficulty in detecting potential CCA is particularly true in patients with PSC. In fact, symptoms of PSC (fatigue, pruritus), or related to its complications, such as acute cholangitis (jaundice, fever, abdominal pain), eventually accompanied by weight loss and worsening of cholestatic laboratory profile, especially a sustained elevation in serum bilirubin and alkaline phosphatase (ALP), can be associated with CCA as well [8, 24].

In this respect, a major concern in PSC is the development of dominant strictures. Dominant strictures are focal high-grade biliary stenoses, generally defined as having a diameter ≤1.5 mm in the common bile duct or ≤1 mm in the right and left hepatic duct [25]. They occur in approximately 50% of patients with PSC and can be difficult to discriminate from CCA, either clinically or morphologically. Typically, recurrent episodes of bacterial cholangitis in a PSC patient are highly suggestive of a dominant stricture and may contribute to disease progression [26]. The relationship between CCA and dominant strictures can be perplexing, since CCA may arise from a dominant stricture, whereas, on the other hand, only 5% of dominant strictures have an underlying malignancy. When associated with a dominant stricture, CCA usually develops in the hilum or in the common bile duct, and, conversely, benign dominant strictures affect mainly the extrahepatic bile ducts [8].

Diagnosis of PSC-Associated CCA: Critical Issues and Multimodal Approach

With the improvement of surgical resection and LT techniques for locally advanced CCA, early detection of this tumor when arising in a PSC background is crucial to improve patient prognosis. As there is no clear relationship between PSC duration and CCA development, patients with a recent PSC diagnosis should be also screened for biliary malignancy with the combined use of laboratory tests, cross-sectional imaging, and endoscopic techniques, along with conventional and, possibly, new biomarkers to be tested in serum and eventually in bile and in other biological fluids [6, 8].

Laboratory Tests and Serum Biomarkers

CCA usually presents with rapid worsening of liver biochemistries (mostly ALP and eventually total bilirubin), eventually leading to clinical deterioration (pruritus, jaundice, weight loss, acute cholangitis) in an otherwise stable PSC patient [27].

Among *conventional* serum biomarkers, carbohydrate antigen (CA) 19-9, a membrane glycolipid expressed by tumoral duct cells, is the most associated with CCA, though studies addressing its role in PSC patients are scarce. In addition, CA19-9 has significant variability in sensitivity and specificity depending on the cutoff value. The optimal cutoff is 129 U/mL, showing a sensitivity of 78% and a specificity of 98%, though 1/3 of PSC patients with increased levels of CA19-9 above this cutoff are not diagnosed with CCA. Importantly, serum levels of CA19-9 are influenced by the allelic variants of fucosyltransferase (FUT). Two different FUT genotypes, 2 and 3, that determine the Lewis blood group, catalyze the final steps of CA19-9 biosynthesis. Based on these genotypes, distinct groups with low, intermediate, and high expression of CA19-9 can be identified, indicating FUT2/3 genotype-dependent cutoff values for CA19-9 as a means to improve its sensitivity by reducing the false positives [27–29]. Noteworthy is the observation that 7–10% of the general population is Lewis blood antigen-negative and lacks expression of CA19-9 [30]; thus, normal or undetectable levels of CA19-9 do not effectively rule out the possibility of CCA. Another factor that can limit the clinical usefulness of CA19-9 in PSC patients is bacterial cholangitis, which is responsible for marked though transient increase in CA19-9 serum levels [31], while dominant strictures seem to have less effect on biomarker expression [32].

Serum CEA is another biomarker of interest, as it is not influenced by bacterial cholangitis and dominant strictures, possesses a higher specificity than CA19-9, and potentially could be used to predict survival after CCA resection. However, compared with CA19-9, CEA has a lower sensitivity, as it is increased, for instance, by cigarette smoking (a well-established risk factor for CCA development). Similar to CA19-9, CEA levels are influenced by FUT genotype. Of note, measurement of both CA19-9 and CEA has been proposed to improve early diagnosis of CCA [8].

Imaging techniques are a critically important asset for CCA diagnosis, as the detection of morphological abnormalities in the biliary tree is a prerequisite for endoscopic procedures, as discussed in detail elsewhere in this book (*Chap. 7, Viragh K et al.*). In brief, ultrasonography (US) is a common first-line test and has a sensitivity of 57% and specificity of 94% in this context. However, while US is particularly useful in detecting mass lesions, the infiltrating or intraductal morphological phenotype of CCA can be difficult to appreciate, especially in a background of PSC [27, 33]. Magnetic resonance imaging (MRI) has a much higher sensitivity than US and has become the technique of choice for both diagnosis and staging of CCA. The combination of MRI with magnetic resonance cholangiopancreatography (MRCP) provides the most accurate noninvasive method to study the biliary tree and to unveil tumoral infiltration. More features suggestive of a neoplastic behavior can be identified by dynamic contrast-enhancement MRI, magnetic resonance angiography, and diffusion-weighted imaging (DWI), which permits recognition of distant metastases, involvement of the vascular bed, and distinction of CCA from HCC [33, 34]. Computed tomography (CT) can characterize mass lesions, investigate tissue invasion with involvement of regional lymph nodes, and detect the presence of extrahepatic dissemination in CCA, but its sensitivity and specificity is reduced in the setting of PSC-associated CCA (75% and 85%, respectively) [27, 33, 35].

^{18}F-Fluoro-deoxyglucose (^{18}F-FDG) positron emission tomography (PET), eventually complemented with CT (PET/CT), can be a valuable approach to detect early, small biliary tumors and metastases. In particular, PET is useful to discriminate CCA from dominant strictures in PSC patients. A high tissue uptake index (SUVmax/liver ≥3.3) is a good parameter for CCA diagnosis, with sensitivity and specificity of both around 90%, while an index <2.4 seems to rule out CCA [36]. Major drawbacks of this technique are (i) the increased number of false positives in conditions of ongoing tissue inflammation due to bacterial cholangitis or intense background disease activity and (ii) the lack of accuracy in detecting perihilar tumors, both of which are unfortunately common events in PSC.

Endoscopic procedures such as endoscopic retrograde cholangiopancreatography (ERCP) remain an important part of PSC management, in particular when imaging results are uncertain or tissue sampling is needed [37]. Dominant strictures represent the most common indication for endoscopic biliary procedures in PSC, as these lesions require careful exclusion of malignancy along with local treatment via balloon dilation and/or stenting [37, 38]. Biliary intraductal brushing can be performed during ERCP to evaluate for possible malignancy; despite a high specificity (>95%), however, it has poor sensitivity (5–40%) [39]. Thus, to improve diagnostic accuracy of conventional cytology, biliary brushing has been coupled with fluorescence in situ hybridization (FISH) assessing for chromosomal instability [39, 40], resulting in a specificity of nearly 100% and an increase in sensitivity up to 45–49% [41]. Of note, sensitivity can reach 76–89% if supported by analysis of the tumor suppressor gene *p16* (by evaluating the deletion of the 9p21 locus) [41, 42]. Detection of polysomy by FISH either in multiple areas of the biliary tree (multifocal) or in consecutive endoscopic procedures (serial) has been associated with a higher risk of CCA than when detected in unifocal or single samples [43, 44].

Endoscopic ultrasound (EUS) is another available technique to evaluate dominant strictures (as well as lymphadenopathy), having the advantage of lower morbidity than ERCP [39]. A meta-analysis performed in biliary obstructions of different etiologies showed that EUS had an overall sensitivity of 78% and a specificity of 84% in detecting malignancy [45]. Sensitivity and specificity could be further improved by combining EUS with fine needle aspiration (FNA), though patients who underwent EUS-FNA would be excluded from LT according to the Mayo Clinic protocol because of the risk of tumor seeding [46]. Additional studies are needed to better understand the role of EUS in this setting [39].

Another useful technique that has drawn increasing interest is cholangioscopy, as it allows direct visualization of the biliary mucosa to detect suspicious lesions such as nodules, ulcers, polyps, or projections and to collect tissue samples [47]. A cholangioscopic finding of dilated, tortuous subepithelial vessels is a highly suggestive feature of malignancy, though it can also be present in PSC without dysplasia [40]. Similarly, cholangioscopic biopsies are relatively limited by their small size. Notably, it is important to recognize that most studies have been conducted so far with the first-generation devices. Given the introduction of the new (third-generation) high-resolution cholangioscope (Spyglass DS™, Boston Scientific Corp., Natick, MA, USA) that provides a more thorough inspection of the mucosal profile, further studies will be needed to reassess the diagnostic accuracy of this technique, its cost-efficacy, and the rate of adverse events [39].

Novel Tumoral Biomarkers

Given the limitations of conventional serum biomarkers and noninvasive techniques, there is a need to identify novel disease biomarkers aimed at improving the early detection of CCA, eventually beyond serum sampling. These include anti-glycoprotein 2 (GP2), bile and urine biomarkers, and extracellular vesicles.

Anti-GP2 is a secretory IgA autoantibody targeting proteins predominantly expressed by exocrine pancreatic cells that can be found in PSC patients, especially those with the classic variant involving the large bile ducts, where it likely associates with poor outcomes (meaning early death or shorter LT-free survival), and this effect was primarily dependent upon development of CCA. Among the several isoforms, the combined use of anti-$GP2_1$ and anti-$GP2_4$ IgA seems more sensitive than using only one isoform, and the detection of anti-$GP2_3$ IgG seems related with a higher risk of CCA development in PSC patients. Notably, the presence of anti-GP2 IgA could identify a subset of PSC patients with a severe disease phenotype, as its association with PSC/CCA is not related with duration of disease, older age at diagnosis, and serum levels of bilirubin [8, 48]. Thus, anti-GP2 IgA may be regarded as novel tool enabling early diagnosis of PSC-associated CCA, but further studies are awaited to figure out its possible role for prioritizing LT in high-risk PSC patients [8, 48]. Another panel that has been proposed with the aim of discriminating benign from malignant biliary strictures includes pyruvate kinase M2, cytokeratin 19 fragment, mucin 5 AC, and gamma glutamyl-transferase [8].

Another biological sample that can be harnessed for prognostic/diagnostic purposes in PSC is bile [28]. Bile and urine proteome analysis have shown interesting results, with combined analysis having a sensitivity of 72% and a specificity of 96% [8]. One fundamental issue with bile collection is that it requires ERC (or other invasive means of biliary access). This is a subject of active investigation deserving consideration in future studies [28, 49].

In addition to soluble factors, cholangiocytes may secrete extracellular vesicles (EVs) as a means of cell-to-cell communication. EVs contain proteins, lipids, and nucleic acids, such as micro-ribonucleic acids (miRNAs) and long noncoding RNAs (lncRNAs). In malignant cholangiocytes, a miRNA of interest is miRNA-195, which is mutually exchanged by neoplastic and stromal cells, as it is constitutionally downregulated in both cell types and, thus, could be involved in tumorigenesis. On the other hand, trafficking of lncRNA seems related more with CCA progression. EVs produced by cancer cells contain a range of pro-invasive factors normally not released by healthy cholangiocytes. Their assessment in the so-called liquid biopsy might provide a novel noninvasive tool for early detection of CCA [49, 50].

Surveillance Programs: Still Searching for the Way to Go

One of the main issues concerning the risk of CCA in PSC has been the lack of an effective evidence-based surveillance protocol to monitor these patients. There are a number of questions that must be addressed before establishing an effective program, including (a) how frequently surveillance should be performed, (b) the tools (radiological and laboratory) with which surveillance should be conducted, and (c) how to risk stratify patients for tumor development (e.g., are there some patients who need not undergo CCA surveillance or who need it more frequently than other PSC patients?) [27].

To help address this uncertainty, a study was undertaken in a large population of PSC patients undergoing annual imaging with US, CT, or MRI/MRCP coupled with annual CA19-9 testing, with further evaluation by MRI/MRCP and/or ERCP if any newly identified biliary lesion. Taking this approach, PSC patients in the surveillance group were found to have a significantly higher 5-year overall survival (68% vs 20%, $p < 0.001$) and a significantly lower rate of CCA-related adverse events (32% vs 75%, $P < 0.001$) compared to those without a regular surveillance [51]. Based primarily on the findings of this study, published in 2018, a CCA surveillance protocol was published in 2019 by the American Gastroenterological Association recommending the combination of imaging and CA19-9 for CCA surveillance [27]. Of the imaging modalities available, MRCP (with intravenous contrast, if possible) and US appeared to have the best performance characteristics [51]. Further considerations regarding cancer surveillance in PSC are discussed elsewhere [5, 8, 27]. Large prospective studies would be useful to identify the best surveillance strategy, with the ultimate goal of improving early diagnosis when CCA is more likely to be eligible for curative treatment (e.g., surgery, LT) [27, 51].

Treatment: LT Is Often the Most Convenient Approach for PSC-Associated CCA

PSC patients with a new CCA diagnosis should undergo a multidisciplinary evaluation to choose the best treatment option based on the tumor stage. Surgical resection and LT are the only potentially curative options for early-stage CCA. If the patient is eligible for resection, surgery is the first-line approach in all CCA subtypes. Patients with intrahepatic CCA can undergo resection of the involved segments or lobe, whereas distal CCA usually involves a pancreatoduodenectomy. In pCCA, based on tumor extension, resection can involve the intra- and extrahepatic bile ducts and the ipsilateral liver, the gallbladder, and the involved regional lymph nodes. Unfortunately, the 3-year survival rate is still quite low (<20%), even when a resection with negative tumor margins is achieved. Moreover, PSC-associated CCAs are rarely diagnosed at an early stage, with most patients presenting with advanced and unresectable disease and reduced functional liver mass caused by the underlying disease.

LT is an option for patients with unresectable disease, and it is particularly attractive in PSC patients as it removes the "oncogenic field effect" exerted by the underlying chronic fibroinflammation. In this regard, patient selection is crucial to achieve the best possible outcomes and to ensure the optimal organ allocation. Data from the Nordic Liver Transplant Center based on a cohort of 53 CCA patients (34 with PSC/CCA) shows a 5-year survival of 58% when patients were selected based on a TNM stage ≤2 and a CA19-9 level ≤100 U/mL, regardless of tumor localization [52]. A 5-year survival rate up to 70% can be achieved in patients with early-stage pCCA if neoadjuvant chemoradiation is performed, although less than 10% of patients are indeed eligible candidates [53]. Another procedure for patients with unresectable pCCA eventually eligible for LT is the Mayo Clinic protocol. In this multimodal approach, patients undergo external beam radiation therapy, followed by 2 weeks of brachytherapy and then abdominal exploration for staging. Intravenous 5-fluorouracil is administered for chemosensitization during radiotherapy, and capecitabine is administered afterward until LT is performed. Following this protocol, a 5-year survival of 74% was reported in the first study [53], and similar results were reproduced in a larger multicenter study in which, notably, more than two thirds of patients had a PSC-associated CCA [54].

Beyond surgery, there are currently no data regarding specific treatment of PSC/CCA in more advanced stages, and the reader may refer to the relative chapters discussed elsewhere in the present book. Whether PSC/CCA harbors specific molecular signatures possibly behaving as actionable targets is a subject deserving attention by future studies. In fact, given the growing number of potential targets emerging in CCA, patients with unresectable PSC/CCA can be an ideal subset to be considered for enrolment in clinical trials [54, 55].

Summary and Future Directions

The close association of CCA with PSC provides a unique opportunity to unravel the intricate mechanisms by which a chronic inflammatory epithelial lesion with prominent scarring progresses through dysplasia and, in some cases, carcinoma. Although this area has been actively investigated in the past few decades, several challenges remain. For instance, the approach to surveillance remains an area of uncertainty, and discriminating CCA from a DS still often poses a diagnostic conundrum. From a therapeutic perspective, LT remains the most definitive treatment for CCA, but in some cases, this is not an option, in part because PSC-associated CCA is a difficult-to-diagnose disease in early stages. Future efforts are eagerly awaited to identify reliable predictive biomarkers of PSC progression and associated carcinogenesis as well as effective tailored therapies.

References

1. Lazaridis KN, LaRusso NF. Primary Sclerosing Cholangitis. N Engl J Med. 2016 Sep 22;375(12):1161–70;
2. Lindor KD, Kowdley KV, Harrison ME. ACG clinical guideline: primary sclerosing cholangitis. Am J Gastroenterol. 2015;110:646–59.
3. Boonstra K, Van Erpecum KJ, Van Nieuwkerk KMJ, Drenth JPH, Poen AC, Witteman BJM, Tuynman HARE, Beuers U, Ponsioen CY. Primary sclerosing cholangitis is associated with a distinct phenotype of inflammatory bowel disease. Inflamm Bowel Dis. 2012;18:2270–6.
4. Karlsen TH, Folseraas T, Thorburn D, Vesterhus M. Primary sclerosing cholangitis – a comprehensive review. J Hepatol. 2017;67:1298–323.
5. Fung BM, Lindor KD, Tabibian JH. Cancer risk in primary sclerosing cholangitis: Epidemiology, prevention, and surveillance strategies. World J Gastroenterol. 2019 Feb 14;25(6):659-671.
6. Bonato G, Cristoferi L, Strazzabosco M, Fabris L. Malignancies in primary sclerosing cholangitis--a continuing threat. Dig Dis. 2015;33:140–8.
7. Zenouzi R, Weismüller TJ, Hübener P, et al. Low risk of hepatocellular carcinoma in patients with primary sclerosing cholangitis with cirrhosis. Clin Gastroenterol Hepatol. 2014;12:1733–8.
8. Song J, Li Y, Bowlus CL, Yang GX, Leung PSC, Gershwin ME. Cholangiocarcinoma in patients with primary sclerosing cholangitis (PSC): a comprehensive review. Clin Rev Allergy Immunol. 2019; https://doi.org/10.1007/s12016-019-08764-7.
9. Rizvi S, Gores GJ. Pathogenesis, diagnosis, and management of cholangiocarcinoma. Gastroenterology. 2013;145:1215–29.
10. Burak K, Angulo P, Pasha TM, Egan K, Petz J, Lindor KD. Incidence and risk factors for cholangiocarcinoma in primary sclerosing cholangitis. Am J Gastroenterol. 2004;99:523–6.
11. Claessen MMH, Vleggaar FP, Tytgat KMAJ, Siersema PD, van Buuren HR. High lifetime risk of cancer in primary sclerosing cholangitis. J Hepatol. 2009;50:158–64.
12. Quinn KP, Tabibian JH, Lindor KD. Clinical implications of serial versus isolated biliary fluorescence in situ hybridization (FISH) polysomy in primary sclerosing cholangitis. Scand J Gastroenterol. 2017;52:377–81.
13. Chung BK, Karlsen TH, Folseraas T. Cholangiocytes in the pathogenesis of primary sclerosing cholangitis and development of cholangiocarcinoma. BBA - Mol Basis Dis. 2018;1864:1390–400.
14. Singal AK, Stanca CM, Clark V, Dixon L, Levy C, Odin JA, Fiel MI, Friedman SL, Bach N. Natural history of small duct primary sclerosing cholangitis: a case series with review of the literature. Hepatol Int. 2011;5:808–13.
15. Mederacke I, Hsu CC, Troeger JS, Huebener P, Mu X, Dapito DH, Pradere J-P, Schwabe RF. Fate tracing reveals hepatic stellate cells as dominant contributors to liver fibrosis independent of its aetiology. Nat Commun. 2013;4:2823.
16. Fabris L, Cadamuro M, Cagnin S, Strazzabosco M, Gores GJ. Liver matrix in benign and malignant biliary tract disease. Semin Liver Dis. 2020; https://doi.org/10.1055/s-0040-1705109.

17. O'Hara SP, Karlsen TH, NF LR. Cholangiocytes and the environment in primary sclerosing cholangitis: where is the link? Gut. 2017;66:1873 LP–1877.
18. Kamihira T, Shimoda S, Nakamura M, Yokoyama T, Takii Y, Kawano A, Handa M, Ishibashi H, Gershwin ME, Harada M. Biliary epithelial cells regulate autoreactive T cells: implications for biliary-specific diseases. Hepatology. 2005;41:151–9.
19. Xu B, Broome U, Ericzon BG, Sumitran-Holgersson S. High frequency of autoantibodies in patients with primary sclerosing cholangitis that bind biliary epithelial cells and induce expression of CD44 and production of interleukin 6. Gut. 2002;51:120–7.
20. Takeda K, Kojima Y, Ikejima K, et al. Death receptor 5 mediated-apoptosis contributes to cholestatic liver disease. Proc Natl Acad Sci. 2008;105:10895–900.
21. Yoon JH, Canbay AE, Werneburg NW, Lee SP, Gores GJ. Oxysterols induce cyclooxygenase-2 expression in cholangiocytes: implications for biliary tract carcinogenesis. Hepatology. 2004;39:732–8.
22. Yoon JH, Gwak GY, Lee HS, Bronk SF, Werneburg NW, Gores GJ. Enhanced epidermal growth factor receptor activation in human cholangiocarcinoma cells. J Hepatol. 2004;41:808–14.
23. Cadamuro M, Stecca T, Brivio S, Mariotti V, Fiorotto R, Spirli C, Strazzabosco M, Fabris L. The deleterious interplay between tumor epithelia and stroma in cholangiocarcinoma. Biochim Biophys Acta Mol basis Dis. 2018;1864:1435–43.
24. Dyson JK, Beuers U, Jones DEJ, Lohse AW, Hudson M. Seminar primary sclerosing cholangitis. Lancet. 2018;391:2547–59.
25. Hilscher MB, Tabibian JH, Carey EJ, Gostout CJ, Lindor KD. Dominant strictures in primary sclerosing cholangitis: a multicenter survey of clinical definitions and practices. Hepatol Commun. 2018;2:836–44.
26. Pohl J, Ring A, Stremmel W, Stiehl A. The role of dominant stenoses in bacterial infections of bile ducts in primary sclerosing cholangitis. Eur J Gastroenterol Hepatol. 2006;18:69–74.
27. Bowlus CL, Lim JK, Lindor KD. AGA clinical practice update on surveillance for hepatobiliary cancers in patients with primary sclerosing cholangitis: expert review. Clin Gastroenterol Hepatol. 2019;17:2416–22.
28. Wannhoff A, Gotthardt DN. Recent developments in the research on biomarkers of cholangiocarcinoma in primary sclerosing cholangitis. Clin Res Hepatol Gastroenterol. 2019 Jun;43(3):236–243.
29. Wannhoff A, Hov JR, Folseraas T, et al. FUT2 and FUT3 genotype determines CA19-9 cut-off values for detection of cholangiocarcinoma in patients with primary sclerosing cholangitis. J Hepatol. 2013;59:1278–84.
30. Nehls O, Gregor M, Klump B. Serum and bile markers for cholangiocarcinoma. Semin Liver Dis. 2004;24:139–54.
31. Sinakos E, Saenger AK, Keach J, Kim WR, Lindor KD. Many patients with primary sclerosing cholangitis and increased serum levels of carbohydrate antigen 19-9 do not have cholangiocarcinoma. Clin Gastroenterol Hepatol. 2011;9:434–9.
32. Wannhoff A, Rupp C, Friedrich K, et al. Inflammation but not biliary obstruction is associated with carbohydrate antigen 19-9 levels in patients with primary sclerosing cholangitis. Clin Gastroenterol Hepatol. 2015;13:2372–9.
33. Jhaveri KS, Hosseini-Nik H. MRI of cholangiocarcinoma. J Magn Reson Imaging. 2015;42:1165–79.
34. Chapman R, Fevery J, Kalloo A, Nagorney DM, Boberg KM, Shneider B, Gores GJ; American Association for the Study of Liver Diseases. Diagnosis and management of primary sclerosing cholangitis. Hepatology. 2010 Feb;51(2):660–78.
35. Charatcharoenwitthaya P, Enders FB, Halling KC, Lindor KD. Utility of serum tumor markers, imaging, and biliary cytology for detecting cholangiocarcinoma in primary sclerosing cholangitis. Hepatology. 2008;48:1106–17.
36. Sangfelt P, Sundin A, Wanders A, Rasmussen I, Karlson BM, Bergquist A, Rorsman F. Monitoring dominant strictures in primary sclerosing cholangitis with brush cytology and FDG-PET. J Hepatol. 2014;61:1352–7.

37. Aabakken L, Karlsen TH, Albert J, et al. Role of endoscopy in primary sclerosing cholangitis: European Society of Gastrointestinal Endoscopy (ESGE) and European Association for the Study of the Liver (EASL) clinical guideline. Endoscopy. 2017;49:588–608.
38. European Association for the Study of the Liver. EASL clinical practice guidelines: management of cholestatic liver diseases. J Hepatol. 2009;51:237–67.
39. Fung BM, Tabibian JH. Biliary endoscopy in the management of primary sclerosing cholangitis and its complications. Liver Res. 2019;3:106–17.
40. Tabibian JH. Advanced endoscopic imaging of indeterminate biliary strictures. World J Gastrointest Endosc. 2015;7:1268.
41. Gonda TA, Glick MP, Sethi A, et al. Polysomy and p16 deletion by fluorescence in situ hybridization in the diagnosis of indeterminate biliary strictures. Gastrointest Endosc. 2012;75:74–9.
42. Boldorini R, Paganotti A, Andorno S, Orlando S, Mercalli F, Orsello M, Ballarè M, Magnani C, Sartori M. A multistep cytological approach for patients with jaundice and biliary strictures of indeterminate origin. J Clin Pathol. 2015;68:283–7.
43. Fritcher EGB, Kipp BR, Voss JS, Clayton AC, Lindor KD, Halling KC, Gores GJ. Primary sclerosing cholangitis patients with serial polysomy fluorescence in situ hybridization results are at increased risk of cholangiocarcinoma. Am J Gastroenterol. 2011;106:2023–8.
44. Eaton JE, Barr Fritcher EG, Gores GJ, Atkinson EJ, Tabibian JH, Topazian MD, Gossard AA, Halling KC, Kipp BR, Lazaridis KN. Biliary multifocal chromosomal polysomy and cholangiocarcinoma in primary sclerosing cholangitis. Am J Gastroenterol. 2015;110:299–309.
45. Garrow D, Miller S, Sinha D, Conway J, Hoffman BJ, Hawes RH, Romagnuolo J. Endoscopic ultrasound: a meta-analysis of test performance in suspected biliary obstruction. Clin Gastroenterol Hepatol. 2007; https://doi.org/10.1016/j.cgh.2007.02.027.
46. Navaneethan U, Njei B, Venkatesh P, et al. Endoscopic ultrasound in the diagnosis of cholangiocarcinoma as the etiology of biliary strictures: a systematic review and meta-analysis. Gastroenterol Rep. 2015; https://doi.org/10.1093/GASTRO/GOU057.
47. Seo DW, Lee SK, Yoo KS, Kang GH, Kim MH, Suh DJ, Il MY. Cholangioscopic findings in bile duct tumors. Gastrointest Endosc. 2000;52:630–4.
48. Jendrek ST, Gotthardt D, Nitzsche T, et al. Anti-GP2 IgA autoantibodies are associated with poor survival and cholangiocarcinoma in primary sclerosing cholangitis. Gut. 2017;66:137–44.
49. Rizvi S, Eaton J, Yang JD, Chandrasekhara V, Gores GJ. Emerging technologies for the diagnosis of perihilar cholangiocarcinoma. Semin Liver Dis. 2018;38:160–9.
50. Arbelaiz A, Azkargorta M, Krawczyk M, et al. Serum extracellular vesicles contain protein biomarkers for primary sclerosing cholangitis and cholangiocarcinoma. Hepatology. 2017;66:1125–43.
51. Ali AH, Tabibian JH, Nasser-Ghodsi N, Lennon RJ, DeLeon T, Borad MJ, Hilscher M, Silveira MG, Carey EJ, Lindor KD. Surveillance for hepatobiliary cancers in patients with primary sclerosing cholangitis. Hepatology. 2018;67:2338–51.
52. Friman S, Foss A, Isoniemi H, Olausson M, Höckerstedt K, Yamamoto S, Karlsen TH, Rizell M, Ericzon B-G. Liver transplantation for cholangiocarcinoma: Selection is essential for acceptable results. Scand J Gastroenterol. 2011;46:370–5.
53. Rosen CB, Heimbach JK, Gores GJ. Liver transplantation for cholangiocarcinoma. Transpl Int. 2010;23:692–7.
54. Darwish Murad S, Kim WR, Harnois DM, et al. Efficacy of neoadjuvant chemoradiation, followed by liver transplantation, for perihilar cholangiocarcinoma at 12 US centers. Gastroenterology. 2012;143:88–98.
55. Rizvi S, Khan SA, Hallemeier CL, Kelley RK. Cholangiocarcinoma — evolving concepts and therapeutic strategies. Nat Rev Clin Oncol. 2017;15:95–111.
56. Hirschfield GM, Karlsen TH, Lindor KD, Adams DH. Primary sclerosing cholangitis. Lancet. 2013;382:1587–99.

Chapter 11
Fluke-Associated Cholangiocarcinoma: A Regional Epidemic

Sakda Waraasawapati, Raksawan Deenonpoe, Prakasit Sa-ngiamwibool, Yaovalux Chamgramol, and Chawalit Pairojkul

Abbreviations

5-FU	5-Fluorouracil
BilIN	Biliary intraepithelial neoplasia
C. sinensis	Clonorchis sinensis
CCA	Cholangiocarcinoma
dCCA	Distal cholangiocarcinoma
eCCA	Extrahepatic cholangiocarcinoma
ELISA	Enzyme-linked immunosorbent assay
HBsAg	Hepatitis B surface antigen
HBV	Hepatitis B virus
HCV Ab	Hepatitis C antibody
HCV	Hepatitis C virus
iCCA	Intrahepatic cholangiocarcinoma
ID	Intraductal-growing intrahepatic cholangiocarcinoma
IL-1	Interleukin-1
IL-1β	Interleukin-1β
IL-6	Interleukin-6
IPNB	Intraductal papillary neoplasm of bile duct
KKCR	Khon Kaen Cancer Registry
KKH	Khon Kaen University Hospital
MF	Mass-forming intrahepatic cholangiocarcinoma
NF-κB	Nuclear factor-κB
O. felineus	Opisthorchis felineus
O. viverrini	Opisthorchis viverrini
PBG	Peribiliary gland
pCCA	Perihilar cholangiocarcinoma

S. Waraasawapati · R. Deenonpoe · P. Sa-ngiamwibool · Y. Chamgramol · C. Pairojkul (✉)
Department of Pathology, Faculty of Medicine, Khon Kaen University, Khon Kaen, Thailand
e-mail: sakdawa@kku.ac.th; raksde@kku.ac.th; prakasa@kku.ac.th; cyaova@kku.ac.th; chawpa@kku.ac.th

J. H. Tabibian (ed.), *Diagnosis and Management of Cholangiocarcinoma*,
https://doi.org/10.1007/978-3-030-70936-5_11

PI	Periductal-infiltrating intrahepatic cholangiocarcinoma
TNF	Tumor necrosis factor

Introduction

In the northeast of Thailand, a cultural habit of eating raw fish on a daily basis results in a local population being repeatedly exposed to liver fluke (*O. viverrini*) infection and having the highest incidence of cholangiocarcinoma (CCA) worldwide [1, 2]. There is substantial evidence from animal models that liver flukes are a CCA risk factor which exert carcinogenic effects by inducing chronic inflammation of bile ducts during the course of persistent infestation [3–6]. The morphology and histology of CCA in regions endemic of liver fluke or hepatolithiasis are similar to sporadic CCA [7, 8], with the majority of tumors arising from large bile ducts, and specifically perihilar CCA (pCCA) being the most common [9, 10]. However, in fluke-related CCA, intrahepatic CCA (iCCA) [1, 2] and the papillary CCA phenotype are more common than in sporadic CCA [10–12]. The peak age incidence of fluke-related CCA is in the sixth decade, about 5–10 years younger than sporadic CCA. This chapter provides an overview of the geographical distribution and pathology of liver flukes, the spectrum of CCA, treatment outcomes, and the prevention of endemic fluke-related CCA in Thailand.

The Parasites and Their Associated Illnesses

Fascioliasis and opisthorchiasis are two food-borne trematode zoonoses, causing hepatobiliary diseases in humans. As the former is not a chronic zoonosis or risk factor for CCA, it will be only briefly discussed, with the major focus of the chapter being on opisthorchiasis, a major risk factor for CCA in endemic regions.

Fascioliasis

Fascioliasis is a parasitic infection of ruminants, caused by *Fasciola hepatica* or *Fasciola gigantica*, also known as "the liver fluke of sheep and cattle" (Fig. 11.1a). Fascioliasis is a global veterinary problem, though an increasing number of human cases, estimated to be exceeding 2.4 million people worldwide, have been reported in several regions of the Middle East, Asia, Latin America, and Africa [13–15]. People are accidental hosts that become infected by eating raw watercress or other water plants contaminated with parasite larvae. The young worms move through the intestinal wall, the abdominal cavity, and the liver tissue, into the bile ducts, where

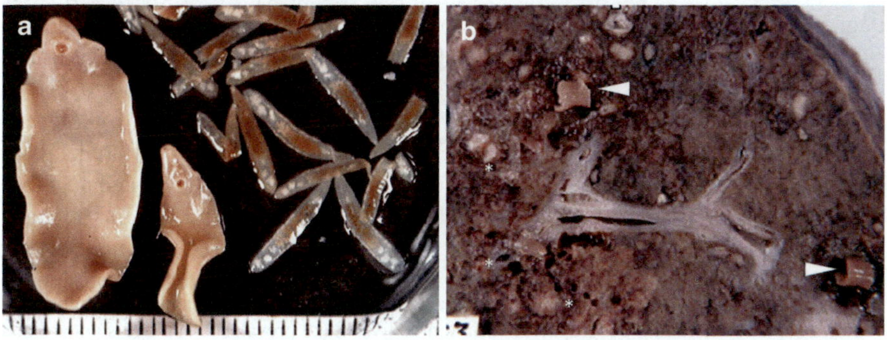

Fig. 11.1 Fascioliasis. (**a**) Two types of liver fluke, adult *Fasciola* (left) and adult *Opisthorchis* (right); (**b**) adult *Fasciola* (arrowhead) migration out of bile ducts causing liver parenchyma necrosis (asterisk)

they develop into adult flukes, which are larger than human bile ducts. The pathology is pronounced in the bile ducts and liver, causing (i) bile duct obstruction and liver necrosis (rotted liver disease) (Fig. 11.1b) or (ii) parasitic pseudotumor, which may also occur in ectopic sites [14, 16]. *Fasciola* infection is transient and noncarcinogenic in humans.

Opisthorchiasis

Geographical Distribution and Mode of Transmission

Opisthorchiasis is a freshwater fish-borne disease caused by the liver flukes, *Opisthorchis viverrini* (Fig. 11.1a), *Opisthorchis felineus,* and its closely related *Clonorchis sinensis* (clonorchiasis). *O. viverrini* is prevalent mainly in the lower Mekong subregion countries including Thailand, Laos, Cambodia, and Vietnam (Fig. 11.2a). *O. felineus* occurs in Ukraine, Kazakhstan, and Russia. *C. sinensis* is endemic in China, Korea, and Taiwan [17–19]. Infection with the liver flukes *O. viverrini* and *C. sinensis* persists as a major public health problem in Asia. Recent estimates suggest that about 35 million people are infected by *C. sinensis* worldwide, and in China alone, it could reach 15 million people [20]. Current reports of *O. viverrini* infection reach over ten million people, with approximately six million in Thailand alone [21]. The geographical pattern of liver fluke infection is not uniform; it depends on local habits of eating raw fish and presence of the first intermediate host, e.g., the sand snail (*"Bithynia siamensis"*). Moreover, in endemic areas, prevalence and intensity of infection are higher in rural riparian communities (as compared to urban communities), being relatively common along the tributaries of rivers and in the vicinity of natural water sources.

In China, *C. sinensis* is found mainly in South China, e.g., Guangdong, Guangxi, and Sichuan [20]. In Thailand, the distribution of *O. viverrini* is endemic in the

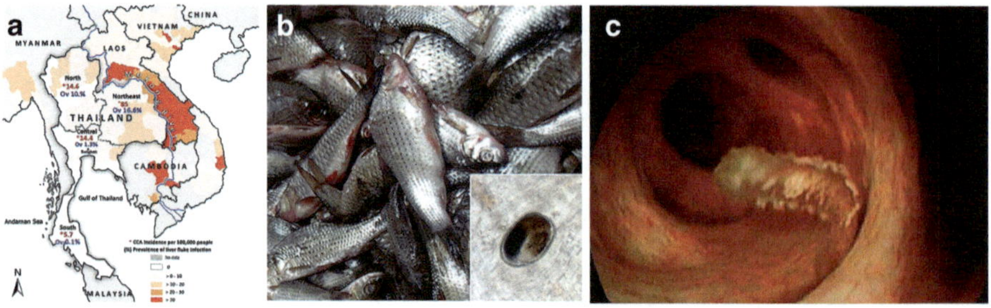

Fig. 11.2 (**a**) The estimated percentages of prevalence of liver fluke infection in the Mekong subregion countries, including geographical variation of liver fluke prevalence and age-standardized incidence rates of cholangiocarcinoma (CCA) in Thailand (Adapted from Bragazzi M et al. (2012) & Sripa B et al. (2011)) [2, 135]. (**b**) Freshwater crypinids, second intermediate host, inset a metacercaria of *O. viverrini* in fish fresh (200 μm). (**c**) Cholangioscopic picture of adult *Opisthorchis* inhabiting inside a lumen of the large intrahepatic bile duct. *Cr. Ake Pugkhem (MD), KKU*

northeast followed by the north and the central region, with virtually no infection in the south of the country (Fig. 11.2a) [22]. Interestingly, the age-standardized incidences rates of CCA are 15 times higher in highly endemic regions of liver fluke infection compared to regions where infection is rare (Fig. 11.2a) [23].

In Northeastern Thailand, liver fluke infection is induced by eating popular simple dishes: marinated chopped raw fish ("Koi Pla") or a short-pickled fish ("PlaSom"), preparations from freshwater fish (a second intermediate host in the life cycle of liver fluke) which contains the infective metacercaria in tissue (Fig. 11.2b) [24, 25]. The metacercaria excysts to become a juvenile worm in the duodenum and then migrates to the intrahepatic bile ducts via the common bile duct, and the hermaphroditic adult flukes (Figs. 11.1a and 11.2c) produce eggs that are excreted in the feces [26]. The egg develops into larva in the *Bithynia* spp. snail (the first intermediated host), which then releases the free-swimming cercaria which penetrates into fish tissue, encyst, and develop into infective metacercaria [24]. Although poor sanitation may be a major cause of human fecal contamination of community water, improvements in sanitation will likely not completely prevent the continuation of *O. viverrini* transmission, as the feline and canine reservoir hosts will continue to pass on the eggs [27].

Diagnosis and Treatment

Fecal analysis and enzyme-linked immunosorbent assay (ELISA) testing are used to diagnose opisthorchiasis. Presence of adult flukes during laparotomy or at autopsy and microscopic demonstration of eggs present in the feces or bile specimens, either by simple smear or concentration techniques, are the gold standard for diagnosing fluke infestation. The modified formalin-ethyl acetate concentration technique can quantify the intensity of infection into number of egg counts per gram of stool [28]. The immunodiagnosis via serologic detection of anti-parasitic antibody for assessment of previous exposure to infection and detection of parasitic antigen using mAb detection in stool for determining current infection is also employed. While mAb ELISA detects *O. viverrini* antigens or copro-antigens in stool, it only detects current infections, whereas the indirect antibody ELISA can detect past infections, as antibodies persist in body fluids following treatment. However, use of the indirect antibody ELISA in epidemiological studies is limited because of cross-reaction with other parasites and inability to differentiate between present and past exposure to infection [29].

Praziquantel is cheap, inexpensive, and effective anti-helminthic treatment for *O. viverrini* infection and has been used in Thailand since the early 1980s. This drug reduced the prevalence of *O. viverrini* infection in Thailand from 80% to 15–20% in 1997 [21]. Despite the high effectivity of anti-parasitic treatments, the prevalence and reinfection rates for liver fluke remain considerable [30], and cholestasis from inflammation and fibrosis of the bile duct persists as a risk factor for CCA development [31].

Pathology of Opisthorchiasis and Cholangiocarcinogenesis

The precise mechanisms of CCA are not completely understood; however, several recognized risk factors share common features: cholestasis; infection; and inflammation. The known reported risk factors for CCA include primary sclerosing cholangitis [32], hepatolithiasis [33], unresected choledochal cyst, chronic hepatitis virus infection [34], *Helicobacter pylori* infection [35], and liver fluke infestation with *O. viverrini* and *C. sinensis* [17, 24, 36]. Based on case series, epidemiological, and experimental animal models, the International Agency for Research on Cancer [37] classified *O. viverrini* and *C. sinensis* as class 1 and 2A carcinogens in humans. Nevertheless, and despite health education efforts, enduring eating habits continue to enable liver flukes to pose a persistent health problem in Asian countries.

Pathology of Opisthorchiasis

Infestation with liver flukes is usually neglected because of a lack of or only nonspecific symptoms. Only small fraction of individuals with liver fluke infection (typically those with heavy infection burden) have symptoms of abdominal pain, flatulence, or dyspepsia [38, 39]. Infestation is occasionally also associated with development of secondary hepatobiliary diseases, e.g., suppurative cholangitis and cholelithiasis [40–44].

In humans, *O. viverrini* inhabits the lumen of the intra- and extrahepatic bile ducts (Fig. 11.2c) and rarely the gallbladder and pancreatic duct [26]. The pathologic consequences of infection occur mainly in the biliary tree, and severity appears to be associated with both intensity and duration of infection.

In early stages of infection, the biliary mucosa in proximity of a fluke becomes edematous or desquamated, with inflammatory cell infiltration in ductal walls. In heavy infection, chronic and repeated mechanical injury by fluke bodies and suckers results in a periductal mononuclear infiltration response to mucosal trauma and fluke antigens, regenerative hyperplasia with or without goblet cell metaplasia of biliary epithelia, and proliferation of submucosal peribiliary glands (PBGs) [44–46] (Fig. 11.3a). Chronic and persistent infection result in increasing fibrosis in periductal tissue and the bile duct wall, and the fibrotic bile ducts compress and narrow the lumen, leading to cholestasis (Fig. 11.3b) [43, 44]. Biliary pathology of opisthorchiasis is similar in adults and children, and the changes are established within 7–15 years after fluke infestation [47].

A distinct gross pathological finding in chronic and heavy infection is white fibrotic lines or nodules that appear on the capsular surface of the liver (Fig. 11.4a) [43, 48, 49]. The bile ducts on cut surfaces of the liver and the extrahepatic bile duct may show slight thickening (Fig. 11.4b). The gallbladder may have mild mural thickening and contain sludge [40, 50]. The other organs are unremarkable.

While opisthorchiasis has mostly nonspecific symptoms, occasional complications do occur. Patients may present with high fever with chills, right subcostal pain from bile sludge or pigment stone obstructing the cystic duct leading to acute cholecystitis, or secondary infection from bacteria in bile on minute ulcers from fluke suckers resulting in a suppurative cholangitis [43, 51].

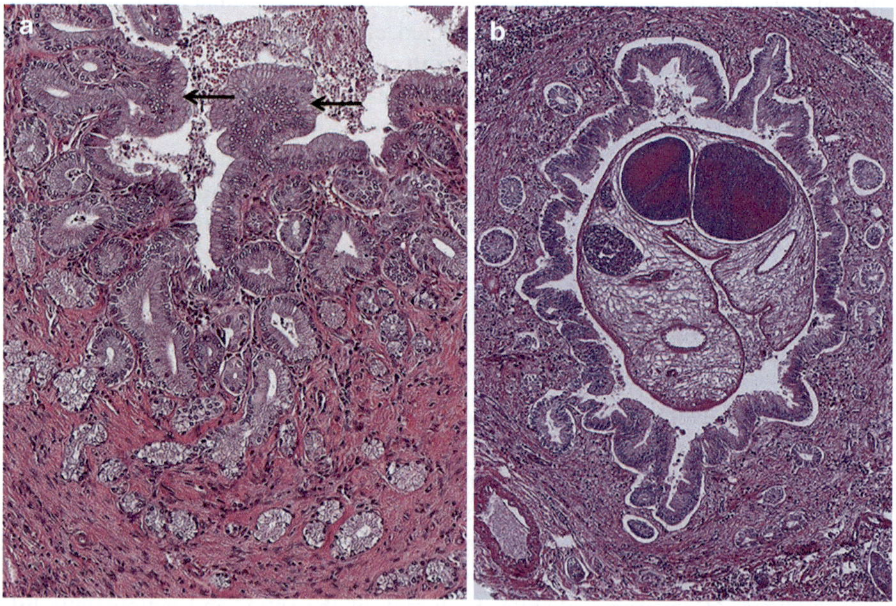

Fig. 11.3 Histopathology of large intrahepatic bile ducts in chronic opisthorchiasis. (**a**) Biliary epithelial and peribiliary gland (PBG) hyperplasia, focal nuclear stratification of biliary epithelial hyperplasia (black arrow), with PBGs and conduits proliferation in the submucosa noted. (**b**) Periductal fibrosis, fibrosis at bile duct wall, with remnant PBGs is focally seen. Focal hyperplasia of biliary epithelium and a fluke in a narrowing bile duct lumen are evidence

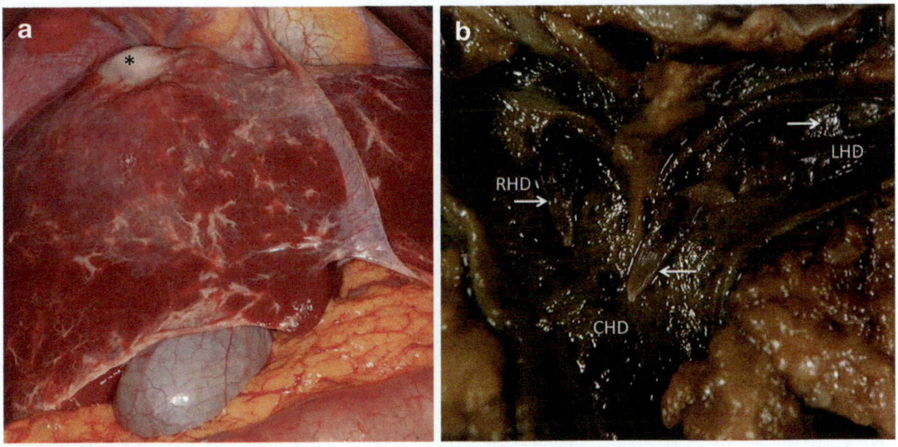

Fig. 11.4 Pathology of the liver and perihilar bile duct in chronic opisthorchiasis. (**a**) Evidence of liver fluke infestation in liver with cholangiocarcinoma (CCA): white streaks and nodules of fibrotic bile ducts at capsular surface on both lobes of liver; note a CCA mass [asterisk] at segment VIII of right lobe; (**b**) few adult *Opisthorchis* [arrow] in lumen of thick-walled bile duct at hepatic hilum [RHD, right hepatic duct; LHD, left hepatic duct; and CHD, common hepatic duct]

Liver Fluke-related Cholangiocarcinogenesis

Carcinogenesis is a multistage process driven by carcinogens which induce genetic and epigenetic damage in susceptible cells that gain a selective growth advantage and undergo clonal expansion as the result of activation of oncogenes and/or inactivation of tumor suppressor genes [51, 52]. In cholangiocarcinogenesis associated with liver fluke infection, the chronic inflammation process plays a key role, and hyperplasia of PBGs and regenerative hyperplasia of the biliary epithelium are thought to be sources of cancer susceptibility.

PBGs are tubular-alveolar glands with serous and mucinous acini embedded in a submucosa and fibromuscular bed which connect to bile duct lumina by small conduits (Fig. 11.5). Human PBGs contain biliary stem/progenitor cells within extrahepatic and large intrahepatic bile ducts [53–55] and are able to respond to bile duct epithelial loss with proliferation, differentiation, and maturation to restore epithelial integrity [56–58]. PBGs may undergo hyperplastic changes, as can be seen in the setting of chronic bile duct inflammation in hepatolithiasis and those with liver fluke infestation (Fig. 11.3a) [59, 60]. Chronic inflammation is a risk factor for the development of numerous cancers. In the case of CCA, several lines of evidence exist. For example, a series of experimental studies of *O. viverrini* infection in hamster models demonstrate this relationship [61–63]. In response to *O. viverrini* infection, macrophages and other inflammatory cells are activated by proinflammatory cytokines (IL-1β, TNF, IL-6). The proinflammatory cytokines (e.g., IL-1, TNF) are capable of stimulating NF-κB transcription factors-mediated induction of oxidative stress response enzymes, thus generating reactive oxygen and nitrogen species.

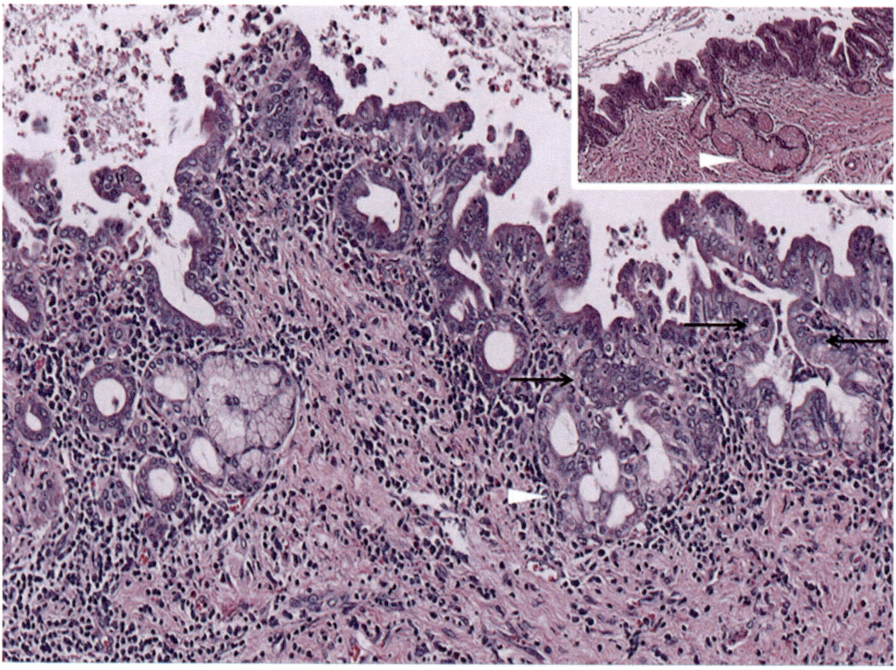

Fig. 11.5 Biliary epithelium dysplasia (note stratification and enlarged nuclei) of flat precursor lesion, now termed biliary intraepithelial neoplasia (BilIN) of the extrahepatic bile duct (large bile duct). Note the dysplasia is also seen at epithelial lining of peribiliary gland (PBG) conduits (black arrow) that continue to BilIN lesion. Inset is normal extrahepatic bile duct, showing normal PBG (arrowhead) and a tubular conduit (white arrow) connecting to bile duct lumen

Nitric oxide is generated by inducible nitric oxide synthase and can cause damage to DNA and proteins resulting in mutagenic changes [64]. During these processes, proinflammatory cytokines can also stimulate cyclooxygenase-2 expression, which can promote PBGs and biliary epithelium growth via activation of growth factors such as epidermal growth factor receptor and mitogen-activated protein kinases [65, 66]. Moreover, during the repair process, PBGs react to maintain bile duct integrity with proliferation and regeneration of the epithelial lining, paralleled by stromal remodeling via myofibroblasts. Myofibroblasts are generated from a variety of sources including resident mesenchymal cells, epithelial and endothelial. These processes are termed epithelial-mesenchymal transition that results in an increase in fibrosis of the bile ducts and nearby tissue (Figs. 11.3b and 11.4) [67–69]. Periductal fibrosis leads to cholestasis, which fosters an environment in which repeated bacterial infection, continued cell death, and compensatory regeneration might act as nonspecific enhancing stimuli and increase susceptibility to carcinogens in bile. Chronic bile duct damage induced by persistent fluke infestation and inflammatory cytokines can result in genetic mutations of regenerative epithelium and expansion of initiated cells, eventually leading to CCA.

It is important to note that that CCA develops only in a small percentage of definitive hosts (e.g., humans, cats, dogs) with chronic liver fluke infection, implying that other factors or an additional pathological process may be necessary for malignant transformation. Most epithelial cancers develop in a stepwise progression from normal mucosal cells to epithelial hyperplasia or adenomatous hyperplasia, dysplasia, carcinoma in situ, and eventually invasive cancer (see also *Chaps 3 and 4*). Marked hyperplasia of PBGs, in part associated with dysplasia, is observed in patients with hepatolithiasis and those with liver fluke infestation [59, 60]. Biliary epithelial hyperplasia precedes biliary epithelial dysplasia [33, 49, 70] (Fig. 11.5), now termed biliary intraepithelial neoplasia (BilIN) [71, 72] (Fig. 11.6a), a flat precursor lesion of large bile duct CCA which progresses to tubular adenocarcinoma via the hyperplasia-dysplasia-carcinoma sequence (Fig. 11.6a, c) [73, 74]. PBG hyperplasia can develop into intraductal papilloma (adenoma), now termed intraductal papillary neoplasm of bile duct (IPNB) (Fig. 11.6b) [59, 75–77], a nodular precursor lesion of papillary carcinoma (of the large bile duct) which

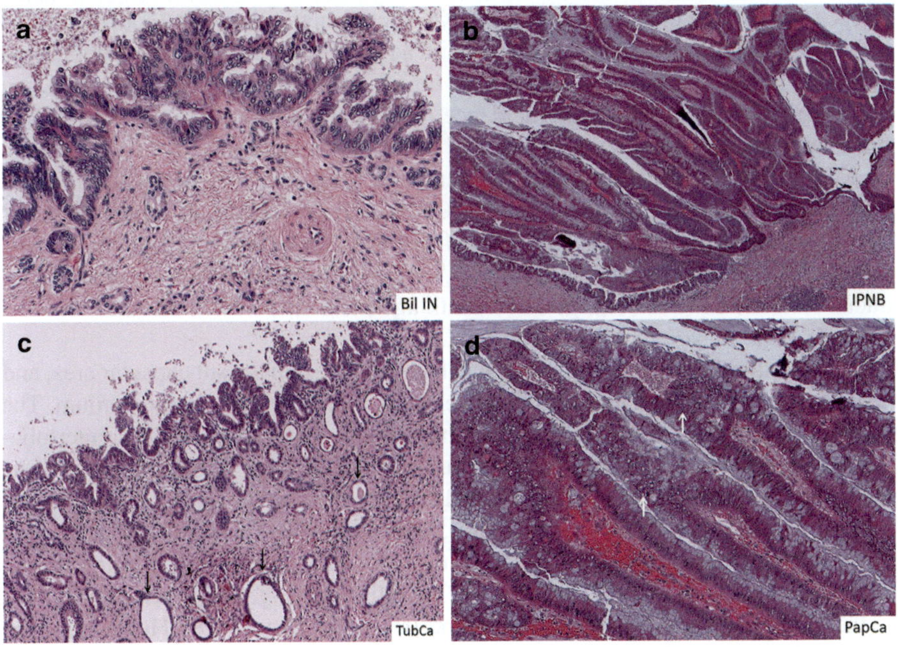

Fig. 11.6 Precursor lesions and carcinogenesis of large bile duct cholangiocarcinoma (CCA). (**a**) Flat precursor lesion: biliary intraepithelial neoplasia [BilIN]. A micropapillary growth of atypical biliary epithelium. (**b**) Nodular precursor lesion: intraductal papillary neoplasm of bile duct [IPNB], a macroscopic lesion with prominent papillary growth of atypical biliary epithelium with fibrovascular core. (**c**) Tubular adenocarcinoma [TubCa] (black arrow); the invasive lesion proceeds from high-grade BilIN lesion and carcinoma in situ at mucosa lining lumen. This carcinogenesis process termed "hyperplasia-dysplasia-carcinoma sequence." (**d**) Papillary carcinoma [PapCa], with early invasive foci (white arrow), wherein the malignant lesion progresses from an IPNB. This carcinogenesis process is named "adenoma-carcinoma sequence"

undergoes malignant transformation by way of adenoma-carcinoma sequence (Fig. 11.6b, d) [78–80]. Thus, bile duct changes in chronic liver fluke infection can progress to precancerous lesions and ultimately transform into CCA.

Cholangiocarcinoma in Thailand

Spectrum of Cholangiocarcinoma

CCA is a heterogeneous group of malignancies arising from hepatic progenitor cells, biliary epithelial cells, or PBGs of the intrahepatic and extrahepatic bile ducts [78, 81, 82]. In 2010, the American Joint Committee on Cancer reclassified CCAs into intrahepatic CCA (iCCA) and extrahepatic CCA (eCCA), using hepatic ducts as the separation point. The latter (eCCA) is further subdivided into perihilar CCA (pCCA) and distal CCA (dCCA) at the level of the cystic duct [83–85]. Using this proposed classification, CCA case distribution is as follows: 60–70% pCCA, 20–30% dCCA, and 8–10% iCCA. CCA arising from the intrahepatic bile ducts accounts for only 10% of cases.

Khon Kaen is a city in NE Thailand, with a population of 1.7 million people, and an endemic area of the liver fluke *O. viverrini*. CCA is highly prevalent in Khon Kaen, with an age-standardized incidence rate (ASR) of 58.8 and 23.6 per 100,000 males and females, respectively [86]. Of 221 patients operated on with a curative intent for CCA between 2011 and 2014 at Khon Kaen University Hospital (KKH), employing the AJCC-2010 subtypes, pCCA was the most common type with 117 (52.9%), followed by iCCA 82 (37.1%), dCCA 9 (4.1%), and combined type (skipped intra- and extrahepatic tumors arising from multifocal or diffuse intraductal lesions) 13 (5.8%) (Fig. 11.7). Peak age incidence was in the sixth decade, about 5–10 years younger than sporadic CCA [10].

iCCA is divided into peripheral type, which is located in the subcapsular area, and central type, which presents as a focal liver mass proximal to the hepatic hilum. The former usually arises from the small intrahepatic bile ducts (bile ductules, interlobular and septal bile ducts), while the latter arises from the large intrahepatic bile ducts (segmental and area ducts) [87, 88]. In addition to their anatomical location, CCAs are also classified by their gross features, which relate to their growth and spread patterns [89, 90]. iCCAs are classified into mass-forming (MF), periductal-infiltrating (PI), and intraductal-growing (ID) types. The MF type (Fig. 11.7a) usually belongs to the peripheral type of iCCA while PI and ID to central type [78]. However, in the advanced stages, iCCA of the PI type and those of IG type invade the liver parenchyma, termed as PI+MF and ID+MF types and manifested as MF type (Fig. 11.8) [88, 90, 91]. These were the cases, found in liver fluke-related CCA; among 82 cases of iCCAs, 71 (86.5%) were MF, and 10 (12.2%) were ID, and PI was 1 (1.2%) case. The gross classification of iCCA is relatively comparable with the grouping of eCCAs (pCCA and dCCA) into nodular-infiltrating (Fig. 11.7b), flat, or scirrhous and polyploid types (Fig. 11.7c) [78]. Among the 117 cases of pCCA in the Khon Kaen University Hospital surgical series, 51 (43.6%) were scirrhous type, 47 (40.2%) were nodular-infiltrating type, and 19 (16.2%) were polypoid type.

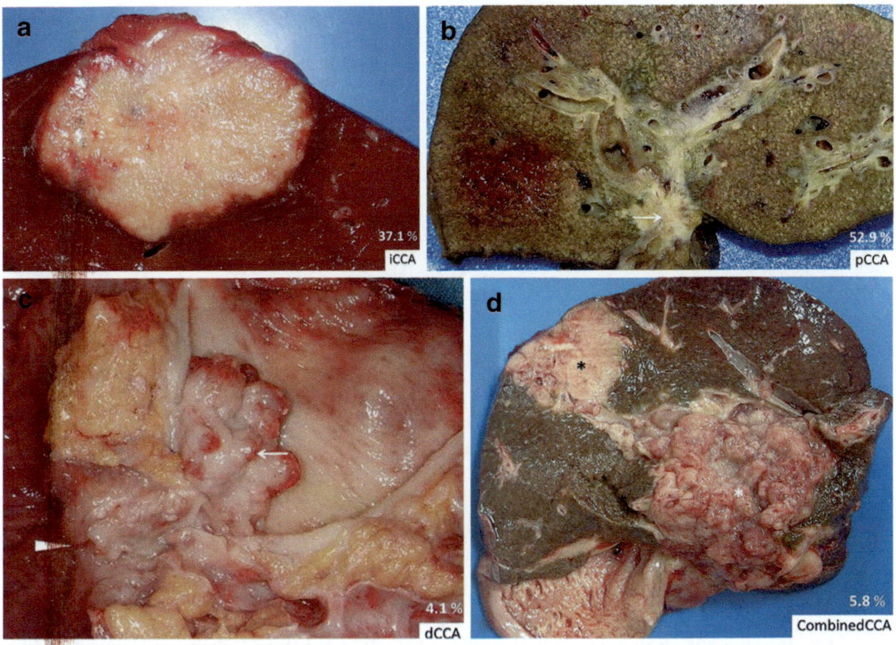

Fig. 11.7 Spectrum of prevalence and subtypes of 221 cholangiocarcinoma (CCA) cases in Thailand, display on each representative of subtype. (**a**) Intrahepatic CCA 82 (37.1%). (**b**) Perihilar CCA 117 (52.9%), the arrow points to the primary site at proximal extrahepatic bile duct. (**c**) Distal CCA 9 (4.1%); the arrowhead indicates the ampulla of Vater and the intraductal polypoid lesion pointed out by arrow. (**d**) Combined CCA 13 (5.8%), skipped intrahepatic and extrahepatic lesions, marked by black and white asterisks, respectively

Histologically, CCAs are adenocarcinomas whose major phenotypes are tubular and papillary, and additionally rare variants (*Chap. 3, Nakanuma et al.*) [78, 89]. With regard to the histological phenotypes in the aforementioned 221 cases, overall incidence of the tubular type (Fig. 11.6c) was 143 (64.7%), the papillary type (Fig. 11.6d) was 62 (28.1%), and variant types was 16 (7.2%).

Risk Factors and CCA Subtypes

CCAs are a heterogeneous group of bile duct cancers. The different CCA subtypes might reflect the diverse underlying risk factors. In Thailand, people are exposed to a number of risk factors for CCA – e.g., infestation with the liver fluke *O. viverrini*, infection with HBV and HCV, and nitrosamine in traditional fermented dishes [3, 6, 49]. Chronic inflammation associated with fluke infestation primarily affects large intrahepatic bile ducts near the hepatic hilum and the proximal extrahepatic bile duct [6, 49], which likely contributes to the high incidence of iCCA and pCCA. A case-control study showed a significant association between papillary iCCA and repeated use of praziquantel [92], findings which support the hypothesis that

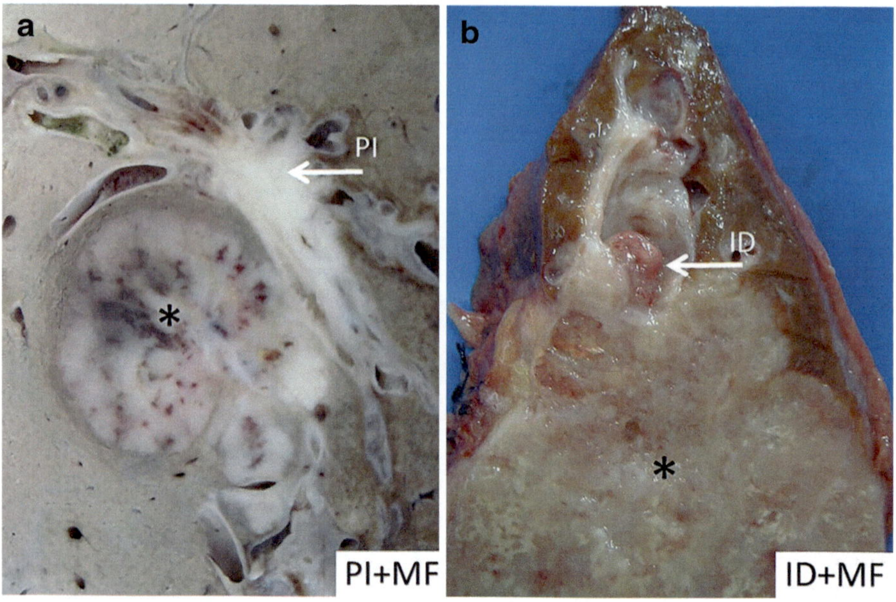

Fig. 11.8 Intrahepatic cholangiocarcinoma (iCCA) at advanced stages when tumor invading liver parenchyma, both periductal-infiltrating (PI) and intraductal-growing (ID) types, can manifest as a focal liver mass akin to the mass-forming (MF) type of CCA. (**a**) MF tumor from advanced PI (PI+MF) iCCA, arrow points to primary lesion. (**b**) MF tumor from advanced ID (ID+MF), arrow points to primary lesion

papillary CCA is more common in chronic inflammation-related CCA, as observed in CCA associated with hepatolithiasis and clonorchiasis in Japan and Korea [93, 94].

Chronic viral hepatitis are the other prevalent risk for CCA in Thailand. The prevalence of HBsAg and HCV infection in Thailand is 10% and 1–3%, respectively. However, a study that compared prevalence of HBsAg and HCV Ab in 295 CCA patients showed no significant difference compared to the general population [95]. Chronic hepatitis or cirrhosis was rare in livers with iCCA, and cholangiocellular carcinoma, a phenotype related to chronic hepatitis-associated CCA, accounts for only 1–2% of cases [96, 97].

Survival Studies of CCA in the Endemic Area of Liver Fluke

A 3-Month Prospective Study

KKH is an academic tertiary care institution. Many patients referred to KKH are diagnosed as CCA on clinical suspicion, and most of the confirmed CCA patients are late clinical cases. In a study including 270 patients (123 referral cases) who were seen at KKH in May–July 2010 for suspicion of CCA, 163 patients were ultimately diagnosed with CCA [98]. The median age was 62 years (53.2–70.8), and M/F ratio was 2/1. Diagnosis was made from radiologic imaging in 84%, and 78.8% of patients had elevated tumor markers. Histopathology confirmation of primary tumor was obtained in only 8.6%. Of the 163 patients, 59% were diagnosed with iCCA and 41% with eCCA. The majority of patients (61.3%) had stage IV disease, and 107 (65.6%) received only supportive care; curative resection was performed for only 6.1% of patients. Overall median survival was 4 months, and 2-year survival was 8.1%. There was no statistically significant difference ($p > 0.05$) in median survival among the symptomatic treatment groups, the biliary drainage group, or the chemotherapy group (Fig. 11.9). Most CCA patients already had unresectable disease at their first visit and received only symptom-based care. These results were comparable with the survival of advanced CCA patients in other Asian countries [99, 100].

A Retrospective Study of Resectable, Mass-Forming iCCA

The MF type is the most common type of iCCA, usually presenting as a non-capsulated firm white mass in the liver, though an advanced MF iCCA lesion cannot be differentiated from the advanced PI type (PI + MF) or advanced ID type (ID + MF) (Fig. 11.8). The mainstay of treatment of iCCA is surgical resection [101, 102], though not all patients are candidates, depending on their stage of disease (*Chap. 14, Gholami et al.*); in addition, many patients experience recurrence despite complete removal of the tumor [102, 103], and the subsequence prognosis is poor.

A retrospective study was performed in which 50 MF iCCA cases underwent hepatic resection at KKH between January 2004 and December 2009 [104]. The median age at diagnosis was 57.2 years (32–72), and the patients were 26 males and 24 females. The mean tumor size was 6.49 cm, and 86% were single masses. Most patients had stage IV disease, and lymph node involvement was noted in 64%. A

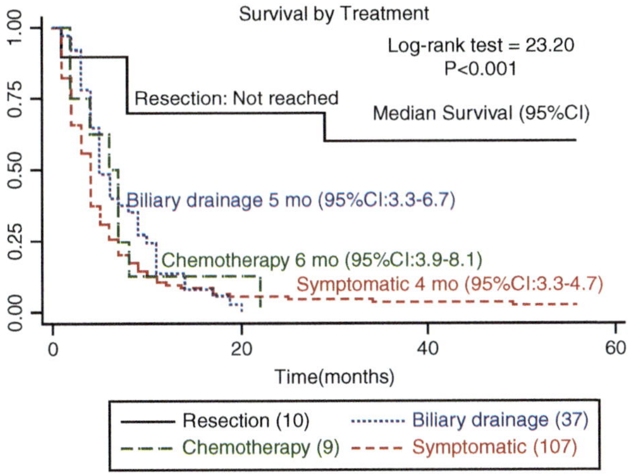

Fig. 11.9 Kaplan-Meier survival curves of the four treatment groups were compared; the surgical resection group had best 2-year survival, 70% (95% CI, 32.9–89.3), $P < 0.001$. Others had similar median survival without statistical difference ($p = 0.37$): biliary drainage 5 months, chemotherapy 6 months, symptomatic treatment 4 months (Adapted from Luvira V. et al. (2016)) [98]

disease-free surgical margin was achieved in half of the patients. The median recurrence-free survival time was 188 days. The most frequent recurrence site was the surgical margin (45%), regional lymph nodes (42.5%), and the liver remnant (37.5%). The respective 1-, 2-, and 3-year recurrence-free survival rates were 16.2%, 5.4%, and 2.7% [104]. The current study had high prevalence of lymph node involvement, leading to recurrences within 2 years after surgery. Lymph node involvement of iCCA represents systemic disease [105, 106], and adjuvant chemotherapy may add benefit in affected patients.

A Twofold Improved Survival in a Subset of Curative Resection for pCCA

Accounting for approximately half of all CCA cases, pCCA is a tumor located in the extrahepatic biliary tree proximal to the origin of the cystic duct. In early stages, it is treated with partial hepatectomy with hilar bile duct resection [107, 108]; however, the perioperative management and surgical procedures are complicated because of the tumor location, and in some instances liver transplantation may be required (*Chap. 15, Agopian et al.*). Previous reports of curative resection of pCCA in Thailand were unsatisfactorily low (0–10.8%) [104, 105].

Multivariate analyses were carried out based on the survival data of 153 patients who underwent curative resection of pCCA at KKH from January 2006 to December 2011. Among these 153 patients, the mean age was 56.8 years (56.8 ± 2), M/F ratio was 3/1, and 66 (43.1%) cases were R0 resection (tumor-free resection margin) and 87 (56.9%) R1 resection (microscopically margin-positive resection). Histological findings showed that 91 (59.4%) were papillary carcinoma and 62 (51.6%) were tubular adenocarcinoma and 50 cases (32.7%) had lymph node metastasis. The overall 5-year survival rate was 20.6%. Patients with R0 and R1 resection had a median survival time of 40.2 and 14.6 months and 5-year survival rate of 35.6% and 6.4%, respectively. Papillary carcinoma had a median survival time of 23.4 months, while tubular adenocarcinomas had a median survival of 16.3 months. Independent factors that were associated with improved survival outcome were R0 resection, no lymph node metastasis, and papillary histology [9]. Radical surgical technique combined with early-stage diagnosis can lead to a substantially improved prognosis and 5-year survival in pCCA patients [9].

Long-Term Follow-Up Intraductal Papillary Neoplasm of the Bile Duct (IPNB)

IPNB is an intraductal papillary tumor of the bile duct with a fine fibrovascular core. It represents a preinvasive lesion of IG type iCCA and polyploid type eCCA (Fig. 11.6b, d) [80, 88]. IPNBs are multifocal lesions (Fig. 11.7d), undergo malignant transformation by adenoma-carcinoma sequence [78, 88], and in general have a better prognosis than conventional CCA, tubular adenocarcinoma [111–113]. A retrospective study was conducted of the prognosis of 148 IPNB patients who underwent curative resection between January 2005 and December 2011. The median age at diagnosis was 60 years (35–76), and the male/female ratio was 2/1. Most tumors (62%) were the intrahepatic type, 27% the extrahepatic type, and 11% the combined type. Microinvasive carcinoma was seen in 50 cases (34%) and was the most common level of invasiveness. The survival of patients with benign IPNB was 3064 days, significantly greater than the 1422 days for malignant IPNB ($p < 0.001$). The respective median survival time for dysplasia, carcinoma in situ, microinvasive carcinoma, and macro-invasive carcinoma was 3064 days, 2034 days, 1483 days, and 730 days, respectively. The 5-year survival of patients undergoing R0 resection approached 59.7% (Fig. 11.10) [11]. This study lends support to the notion that IPNB has more favorable prognosis than conventional CCA. The survival after 5 years decreased from adenoma to dysplasia and carcinoma in situ to invasive carcinoma, confirming the adenoma-carcinoma sequence in carcinogenesis [80, 88]. There was no difference in mean age between groups, suggesting the intraductal tumors might require a short time to evolve into invasive lesions. Thus, performing early surgical intervention was recommended [11].

Adjuvant Chemotherapy Improves Survival Time in Resectable Patients

CCA patients are known to have poor treatment outcomes. Surgery is the best option for all subtypes of CCA with local, resectable disease. Chemotherapy and radiotherapy are relatively ineffective in treating non-operable CCA. Single-agent chemotherapy (mitomycin C, fluorouracil (5-FU), cisplatin) for unresectable CCA

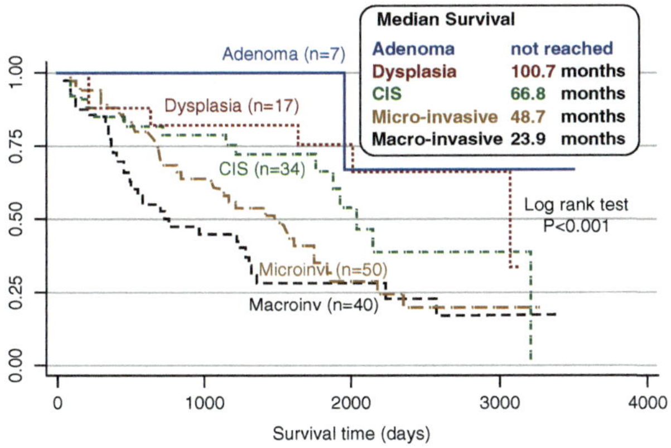

Fig. 11.10 Kaplan-Meier survival curves of intraductal papillary neoplasm of bile duct (IPNB) patients treated by hepatic resection stratified by benign (n = 24) and malignant IPNB (n = 124). The survival of patients with benign IPNB was significantly greater than malignant IPNB ($P < 0.001$). The respective median survival time for dysplasia, carcinoma in situ, microinvasive carcinoma, and macro-invasive carcinoma was 3064 days (95% CI: 2329–3798), 2034 days (95% CI: 1761–2306), 1483 days (95% CI: 1032–1933), and 730 days (95% CI: 205–1254) (Adapted from Luvira V. et al. (2017)) [12]

yields a poor response rate of 8–10% [114–116]; combined gemcitabine and capecitabine yields a median survival of 12–14 months [116, 117]. Benefits of adjuvant therapy in achieving long-term survival in resectable CCA patients are controversial [118]. Adjuvant chemotherapy is discussed in greater detail elsewhere in this book (*Chap. 16, Kirks and Rocha*), as are palliative chemotherapy (*Chap. 17, Hessey and Bridgewater*) and interventional radiologic therapies (*Chap. 18, An and Wehrenberg-Klee*).

A retrospective study was done to evaluate benefits of adjuvant chemotherapy which included 263 patients who underwent curative resection in KKH. These patients had pathological reports showing a clear margin (R0) or microscopic margin (R1) of lesion-free tissue. There were 138 patients who received adjuvant chemotherapy. This group had a significantly lower mean age than patients not receiving adjuvant chemotherapy (57.7 vs 60.4 years, $p = 0.01$). A serum albumin level above 3 g/dL was more common in the adjuvant chemotherapy group than in the no adjuvant chemotherapy group (87.7% vs 79.2%, $P = 0.04$). Patients who received adjuvant chemotherapy had significantly longer overall median survival time (21.6 vs 13.4 months, $p = 0.01$). Patients who received a combination of gemcitabine and capecitabine regimen had the longest survival time (median survival time of gemcitabine and capecitabine 31.5 months, 5-fluorouracil and mitomycin 17.3 months, 5-fluorouracil alone 22.2 months, capecitabine alone 21.6 months, and gemcitabine alone 7.9 months, $p = 0.02$) [119]. This large study shows that adjuvant chemotherapy significantly improves survival time in resectable surgical patients. The possible mechanism of benefit of adjuvant chemotherapy in CCA is prevention of outgrowth of micrometastatic disease, which consequently prolongs disease-free survival [120, 121].

Cancer Control for Cholangiocarcinoma in Thailand

Primary Prevention: Liver Fluke Control

Over the last four decades, animal models have revealed substantial evidence that chronic liver fluke infestation is a strong risk factor for endemic fluke-associated CCA [3, 4, 61, 62]. Thus, the prevention of CCA has largely been centered around control of the liver fluke by anti-parasitic drugs and a campaign to refrain from eating raw fish [122–124].

Khon Kaen Cancer Registry (KKCR) reported the ASR of CCA in Khon Kaen over three decades, from 1989 to 2013 [86] (Fig. 11.11a). Most patients presented at late stages, and 5-year survival is only 3.1% (CI 2.4–10.4). However, the KKCR data showed that there was a decreased trend in CCA incidence occurring since 2002 through 2013 and that the incidence was projected to stabilize by 2025 [86]. Of note, the declining incidence was in parallel with the prevalence of *O. viverrini* both at local and national levels, which decreased over time from >60% in 1984 to

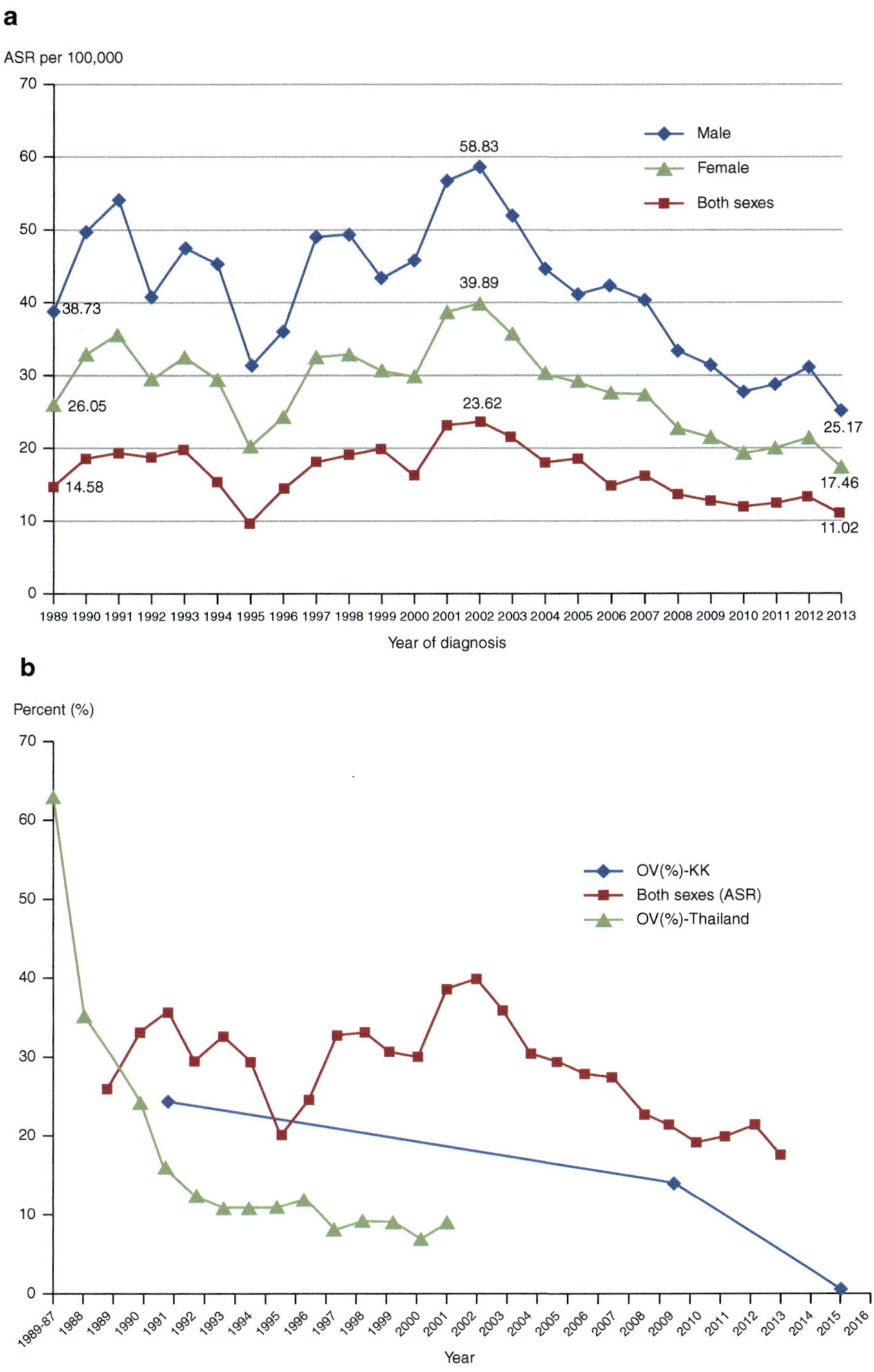

Fig. 11.11 (**a**) Incidence rates (per 100,000 per year) for cholangiocarcinoma (CCA) by sex in Khon Kaen Province from 1989 to 2013, showing trend downward since 2002 through 2013. (**b**) The incidence of CCA was declining, in parallel with the prevalence of *O. viverrini* both at local and national levels (Adapted from Kamsa-Ard et al. (2019)) [86]

<10% after 1997 [86] (Fig. 11.11b). The explanations behind the decrease in the incidence of CCA are far from conclusive given the multifactorial risk factors involved and the complex nature of carcinogenesis; nevertheless, it is conceivable that the decrease in fluke burden could have been a contributing factor. It should be noted, though, that these trends are not solely based on liver fluke control programs but also general extensive improvements in the healthcare system and socioeconomic development in the region. In fact, the incidence of CCA in the region remains high and still largely confined to a restricted group of people, wherein lifestyles and/or environmental carcinogenesis factors are likely issues. Indeed, a recent systemic review and meta-analysis reported numerous risk factors which were grouped into behaviors, socioeconomics, diet, genetics, gender, immune response, treatment for *O. viverrini*, and other infections [118, 125].

In addition, the combination of alcohol and smoking is significantly associated with an increased risk of CCA and is an even greater risk factor than *O. viverrini* exposure [125, 126]. These findings indicate continuous education of the public aiming not only for the next generation without fluke infestation but also acquisition of appropriate health behaviors.

Secondary Prevention: Ultrasonography Screening for Early CCA

CCA in the early stage of disease has no specific symptoms and clinical signs, and noninvasive biomarkers are not always reliable, especially in subclinical cases [127] (see also *Chap. 6, Luang et al.*). In addition, chronic infestation of liver fluke infection has nonspecific symptoms, as mentioned previously; thus to identify risk groups among a high-prevalence community adds further difficulty [128, 129]. In 2014, a preliminary study for early CCA detection using transabdominal ultrasonography screening at an endemic community on the *outskirts* of Khon Kaen was reported. Ultrasonography was used to detect small masses, bile duct segmental dilatation, or abnormally thickened bile duct echo patterns (fibrotic thickening ducts, a stigmata of chronic liver fluke infestation) [128, 130–132]. Suspicious lesions required further imaging for characterization, including computerized tomography (CT) or magnetic resonance imaging (MRI) [130, 133]. Two of eight suspected cases of early CCA consented to operation. Pathological diagnosis revealed that both had CCA: Case 1 was a 67-year-old women with papillary carcinoma in situ of iCCA (IPNB with carcinoma in situ of superficial spreading type) (Fig. 11.12a, c) [71] in whom diagnostic imaging had demonstrated a thickening and dilatation of bile duct in left lobe of the liver. Case 2 was a 57-year-old male in whom ultrasound showed an ill-defined outline mass lesion in the right liver lobe with a mild degree of dilatation of intrahepatic ducts; MRI showed a 2 cm mass lesion in segment 8. The pathological diagnosis was a subclinical advanced tubular adenocarcinoma of pCCA (T3N1M0, stage 3B) [71], with tumor arising from the

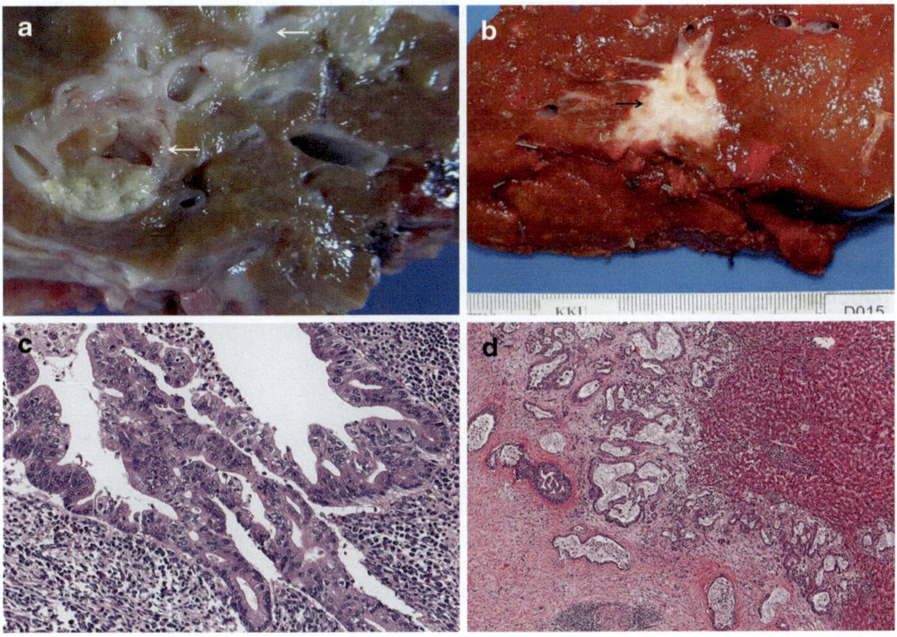

Fig. 11.12 Two cholangiocarcinoma (CCA) cases from ultrasonographic screening. (**a**) Case 1. Intrahepatic CCA, papillary carcinoma in situ, displayed thickening, and dilatation of the large intrahepatic bile ducts (white arrow) at left lobe of the liver. (**b**) Case 2. Tubular adenocarcinoma of perihilar CCA, a 2 cm focal mass lesion at hepatic hilum. Tumor arising from the proximal extrahepatic bile duct (black arrow). (**c**) A micrograph from (**a**) showing an intraductal papillary carcinoma of bile duct, superficial spreading type. (**d**) A micrograph from (**b**) showing tubular adenocarcinoma (mucin-producing), infiltrating at perihilar soft tissue and liver parenchyma

proximal extrahepatic bile duct, invading transmurally, and then periductal infiltrating with vascular and liver parenchymal involvement forming a liver mass (Fig. 11.12b, d) [134]. Overall, the study findings indicate that transabdominal ultrasonography has a potential role as a routine surveillance modality in an endemic area of liver fluke; however, unexpected subclinical advanced cases or misdiagnosis could occur; thus tissue diagnosis prior to complete surgical resection is mandatory.

Conclusion

Despite increased awareness and steady progress with regard to liver fluke control, while there has been a decreased trend in CCA incidence, prognosis in those who do develop CCA has not improved substantially. A majority of patients receive only palliative treatment due to their advanced stage of disease, with only 10–15% of patients being considered surgical candidates. Papillary carcinoma is common in the east, accounting for a third or more of large bile duct CCA cases, and has a better prognosis than the tubular adenocarcinoma (i.e., conventional) phenotype of CCA. The pathogenesis of tubular and papillary CCA is different; studies regarding the risk factors and therapeutic outcomes of these two CCA phenotypes should be performed separately. Bile duct stem cells are endodermal stem cells like the stem cells of the pancreas and gallbladder. Malignant tumorigenesis of these three organs may share benefits from future biomarkers for diagnosis, chemoprevention, chemotherapy, and targeted treatments. Taken together, such advancements could help decrease the incidence and public health burden of CCA and improve prognosis in patients suffering from it.

References

1. Khan SA, Tavolari S, Brandi G. Cholangiocarcinoma: epidemiology and risk factors. Liver Int. 2019;39:19–31.
2. Bragazzi MC, et al. Cholangiocarcinoma: epidemiology and risk factors. Transl Gastrointest Cancer. 2011;1(1):21–32.
3. Thamavit W, et al. Effects of dimethylnitrosamine on induction of cholangiocarcinoma in *Opisthorchis viverrini*-infected Syrian golden hamsters. Cancer Res. 1978;38(12):4634–9.
4. Flavell DJ, Lucas SB. Potentiation by the human liver fluke, *Opisthorchis viverrini*, of the carcinogenic action of N-nitrosodimethylamine upon the biliary epithelium of the hamster. Br J Cancer. 1982;46(6):985–9.
5. Lee JH, Rim HJ, Bak UB. Effect of *Clonorchis sinensis* infection and dimethylnitrosamine administration on the induction of cholangiocarcinoma in Syrian golden hamsters. Korean J Parasitol. 1993;31(1):21–30.
6. Sripa B, Tangkawattana S, Brindley PJ. Update on pathogenesis of opisthorchiasis and cholangiocarcinoma. Adv Parasitol. 2018;102:97–113.
7. Nakajima T, et al. A histopathologic study of 102 cases of intrahepatic cholangiocarcinoma: histologic classification and modes of spreading. Hum Pathol. 1988;19(10):1228–34.
8. Shirai T, et al. Histomorphological characteristics of cholangiocellular carcinomas in northeast Thailand, where a region infection with the liver fluke, *Opisthorchis viverrini* is endemic. Acta Pathol Jpn. 1992;42(10):734–9.
9. Titapun A, et al. Outcome of curative resection for perihilar cholangiocarcinoma in Northeast Thailand. World J Gastrointest Oncol. 2015;7(12):503–12.
10. Pairojkul C. Liver fluke and cholangiocarcinoma in Thailand. Pathology. 2014;46(Suppl 2):24.
11. Luvira V, et al. Long-term outcome of surgical resection for intraductal papillary neoplasm of the bile duct. J Gastroenterol Hepatol. 2017;32(2):527–33.
12. Luvira V, et al. Morphological classification of intraductal papillary neoplasm of the bile duct with survival correlation. Asian Pac J Cancer Prev. 2017;18(1):207–13.
13. Mas-Coma S, Valero MA, Bargues MD. Fascioliasis. Adv Exp Med Biol. 2014;766:77–114.
14. Farag HF, el Sayad MH. Biomphalaria alexandrina naturally infected with *Fasciola gigantica* in Egypt. Trans R Soc Trop Med Hyg. 1995;89(1):36.
15. Mas-Coma S, Bargues MD. Human liver flukes: a review res. Rev Parasitol. 1997;57(3–4):145–218.
16. Chen MGM, Mott KE. Progress in assessment of morbidity due to *Fasciola hepatica* infection: a review of recent literature. World Health Organization. 1990. Unpublished: 44.
17. Shin HR, et al. Epidemiology of cholangiocarcinoma: an update focusing on risk factors. Cancer Sci. 2010;101(3):579–85.

18. Suwannatrai A, Saichua P, Haswell M. Epidemiology of *Opisthorchis viverrini* infection. Adv Parasitol. 2018;101:41–67.
19. Rollinson D. Control of foodborne trematode infections. Report of a WHO Study Group. Trans R Soc Trop Med Hyg. 1995;89(6):704.
20. Lun ZR, et al. Clonorchiasis: a key foodborne zoonosis in China. Lancet Infect Dis. 2005;5(1):31–41.
21. Jongsuksuntigul P, Imsomboon T. Opisthorchiasis control in Thailand. Acta Trop. 2003;88(3):229–32.
22. Preuksaraj S. Public health aspects of opisthorchiasis in Thailand. Arzneimittelforschung. 1984;34(9B):1119–20.
23. Srivatanakul P, et al. Liver cancer in Thailand: temporal and geographic variations. J Gastroenterol Hepatol. 1988;3(5):413–20.
24. Sripa B, et al. Liver fluke induces cholangiocarcinoma. PLoS Med. 2007;4(7):e201.
25. Sithithaworn P, et al. The current status of opisthorchiasis and clonorchiasis in the Mekong Basin. Parasitol Int. 2012;61(1):10–6.
26. Harinasuta T, Riganti M, Bunnag D. *Opisthorchis viverrini* infection: pathogenesis and clinical features. Arzneimittelforschung. 1984;34(9B):1167–9.
27. Enes JE, et al. Prevalence of *Opisthorchis viverrini* infection in the canine and feline hosts in three villages, Khon Kaen Province, northeastern Thailand. Southeast Asian J Trop Med Public Health. 2010;41(1):36–42.
28. Johansen MV, Lier T, Sithithaworn P. Towards improved diagnosis of neglected zoonotic trematodes using a one health approach. Acta Trop. 2015;141(Pt B):161–9.
29. Jamornthanyawat N. The diagnosis of human opisthorchiasis. Southeast Asian J Trop Med Public Health. 2002;33(Suppl 3):86–91.
30. Prakobwong S, et al. A large scale study of the epidemiology and risk factors for the carcinogenic liver fluke *Opisthorchis viverrini* in Udon Thani Province, Thailand. Asian Pac J Cancer Prev. 2017;18(10):2853–60.
31. Hughes T, et al. Opisthorchiasis and cholangiocarcinoma in Southeast Asia: an unresolved problem. Int J Gen Med. 2017;10:227–37.
32. Boonstra K, et al. Population-based epidemiology, malignancy risk, and outcome of primary sclerosing cholangitis. Hepatology. 2013;58(6):2045–55.
33. Nakanuma Y, et al. Are hepatolithiasis and cholangiocarcinoma aetiologically related? A morphological study of 12 cases of hepatolithiasis associated with cholangiocarcinoma. Virchows Arch A Pathol Anat Histopathol. 1985;406(1):45–58.
34. Matsumoto K, et al. Hepatitis B and C virus infection is a risk factor for the development of cholangiocarcinoma. Intern Med. 2014;53(7):651–4.
35. Segura-Lopez FK, Guitron-Cantu A, Torres J. Association between Helicobacter spp. infections and hepatobiliary malignancies: a review. World J Gastroenterol. 2015;21(5):1414–23.
36. Kim TS, et al. *Clonorchis sinensis*, an oriental liver fluke, as a human biological agent of cholangiocarcinoma: a brief review. BMB Rep. 2016;49(11):590–7.
37. IARC. Infection with liver flukes *Opisthorchis viverrini*, *Opisthorchis felineus* and *Clonorchis sinensis*. IARC Monogr Eval Carcinog Risks Hum. 1994;61:121–75.
38. Upatham ES, et al. Morbidity in relation to intensity of infection in Opisthorchiasis viverrini: study of a community in Khon Kaen, Thailand. Am J Trop Med Hyg. 1982;31(6):1156–63.
39. Upatham ES, et al. Relationship between prevalence and intensity of *Opisthorchis viverrini* infection, and clinical symptoms and signs in a rural community in north-east Thailand. Bull World Health Organ. 1984;62(3):451–61.
40. Riganti M, et al. *Opisthorchis viverrini* eggs and adult flukes as nidus and composition of gallstones. Southeast Asian J Trop Med Public Health. 1988;19(4):633–6.
41. Sripa B, et al. The tumorigenic liver fluke *Opisthorchis viverrini*–multiple pathways to cancer. Trends Parasitol. 2012;28(10):395–407.
42. Lim JH. Liver flukes: the malady neglected. Korean J Radiol. 2011;12(2):269–79.

43. Sorvillo FJ. Food-borne parasitic zoonoses fish and plant-borne parasites (world class parasites). Emerg Infect Dis. 2008;14(9):1503a–1503.
44. Hou PC. The pathology of *Clonorchis sinensis* infestation of the liver. J Pathol Bacteriol. 1955;70(1):53–64.
45. Bhamarapravati N, Thammavit W, Vajrasthira S. Liver changes in hamsters infected with a liver fluke of man, *Opisthorchis viverrini*. Am J Trop Med Hyg. 1978;27(4):787–94.
46. Kim YI. Liver carcinoma and liver fluke infection. Arzneimittelforschung. 1984;34(9B):1121–6.
47. Riganti M, et al. Human pathology of *Opisthorchis viverrini* infection: a comparison of adults and children. Southeast Asian J Trop Med Public Health. 1989;20(1):95–100.
48. Rim HJ. Clonorchiasis: an update. J Helminthol. 2005;79(3):269–81.
49. Pairojkul C, et al. Multistage carcinogenesis of liver-fluke-associated cholangiocarcinoma in Thailand. Princess Takamatsu Symp. 1991;22:77–86.
50. Sripa B, et al. Opisthorchiasis-associated biliary stones: light and scanning electron microscopic study. World J Gastroenterol. 2004;10(22):3318–21.
51. Verweij KE, van Buuren H. Oriental cholangiohepatitis (recurrent pyogenic cholangitis): a case series from the Netherlands and brief review of the literature. Neth J Med. 2016;74(9):401–5.
52. Harris CC. Chemical and physical carcinogenesis: advances and perspectives for the 1990s. Cancer Res. 1991;51(18 Suppl):5023s–44s.
53. Cardinale V, et al. Multipotent stem/progenitor cells in human biliary tree give rise to hepatocytes, cholangiocytes, and pancreatic islets. Hepatology. 2011;54(6):2159–72.
54. Carpino G, et al. Biliary tree stem/progenitor cells in glands of extrahepatic and intrahepatic bile ducts: an anatomical in situ study yielding evidence of maturational lineages. J Anat. 2012;220(2):186–99.
55. Bragazzi MC, et al. New insights into cholangiocarcinoma: multiple stems and related cell lineages of origin. Ann Gastroenterol. 2018;31(1):42–55.
56. Sutton ME, et al. Regeneration of human extrahepatic biliary epithelium: the peribiliary glands as progenitor cell compartment. Liver Int. 2012;32(4):554–9.
57. Lanzoni G, Cardinale V, Carpino G. The hepatic, biliary, and pancreatic network of stem/progenitor cell niches in humans: a new reference frame for disease and regeneration. Hepatology. 2016;64(1):277–86.
58. De Jong IEM, et al. Repopulating the biliary tree from the peribiliary glands. Biochim Biophys Acta Mol basis Dis. 2018;1864(4 Pt B):1524–31.
59. Nakanuma Y, et al. Intrahepatic peribiliary glands of humans. II. Pathological spectrum. J Gastroenterol Hepatol. 1994;9(1):80–6.
60. Hughes NR, et al. Liver fluke-associated and sporadic cholangiocarcinoma: an immunohistochemical study of bile duct, peribiliary gland and tumour cell phenotypes. J Clin Pathol. 2006;59(10):1073–8.
61. Pinlaor S, et al. iNOS-dependent DNA damage via NF-kappaB expression in hamsters infected with Opisthorchis viverrini and its suppression by the antihelminthic drug praziquantel. Int J Cancer. 2006;119(5):1067–72.
62. Pinlaor S, et al. Mechanism of NO-mediated oxidative and nitrative DNA damage in hamsters infected with *Opisthorchis viverrini*: a model of inflammation-mediated carcinogenesis. Nitric Oxide. 2004;11(2):175–83.
63. Pinlaor S, et al. 8-nitroguanine formation in the liver of hamsters infected with *Opisthorchis viverrini*. Biochem Biophys Res Commun. 2003;309(3):567–71.
64. Kawanishi S, et al. Oxidative and nitrative DNA damage in animals and patients with inflammatory diseases in relation to inflammation-related carcinogenesis. Biol Chem. 2006;387(4):365–72.
65. Sia D, et al. Intrahepatic cholangiocarcinoma: pathogenesis and rationale for molecular therapies. Oncogene. 2013;32(41):4861–70.

66. Endo K, et al. ERBB-2 overexpression and cyclooxygenase-2 up-regulation in human cholangiocarcinoma and risk conditions. Hepatology. 2002;36(2):439–50.
67. Thiery JP. Epithelial-mesenchymal transitions in development and pathologies. Curr Opin Cell Biol. 2003;15(6):740–6.
68. Kalluri R, Neilson EG. Epithelial-mesenchymal transition and its implications for fibrosis. J Clin Invest. 2003;112(12):1776–84.
69. Guarino M, Tosoni A, Nebuloni M. Direct contribution of epithelium to organ fibrosis: epithelial-mesenchymal transition. Hum Pathol. 2009;40(10):1365–76.
70. Sripa B, Pairojkul C. Cholangiocarcinoma: lessons from Thailand. Curr Opin Gastroenterol. 2008;24(3):349–56.
71. Zen Y, et al. Proposal of histological criteria for intraepithelial atypical/proliferative biliary epithelial lesions of the bile duct in hepatolithiasis with respect to cholangiocarcinoma: preliminary report based on interobserver agreement. Pathol Int. 2005;55(4):180–8.
72. Zen Y, et al. Biliary intraepithelial neoplasia: an international interobserver agreement study and proposal for diagnostic criteria. Mod Pathol. 2007;20(6):701–9.
73. Holzinger F, Graggen KZ, Buchler MW. Mechanisms of biliary carcinogenesis: a pathogenetic multi-stage cascade towards cholangiocarcinoma. Ann Oncol. 1999;10(Suppl 4):122–6.
74. Nagtegaal ID, et al. The 2019 WHO classification of tumours of the digestive system. Histopathology. 2020;76(2):182–8.
75. Miyata T, Uesaka K, Nakanuma Y. Cystic and papillary neoplasm at the hepatic hilum possibly originating in the peribiliary glands. Case Rep Pathol. 2016;2016:9130754.
76. Nakanishi Y, et al. Intraductal oncocytic papillary neoplasm of the bile duct: the first case of peribiliary gland origin. J Hepato-Biliary-Pancreat Surg. 2009;16(6):869–73.
77. Nakanishi Y, et al. Intraductal papillary neoplasm arising from peribiliary glands connecting with the inferior branch of the bile duct of the anterior segment of the liver. Pathol Int. 2011;61(12):773–7.
78. Nakanuma Y, Kakuda Y. Pathologic classification of cholangiocarcinoma: new concepts. Best Pract Res Clin Gastroenterol. 2015;29(2):277–93.
79. Aishima S, et al. Histological features of precancerous and early cancerous lesions of biliary tract carcinoma. J Hepatobiliary Pancreat Sci. 2014;21(7):448–52.
80. Schlitter AM, et al. Intraductal papillary neoplasms of the bile duct: stepwise progression to carcinoma involves common molecular pathways. Mod Pathol. 2014;27(1):73–86.
81. Banales JM, et al. Expert consensus document: Cholangiocarcinoma: current knowledge and future perspectives consensus statement from the European Network for the Study of Cholangiocarcinoma (ENS-CCA). Nat Rev Gastroenterol Hepatol. 2016;13(5):261–80.
82. Sia D, et al. Liver cancer cell of origin, molecular class, and effects on patient prognosis. Gastroenterology. 2017;152(4):745–61.
83. Edge SB, Compton CC. The American Joint Committee on Cancer: the 7th edition of the AJCC cancer staging manual and the future of TNM. Ann Surg Oncol. 2010;17(6):1471–4.
84. Blechacz B, et al. Clinical diagnosis and staging of cholangiocarcinoma. Nat Rev Gastroenterol Hepatol. 2011;8(9):512–22.
85. Krasinskas AM. Cholangiocarcinoma. Surg Pathol Clin. 2018;11(2):403–29.
86. Kamsa-Ard S, et al. Cholangiocarcinoma trends, incidence, and relative survival in Khon Kaen, Thailand from 1989 through 2013: a population-based cancer registry study. J Epidemiol. 2019;29(5):197–204.
87. Aishima S, et al. Proposal of progression model for intrahepatic cholangiocarcinoma: clinicopathologic differences between hilar type and peripheral type. Am J Surg Pathol. 2007;31(7):1059–67.
88. Nakanuma Y, Miyata T, Uchida T. Latest advances in the pathological understanding of cholangiocarcinomas. Expert Rev Gastroenterol Hepatol. 2016;10(1):113–27.
89. Uchida T, et al. Cystic micropapillary neoplasm of peribiliary glands with concomitant perihilar cholangiocarcinoma. World J Gastroenterol. 2016;22(7):2391–7.

90. Kudo M, et al. general rules for the clinical and pathological study of primary liver cancer, nationwide follow-up survey and clinical practice guidelines: the outstanding achievements of the Liver Cancer Study Group of Japan. Dig Dis. 2015;33(6):765–70.
91. Isaji S, et al. Clinicopathological features and outcome of hepatic resection for intrahepatic cholangiocarcinoma in Japan. J Hepato-Biliary-Pancreat Surg. 1999;6(2):108–16.
92. Luvira V, et al. Association between repeated praziquantel treatment and papillary, and intrahepatic cholangiocarcinoma. Ann Hepatol. 2018;17(5):802–9.
93. Chen TC, et al. Intraductal papillary neoplasia of the liver associated with hepatolithiasis. Hepatology. 2001;34(4 Pt 1):651–8.
94. Nakanuma Y, et al. Biliary papillary neoplasm of the liver. Histol Histopathol. 2002;17(3):851–61.
95. Barusrux S, et al. Viral hepatitis B, C infection and genotype distribution among cholangiocarcinoma patients in northeast Thailand. Asian Pac J Cancer Prev. 2012;13(Suppl):83–7.
96. Ariizumi S, Yamamoto M. Intrahepatic cholangiocarcinoma and cholangiolocellular carcinoma in cirrhosis and chronic viral hepatitis. Surg Today. 2015;45(6):682–7.
97. Aishima S, Oda Y. Pathogenesis and classification of intrahepatic cholangiocarcinoma: different characters of perihilar large duct type versus peripheral small duct type. J Hepatobiliary Pancreat Sci. 2015;22(2):94–100.
98. Luvira V, et al. Cholangiocarcinoma patient outcome in Northeastern Thailand: single-center prospective study. Asian Pac J Cancer Prev. 2016;17(1):401–6.
99. Park J, et al. Natural history and prognostic factors of advanced cholangiocarcinoma without surgery, chemotherapy, or radiotherapy: a large-scale observational study. Gut Liver. 2009;3(4):298–305.
100. Yusoff AR, et al. Survival analysis of cholangiocarcinoma: a 10-year experience in Malaysia. World J Gastroenterol. 2012;18(5):458–65.
101. Bridgewater J, et al. Guidelines for the diagnosis and management of intrahepatic cholangiocarcinoma. J Hepatol. 2014;60(6):1268–89.
102. Konstantinidis IT, Arkadopoulos N, Ferrone CR. Surgical management of intrahepatic cholangiocarcinoma in the modern era: advances and challenges. Chin Clin Oncol. 2016;5(1):9.
103. Spolverato G, et al. Management and outcomes of patients with recurrent intrahepatic cholangiocarcinoma following previous curative-intent surgical resection. Ann Surg Oncol. 2016;23(1):235–43.
104. Luvira V, et al. Patterns of recurrence after resection of mass-forming type intrahepatic cholangiocarcinomas. Asian Pac J Cancer Prev. 2016;17(10):4735–9.
105. Adachi T, Eguchi S. Lymph node dissection for intrahepatic cholangiocarcinoma: a critical review of the literature to date. J Hepatobiliary Pancreat Sci. 2014;21(3):162–8.
106. Morine Y, Shimada M. The value of systematic lymph node dissection for intrahepatic cholangiocarcinoma from the viewpoint of liver lymphatics. J Gastroenterol. 2015;50(9):913–27.
107. Igami T, et al. Surgical treatment of hilar cholangiocarcinoma in the "new era": the Nagoya University experience. J Hepatobiliary Pancreat Sci. 2010;17(4):449–54.
108. Neuhaus P, et al. Oncological superiority of hilar en bloc resection for the treatment of hilar cholangiocarcinoma. Ann Surg Oncol. 2012;19(5):1602–8.
109. Yeh TS, et al. Characterization of intrahepatic cholangiocarcinoma of the intraductal growth-type and its precursor lesions. Hepatology. 2005;42(3):657–64.
110. Yeh TS, et al. Cholangiographic spectrum of intraductal papillary mucinous neoplasm of the bile ducts. Ann Surg. 2006;244(2):248–53.
111. Jarnagin WR, et al. Papillary phenotype confers improved survival after resection of hilar cholangiocarcinoma. Ann Surg. 2005;241(5):703–12. discussion 712-4.
112. Jan YY, et al. Prognostic analysis of surgical treatment of peripheral cholangiocarcinoma: two decades of experience at Chang Gung Memorial Hospital. World J Gastroenterol. 2005;11(12):1779–84.
113. Yeh CN, et al. Hepatic resection for hepatocellular carcinoma in elderly patients. Hepato-Gastroenterology. 2004;51(55):219–23.

114. Taal BG, et al. Phase II trial of mitomycin C (MMC) in advanced gallbladder and biliary tree carcinoma. An EORTC Gastrointestinal Tract Cancer Cooperative Group Study. Ann Oncol. 1993;4(7):607–9.
115. Okada S, et al. A phase II study of cisplatin in patients with biliary tract carcinoma. Oncology. 1994;51(6):515–7.
116. Okusaka T, et al. Gemcitabine alone or in combination with cisplatin in patients with biliary tract cancer: a comparative multicentre study in Japan. Br J Cancer. 2010;103(4):469–74.
117. Valle J, et al. Cisplatin plus gemcitabine versus gemcitabine for biliary tract cancer. N Engl J Med. 2010;362(14):1273–81.
118. Skipworth JR, et al. Review article: surgical, neo-adjuvant and adjuvant management strategies in biliary tract cancer. Aliment Pharmacol Ther. 2011;34(9):1063–78.
119. Wirasorn K, et al. Adjuvant chemotherapy in resectable cholangiocarcinoma patients. J Gastroenterol Hepatol. 2013;28(12):1885–91.
120. Ringborg U. Adjuvant chemotherapy. a discussion of some basic principles. Acta Oncol. 1991;30(2):251–3.
121. Epstein RJ. Maintenance therapy to suppress micrometastasis: the new challenge for adjuvant cancer treatment. Clin Cancer Res. 2005;11(15):5337–41.
122. Bunnag D, Harinasuta T. Studies on the chemotherapy of human opisthorchiasis in Thailand: I. Clinical trial of praziquantel. Southeast Asian J Trop Med Public Health. 1980;11(4):528–31.
123. Upatham ES, et al. Rate of re-infection by *Opisthorchis viverrini* in an endemic northeast Thai community after chemotherapy. Int J Parasitol. 1988;18(5):643–9.
124. Jongsuksuntigul P, Imsomboon T. Epidemiology of opisthorchiasis and national control program in Thailand. Southeast Asian J Trop Med Public Health. 1998;29(2):327–32.
125. Steele JA, et al. Thinking beyond *Opisthorchis viverrini* for risk of cholangiocarcinoma in the lower Mekong region: a systematic review and meta-analysis. Infect Dis Poverty. 2018;7(1):44.
126. Kamsa-ard S, et al. Association between praziquantel and cholangiocarcinoma in patients infected with *Opisthorchis viverrini*: a systematic review and meta-analysis. Asian Pac J Cancer Prev. 2013;14(11):7011–6.
127. Weber A, Schmid RM, Prinz C. Diagnostic approaches for cholangiocarcinoma. World J Gastroenterol. 2008;14(26):4131–6.
128. Mairiang E, et al. Ultrasonography assessment of hepatobiliary abnormalities in 3359 subjects with *Opisthorchis viverrini* infection in endemic areas of Thailand. Parasitol Int. 2012;61(1):208–11.
129. Mairiang E, et al. Relationship between intensity of *Opisthorchis viverrini* infection and hepatobiliary disease detected by ultrasonography. J Gastroenterol Hepatol. 1992;7(1):17–21.
130. Weill F, Eisencher A, Zeltner F. Ultrasonic study of the normal and dilated biliary tree. The "shotgun" sign. Radiology. 1978;127(1):221–4.
131. Catalano OA, et al. Biliary infections: spectrum of imaging findings and management. Radiographics. 2009;29(7):2059–80.
132. Sripa B, et al. Advanced periductal fibrosis from infection with the carcinogenic human liver fluke *Opisthorchis viverrini* correlates with elevated levels of interleukin-6. Hepatology. 2009;50(4):1273–81.
133. Karcaaltincaba M, et al. Multidetector CT and MRI findings in periportal space pathologies. Eur J Radiol. 2007;61(1):3–10.
134. Chamadol N, et al. Histological confirmation of periductal fibrosis from ultrasound diagnosis in cholangiocarcinoma patients. J Hepatobiliary Pancreat Sci. 2014;21(5):316–22.
135. Sripa B, et al. Opisthorchiasis and Opisthorchis-associated cholangiocarcinoma in Thailand and Laos. Acta Trop. 2011;120(Suppl 1):S158–68.

Chapter 12
Endoscopic Management of Cholangiocarcinoma

Rodrigo Mansilla-Vivar, Camila Bahamonde-Ovando, and Renato Carrasco-Farias

Abbreviations

AJCC	American Joint Committee on Cancer
CCA	Cholangiocarcinoma
CT	Computerized tomography
dCCA	Distal cholangiocarcinoma
ERCP	Endoscopic retrograde cholangiopancreatography
FNA	Fine-needle aspiration
iCCA	Intrahepatic cholangiocarcinoma
MRCP	Magnetic resonance cholangiopancreatography
MRI	Magnetic resonance imaging
pCCA	Perihilar cholangiocarcinoma
PDT	Photodynamic therapy
PTC	Percutaneous transhepatic cholangiography
RFA	Radiofrequency ablation
SEMS	Self-expanding metallic stent
SOCP	Single operatory cholangiopancreatoscope
TNM	Tumor-node-metastasis classification

R. Mansilla-Vivar (✉)
Digestive Endoscopy Unit, Hospital Puerto Montt, University San Sebastian, Puerto Montt, Chile

C. Bahamonde-Ovando
Department of Internal Medicine, Hospital Puerto Montt, Puerto Montt, Chile

R. Carrasco-Farias
Digestive Endoscopy Unit, Hospital Puerto Montt, Puerto Montt, Chile

J. H. Tabibian (ed.), *Diagnosis and Management of Cholangiocarcinoma*,
https://doi.org/10.1007/978-3-030-70936-5_12

Background

Cholangiocarcinoma (CCA) is the most frequent and aggressive malignant tumor of the biliary tract [1] and the second most common hepatic malignancy (after hepatocellular carcinoma). The first reported case of CCA was described by Durand-Fardel in 1840 [2].

CCAs represent a heterogeneous group of intrahepatic and extrahepatic epithelial cell malignancies with features of cholangiocyte differentiation [3–5]. Cholangiocarcinogenesis is a multistep process which progresses in a background of chronic bile duct inflammation, cholangiocyte damage, and bile stasis [6–9].

In addition, CCAs are extensively supported by a highly desmoplastic tumor microenvironment and have profound genetic heterogeneity, both of which contribute to therapeutic resistance [10].

CCAs are classified anatomically as intrahepatic (iCCA), perihilar (pCCA), and distal (dCCA), as discussed in greater detail elsewhere in this book (Chap. 2) [11]. Among these, pCCA is the most common subtype, representing 50% of CCA cases [12]. Endoscopic management plays a major role in pCCA and dCCA, as will be discussed in this chapter, whereas the role of endoscopy in iCCA is minimal, though there is a growing role for endoscopic ultrasound (EUS) (Chap. 13).

Classification and Staging

pCCA

The Bismuth classification, later modified by Corlette, is the best known and most used classification system for pCCA. It is used to try to define the correct therapeutic approach and is based on macroscopic tumor appearance on pre-surgical imaging and/or endoscopic data (Fig. 12.1). This classification [13, 14] provides preoperative assessment of local spread and classifies Klatskin tumors as Type I (below the confluence of the left and right hepatic ducts), Type II (reaching the confluence), Types IIIA and IIIB (occluding the common hepatic duct and the right or left hepatic ducts, respectively), and Type IV (involving the confluence and both the right and left hepatic ducts). Despite its worldwide application and large use in literature, it has some limitations: the absence of longitudinal description of the cancer extension, no relation with prognostic data, and no clearly defined resectability criteria [15].

Since the 7th edition of American Joint Committee on Cancer (AJCC) classification, pCCA has been recognized as a separate disease from the distal CCA. Unfortunately, histopathological evaluation of surgical specimens, together with preoperative imaging data, is needed to define the correct TNM classification.

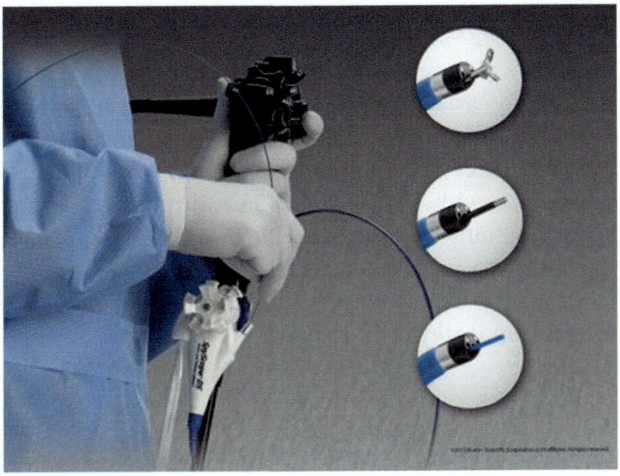

Fig. 12.1 SpyGlass system fastened to and inserted through the duodenoscope

For these reasons, it cannot be used to define resectability during the diagnostic phase. At the end of 2016, the AJCC classification was revised, and the 8th edition of TNM classification was published. Some main changes were introduced in the 8th edition to improve tumor description [16]. T4 stage is no longer linked to Bismuth-Corlette Type IV pCCA, as underlined by Ebata et al. [17]. T4 pCCA is now defined as a tumor invading the main portal vein or its branches bilaterally, or the common hepatic artery, or unilateral second-order biliary radicals with contralateral portal or hepatic artery involvement. According to the current TNM classification, N stage depends on the number of locoregional lymph nodes involved. Furthermore, stage IIIC category was introduced in TNM staging.

In selected pCCA cases, diagnosis should rely on invasive examinations: endoscopic retrograde cholangiopancreatography (ERCP), percutaneous transhepatic cholangiography (PTC), cholangioscopy, and EUS. They should be addressed to clarify the nature of a stenosis (biopsy) or to drain bile ducts [16, 18, 19]. Indeed, ERCP and PTC are not more relevant than MRCP images in visualizing complete biliary tree [20, 21], hence the need for a clear and objective planning of the study ahead for the patient.

CCA in General

Other classifications have been proposed (e.g., Memorial Sloan Kettering Cancer Center), but none of them have supplanted the use of the Bismuth-Corlette. In oncology, tumor-node-metastasis (TNM) classification is accepted worldwide to define CCA stage and prognosis, regardless of anatomical location [4].

Endoscopic Management

Endoscopy, as a diagnosis tool, is indicated in patients with indeterminate biliary strictures (classically defined as strictures for which a definitive diagnosis is not available after imaging and biliary cytology). In these cases of biliary dilation/obstruction without an obvious mass lesion seen on cross-sectional imaging, endoscopic modalities, such as EUS (discussed in detail in Chap. 13) and ERCP, offer the ability to further characterize indeterminate biliary strictures (location, length, etc.), assess for presence of biliary mass, and assist with staging by identifying lymphadenopathy or liver lesions [4].

Endoscopic Retrograde Cholangiopancreatography

Biliary endoscopy plays a major role in the diagnosis of CCA. Endoscopic techniques have become the primary modality to obtain samples for cytology and/or histology, though the diagnostic yield with traditional methods has remained modest (Fig. 12.1). There are several factors that contribute to this: small lesion size, lack of direct endoscopic (i.e., cholangioscopic) visualization, and significant desmoplastic reaction surrounding the tumor [4].

ERCP has an integral role in pCCA management by enabling not only the detection of malignant biliary strictures but also the acquisition of biliary brushing samples for cytological and genetic assessment. A number of emerging cytological techniques have potential clinical utility in pCCA diagnosis. Conventional biliary cytology has a high specificity (97%) in the detection of pCCA but limited sensitivity (43%) [22], predominantly because CCAs are desmoplastic, paucicellular tumors potentially located in inaccessible regions of the biliary tree, causing difficulties in adequate specimen retrieval.

Endoscopy-Guided Therapy

Cholangioscopy (SpyGlass)

Biliary strictures are the second most frequent indication for ERCP. Biliary stricture diagnosis (i.e., stricture etiology) using either biliary brush cytology or forceps biopsies cannot distinguish between malignant and benign etiologies in around 50% of cases [23, 24]. Smaller-caliber endoscopic equipment has been developed to enter into small ducts. In 1975, peroral cholangiopancreatoscopy began with the mother-baby system. This endoscopic technique enabled direct visual examination of the pancreatobiliary tree, tissue sampling, and treatment of difficult biliary and pancreatic stones [25, 26]. Nevertheless, the use of this device has some limitations [24, 27]. The SpyGlass™ Direct Visualization System, a single-operator cholangio-pancreatoscope (SOCP) for peroral cholangiopancreatoscopy, was released in 2006 [28]. The system includes a reusable optical probe and a small 3.3 mm catheter (SpyScope™) with four-way tip deflection and a separate irrigation and working channel; while an important development, it also had various limitations [29, 30]. In 2015, the upgraded SpyGlass™ Digital System was released. Compared to its legacy version, the Digital System has a digital sensor with a higher resolution, wider field of view, automatic light control, and LED illumination. In the last years, SpyGlass has opened new opportunities for the management of biliopancreatic diseases (Fig. 12.2). The endoscopic sensitivity, specificity, and diagnostic accuracy for the detection of malignancy using this system have been reported to be up to 88%, 80%, and 83%, respectively (Figs. 12.1 and 12.2).

The other importance of SpyGlass is to confirm malignant diagnosis in patients with indeterminate biliary stenosis. Many patients with benign biliary strictures are wrongly diagnosed only by ERCP. In our experience, with SpyGlass we can reliably obtain samples having a bile duct malignancy discovered by further histopathological analysis. In this scenario, many of them are good candidates for surgical curative treatment. In one of our studies, we estimated that four or more biopsies per patient are considered as adequate to obtain a sensitivity and specificity of 54% and 87.5% [29]

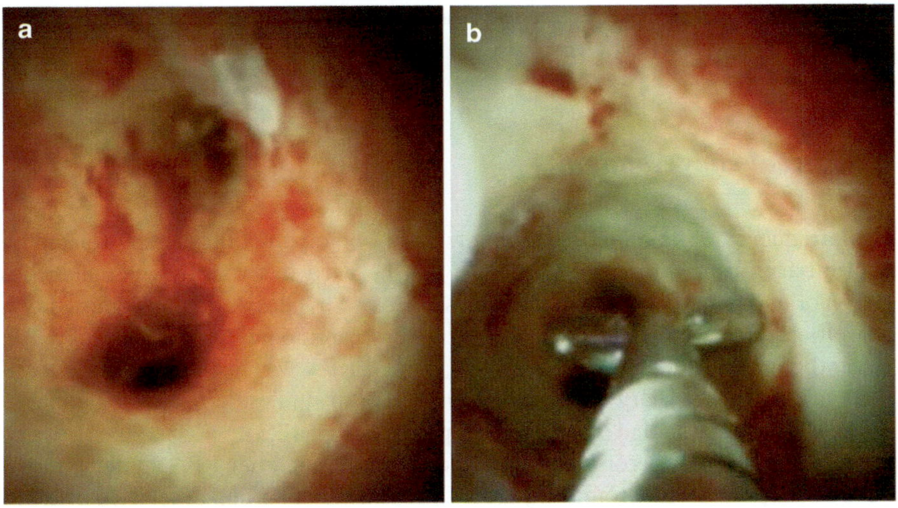

Fig. 12.2 (**a**) An indeterminate biliary stricture visualized by SpyGlass cholangioscopy with spontaneous bleeding and tortuous vessels, suggestive of a cholangiocarcinoma. (**b**) Biopsies taken at the site of a biliary stricture with cholangioscopic forceps (SpyBite™)

Endosonography

Presently, the use of EUS alone is associated with a high tumor detection rate compared with the use of CT or MRI, with better performance in the detection of dCCA versus pCCA (100% versus 83%, respectively) [29]. Fine-needle aspiration (FNA) during EUS carries a high risk of tumor seeding: among 191 patients with pCCA, 5 of 6 patients (83%) who underwent a transperitoneal primary tumor biopsy developed peritoneal metastases compared to 14 of 175 (8%) of those who did not undergo a transperitoneal biopsy [30].

Photodynamic Therapy

As CCAs often spreads along the biliary tree, local treatment for patency of the common bile duct and the hilum is of crucial interest [31]. PDT acts by creating free radicals-associated tumor cell destruction due to porfimer enrichment in CCA cells. Usually, porfimers are injected intravenously followed by intraluminal photoactivation through cholangioscopy.

Effectiveness of photodynamic therapy (PDT) has been demonstrated in two randomized controlled and a few controlled studies [32–37]. Today, endoscopic drainage in combination with intraluminal PDT is arguably the best palliative concept that patients can be offered. Mean survival can be prolonged from 6 months to approximately 14 months by adding PDT to sufficient endoscopic drainage. A burden associated with PDT for patients is the increased phototoxicity of the photosensitizer for 3–4 weeks [38].

Radiofrequency Ablation

Radiofrequency ablation (RFA) is a new endoscopic palliation therapy for malignant biliary obstruction. This technique can be used in two ways; percutaneous (PTC) or endoscopic (via small duodenoscopes or SpyGlass). Percutaneous RFA is a well-established therapy for hepatocellular carcinoma and iCCA [57, 58]. Recently, in two studies, endoscopically applied RFA was evaluated for the treatment of malignant biliary obstruction [39, 40]. Both studies demonstrated immediate and 30-day safety and 90-day biliary patency (Fig. 12.3).

The utilization of peroral cholangioscopy before and after RFA application has been also reported with promissory results [41]. In a small group of selected patients, including some randomized controlled trials, pre and post-cholangioscopy RFA treatment was demonstrated to be feasible including cases with previously SEMS placement (confirmed with the presence of the neoplastic tissue) to achieve tumor ablation [42, 43]. However, the value of peroral cholangioscopy in directing the

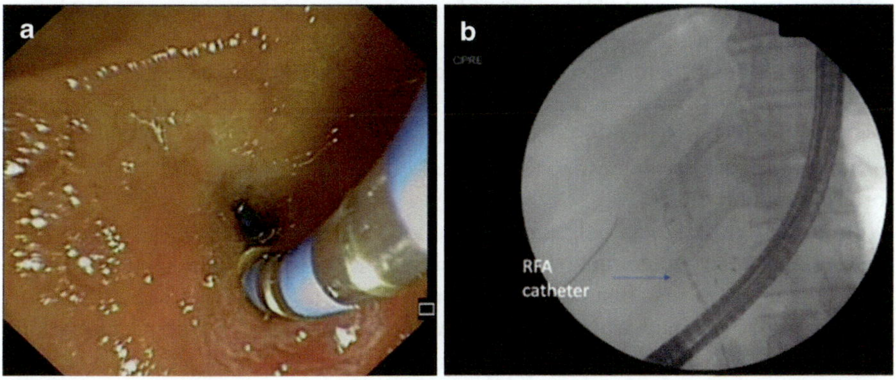

Fig. 12.3 (**a**) Endoscopic view of radiofrequency ablation therapy catheter insertion through duodenoscope working channel. (**b**) Fluoroscopic view of radiofrequency ablation therapy catheter within the distal common bile duct

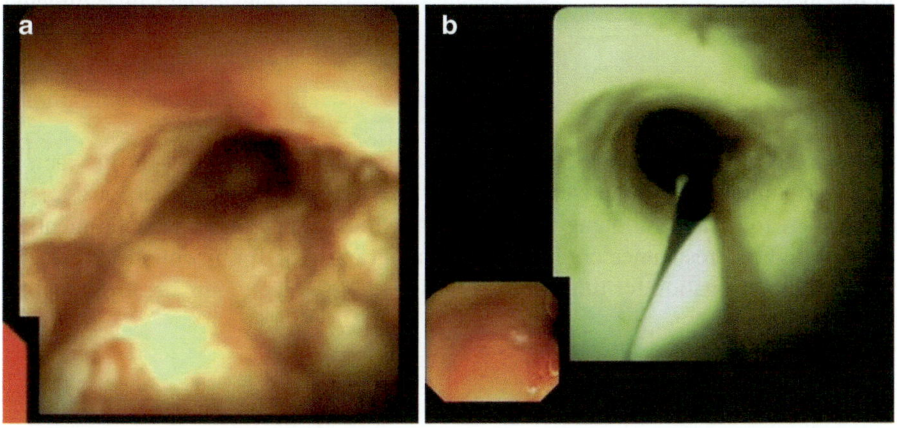

Fig. 12.4 (**a**) Cholangioscopy pre-radiofrequency ablation (RFA). (**b**) Cholangioscopy post-RFA, with therapeutic ductal changes noted

RFA biliary application still remains to be established. Our group recommends the use of RFA with cholangioscopy to have more intraductal details of results.

Biliary RFA can significantly alleviate jaundice, reduce the thickness of tumor lesions, prolong stent patency, and improve survival and quality of life with pCCA and dCCA (Fig. 12.5) [39]. Adverse events, as reported by some multicenter trials conducting RFA, are residual intraductal adenoma after papillectomy, comprised hemorrhage, pancreatitis, paraduodenal abscess, and post-RFA biliary strictures necessitating biliary drainage [44, 45] (Fig. 12.4). Of note, hepatobiliary lesions are usually surrounded by normal parenchyma, and thermal injury beyond the neoplasia does not usually affect important structures, whereas pancreatic tumors often encase vessels and the distal bile duct or are in contact with the gastric or duodenal wall. Some studies reported frequent and severe adverse events in pancreatic tumors with biliary extension [46].

At the moment there is no consensus on the optimal frequency and interval of RFA therapy. In most studies, RFA therapy was performed regularly every 3–4 months [47]. Because of inter-individual differences in tumor growth rate, it is difficult to accurately determine the time and frequency of RFA treatment required for each patient.

Importantly, RFA acts only on local tumors, indicating that this treatment may not have the ability to completely destroy a tumor mass. Cisplatin and gemcitabine have been used as first-line chemotherapies in advanced CCA. However, the efficacy of RFA combined with palliative chemotherapy for the treatment of extrahepatic CCA is not clear [48].

Biliary RFA treatment appears to be a promising adjuvant therapy in patients with malignant biliary obstruction. In these patients, the procedure is safe and well tolerated and improves stent patency and survival [9]. More data on larger patient population is needed, but this step is progressively achieved with cumulative articles in recent years.

Endoscopic Palliation

Before planning any palliative drainage, either by ERCP or percutaneously, it is mandatory to obtain a cholangiogram to define the extent of biliary ductal involvement. Magnetic resonance cholangiopancreatography (MRCP) continues to be the preferred investigation for this purpose.

Endoscopic Stenting Technique

Stents for palliation of biliary obstruction due to CCA are mostly placed via ERCP [49]. In a recent consensus, the American Society for Gastrointestinal Endoscopy graded endoscopic hilar stenting as a level 3 ERCP procedure in terms of complexity, with level 1 being the simplest and level 4 being most complex [50]. In general, a higher level of complexity is associated with a lower success rate and a higher adverse event rate [51]. Therefore, hilar stenting should be practiced only by experienced therapeutic endoscopists.

In general, there are two types of biliary stents: plastic and metallic stents. The design and coating of plastic stents may differ between producers, but do not differ largely in terms of clinical success or adverse events [52, 53]. The main adverse event of plastic stents is early clogging or stent migration. Therefore, the diameter of plastic stents with the best clinical patency rate is 10 Fr, whereas a diameter >11.5 Fr does not add any advantage [54, 55]. Different plastic designs with coating and antireflux valve mechanisms have been introduced to the market. They seem to show higher patency rates compared to standard polyethylene stents [56]. Larger studies need to confirm this effect. The need for stent exchange after 3–4 months or due to clogging or infection is considered to be one of the major drawbacks of plastic stents. Multiple plastic stent insertion may lead to better biliary drainage but can be technically challenging and time-consuming. Self-expanding metallic stents (SEMS) are differentiated into uncovered, partially covered, and covered. Covered SEMS are normally used when the stent might need to be retrieved later on. Uncovered SEMS show a lower cholecystitis rate but a higher rate of tissue ingrowth and therefore stenosis [57, 58]. Stent-in-stent insertion may be performed to address the latter. The effectiveness of such techniques has not been rigorously evaluated to date. Because of tissue ingrowth, uncovered SEMS are also hardly removable; thus stent migration occurs significantly more often with covered SEMS [59, 60]. A recent meta-analysis by Moole et al. [61] comparing covered and uncovered SEMS found that covered SEMS come along with higher patency rates.

A variety of plastic stents and SEMS are available and have been used for the stenting in CCA. In general, 10 Fr plastic stent and uncovered SEMS are preferred. The distal end of stents may be left in the duodenum or in distal bile duct, but the later situation may make reintervention more difficult. When more than one stent (plastic or SEMS) is to be placed, the stents are usually placed side by side (Fig. 12.2). However, in the last few years, a new dual stent design called "stent-in-stent" has been developed for metal stenting [62, 63]. In this technique, the first stent has an open-cell design, allowing the second stent to pass easily through the first stent.

In a recent study by Lee et al. [64] from South Korea, the stent-in-stent technique for bilateral stenting was evaluated in 84 patients with inoperable CCA. Technical and clinical success was achieved in 95.2% and 92.9% of patients, respectively. The median survival and patency were noted to be 256 days and 239 days, respectively. Still, this new stent design can be problematic if the first stent becomes occluded. In the study by Lee et al. [64], 30.8% patients had an obstruction of the primary biliary stent. For revision stenting, bilateral metal stents could be placed in 55%, while plastic stents were placed in the remaining patients [64].

When survival is estimated to be <4 months, 10 Fr plastic stents are recommended, even if recommendation grade Ic was given [65]. In former guidelines SEMS showed higher effectiveness in patients with an overall survival estimated to be >4 months. In patients with a life expectancy of up to 1 month, no clear indication for either plastic or SEMS exists [65]. The concept of best supportive care should be followed in these cases. The new ESGE guidelines instead recommend a covered 10 mm SEMS placement at first intervention, regardless of general life expectancy [9]. The former argument of better cost-effectiveness in plastic stents is now proven not to be true. Uncovered SEMS should normally be used only in histologically confirmed hilar or distal obstruction by CCA, as retrieval is difficult or impossible afterward [9]. The number of stents depends of the location of the obstruction and the efficacy of the drainage. In patients with distal obstruction, single stent insertion is the standard of care. The question of uni or bilateral stent insertion only becomes important in hilar obstruction. Several meta-analyses have discussed the role of uni and bilateral drainage. Unilateral drainage seems to be equally efficient to bilateral drainage for bilirubin regression and diminution of patients' symptoms with no statistical difference in occlusion rate, therapeutic failure, or cholangitis. SEMS placement is clearly favored [66, 67]. The objective of ERCP should be drainage of at least 50% of all liver sectors as it provides better overall survival [68]. In general, endoscopic bile duct decompression should not only relieve jaundice or treat cholangitis, it should also allow for readministration of chemotherapy. Up to now, no clear data exist on how many patients are able to resume chemotherapy after bile duct decompression. The advantages of endoscopic decompression on patient survival of this highly morbid patient cohort are neither studied nor subclassified for distal, hilar, or intrahepatic CCs. Clinically, the main advantage of endoscopic instead of percutaneous bile duct compression is a higher quality of life with less need for technical surveillance in patients receiving ERCP. In terms of morbidity/mortality after endoscopic or percutaneous bile duct decompression, the center's experience is crucial for choosing the right method.

The total failure rate of ERCP-guided drainage in CC is 6–7%. Therefore, other drainage possibilities such as PTBD and EUS/computed tomography-guided transhepatic or EUS-guided transduodenal drainage need to be considered. The technique of EUS-BD is being increasingly investigated in cases of ERCP failure. Up to now, it is mostly performed at centers with high experience for interventional EUS. In EUS-BD, a transgastric hepatic EUS is performed in order to characterize intrahepatic biliary dilation not accessible by ERCP. Then, biliary drainage is ensured by direct transgastric endosonography-guided puncture of the intrahepatic dilated bile ducts and stent insertion [69]. Indications of EUS-BD are insufficient, technically not feasible, or contraindicated PTBD or ERCP. The technical success rate can reach 100% when the procedure is performed by experts. Still, adverse events such as peritonitis, cholangitis, bile leakage, and stent migration may occur in up to 20% [70, 71] (Fig. 12.5).

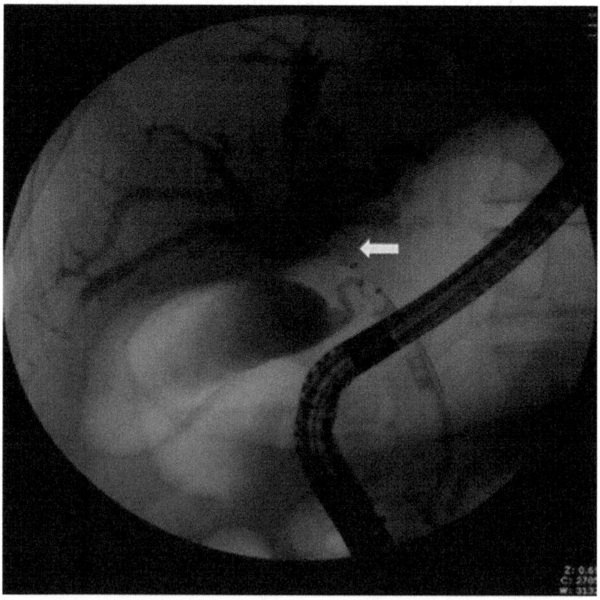

Fig. 12.5 ERCP with hilar biliary stenosis with proximal bile duct dilation suggestive of perihilar cholangiocarcinoma

Conclusion

CCA is characterized by high mortality and low rate of resectable patients. The complete approach to these patients requires multidisciplinary working groups. The best results, with low rates of adverse events, are seen in high-volume centers.

Endoscopy plays a major role in patients with CCA, especially pCCA and dCCA. Biliary tract compression with cholangitis is often the first problem to manage during the subsequent clinical course. Immediate antibiotic therapy is crucial, and ERCP with stent placement should be performed within <48 h after diagnosis of cholangitis to reduce morbidity and mortality. If ERCP fails, repeated ERCP should be considered before switching to other treatment options such as PTBD or EUS-BD. PTBD is often the treatment of choice for decompression in Type III and IV Klatskin tumors. Some new guidelines recommend SEMS placement early on, regardless of the patient's life expectancy. Nutritional care must not be forgotten.

An enduring issue for the medical team is to obtain rapid and accurate diagnosis. New endoscopic modalities and technologies, such as SpyGlass, are occupying an important role in early diagnosis, and in addition, there is a growing role for endoscopic treatment of CCA via advanced stenting and ablative techniques. For this reason, patients must be referred to specialized centers upon a suspected diagnosis of CCA. Endoscopic biliary drainage is an important tool in non-resectable patients and in those that are candidates for two-stage hepatectomy.

References

1. Dondossola D, Ghidini M, Grossi F, Rossi G, Foschi D. Practical review for diagnosis and clinical management of perihilar cholangiocarcinoma. World J Gastroenterol. 2020;26(25):3542–61. https://doi.org/10.3748/wjg.v26.i25.3542.
2. Renshaw K. Malignant neoplasms of the extrahepatic biliary ducts. Ann Surg. 1922;76(2):205–21. https://doi.org/10.1097/00000658-192208000-00008.
3. Rizvi S, Gores GJ. Pathogenesis, diagnosis, and management of cholangiocarcinoma. Gastroenterology. 2013;145(6):1215–29. https://doi.org/10.1053/j.gastro.2013.10.013.
4. Singh A, Siddiqui UD. The role of endoscopy in the diagnosis and management of cholangiocarcinoma. J Clin Gastroenterol. 2015;49(9):725–37. https://doi.org/10.1097/MCG.0000000000000390.
5. Berthiaume EP, Wands J. The molecular pathogenesis of cholangiocarcinoma. Semin Liver Dis. 2004;24(2):127–37. https://doi.org/10.1055/s-2004-828890.
6. Fava G, Lorenzini I. Molecular pathogenesis of cholangiocarcinoma. Int J Hepatol. 2012;2012:630543. https://doi.org/10.1155/2012/630543.
7. Nakanuma Y, Sato Y, Harada K, Sasaki M, Xu J, Ikeda H. Pathological classification of intrahepatic cholangiocarcinoma based on a new concept. World J Hepatol. 2010;2(12):419–27. https://doi.org/10.4254/wjh.v2.i12.419.
8. Blechacz B, Gores GJ. Cholangiocarcinoma: advances in pathogenesis, diagnosis, and treatment. Hepatology. 2008;48(1):308–21. https://doi.org/10.1002/hep.22310.
9. Sirica AE. The role of cancer-associated myofibroblasts in intrahepatic cholangiocarcinoma. Nat Rev Gastroenterol Hepatol. 2011;9(1):44–54. Published 2011 Nov 29. https://doi.org/10.1038/nrgastro.2011.222.

10. Razumilava N, Gores GJ. Cholangiocarcinoma. Lancet. 2014;383(9935):2168–79. https://doi.org/10.1016/S0140-6736(13)61903-0.
11. Rizvi S, Eaton J, Yang JD, Chandrasekhara V, Gores GJ. Emerging technologies for the diagnosis of perihilar cholangiocarcinoma. Semin Liver Dis. 2018;38(2):160–9. https://doi.org/10.1055/s-0038-1655775.
12. DeOliveira ML, Cunningham SC, Cameron JL, et al. Cholangiocarcinoma: thirty-one-year experience with 564 patients at a single institution. Ann Surg. 2007;245(5):755–62. https://doi.org/10.1097/01.sla.0000251366.62632.d3.
13. Bismuth H, Corlette MB. Intrahepatic cholangioenteric anastomosis in carcinoma of the hilus of the liver. Surg Gynecol Obstet. 1975;140:170–8.
14. Bismuth H, Nakache R, Diamond T. Management strategies in resection for hilar cholangiocarcinoma. Ann Surg. 1992;215:31–8.
15. Zervos EE, Osborne D, Goldin SB, Villadolid DV, Thometz DP, Durkin A, Carey LC, Rosemurgy AS. Stage does not predict survival after resection of hilar cholangiocarcinomas promoting an aggressive operative approach. Am J Surg. 2005;190:810–5.
16. Ruzzenente A, Bagante F, Ardito F, Campagnaro T, Scoleri I, Conci S, Iacono C, Giuliante F, Guglielmi A. Comparison of the 7th and 8th editions of the American Joint Committee on Cancer Staging Systems for perihilar cholangiocarcinoma. Surgery. 2018;164:244–50.
17. Ebata T, Kosuge T, Hirano S, Unno M, Yamamoto M, Miyazaki M, Kokudo N, Miyagawa S, Takada T, Nagino M. Proposal to modify the International Union against cancer staging system for perihilar cholangiocarcinomas. Br J Surg. 2014;101:79–88.
18. AI di Oncologia Medica. Linee guida TUMORI DELLE VIE BILIARI. Available from: http://media.aiom.it/userfiles/files/doc/LG/2016_LG_AIOM_Vie_biliari.pdf.
19. Miyazaki M, Yoshitomi H, Miyakawa S, et al. Clinical practice guidelines for the management of biliary tract cancers 2015: the 2nd English edition [published correction appears in J Hepatobiliary Pancreat Sci. 2015;22(6):510. Iasayama, Hiroyuki [corrected to Isayama, Hiroyuki]]. J Hepatobiliary Pancreat Sci. 2015;22(4):249–73. https://doi.org/10.1002/jhbp.233.
20. Vogl TJ, Schwarz WO, Heller M, Herzog C, Zangos S, Hintze RE, Neuhaus P, Hammerstingl RM. Staging of Klatskin tumours (hilar cholangiocarcinomas): comparison of MR cholangiography, MR imaging, and endoscopic retrograde cholangiography. Eur Radiol. 2006;16:2317–25.
21. Jorgensen JE, Waljee AK, Volk ML, et al. Is MRCP equivalent to ERCP for diagnosing biliary obstruction in orthotopic liver transplant recipients? A meta-analysis. Gastrointest Endosc. 2011;73(5):955–62. https://doi.org/10.1016/j.gie.2010.12.014.
22. Meister T, Heinzow HS, Woestmeyer C, Lenz P, Menzel J, Kucharzik T, Domschke W, Domagk D. Intraductal ultrasound substantiates diagnostics of bile duct strictures of uncertain etiology. World J Gastroenterol. 2013;19:874–81.
23. Kahaleh M. Spyglass direct visualization system. Clin Endosc. 2012;45:316–8. https://doi.org/10.5946/ce.2012.45.3.316.
24. Pleskow D, Parsi MA, Chen YK, et al. Biopsy of indeterminate biliary strictures. Does direct visualization help? A multicenter experience. Gastrointest Endosc. 2008;67:AB103. https://doi.org/10.1016/j.gie.2008.03.127.
25. Bhandari S, Bathini R, Sharma A, et al. Usefulness of single-operator cholangioscopy-guided laser lithotripsy in patients with Mirizzi syndrome and cystic duct stones: experience at a tertiary care center. Gastrointest Endosc. 2016;84:56–61. https://doi.org/10.1016/j.gie.2015.12.025.
26. Nakajima M, Akasaka Y, Yamaguchi K, et al. Direct endoscopic visualization of the bile and pancreatic duct systems by peroral cholangiopancreatoscopy (PCPS). Gastrointest Endosc. 1978;24:141–5. https://doi.org/10.1016/S0016-5107(78)73488-7.
27. Chen YK. Preclinical characterization of the Spyglass peroral cholangiopancreatoscopy system for direct access, visualization, and biopsy. Gastrointest Endosc. 2007;65:303–11. https://doi.org/10.1016/j.gie.2006.07.048.

28. Kim HJ, Kim MH, Lee SK, et al. Tumor vessel: a valuable cholangioscopic clue of malignant biliary stricture. Gastrointest Endosc. 2000;52:635–8. https://doi.org/10.1067/mge.2000.108969.
29. Pons-Beltrán V, Alonso-Lázaro N, Mansilla-Vivar R, Sáez-González E, Ponce Romero M, Argüello-Viudez L, Ramos-Soler D, Pérez-Rojas J, Leathers J, Bustamante-Balen M, Grupo de Investigación de Endoscopia Digestiva. IIS Hospital La Fe. Valencia, Spain. Single-operator cholangiopancreatoscopy in pancreatobiliary diseases: clinical experience in a tertiary referral hospital. Rev Esp Enferm Dig. 2018;110(12):748–54.
30. Fung BM, Fejleh MP, Tejaswi S, Tabibian JH. Cholangioscopy and its role in primary sclerosing cholangitis. Eur Med J Hepatol. 2020;8(1):42–53.
31. de Groen PC, Gores GJ, LaRusso NF, Gunderson LL, Nagorney DM. Biliary tract cancers. N Engl J Med. 1999;341(18):1368–78.
32. Ortner ME, Caca K, Berr F, et al. Successful photodynamic therapy for nonresectable cholangiocarcinoma: a randomized prospective study. Gastroenterology. 2003;125:1355–63.
33. Kahaleh M, Mishra R, Shami VM, et al. Unresectable cholangiocarcinoma: comparison of survival in biliary stenting alone versus stenting with photodynamic therapy. Clin Gastroenterol Hepatol. 2008;6:290–7.
34. Witzigmann H, Berr F, Ringel U, et al. Surgical and palliative management and outcome in 184 patients with hilar cholangiocarcinoma: palliative photodynamic therapy plus stenting is comparable to r1/r2 resection. Ann Surg. 2006;244:230–9.
35. Zoepf T, Jakobs R, Arnold JC, et al. Palliation of nonresectable bile duct cancer: improved survival after photodynamic therapy. Am J Gastroenterol. 2005;100:2426–30.
36. Shim CS, Cheon YK, Cha SW, et al. Prospective study of the effectiveness of percutaneous transhepatic photodynamic therapy for advanced bile duct cancer and the role of intraductal ultrasonography in response assessment. Endoscopy. 2005;37:425–33.
37. Schmidt A, Bloechinger M, Weber A, et al. Short-term effects and adverse events of endoscopically applied radiofrequency ablation appear to be comparable with photodynamic therapy in hilar cholangiocarcinoma. United European Gastroenterol J. 2016;4(4):570–9. https://doi.org/10.1177/2050640615621235.
38. Wiedmann M, Berr F, Schiefke I, et al. Photodynamic therapy in patients with non-resectable hilar cholangiocarcinoma: 5-year follow-up of a prospective phase II study. Gastrointest Endosc. 2004;60:68–75.
39. Steel AW, Postgate AJ, Khorsandi S, et al. Endoscopically applied radiofrequency ablation appears to be safe in the treatment of malignant biliary obstruction. Gastrointest Endosc. 2011;73:149–53. https://doi.org/10.1016/j.gie.2010.09.031. PubMed PMID: 21184881.
40. Figueroa-Barojas P, Bakhru MR, Habib NA, et al. Safety and efficacy of radiofrequency ablation in the management of unresectable bile duct and pancreatic cancer: a novel palliation technique. J Oncol. 2013;2013:910897.
41. Mansilla-Vivar R, Argüello-Viúdez L, Sánchez-Montes C, Alonso-Lázaro N, Pons-Beltrán V. Endoluminal radiofrequency ablation with SpyGlass™ in the management of cholangiocarcinoma. Rev Esp Enferm Dig. 2019;111(10):803–5. https://doi.org/10.17235/reed.2019.6230/2019.
42. Ogura T, Onda S, Sano T, Takagi W, Okuda A, Miyano A, Nishioka N, Imanishi M, Amano M, Masuda D, Higuchi K. Evaluation of the safety of endoscopic radiofrequency ablation for malignant biliary stricture using a digital peroral cholangioscope (with videos). Dig Endosc. 2017;29(6):712–7. https://doi.org/10.1111/den.12837. Epub 2017 Mar 16. PubMed PMID: 28181704.
43. Monga A, Gupta R, Ramchandani M, et al. Endoscopic radiofrequency ablation of cholangiocarcinoma: new palliative treatment modality with videos. Gastrointest Endosc. 2011;74(4):935–7. https://doi.org/10.1016/j.gie.2010.10.018. Epub 2010 Dec 18. PubMed PMID: 21168839.
44. Yang J, Wang J, Zhou H, Zhou Y, Wang Y, Jin H, et al. Efficacy and safety of endoscopic radiofrequency ablation for unresectable extrahepatic cholangiocarcinoma: a randomized trial. Endoscopy. 2018;50(8):751–60.

45. Sofi AA, Khan MA, Das A, Sachdev M, Khuder S, Nawras A, et al. Radiofrequency ablation combined with biliary stent placement versus stent placement alone for malignant biliary strictures: a systematic review and meta-analysis. Gastrointest Endosc. 2018;87:944–51.e1.
46. Shariff MI, Khan SA, Westaby D. The palliation of cholangiocarcinoma. Curr Opin Support Palliat Care. 2013;7(2):168–74. https://doi.org/10.1097/SPC.0b013e32835f1e2f. Review. PubMed PMID: 23422512.
47. Sofi AA, Khan MA, Das A, et al. Radiofrequency ablation combined with biliary stent placement versus stent placement alone for malignant biliary strictures: a systematic review and meta-analysis. Gastrointest Endosc. 2018;87(4):944–51.e1. https://doi.org/10.1016/j.gie.2017.10.029. Epub 2017 Nov 3. Review. PubMed PMID: 29108980.
48. Larghi A, Rimbaş M, Tringali A, et al. Endoscopic radiofrequency biliary ablation treatment: a comprehensive review. Dig Endosc. 2018. https://doi.org/10.1111/den.13298. Review. PubMed PMID: 30444547.
49. Khan SA, Davidson BR, Goldin R, Pereira SP, Rosenberg WM, Taylor-Robinson SD, Thillainayagam AV, Thomas HC, Thursz MR, Wasan H. Guidelines for the diagnosis and treatment of cholangiocarcinoma: consensus document. Gut. 2002;51(Suppl 6):VI1–9.
50. Cotton PB, Eisen G, Romagnuolo J, Vargo J, Baron T, Tarnasky P, Schutz S, Jacobson B, Bott C, Petersen B. Grading the complexity of endoscopic procedures: results of an ASGE working party. Gastrointest Endosc. 2011;73:868–74.
51. Ragunath K, Thomas LA, Cheung WY, Duane PD, Richards DG. Objective evaluation of ERCP procedures: a simple grading scale for evaluating technical difficulty. Postgrad Med J. 2003;79:467–70.
52. van Berkel AM, Boland C, Redekop WK, Bergman JJ, Groen AK, Tytgat GN, et al. A prospective randomized trial of Teflon versus polyethylene stents for distal malignant biliary obstruction. Endoscopy. 1998;30(8):681–6.
53. van Berkel AM, Huibregtse IL, Bergman JJ, Rauws EA, Bruno MJ, Huibregtse K. A prospective randomized trial of Tannenbaum-Type Teflon-coated stents versus polyethylene stents for distal malignant biliary obstruction. Eur J Gastroenterol Hepatol. 2004;16(2):213–7.
54. Speer AG, Cotton PB, MacRae KD. Endoscopic management of malignant biliary obstruction: stents of 10 French gauge are preferable to stents of 8 French gauge. Gastrointest Endosc. 1988;34(5):412–7.
55. Kadakia SC, Starnes E. Comparison of 10 French gauge stent with 11.5 French gauge stent in patients with biliary tract diseases. Gastrointest Endosc. 1992;38(4):454–9.
56. Tringali A, Mutignani M, Perri V, Zuccalà G, Cipolletta L, Bianco MA, et al. A prospective, randomized multicenter trial comparing DoubleLayer and polyethylene stents for malignant distal common bile duct strictures. Endoscopy. 2003;35(12):992–7.
57. Dumonceau JM, Tringali A, Papanikolaou IS, Blero D, Mangiavillano B, Schmidt A, et al. Endoscopic biliary stenting: indications, choice of stents, and results: European Society of Gastrointestinal Endoscopy (ESGE) Clinical Guideline – Updated October 2017. Endoscopy. 2018;50(9):910–30.
58. Dumonceau JM, Tringali A, Blero D, Devière J, Laugiers R, Heresbach D, et al. European Society of Gastrointestinal Endoscopy. Biliary stenting: indications, choice of stents and results: European Society of Gastrointestinal Endoscopy (ESGE) clinical guideline. Endoscopy. 2012;44(3):277–98.
59. Saleem A, Leggett CL, Murad MH, Baron TH. Meta-analysis of randomized trials comparing the patency of covered and uncovered self-expandable metal stents for palliation of distal malignant bile duct obstruction. Gastrointest Endosc. 2011;74(2):321–7.e1–3.
60. Li J, Li T, Sun P, Yu Q, Wang K, Chang W, et al. Covered versus uncovered self-expandable metal stents for managing malignant distal biliary obstruction: a meta-analysis. PLoS One. 2016;11(2):e0149066.
61. Moole H, Bechtold ML, Cashman M, Volmar FH, Dhillon S, Forcione D, et al. Covered versus uncovered self-expandable metal stents for malignant biliary strictures: a meta-analysis and systematic review. Indian J Gastroenterol. 2016;35(5):323–30.

62. Park do H, Lee SS, Moon JH, Choi HJ, Cha SW, Kim JH, Seo DW, Lee SK, Park SH, Lee MS. Newly designed stent for endoscopic bilateral stent-in-stent placement of metallic stents in patients with malignant hilar biliary strictures: multicenter prospective feasibility study (with videos). Gastrointest Endosc. 2009;69:1357–60.
63. Chahal P, Baron TH. Expandable metal stents for endoscopic bilateral stent-within-stent placement for malignant hilar biliary obstruction. Gastrointest Endosc. 2010;71:195–9.
64. Lee TH, Moon JH, Kim JH, Park DH, Lee SS, Choi HJ, Cho YD, Park SH, Kim SJ. Primary and revision efficacy of cross-wired metallic stents for endoscopic bilateral stent-in-stent placement in malignant hilar biliary strictures. Endoscopy. 2013;45:106–13.
65. Tyson GL, El-Serag HB. Risk factors for cholangiocarcinoma. Hepatology. 2011;54(1):173–84. https://doi.org/10.1002/hep.24351.
66. Lee TH, Kim TH, Moon JH, Lee SH, Choi HJ, Hwangbo Y, et al. Bilateral versus unilateral placement of metal stents for inoperable high-grade malignant hilar biliary strictures: a multicenter, prospective, randomized study (with video). Gastrointest Endosc. 2017;86(5):817–27.
67. Sawas T, Al Halabi S, Parsi MA, Vargo JJ. Self-expandable metal stents versus plastic stents for malignant biliary obstruction: a meta-analysis. Gastrointest Endosc. 2015;82: 256–67.e7.
68. Vienne A, Hobeika E, Gouya H, Lapidus N, Fritsch J, Choury AD, et al. Prediction of drainage effectiveness during endoscopic stenting of malignant hilar strictures: the role of liver volume assessment. Gastrointest Endosc. 2010;72(4):728–35.
69. Oh D, Park DH, Song TJ, Lee SS, Seo DW, Lee SK, et al. Optimal biliary access point and learning curve for endoscopic ultrasound-guided hepaticogastrostomy with transmural stenting. Ther Adv Gastroenterol. 2017;10(1):42–53.
70. Rerknimitr R, Angsuwatcharakon P, Ratanachu-ek T, Khor CJ, Ponnudurai R, Moon JH, et al. Asia-Pacific Working Group on Hepatobiliary Cancers. Asia-Pacific consensus recommendations for endoscopic and interventional management of hilar cholangiocarcinoma. J Gastroenterol Hepatol. 2013;28(4):593–607.
71. Will U, Thieme A, Fueldner F, Gerlach R, Wanzar I, Meyer F. Treatment of biliary obstruction in selected patients by endoscopic ultrasonography (EUS)-guided transluminal biliary drainage. Endoscopy. 2007;39(4):292–5.

Chapter 13
The Role of Endoscopic Ultrasound in Cholangiocarcinoma

Tarek Sawas, Neil Marya, and Michael Levy

Abbreviations

AE	Adverse event
CCA	Cholangiocarcinoma
CT	Computed tomography
eCCA	Extrahepatic cholangiocarcinoma
ERCP	Endoscopic retrograde cholangiopancreatography
EUS	Endoscopic ultrasound
FNA	Fine needle aspiration
FNB	Fine needle biopsy
HCC	Hepatocellular carcinoma
iCCA	Intrahepatic cholangiocarcinoma
MRCP	Magnetic resonance cholangiopancreatography
MRI	Magnetic resonance imaging
PSC	Primary sclerosing cholangitis
US	Transabdominal ultrasound

Introducstion

Cholangiocarcinoma (CCA) is a biliary tumor that can originate from both the intrahepatic and extrahepatic biliary epithelium. Annually, approximately 5000 new cases of CCA are diagnosed in the United States [1]. Although CCA is a relatively rare cancer, data suggest that the incidence of both intrahepatic and extrahepatic CCA (iCCA and eCCA, respectively) is increasing [2]. Despite advances in chemotherapy regimens and surgical treatments, CCA continues to be an aggressive

Tarek Sawas and Neil Marya contributed equally with all other contributors.

T. Sawas · N. Marya · M. Levy (✉)
Division of Gastroenterology and Hepatology, Mayo Clinic, Rochester, MN, USA
e-mail: Levy.michael@mayo.edu

J. H. Tabibian (ed.), *Diagnosis and Management of Cholangiocarcinoma*,
https://doi.org/10.1007/978-3-030-70936-5_13

cancer with a high mortality rate. Patients with localized iCCA and eCCA have 5-year survival rates of 15% and 30%, respectively, while those with metastatic CCA have a 5-year survival rate of only 2%, regardless of tumor location [3]. Thus, early diagnosis and accurate staging are key to optimizing treatment outcomes and improving survival in patients with CCA.

Currently, diagnostic approaches for patients with suspected CCA involve a combination of imaging modalities (e.g., transabdominal ultrasound [US], computed tomography [CT], and magnetic resonance imaging/cholangiopancreatography [MRI/MRCP]) as well as laboratory markers (e.g., serum liver tests, carbohydrate antigen 19-9) [4]. Endoscopic retrograde cholangiopancreatography (ERCP) is commonly performed along with intraductal brushings and biopsies for a tissue diagnosis of suspicious lesions in cases of eCCA. The role of endoscopic ultrasound (EUS) in CCA, by contrast, is generally less established but continues to evolve. Like other endoscopic procedures, EUS is a minimally invasive procedure that is often performed in the outpatient setting. Due to the proximity of the stomach and duodenum to the extrahepatic and intrahepatic bile ducts, EUS allows for detailed imaging of the biliary tree, liver, regional lymph nodes, surrounding vasculature, and potential sites of regional metastasis.

This chapter focuses on the role of EUS in the diagnosis and staging of CCA and addresses pitfalls and risks associated with the procedure, particularly as it relates to the CCA patient population.

Diagnosis and Staging

Endosonographic Detection of Tumors and Strictures

The evaluation for potential etiologies of biliary obstruction routinely begins with noninvasive imaging (typically US or CT and thereafter MRI/MRCP), which is useful for directing whether more invasive procedures, including ERCP and EUS, are necessary. Occasionally noninvasive imaging modalities are unable to determine the presence and cause of biliary obstruction, in which case EUS has an important and complementary role for identifying the cause of obstruction. Unlike ERCP, which carries risks such as acute pancreatitis due to the invasive nature of cannulation, imaging of the bile duct on EUS has a risk profile akin to traditional upper endoscopy. While EUS is less capable of identifying the etiology of obstruction for many intrahepatic and hilar tumors due to the restricted imaging in these locations, imaging of other local and distant sites, with or without tissue sampling (e.g., fine needle aspiration [FNA] or biopsy [FNB]), often provides additional key staging information.

Zaheer et al. (2013) evaluated the role of EUS in determining the cause of biliary obstruction among 412 consecutive patients who were referred for EUS prior to ERCP. The authors demonstrated that EUS was 99%, 92%, and 90% accurate in

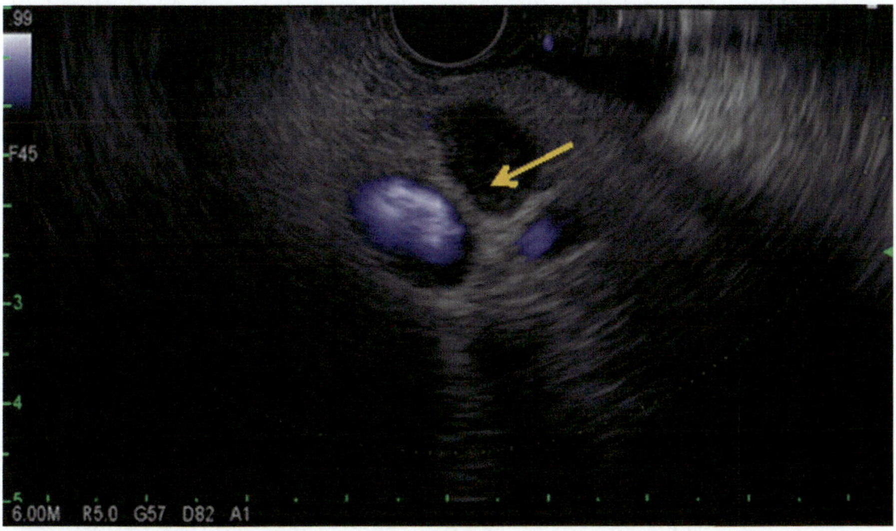

Fig. 13.1 EUS evidence of a biliary stricture and diminutive lumen (arrow) surrounded by marked bile duct wall thickening. The bile duct wall was biopsied and brushed. Findings came back positive for cholangiocarcinoma

detecting choledocholithiasis, benign biliary strictures, and malignant biliary strictures, respectively. The most common sources of malignant biliary obstruction were pancreatic adenocarcinoma, CCA, and ampullary tumors, respectively [5]. This study demonstrated the accuracy of EUS in detecting malignant biliary strictures across an array of tumor sites and pathologies. Similarly, Mohamadnejad et al. (2011) prospectively evaluated 81 patients with CCA and reported an overall primary tumor detection rate of 94% that was significantly greater for eCCA versus iCCA (100% vs. 83%, $p < 0.01$) [6].

These studies and other demonstrate how EUS imaging alone is a powerful tool used to determine the cause and site of biliary obstruction (Fig. 13.1).

Sampling of Strictures via Fine Needle Aspiration

In patients with laboratory and imaging findings concerning for possible CCA, tissue acquisition is generally required to establish a definitive diagnosis prior to initiating therapy. Historically, however, obtaining a definitive histological or cytological diagnosis of CCA has been challenging, in large part due to the desmoplastic nature of these lesions. In patients with suspected eCCA (including perihilar and distal), ERCP is commonly the first modality chosen for tissue acquisition purposes. The preference for ERCP is driven by the ability to sample strictures but to also perform therapeutic interventions, such as balloon dilation and intraductal stenting. ERCP-based tissue acquisition techniques include intraductal brush cytology and intraductal biopsies (guided by either fluoroscopy or cholangioscopy). Studies demonstrate that the sensitivity of ERCP-based tissue acquisition for indeterminate biliary strictures ranges from only 35% to 75% [7–11].

Multiple studies have shown that EUS-FNA has superior sensitivity compared to ERCP-based tissue acquisition techniques. While FNA should not be performed for strictures that represent potentially resectable or transplantable perihilar tumors, Weilert et al. (2014) compared the sensitivity and accuracy of primary tumor EUS-FNA to ERCP with brushings in 51 patients with malignant and benign biliary strictures. The authors found that compared to ERCP, EUS-FNA was significantly more sensitive (94% versus 50%, $p < 0.001$) and significantly more accurate (94% versus 53%, $p < 0.001$). A recent meta-analysis by De Moura et al. (2018) compared yields of EUS-FNA and ERCP with brushings in 294 patients presenting with indeterminate biliary strictures. The study demonstrated that the mean sensitivity of EUS-FNA was greater than ERCP with brushings (75% versus 49%) [12].

The diagnostic yield of EUS-FNA of biliary tract lesions is expected to increase substantially as novel genetic analysis techniques for biliary tract specimens expand. The feasibility of applying targeted next-generation sequencing for EUS-FNA samples obtained from various other organ systems has already been demonstrated [13–16]. A recent study by Hirata et al. (2019) evaluated whether targeted amplicon sequencing of biliary tract tumors specimens obtained during EUS-FNA was feasible, demonstrating that targeted amplicon sequencing of EUS-FNA samples of the biliary tract was successful in identifying pathogenic genetic abnormalities in 95% of patients [17]. More work is needed to clarify whether these and other detected molecular changes guide and improve patient management and outcome.

As will be more fully reviewed later, despite the demonstrated utility of EUS-FNA of primary CCA tumors, this practice cannot be routinely advocated due to the risk tumor seeding. In fact, the mere performance of EUS-FNA of primary CCA is considered an absolute contraindication to resection and transplant in most centers.

Staging and Evaluating Resectability

Currently, the only options for curative treatment of CCA are surgical resection or liver transplantation. Preoperative staging of CCA is necessary to optimize treatment options and outcomes. Multiple staging systems have been utilized for CCA, and several factors are considered when determining if a patient has resectable or transplantable disease [18–20]. Factors include the primary tumor location and extent, presence of nodal metastases, atrophic hepatic lobes, tumor invasion of surrounding vasculature, distant metastases, and anticipated residual hepatic function. The gold standard for accurate disease staging is a staging laparoscopy. Enhanced imaging techniques, however, can prevent patients from having to undergo staging laparoscopy.

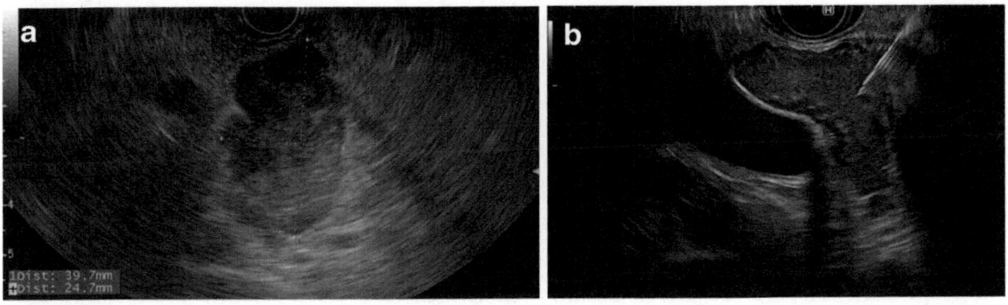

Fig. 13.2 (**a**, **b**) Linear EUS evaluation of two porta hepatis lymph nodes. EUS-FNA of the nodes came back malignant (**a**) and benign (**b**)

Currently, CT and MRI/MRCP are commonly employed noninvasive imaging methods for CCA staging. Fewer data are available to determine the role and utility of EUS in this regard. Mohamadnejad et al. (2011) evaluated EUS among 81 patients who were referred for surgical management of CCA and found EUS to be superior to CT or MRI in identifying patients ultimately deemed to have unresectable disease. In their study, EUS correctly identified unresectable disease in 8 of 15 patients; of these 8 patients identified on EUS as being unresectable, CT/MRI failed to identify unresectable disease in 6 of the patients. Typical sites of disease spread identified on EUS, but not CT or MRI, included hepatic artery invasion, peritoneal involvement, and liver metastases [6].

Additionally, EUS has an essential role in evaluating for locoregional nodal metastases (Fig. 13.2) in CCA patients, which is important given the poor 5-year survival rates of those with nodal disease (0–25%) [21–23]. Thus, correctly identifying nodal metastases in CCA is vital in selecting which patients may reasonably undergo surgical resection or liver transplantation. Gleeson et al. (2008) evaluated the accuracy of EUS-FNA in detecting locoregional nodal metastases in patients with unresectable hilar CCA prior to possible liver transplantation. Given that in our experience the lymph node morphology does not correlate with malignancy in patients with CCA, we sample locoregional lymph nodes whenever identified at EUS, as performed in this study. EUS identified locoregional lymph nodes in all of the included patients, among whom EUS-FNA identified nodal metastases in eight patients (17%). Among the eight patients with malignant lymph nodes on EUS, only two were found to have had suspicious adenopathy on CT and/or MRI. Importantly, among the 22 patients who subsequently underwent exploratory laparotomy, 20 (90.9%) were confirmed to have no nodal metastases as demonstrated on EUS [24]. Thus, the role of EUS-FNA in CCA patients prior to undergoing liver transplant or resection should be considered. It is important to note that the investigators found that sonographic nodal features did not distinguish between malignant and nonmalignant adenopathy, thereby mandating lymph node FNA among CCA patients to make such distinction.

Assessment of Intrahepatic Cholangiocarcinoma

By definition, iiCCA arises above the level of the second-order bile ducts and generally presents as a mass lesion within the hepatic parenchyma [4]. Although iCCA is a rare malignancy, it is the second most common primary hepatic malignancy after hepatocellular carcinoma (HCC) [1]. It is usually detected during routine HCC screening transabdominal US or CT in patients with liver cirrhosis. The enhancement pattern on CT or MRI usually distinguishes iCCA from HCC [24, 25]. However, this can be extremely challenging, and a tissue diagnosis (FNA/B) might be needed for the ultimate diagnosis. Historically, hepatic lesions were sampled percutaneously using US guidance due to easy access and the widespread misconception that hepatic lesions could not be adequately visualized and sampled with EUS. Although the percutaneous approach remains the predominant method for tissue acquisition, the use of EUS-FNA has increased in recent years. EUS provides appropriate assessment of the left lobe and hilum from the gastric body, antrum, and duodenal bulb, whereas portions of the right lobe are best examined from the duodenal bulb or second portion of the duodenum. Unfortunately, published EUS studies excluded patients with iCCA, thereby limiting our knowledge of the role of EUS in the diagnosis and management of iCCA.

Tumor Seeding

Tissue confirmation of suspected CCA is highly desired before proceeding with a complex and high-risk surgical treatment. However, the benefits of primary tumor EUS-FNA (as opposed to lymph node EUS-FNA) must be weighed against the risk of tumor seeding, which is also referred to as needle tract seeding or implantation metastasis. Needle tract seeding is a result of implantation of tumor cells along the FNA (or FNB) needle tract. This occurrence may lead to change of tumor stage and always converts resectable tumors to a non-operable care strategy. In fact, mere performance of EUS-FNA, in the absence of any clear needle tract seeding, and irrespective of the cytological interpretation, designates a tumor as unresectable and non-transplantable in most centers. As a result of these concerns, we avoid EUS-FNA or FNB for potentially resectable or transplantable tumors.

Generally, risk factors for needle tract tumor seeding include larger tumor size and high-grade tumors, large-caliber needles, multiple needle passes, and paucity of normal parenchymal tissue along the needle tract [26]. The reported clinically apparent tumor seeding after FNA is rare, estimated at 1/10,000–40,000 [27]. However, this risk is likely greatly underestimated due to the high mortality among patients who are not surgical or liver transplant candidates [28]. Additionally, tumor seeding might be misinterpreted as a recurrence in patients who undergo curative surgery or liver transplant. Tumor seeding may deposit cells that are undetected in the resected surgical specimen. This would progress over time to an overt clinical disease, which is often misinterpreted as recurrence rather than a disease progression due to a needle tract seeding [28].

In a prospective study by Levy et al. [29], the presence of malignant cells within the gastrointestinal luminal fluid after performing EUS-FNA was evaluated in patients with pancreatic cancer. Post-EUS-FNA luminal fluid cytology was positive in 12% of patients, suggesting translocation of malignant cells from pancreatic cancer tissue into the gastrointestinal lumen due to EUS-FNA. This process likely represents the underlying method by which needle tract seeding develops. In another retrospective cohort study from our institution, Heimbach et al. [30] compared the incidence of peritoneal metastasis between patients who did and did not undergo transperitoneal FNA among 191 liver transplant candidates with locally unresectable perihilar CCA. Among the 16 patients who underwent transperitoneal FNA (13 percutaneous, 3 EUS), 6 were positive for malignancy. During operative staging, peritoneal metastasis were detected in 5/6 (83%) patients who underwent transperitoneal FNA and had positive pathology compared to only 14/175 (8%) in those who did not undergo transperitoneal FNA ($p = 0.0097$). The two groups were similar in terms of CA 19-9 levels, frequency of mass detection, tumor size, and histology, arguing that the transperitoneal tumor sampling itself might be responsible for the higher incidence of peritoneal metastasis from tumor seeding. Therefore, our center adopted a protocol excluding patients with CCA from liver transplant who have had undergone transperitoneal sampling.

This approach poses significant clinical challenges as obtaining tissue diagnosis with traditional ERCP brush cytology and transpapillary biopsy can be extremely difficult and exhaustive. It also poses the challenge of proceeding into a high-risk surgery without a confirmed tissue diagnosis, since 10–20% of patients resected for presumed diagnosis of CCA may be found to have benign disease or another malignancy [31–34]. This diagnostic dilemma has led some to adopt less stringent criteria and reliance on other surrogates such as CA 19-9 levels and/or imaging to provide a presumptive diagnosis in an appropriate clinical presentation. However, this approach might lead to a potential misdiagnosis and unnecessary surgery.

It is important to point out that most studies evaluating needle tract seeding were performed on percutaneous biopsies and that these studies might not reflect the actual risk of tumor seeding after EUS-FNA. Data suggest that percutaneous FNA may carry a higher risk of tumor seeding compared to EUS-FNA. Micames et al. [35] conducted a retrospective study in patients with pancreatic cancer and found a significantly lower incidence of peritoneal metastasis with EUS-FNA 2.2% compared to percutaneous FNA 16.3%, $P = 0.025$. One plausible explanation for these findings is that EUS-FNA has a shorter tract to traverse (and hence lower risk of causing tumor seeding). Another important point is whether EUS-FNA of a primary CCA tumor would worsen survival. In a retrospective single center study [36] of 119 patients with CCA who underwent curative intent surgical resection, preoperative EUS-FNA did not impact overall survival or progression-free survival in the FNA group compared with those without FNA.

Finally, our stringent protocol to avoid EUS-FNA in transplant candidates or surgically resectable tumors pertains to the primary CCA tumor only. In contrast, lymph node EUS-FNA has not been shown to induce tumor seeding, and the findings substantially impact clinical decisions and the disease course. Identifying positive lymph nodes spares patients from undergoing unnecessary neoadjuvant chemotherapy and staging laparotomy [22, 37].

Hindrances of EUS

There are several factors that impact the diagnostic yield of EUS in CCA. First, primary sclerosing cholangitis (PSC) is a major risk factor for CCA. PSC is often associated with multiple biliary strictures, dense fibrosis, and diffuse benign (and sometimes bulky) lymphadenopathy. These features impair the accuracy of the EUS imaging in detecting CCA [6, 38, 39]. Another hindering factor of EUS imaging is the presence of biliary stents that are present in approximately 90% of patients at the time of EUS [6, 40, 41]. Their presence decreases EUS performance by creating acoustic shadowing deep to the stent or from stent-induced sludge. The resulting artifact impairs EUS examination of the bile ducts and surrounding tissues and can prohibit FNA of deep structures [40]. These limitations may be overcome by imaging from various locations (e.g., duodenum and stomach), minimizing air insufflation (which further hinders visualization), and occasionally stent removal prior to EUS [28].

Adverse Events Associated with Hepatic FNA/B

EUS and EUS-FNA/B are generally safe. However, the adverse event (AE) rate following hepatic EUS-FNA is higher than for other sites. In a meta-analysis, Wang et al. [42] reported a 2.3% morbidity after hepatic EUS-FNA. Similarly, in a retrospective international study [43], AEs were encountered in 3.5% of patients; these included abdominal pain, fever, bleeding, and death. The only AE reported in a CCA study was hemobilia following EUS-FNA in 1 of 74 patients [6]. This patient was managed conservatively with observation alone.

Conclusion

The growing role of EUS and EUS-FNA for CCA diagnosis and staging has largely been driven by the limited and not-infrequently suboptimal noninvasive imaging and endoscopic sampling techniques. While primary tumor EUS-FNA is strongly discouraged due to the potential of tumor seeding and potential consequent exclusion from resection and transplant treatment options, EUS-FNA has an important role for detecting malignant lymphadenopathy, which can have considerable impact on staging, prognosis, and management. Critical is the understanding that imaging criteria among suspected CCA patients do not distinguish benign from malignant nodes, thus making tissue sampling (e.g., FNA) necessary for all such patients. We consider EUS necessary regardless of cross-sectional imaging findings (unless unresectable disease is identified) due to the enhanced staging that is primarily associated with nodal assessment. Although PSC, the presence of biliary stents, and other factors can hinder EUS performance, their impact can be greatly minimized by adopting careful examination techniques. Further study is needed to more clearly determine the impact of EUS and EUS-FNA on tumor detection, staging, needle tract seeding, treatment, and long-term outcomes.

References

1. Saha SK, Zhu AX, Fuchs CS, et al. Forty-year trends in cholangiocarcinoma incidence in the U.S.: intrahepatic disease on the rise. Oncologist. 2016;21:594–9.
2. Mukkamalla SKR, Naseri HM, Kim BM, et al. Trends in incidence and factors affecting survival of patients with cholangiocarcinoma in the United States. J Natl Compr Cancer Netw. 2018;16:370–6.
3. Doherty B, Nambudiri VE, Palmer WC. Update on the diagnosis and treatment of cholangiocarcinoma. Curr Gastroenterol Rep. 2017;19:2.
4. Razumilava N, Gores GJ. Cholangiocarcinoma. Lancet. 2014;383:2168–79.
5. Zaheer A, Anwar MM, Donohoe C, et al. The diagnostic accuracy of endoscopic ultrasound in suspected biliary obstruction and its impact on endoscopic retrograde cholangiopancreatography burden in real clinical practice: a consecutive analysis. Eur J Gastroenterol Hepatol. 2013;25:850–7.
6. Mohamadnejad M, DeWitt JM, Sherman S, et al. Role of EUS for preoperative evaluation of cholangiocarcinoma: a large single-center experience. Gastrointest Endosc. 2011;73:71–8.
7. Jailwala J, Fogel EL, Sherman S, et al. Triple-tissue sampling at ERCP in malignant biliary obstruction. Gastrointest Endosc. 2000;51:383–90.
8. Rosch T, Hofrichter K, Frimberger E, et al. ERCP or EUS for tissue diagnosis of biliary strictures? A prospective comparative study. Gastrointest Endosc. 2004;60:390–6.
9. Stewart CJ, Mills PR, Carter R, et al. Brush cytology in the assessment of pancreatico-biliary strictures: a review of 406 cases. J Clin Pathol. 2001;54:449–55.
10. Wakatsuki T, Irisawa A, Bhutani MS, et al. Comparative study of diagnostic value of cytologic sampling by endoscopic ultrasonography-guided fine-needle aspiration and that by endoscopic retrograde pancreatography for the management of pancreatic mass without biliary stricture. J Gastroenterol Hepatol. 2005;20:1707–11.
11. Weilert F, Bhat YM, Binmoeller KF, et al. EUS-FNA is superior to ERCP-based tissue sampling in suspected malignant biliary obstruction: results of a prospective, single-blind, comparative study. Gastrointest Endosc. 2014;80:97–104.
12. De Moura DTH, Moura EGH, Bernardo WM, et al. Endoscopic retrograde cholangiopancreatography versus endoscopic ultrasound for tissue diagnosis of malignant biliary stricture: Systematic review and meta-analysis. Endosc Ultrasound. 2018;7:10–9.
13. Kameta E, Sugimori K, Kaneko T, et al. Diagnosis of pancreatic lesions collected by endoscopic ultrasound-guided fine-needle aspiration using next-generation sequencing. Oncol Lett. 2016;12:3875–81.
14. Gleeson FC, Kipp BR, Voss JS, et al. Endoscopic ultrasound fine-needle aspiration cytology mutation profiling using targeted next-generation sequencing: personalized care for rectal cancer. Am J Clin Pathol. 2015;143:879–88.

15. Gleeson FC, Kipp BR, Kerr SE, et al. Kinase genotype analysis of gastric gastrointestinal stromal tumor cytology samples using targeted next-generation sequencing. Clin Gastroenterol Hepatol. 2015;13:202–6.
16. Gleeson FC, Kerr SE, Kipp BR, et al. Targeted next generation sequencing of endoscopic ultrasound acquired cytology from ampullary and pancreatic adenocarcinoma has the potential to aid patient stratification for optimal therapy selection. Oncotarget. 2016;7:54526–36.
17. Hirata K, Kuwatani M, Suda G, et al. A novel approach for the genetic analysis of biliary tract cancer specimens obtained through endoscopic ultrasound-guided fine needle aspiration using targeted amplicon sequencing. Clin Transl Gastroenterol. 2019;10:e00022.
18. Jarnagin WR, Fong Y, RP DM, et al. Staging, resectability, and outcome in 225 patients with hilar cholangiocarcinoma. Ann Surg. 2001;234:507–17. discussion 517-9.
19. Bismuth H, Nakache R, Diamond T. Management strategies in resection for hilar cholangiocarcinoma. Ann Surg. 1992;215:31–8.
20. Nathan H, Aloia TA, Vauthey JN, et al. A proposed staging system for intrahepatic cholangiocarcinoma. Ann Surg Oncol. 2009;16:14–22.
21. Yamamoto M, Takasaki K, Yoshikawa T. Lymph node metastasis in intrahepatic cholangiocarcinoma. Jpn J Clin Oncol. 1999;29:147–50.
22. Morimoto Y, Tanaka Y, Ito T, et al. Long-term survival and prognostic factors in the surgical treatment for intrahepatic cholangiocarcinoma. J Hepato-Biliary-Pancreat Surg. 2003;10:432–40.
23. Bagante F, Tran T, Spolverato G, et al. Perihilar cholangiocarcinoma: number of nodes examined and optimal lymph node prognostic scheme. J Am Coll Surg. 2016;222:750–759 e2.
24. Gleeson FC, Rajan E, Levy MJ, et al. EUS-guided FNA of regional lymph nodes in patients with unresectable hilar cholangiocarcinoma. Gastrointest Endosc. 2008;67:438–43.
25. Iavarone M, Piscaglia F, Vavassori S, et al. Contrast enhanced CT-scan to diagnose intrahepatic cholangiocarcinoma in patients with cirrhosis. J Hepatol. 2013;58:1188–93.
26. Kim SH, Lee CH, Kim BH, et al. Typical and atypical imaging findings of intrahepatic cholangiocarcinoma using gadolinium ethoxybenzyl diethylenetriamine pentaacetic acid-enhanced magnetic resonance imaging. J Comput Assist Tomogr. 2012;36:704–9.
27. Tyagi R, Dey P. Needle tract seeding: an avoidable complication. Diagn Cytopathol. 2014;42:636–40.
28. Lundstedt C, Stridbeck H, Andersson R, et al. Tumor seeding occurring after fine-needle biopsy of abdominal malignancies. Acta Radiol. 1991;32:518–20.
29. Levy MJ, Heimbach JK, Gores GJ. Endoscopic ultrasound staging of cholangiocarcinoma. Curr Opin Gastroenterol. 2012;28:244–52.
30. Levy MJ, Gleeson FC, Campion MB, et al. Prospective cytological assessment of gastrointestinal luminal fluid acquired during EUS: a potential source of false-positive FNA and needle tract seeding. Am J Gastroenterol. 2010;105:1311–8.
31. Heimbach JK, Sanchez W, Rosen CB, et al. Trans-peritoneal fine needle aspiration biopsy of hilar cholangiocarcinoma is associated with disease dissemination. HPB (Oxford). 2011;13:356–60.
32. Wetter LA, Ring EJ, Pellegrini CA, et al. Differential diagnosis of sclerosing cholangiocarcinomas of the common hepatic duct (Klatskin tumors). Am J Surg. 1991;161:57–62. discussion 62-3.
33. Verbeek PC, van Leeuwen DJ, de Wit LT, et al. Benign fibrosing disease at the hepatic confluence mimicking Klatskin tumors. Surgery. 1992;112:866–71.
34. Vauthey JN, Blumgart LH. Recent advances in the management of cholangiocarcinomas. Semin Liver Dis. 1994;14:109–14.
35. Gerhards MF, Vos P, van Gulik TM, et al. Incidence of benign lesions in patients resected for suspicious hilar obstruction. Br J Surg. 2001;88:48–51.
36. Micames C, Jowell PS, White R, et al. Lower frequency of peritoneal carcinomatosis in patients with pancreatic cancer diagnosed by EUS-guided FNA vs. percutaneous FNA. Gastrointest Endosc. 2003;58:690–5.

37. El Chafic AH, Dewitt J, Leblanc JK, et al. Impact of preoperative endoscopic ultrasound-guided fine needle aspiration on postoperative recurrence and survival in cholangiocarcinoma patients. Endoscopy. 2013;45:883–9.
38. Malikowski T, Levy MJ, Gleeson FC, et al. EUS-FNA is effective for lymph node staging in patients with cholangiocarcinoma. Hepatology. 2020;72(3):940–48.
39. DeWitt J, Misra VL, Leblanc JK, et al. EUS-guided FNA of proximal biliary strictures after negative ERCP brush cytology results. Gastrointest Endosc. 2006;64:325–33.
40. Strongin A, Singh H, Eloubeidi MA, et al. Role of endoscopic ultrasonography in the evaluation of extrahepatic cholangiocarcinoma. Endosc Ultrasound. 2013;2:71–6.
41. Lee JH, Salem R, Aslanian H, et al. Endoscopic ultrasound and fine-needle aspiration of unexplained bile duct strictures. Am J Gastroenterol. 2004;99:1069–73.
42. Eloubeidi MA, Chen VK, Jhala NC, et al. Endoscopic ultrasound-guided fine needle aspiration biopsy of suspected cholangiocarcinoma. Clin Gastroenterol Hepatol. 2004;2:209–13.
43. Wang KX, Ben QW, Jin ZD, et al. Assessment of morbidity and mortality associated with EUS-guided FNA: a systematic review. Gastrointest Endosc. 2011;73:283–90.

Chapter 14
Surgical Approach to the Treatment of Cholangiocarcinoma

Sean J. Judge, Thomas W. Loehfelm, and Sepideh Gholami

Abbreviations

AFP	Alpha fetoprotein
AJCC	American Joint Committee on Cancer
BSA	Body surface area
CCA	Cholangiocarcinoma
CEA	Carcinoembryonic antigen
CT	Computed tomography
dCCA	distal cholangiocarcinoma
eCCA	extrahepatic cholangiocarcinoma
ERC	Endoscopic retrograde cholangiography
FGFR	Fibroblast growth factor receptor
FLR	Future liver remnant
GEMOX	Gemcitabine with oxaliplatin
iCCA	intrahepatic cholangiocarcinoma
IDH	Isocitrate dehydrogenase
KGR	Kinetic growth rate
NCCN	National Comprehensive Cancer Network
OLT	Orthotopic liver transplantation
pCCA	perihilar cholangiocarcinoma
PET	Positron emission tomography
PVE	Portal vein embolization

S. J. Judge
Department of Surgery, University of California, Davis, Sacramento, CA, USA
e-mail: sjjudge@ucdavis.edu

T. W. Loehfelm
Department of Radiology, University of California, Davis, Sacramento, CA, USA
e-mail: twloehfelm@ucdavis.edu

S. Gholami (✉)
Division of Surgical Oncology, Department of Surgery, University of California, Davis, Sacramento, CA, USA
e-mail: sgholami@ucdavis.edu

J. H. Tabibian (ed.), *Diagnosis and Management of Cholangiocarcinoma*,
https://doi.org/10.1007/978-3-030-70936-5_14

RLV	Remnant liver volume
SEER	Surveillance, Epidemiology, and End Results
TFLV	Total functional liver volume
TLV	Total liver volume
TNM	Tumor Node Metastasis

Introduction

Cholangiocarcinomas (CCAs) are a rare and heterogeneous group of malignancies arising from the biliary ductal epithelium. It can be classified based on histopathology, gross pathology, and anatomic location, though from a surgical perspective, the anatomic classification has the greatest impact on management considerations. Histopathologically, the vast majority of CCAs are adenocarcinomas (>90%), followed by squamous cell carcinomas, and rarely adenosquamous carcinomas. For intrahepatic CCA (iCCA), the disease can also be classified based on the gross histologic appearance of lesions. Specifically, intrahepatic CCA occurs as mass forming, periductal infiltrating, or intraductal [1]. This gross appearance classification does not pertain to extrahepatic cholangiocarcinoma (eCCA), which tends to have less uniform morphology. Morphologic variation has implications for local structure invasion and prognosis but typically does not alter medical or surgical treatment considerations. Anatomically, CCA is most commonly divided into iCCA and eCCA, with extrahepatic CCA being subdivided into hilar CCA and distal CCA, a delineation which helps determine options for therapy [2]. Using a modified anatomic classification, CCA may be more appropriately divided into three subsets: iCCA, perihilar (pCCA), and distal CCA (dCCA) [3].

In this chapter, we will discuss the evaluation and surgical management of patients presenting with CCA, with an emphasis on anatomic considerations, surgical technique, and postoperative outcomes, including morbidity, mortality, and long-term survival.

Anatomic Distribution

The anatomic landmarks that discern the modified anatomic classification of CCA are as follows: iCCA occurs proximal to the confluence of the left and right hepatic ducts; pCCA occurs between the common hepatic duct and insertion of the cystic duct into the common hepatic duct; dCCA occurs down to the ampulla of Vater (Fig. 14.1) [4]. Klatskin tumors, a subtype of pCCA, occur at the junction of the left and right hepatic ducts within the porta hepatis, as originally described by G. Klatskin [5]. The relative anatomic distribution of CCAs does appear to have geo-regional differences, with potential impact on mortality [6]. In the United

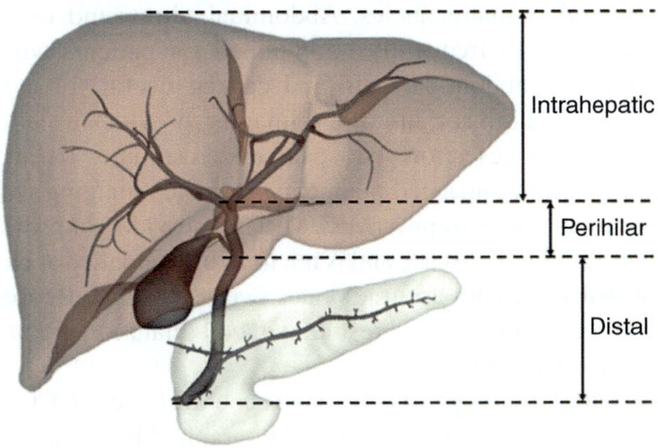

Fig. 14.1 Anatomic classification of cholangiocarcinoma. Intrahepatic CCA occurs proximal to the joining of the left and right hepatic ducts, perihilar CCA occurs between the formation of the main hepatic duct and the insertion of the cystic duct, and distal CCA occurs distal to the insertion of the cystic duct up to the ampulla of Vater

States, the anatomic distribution of CCA has been well-described, with approximately 67% of cases as perihilar, 27% distal, and 6% intrahepatic as described in one of the early, seminal studies of a single institution experience of 294 patients [3]. On follow-up analysis of 564 patients, a relative increase in dCCA was found (42%), while 50% of cases were perihilar and 8% were intrahepatic [7]. A more recent analysis of the Surveillance, Epidemiology, and End Results (SEER) data shows that the incidence of iCCA has been increasing in the United States, whereas the incidence of extrahepatic CCA appears relatively stable [8], though this could be related to changes in classification and coding. On a global scale, a recent report examining World Health Organization and Pan American Health Organization databases also identified a rise in iCCA incidence with associated increase in mortality [9].

Preoperative Evaluation of Cholangiocarcinoma

The workup and evaluation of CCA begins with the clinical presentation as patients presenting with signs or symptoms of biliary obstruction may need intervention prior to a more definitive diagnosis. It is estimated that approximately 90% of patients with pCCA will have signs or symptoms of biliary obstruction and up to 10% will have cholangitis [10]. For those patients presenting with cholangitis, immediate attention needs to be made toward decompression of the biliary system and management of the acute infection. Decompression can be achieved via endoscopic retrograde cholangiography (ERC) or transhepatic biliary drainage, with pros and cons to each approach in the setting of potential underlying CCA.

For patients with *incidental* hepatobiliary lesions on imaging or abnormalities in laboratory values, the initial workup includes measurement of serum liver tests and tumor markers, including CA19-9, AFP, and CEA. There are limitations to these tumor markers, however. Notably, CA19-9 is elevated with biliary (or pancreatic ductal) obstruction of any etiology, and CEA is less specific and can be increased with other malignancies. Abdominal ultrasound or computed tomography (CT) imaging will frequently be obtained for patients with abnormal serum liver test values or abdominal pain and can be useful for evaluation of CCA. Contrast-enhanced high-resolution CT imaging provides excellent diagnostic and anatomic detail for resection but can underestimate intrahepatic tumor extent [11]. Gadolinium-enhanced magnetic resonance imaging with magnetic resonance cholangiopancreatography (MRI/MRCP) provides improved resolution of the intrahepatic extent of disease and is the imaging modality of choice for evaluation of biliary obstruction, with accuracy rates over 80% [11]. Representative illustrations of the anatomic subtypes and resultant ductal dilatation as may be seen on imaging studies are shown in Fig. 14.2.

Other imaging tests that have been evaluated in CCA include duplex ultrasonography and positron emission tomograph (PET) imaging. Although duplex ultrasonography has a role in providing additional information regarding vascular involvement, the role for PET imaging is less clear. For pCCA, PET imaging has not been shown to add additional diagnostic or prognostic benefit over other high-quality cross-sectional imaging modalities [10], though there is some debate regarding its utility in iCCA, especially when combined with CT imaging [12]. Additional information regarding imaging of cholangiocarcinoma is presented elsewhere in this book (*Chap. 7, Viragh et al*).

In addition to the items discussed above, per 2019 NCCN guidelines [2], the complete workup for iCCA and eCCA is similar with a notable difference of upper and lower endoscopy for patients with iCCA to evaluate for primary malignancies that may be the source of hepatic metastatic disease masquerading as CCA. Additional imaging to complete the workup and staging should include CT imaging of the thorax to rule out metastatic disease.

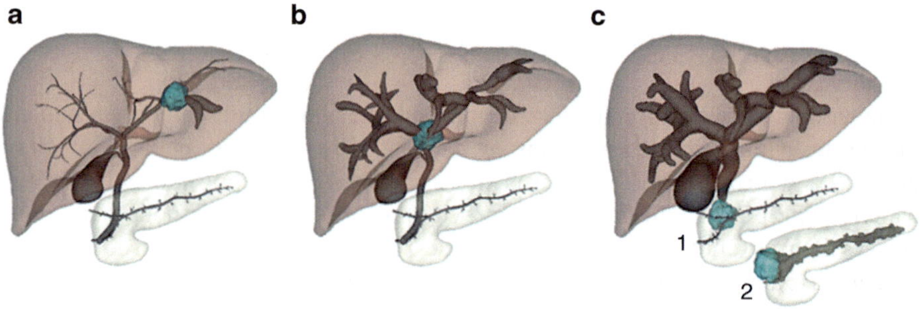

Fig. 14.2 3D modelling illustrations of cholangiocarcinoma anatomic subtypes (green mass) and radiographic sequelae based on tumor location. (**a**) Intrahepatic cholangiocarcinoma in the left lobe with resultant dilatation of the proximal left lobe ducts. (**b**) Klatskin tumor or perihilar cholangiocarcinoma at the bifurcation of the left and right hepatic ducts with bilateral proximal ductal dilatation. (**c**) Distal cholangiocarcinoma leading to intrahepatic and extrahepatic ductal dilatation occurring (c1) without or (c2) with pancreatic ductal dilatation, depending on tumor location

Anatomic Classification and Initial Staging

Following initial evaluation, anatomic disease classification can be assigned (iCCA, pCCA, or dCCA), and patients can then be clinically staged accordingly, keeping in mind that tissue diagnosis is not required for proceeding with definitive surgical treatment. For all CCA subtypes, staging can be performed according to the AJCC eighth edition (Table 14.1). Additionally, other staging adjuncts and modalities exist and can be helpful for staging iCCA (Liver Cancer Study Group of Japan [1], National Cancer Center of Japan Staging System [13]), pCCA (Bismuth-Corlette Classification [14], Jarnagin-Blumgart Classification [15, 16]), and dCCA (US Extrahepatic Biliary Malignancy Consortium [17]). Most typically in the United States, clinical staging follows the AJCC TNM system, with notable differences in staging between the CCA subtypes based on T stage (Table 14.1). For iCCA, size and depth of invasion dictate T stage. This slightly differs from pCCA in which depth of invasion and invasion of surrounding structures are critical determinations of T stage. The Jarnagin-Blumgart Classification of T stage in pCCA expands on this by utilizing a more complete assessment of the extent of tumor invasion and anatomic sequelae (i.e., vascular occlusion and liver atrophy), adding predictive and prognostic value to pCCA staging [16]. Lastly, determining clinical T stage for dCCA is currently based on measured depth of invasion (if not invading major

Table 14.1 TNM staging for site-specific cholangiocarcinoma based on AJCC eighth edition

Tumor	Intrahepatic	Perihilar	Distal
Tis	Intraductal	In situ or high-grade dysplasia	In situ or high-grade dysplasia
T1	T1a: ≤5 cm, no vascular invasion T1b: >5 cm, no vascular invasion	Confined to bile duct	<5 mm bile duct wall invasion
T2	Single tumor with vascular invasion, or ≥2 tumors ± vascular invasion	T2a: invades periductal adipose tissue T2b: invades liver	5–12 mm bile duct wall invasion
T3	Perforates visceral peritoneum	Invades portal vein or hepatic artery (unilateral involvement)	>12 mm bile duct wall invasion
T4	Invades extrahepatic structures	Complete invasion of portal vein or CHA	Invades major vascular structures
Node	*Intrahepatic*	*Perihilar*	*Distal*
N0	Absent	Absent	Absent
N1	Present	1–3 LN+	1–3 LN+
N2	N/A	≥4 LN+	≥4 LN+
Metastasis	*Intrahepatic*	*Perihilar*	*Distal*
M0	Absent	Absent	Absent
M1	Present	Present	Present

CHA common hepatic artery, *LN* lymph node

vascular structures). Recent results from a multi-institution consortium have also expanded the pathologic T-stage classification for dCCA by incorporating tumor size and lymphovascular invasion status as the key criteria for T-stage determination and improved prognostication [17]. While pathologic staging of CCA can only be obtained after resection, assessment of clinical stage based on high-quality imaging allows for the most thorough consideration of resectability and adequate preoperative preparation where applicable. Excluding metastatic disease (most commonly liver, peritoneum, and lung) and extensive nodal involvement, there is no consensus on what disease is "unresectable," and this will be addressed in later Section (*Defining Resectability*).

Future Liver Remnant and Portal Vein Embolization

Surgical management of iCCA and pCCA is unique from dCCA, as an R0 hepatic resection is the cornerstone of surgical therapy. Because iCCA and pCCA involve liver resection, accurate determination of the future liver remnant (FLR) is necessary to minimize the risk of postoperative liver failure. The percent FLR can be calculated using high-quality cross-sectional imaging, typically as remnant liver volume (RLV)/total functional liver volume (TFLV) × 100). Total liver volume (TLV) can be estimated from CT imaging but can also be calculated based on body surface area (BSA) as $-794.41 + 1267.28 \times \text{BSA}$ [18]. In a healthy liver, a FLR $\geq 20\%$ is considered adequate, though this increases to $\geq 40\%$ in patients with intrinsic liver dysfunction [19]. For those patients in whom the projected FLR is inadequate, preoperative portal vein embolization (PVE) of the tumor-bearing liver segment(s) can be selectively performed to induce growth of the contralateral hemiliver and increase the FLR [20].

The principle of PVE in this context involves selective portal venous occlusion to take advantage of the liver's remarkable ability to regenerate as a mechanism of compensation. This phenomenon was first identified in a rabbit model 100 years ago [21]. Following occlusion of the intended segment, an immediate change in portal venous flow occurs, increasing the metabolic demand of the liver and inducing a cascade of downstream signals, ultimately resulting in hepatocyte replication and liver hyperplasia [22]. As these changes begin very early following PVE, studies have examined the timing in which liver changes can be clinically detected [23]. In this study the authors identified a kinetic growth rate (KGR) of approximately 2.4% per week, noting that these patients did not have significant underlying liver dysfunction. The KGR is variable and is typically lower in patients with intrinsic liver dysfunction (e.g., cirrhosis or active inflammation); however, a KGR above 1.5% per week is considered adequate for resection. In addition to the efficacy of PVE, large studies have also confirmed the safety of the procedure and associated postoperative outcomes. A meta-analysis evaluating the impact of preoperative PVE in

1088 patients [24] demonstrated the relative safety of PVE with a morbidity rate of 2.2% and no mortality reported. Moreover, of the patients that underwent PVE, 85% underwent the planned operation after 4 weeks, and of the 930 patients who underwent resection following PVE, only 23 (2.5%) developed transient liver failure and 7 patients (0.8%) died.

Periampullary Tumors: Distal Cholangiocarcinoma or Pancreatic Ductal Adenocarcinoma?

One challenge in the evaluation of patients presenting with a periampullary mass is the differentiation of dCCA and pancreatic ductal adenocarcinoma (PDAC). Although differences in preoperative laboratory values and imaging characteristics have been described (i.e., CA19-9, pancreatic duct diameter), definitive determination of dCCA vs. PDAC is not made until final pathologic analysis of the resected specimen. Even ERCP-guided biopsies cannot confidently delineate the two pathologies, with reported accuracy ranging from 47% to 95% [25]. For clearly resectable disease, this may not pose a dilemma. In the locally advanced or metastatic setting, however, neoadjuvant and definitive chemotherapeutic regimens differ between the two diseases, and without a definitive tissue diagnosis, inadequate treatment may be given.

Resection for Cholangiocarcinoma

Defining Resectability

The definition of resectability is dependent on the subtype of CCA; however, the presence of metastases and a patient's inability to tolerate a major operation preclude resection for all subtypes. For iCCA, the presence of lymph node metastases outside the regional nodal basin (N2 disease) and invasion of the main hepatic artery or bilateral hepatic arteries are generally considered unresectable. For pCCA, the presence of N2 disease also precludes resection, in addition to specific characteristics of the local tumor invasion, including extension of the tumor into bilateral segmental bile ducts, unilateral hepatic atrophy with contralateral bile duct involvement or vascular involvement, or unilateral bile duct involvement with contralateral vascular involvement [10]. Unresectability for dCCA follows general recommendations for all periampullary tumors, in which unresectable disease is generally considered to be encasement of the hepatic artery or superior mesenteric artery and/or extensive involvement of the portal vein.

Diagnostic Laparoscopy in CCA

Many surgeons begin with a diagnostic laparoscopy, as it has been reported that nearly 30% (6/22) of iCCA patients undergoing curative intent surgery will have occult metastatic disease at the time of surgery [26], and for pCCA, nearly 50% of tumors are unresectable at the time of surgery (of which 58% was due to metastatic disease and 43% due to unresectable local invasion) [27]. This has led most surgeons to suggest the need for staging laparoscopy for all CCA patients with radiologically resectable disease. Although some groups have challenged this with more recent results suggesting decreasing rates of unresectability likely secondary to improvements in imaging technology [28], currently, diagnostic laparoscopy is practiced at many high-volume centers and recommended by the authors.

Resection of iCCA

After determination of resectability, surgical treatment of iCCA involves achieving an R0 liver resection and portal lymphadenectomy. If found to be resectable, most typically, the operation begins with the portal lymphadenectomy followed by major hepatic resection. Major vascular involvement, determined either preoperatively or during surgery, should not preclude resection. Although the negative prognostic impact of major vascular invasion is known, a recent multi-institutional study demonstrated that surgery should proceed if an R0 resection can be obtained [29]. In this retrospective study evaluating over 1000 patients who underwent resection for iCCA, patients were divided into those that did (n = 128) and did not (n = 959) undergo vascular resection. Although the two groups had significantly different clinical and demographic characteristics, the authors showed that the postoperative mortality and complication rate was not significantly different between the two groups. It should be noted, however, that while not statistically significant, the complication rate was nearly 14 percent higher in the vascular resection group (55.5% vs. 41.9%) [29]. A recent review evaluating the literature on minimally invasive resection for CCA highlights the challenges of laparoscopic or robotic approaches and notes that iCCA and dCCA may be most amenable to a minimally invasive approach, though prospective data investigating this question are limited [30].

Resection of pCCA

Similar to the principles of resection for iCCA, surgery for pCCA aims for an R0 resection with adequate biliary drainage, vascular supply, and intrinsic hepatic function. As noted above, a critical difference in pCCA management is the benefit of orthotopic liver transplantation (OLT) in highly selected patients. As most patients are not eligible for LT, critical components of resection are as follows: (1) thorough exploration for metastatic disease, (2) lymphadenectomy, (3) distal biliary transection, (4) arterial and portal venous division, (5) hepatic venous division, (6) partial hepatectomy, and (7) biliary reconstruction. Another caveat to resection for pCCA is the need for routine resection of the caudate lobe; a caudate lobectomy is frequently performed during pCCA resection due to the high rate of pathologic involvement and increased R0 resection rates when caudate lobectomies are performed [10].

The anatomic proximity to critical vascular structures in pCCA increases the risk of portal venous and hepatic arterial invasion. Again, similar to iCCA principles, while major vascular invasion has negative prognostic implications, the need for portal venous resection to achieve complete tumor removal for an R0 resection should not be a contraindication to surgery. Evidence for hepatic arterial resection and reconstruction is less clear, and any oncologic benefits may be limited by increased postoperative complications. A 2018 retrospective analysis of patients with pCCA aimed to answer the question of which vascular involvement has poor prognostic impact for all patients, regardless of future treatments. The authors showed that main portal vein and unilateral or main hepatic artery involvement adversely affected overall survival, whereas unilateral portal vein involvement did not have significant impact on overall survival [31].

Resection for dCCA

The surgical management for dCCA does not involve hepatic resection but rather most commonly involves pancreaticoduodenectomy (e.g., Whipple procedure). Rarely, if disease is limited to the proximal bile duct, an R0 resection can be achieved with biliary resection and hepaticojejunostomy reconstruction (i.e., without pancreatic head resection). During pancreaticoduodenectomy for dCCA, there is debate over the benefit of portal venous resection to increase R0 resection rates and improve survival [32, 33]. For pancreatic adenocarcinoma (PDAC) outcomes, the role of portal venous resection is similarly controversial, despite being more extensively investigated. For example, a recent meta-analysis evalsuated 30 articles pertaining to PDAC and concluded that the addition of venous resection (portal and/or superior mesenteric vein) was associated with increased complications and mortality and decreased R0 resection rates [34]. These conclusions are challenged by results from the MD Anderson group showing that in a high-volume specialty center, venous resection and reconstruction are not independently associated with worse outcomes and are beneficial with appropriate PDAC patient selection [35].

Although this subject has not been investigated in dCCA to the extent of PDAC, retrospective data suggest that combined vascular resection and pancreaticoduodenectomy for dCCA did not increase R0 resection rates or improve survival and were associated with increased blood transfusions and length of surgery [33]. As the evidence for vascular resection and reconstruction continue to develop for all CCA subtypes, the boundaries of anatomic resectability will continue to evolve.

Transplantation for CCA

The goal of surgical management of CCA, regardless of anatomic classification, is complete removal of the tumor resulting in an R0 resection, with adequate biliary drainage, vascular supply, and intrinsic hepatic function. Options for locally advanced, unresectable tumors are limited, and OLT has been extensively evaluated as a treatment for CCA in this population and is further discussed in this text (*Agopian et al., Chap. 15*). Reports on the early experience of transplantation for unresectable iCCA and pCCA were disappointing and did not support the use of transplantation [36]. High postoperative mortality and recurrence rates significantly limited the use of OLT for CCA.

For transplantation to be effective in CCA, there was a clear need for improved patient selection and neoadjuvant therapies to mitigate systemic microscopic disease and thus recurrence rates. This was addressed by the Mayo Clinic Rochester group beginning in 1993 with a novel protocol for pCCA. Using strict inclusion and exclusion criteria, appropriately selected patients underwent extensive neoadjuvant therapy and then were maintained on capecitabine while awaiting transplantation [37]. The results of this protocol were very encouraging with 5-year survival rates of 56% in de novo CCA patients and 76% in patients with primary sclerosing cholangitis (PSC). These results were corroborated in a large, retrospective multicenter cohort study examining outcomes for pCCA treated with either resection or transplantation (many in accordance with the aforementioned Mayo Clinic protocol). In the intention-to-treat analysis, 5-year overall survival for patients undergoing resection and transplantation was 17% and 53%, respectively, and this difference was maintained when the data were stratified for tumors size less than 3 cm and negative lymph node status [38]. Although transplantation appears to provide a significant benefit to the few selected patients with locally advanced pCCA, the majority of CCA patients do not meet the strict eligibility criteria due to disease burden or tumor location. Resection remains the only chance for cure for those patients with localized disease.

Postoperative Morbidity and Mortality

The rate, severity, and types of postoperative complications following resection of CCA are dependent on disease location and extent of surgery, among other factors (e.g., baseline patient comorbidities). Table 14.2 highlights postoperative outcomes for CCA based on anatomic location. The current overall postoperative complication rate is around 40%, and postoperative mortality ranges from 0% to 4%. Types of complications are dependent on disease location, with iCCA and pCCA having increased rates of pleural effusions, bile leaks, and hepatic insufficiency, while dCCA is complicated by pancreatic fistulae and delayed gastric emptying. While the association between location of resected disease and type of complication may

Table 14.2 Postoperative morbidity and mortality rates for resection of cholangiocarcinoma from selected publications

Intrahepatic cholangiocarcinoma (iCCA)					
Author[a]	Study period	Total patients	Morbidity[n]	Mortality	Complications
Spolverato et al. [39]	1990–2013	583	44.4% overall 15.6% major 26.2% minor	90-day: 3.5%	Pleural effusion (20%) Fluid collection/biloma (19%) Intra-abdominal abscess (10%) Wound infection (8%) Hepatic insufficiency (7%)
Ali et al. [40]	1997–2011	121	43% overall 17% major	90-day: 1%	Not described
DeOliveira et al. [7]	1973–2004	44	35% overall	30-day: 4.5%	Abscess (9%) Respiratory (7%) Wound infection (5%) MOSF (5%) Sepsis (5%)
Ohtsuka et al. [41]	1984–2001	64	50%	30-day: 4% In-hospital: 8%	Pleural effusion (16%) Wound infection (16%) Liver failure (10%)
Perihilar cholangiocarcinoma (pCCA)					
Author	*Study period*	*Total patients*	*Morbidity*	*Mortality*	*Complications*
Allen et al. [42]	1987–2005	106	Not reported	30-day: 3.8%	
DeOliveira et al. [7]	1973–2004	281	35% overall	30-day: 5.4%	Wound infection (16%) Sepsis (10%) Abscess (8%) Bile leak (7%) Respiratory (5%) GI bleed (5%)
Hasegaqa et al. [43]	1990–2003	49	46.8% major	In-hospital: 2%	Bile leak (26%) Cholangitis (10%) Abscess (8%)
Nagino et al. [44]	1990–1999	105	37.1% minor 43.8% major	30-day: 3.8% 90-day: 9.5%	Pleural effusion (63%) Wound sepsis (37%) Liver failure (28%) Intra-abdominal abscess (12%)
Gerhards et al. [45]	1983–1998	112	65%	30-day: 14% In-hospital: 18%	Liver or intra-abdominal abscess (25%) Bile leak (22%) Bleeding (intra-abdominal or GI) (18%) Liver failure/necrosis (12%) Cholangitis (10%)

(continued)

Table 14.2 (continued)

Intrahepatic cholangiocarcinoma (iCCA)					
Author[a]	Study period	Total patients	Morbidity[n]	Mortality	Complications
Distal cholangiocarcinoma (dCCA)					
Author	*Study period*	*Total patients*	*Morbidity*	*Mortality*	*Complications*
Andrianello et al. [46]	2000–2013	46	76.1% overall	0%	Pancreatic fistula (48%) Abdominal collections (35%) Respiratory (24%) Hemorrhage (22%) Delayed gastric emptying (11%)
Allen et al. [42]	1987–2005	98	Not reported	30-day: 3.1%	
DeOliveira et al. [7]	1973–2004	239	35% overall	30-day: 3%	Pancreatic leak (13%) Wound infection (11%) Delayed gastric emptying (11%) Abscess (7%)

[a]DeOliveira et al. (2007) include 564 total patients, and results are divided by anatomic classification. Allen et al. (2008) include 204 total patients and results are divided by anatomic classification
[b]Major and minor morbidity determined by Clavien-Dindo classification (≥3 for major) or at discretion of author(s)

seem obvious to the experienced hepatopancreatobiliary surgeon, this may be less clear to other nonsurgical members of the patient care team. Specifications on the anatomic location and extent of resection are critical details to all healthcare professionals involved in the perioperative care of patients with CCA, as these details guide differential diagnoses, management, and intervention strategies.

Adjuvant Therapy and Outcomes Following Surgery

Outside of the Mayo Clinic protocol for transplantation for pCCA, the role of neoadjuvant therapy for CCA is unclear. Due to the high postoperative recurrence rates of CCA, efforts have focused on adjuvant therapies (Table 14.3). For locally advanced or metastatic CCA, the ABC-02 trial established cisplatin plus gemcitabine as the optimal regimen [47]. For resectable disease, current standard of care is surgery (with goal of R0 resection) followed by observation alone. A few larger trials have investigated the role of adjuvant chemotherapy with varying results. The BCAT trial, a phase II randomized trial, compared gemcitabine (n = 117) to observation (n = 108) in patients with eCCA [48]. Results from this trial found no difference in median overall survival between the treated and untreated groups (62.3 vs. 63.8 months) or relapse-free survival (36.0 vs. 39.9 months) and no differences on

Table 14.3 Results from clinical trials evaluating adjuvant therapy for resected cholangiocarcinoma

Study	Year	Cancer	Treatment	Total patients	CCA patients	Overall outcomes	CCA outcomes
SWOG S0809	2015	Extrahepatic CCA, GBCA	Gemcitabine and capecitabine, then capecitabine and radiation therapy	79	54[a] 13 distal 38 hilar	Median survival: 35 mo. 2-year OS: 65%	Median survival: ~35 months 2-year OS: 68%
BCAT	2018	Extrahepatic CCA	Gemcitabine vs. observation	225	225 123 distal 102 perihilar	Median survival: 62.3 vs. 63.8 months (HR 1.01, $P = 0.964$)	Median survival: Distal: 62.3 vs. 67.2 months (HR 1.07, $P = 0.790$) Perihilar: NR vs. 61.5 months (HR 0.97, $P = 0.915$)
PRODIGE 12-ACCORD	2019	CCA, GBCA	Gemcitabine and oxaliplatin vs. observation	196	156 55 distal 15 perihilar 86 intrahepatic	Median survival: 75.8 vs. 50.8 months (HR 1.08, $P = 0.74$)	No difference in subpopulation of cholangiocarcinoma
BILCAP	2019	CCA, GBCA	Capecitabine vs. observation	447	368 156 distal 128 perihilar 84 intrahepatic	Intention-to-treat analysis Median survival: 51.1 vs. 36.4 months (HR 0.81, $P = 0.097$ Per-protocol analysis Median survival: 52.7 vs. 36 months (HR 0.75, $P = 0.028$)	

Abbreviations: *CCA* cholangiocarcinoma, *GBC* gallbladder carcinoma, *NR* not reached
[a]Three CCA patients without central pathologic review

subset analysis based on lymph node status or anatomic classification. Similar results were obtained from the recently published PRODIGE 12-ACCORD trial evaluating the effects of adjuvant gemcitabine with oxaliplatin (GEMOX) compared to observation alone [49]. In this randomized, multicenter trial, 196 total patients were evaluated (156 patients with CCA), and those patients receiving GEMOX had a median survival of 75.8 months compared to 50.8 months in the observation group (HR 1.08, $p = 0.74$). No differences were identified in recurrence-free survival between the treatment groups or within disease subsets, although adverse events were significantly higher in the group receiving GEMOX (GEMOX with 62% grade 3, 11% grade 4 vs. observation with 18% grade 3, 3% grade 4).

In contrast to these negative trials, the recently published BILCAP trial showed a trend toward a survival benefit for patients receiving adjuvant capecitabine [50]. The BILCAP trial included 447 patients randomly assigned to either adjuvant capecitabine or observation, of which 368 patients had pathologically proven CCA (including intrahepatic, perihilar, and distal). Patients underwent curative intent surgery and after 16 weeks underwent randomization. The primary outcome was overall survival in the intention-to-treat group, and secondary outcomes were overall survival in the per-protocol group. The intention-to-treat group trended toward increased overall survival but did not reach statistical significance. In the per-protocol analysis, however, median survival was 53 months in the capecitabine arm compared to 36 months in the observation arm (HR 0.75, $P = 0.028$), suggesting a benefit of adjuvant therapy for all CCA subtypes. Although the results of this trial did not reach statistical significance in intention-to-treat analysis, they have become the new standard by most physicians. Currently, updated American Society of Clinical Oncology (ASCO) guidelines recommend 6 months of adjuvant capecitabine for resected biliary tract cancer [51].

The role of combined chemotherapy and radiation therapy has also been investigated as adjuvant therapy for CCA. Published in 2015, the SWOG S0809 trial was a phase II trial examining the role of adjuvant chemoradiotherapy for extrahepatic CCA. The investigators utilized a non-random cohort of patients who received capecitabine and gemcitabine followed by capecitabine and external-beam radiation [52]. This trial included patients with pCCA and dCCA as well as gallbladder carcinoma. Two-year overall survival was 67% for patients with an R0 resection and 60% for R1 resection, respectively. Compared to historic controls, these results were quite encouraging and suggested a role for adjuvant chemoradiation in patients where an R0 resection could not be obtained. These results have also been incorporated into the ASCO guidelines, wherein it is recommended that patients with an R1 resection receive adjuvant chemoradiation under the guidance of a multidisciplinary team [51].

Results from the described clinical trials investigating adjuvant therapy for CCA highlight some of the challenges in making progress in this field. CCA is a relatively rare and heterogenous disease. To attain adequate enrollment to detect clinically meaningful results, there is often a need to combine anatomic disease subtypes. While this increases the heterogeneity of the study population, it also allows for more generalizability of the results (as seen with the BILCAP trial). The positive trials to date provide great inspiration that, through international collaboration and thoughtful trial design, further advances can be made in adjuvant and neoadjuvant therapies for CCA. This approach is highlighted by the increasing understanding of the molecular heterogeneity of CCA and use of targeted therapies [53].

Postoperative Surveillance

The NCCN guidelines propose a similar surveillance algorithm for both iCCA and eCCA [2]. Specifically, following resection, both iCCA and eCCA patients may undergo high-quality cross-sectional imaging of the chest and abdomen every 6 months for the first 2 years, followed by yearly imaging for up to 5 years. In many high-volume centers, these patients may undergo extended surveillance as site and timing of disease recurrence are quite variable, and the majority of resected patients will ultimately experience recurrence [54, 55].

Future Directions in Surgery for Cholangiocarcinoma

Future directions and advancements in the treatment of CCA fall into three broad categories – patient selection, operative techniques, and adjuvant therapies. Selecting the patients who will most benefit from resection has been an area of extensive investigation. The principle of neoadjuvant therapy is based on the assumption that even in localized disease there is already micrometastases present; therefore upfront surgery is not optimal as it may delay more important systemic therapies. Another benefit of neoadjuvant therapy is the selection of patients with both preferable tumor biology and performance status. Efforts are then placed on stratifying patients with localized disease into who benefits most from upfront surgery vs. neoadjuvant systemic treatment. Extensive research is being conducted into biomarkers, such as the use of circulating tumor DNA, to help identify these patients and track response to therapies to help guide these clinical decisions.

Improvement in operative techniques and vascular reconstruction have greatly expanded the "resectability" of CCA, but significant limitations remain for advancing minimally invasive approaches to CCA. Currently, either a laparoscopic or robotic approach to CCA is limited to select cases but can include all anatomic variants (iCCA, pCCA, dCCA). A minimally invasive approach to pCCA can be technically difficult, though, due to challenges in caudate lobectomy and vascular reconstruction. As experience and advances in robotic technology increase, complete minimally invasive approaches to all forms of CCA may be more common, with the resultant improvement in length of stay and complications and without compromising oncologic outcomes [56, 57]. Given the expertise required and steep learning curve associated with minimally invasive hepatic resection, it is likely that these operations will be appropriately limited to high-volume, specialized centers.

Results of clinical trials investigating adjuvant therapy in CCA highlight the urgent need for improved therapies. This is being addressed through novel trials attempting to match susceptible tumors to specific therapies. The MOSCATO-1 trial aims to direct specific tumors to targeted agents via high-throughput tumor sequencing [58]. Through this technique, the authors have identified a subset of CCA patients who appear to benefit from novel therapies that may otherwise not be addressed in larger clinical trials [59]. Several targetable pathways and therapies for CCA have been investigated to date [53, 60], but the fibroblast growth factor receptor (FGFR) and isocitrate dehydrogenase (IDH) pathways have yielded encouraging early results. FGFR inhibitors are being used to target CCA subtypes with *FGFR* translocations and resultant fusion proteins, which is present at varying proportions depending on anatomic subtype (higher in iCCA) [61]. *IDH1/IDH2* are commonly mutated genes in CCA (also occurring more frequently in iCCA) but are also present in other GI cancers [62]. Ivosidenib, an IDH1 inhibitor, is currently being investigated in the multi-institutional ClarIDHy trial, and an updated analysis was recently presented [63]. Early results showed that nearly 22% of patients in the treatment arm were progression-free at 12 months, while all patients recurred within 12 months in the placebo arm. These encouraging results for FGFR and IDH inhibition highlight the potential for improved outcomes with targeted therapy in appropriately selected patients.

Conclusion

The success of surgical management for CCA heavily relies on advances in patient selection, operative technique, and novel therapies. Significant progress has already been achieved in CCA treatment through improvements in disease classification, expanding criteria for resection, selection of those who may benefit from transplantation, and molecular and genomic analysis of tumors. These advances highlight the burgeoning recognition of the vast heterogeneity underlying a single diagnosis of "cholangiocarcinoma." As this appreciation for the heterogeneity of CCA continues to grow, the role for surgery in the management of CCA is likely to change. This will include clearer identification of which patients will benefit from surgery early in their management and which patients require neoadjuvant chemotherapy or targeted therapies. And although there are advances in transplantation and novel targeted therapies, surgery has been and will continue to be the cornerstone of therapy for CCA.

References

1. Yamasaki S. Intrahepatic cholangiocarcinoma: macroscopic type and stage classification. J Hepato-Biliary-Pancreat Surg. 2003;10:288–91.
2. National Comprehensive Cancer Network. 2019. Hepatobiliary cancers.

3. Nakeeb A, Pitt HA, Sohn TA, Coleman J, Abrams RA, Piantadosi S, Hruban RH, Lillemoe KD, Yeo CJ, Cameron JL. Cholangiocarcinoma. A spectrum of intrahepatic, perihilar, and distal tumors. Ann Surg. 1996;224:463–75.
4. de Groen PC, Gores GJ, LaRusso NF, Gunderson LL, Nagorney DM. Biliary tract cancers. N Engl J Med. 1999;341:1368–78.
5. Klatskin G. Adenocarcinoma of the hepatic duct at its bifurcation within the porta hepatis: an unusual tumor with distinctive clinical and pathological features. Am J Med. 1965;38:241–56.
6. Patel T. Worldwide trends in mortality from biliary tract malignancies. BMC Cancer. 2002;2:10.
7. DeOliveira ML, Cunningham SC, Cameron JL, Kamangar F, Winter JM, Lillemoe KD, Choti MA, Yeo CJ, Schulick RD. Cholangiocarcinoma: thirty-one-year experience with 564 patients at a single institution. Ann Surg. 2007;245:755–62.
8. Saha SK, Zhu AX, Fuchs CS, Brooks GA. Forty-year trends in cholangiocarcinoma incidence in the u.s.: intrahepatic disease on the rise. Oncologist. 2016;21:594–9.
9. Bertuccio P, Malvezzi M, Carioli G, Hashim D, Boffetta P, El-Serag HB, La Vecchia C, Negri E. Global trends in mortality from intrahepatic and extrahepatic cholangiocarcinoma. J Hepatol. 2019;71:104–14.
10 Mansour JC, Aloia TA, Crane CH, Heimbach JK, Nagino M, Vauthey J-N. Hilar Cholangiocarcinoma: expert consensus statement. HPB. 2015;17:691–9.
11. Vilgrain V. Staging cholangiocarcinoma by imaging studies. HPB (Oxford). 2008;10:106–9.
12. Breitenstein S, Apestegui C, Clavien P-A. Positron emission tomography (PET) for cholangiocarcinoma. HPB (Oxford). 2008;10:120–1.
13. Okabayashi T, Yamamoto J, Kosuge T, Shimada K, Yamasaki S, Takayama T, Makuuchi M. A new staging system for mass-forming intrahepatic cholangiocarcinoma. Cancer. 2001;92:2374–83.
14. Bismuth H, Corlette M. Intrahepatic cholangioenteric anastomosis in carcinoma of the hilus of the liver. Surgery. Gynecol Obstet. 1975;140:170–8.
15. Burke EC, Jarnagin WR, Hochwald SN, Pisters PW, Fong Y, Blumgart LH. Hilar Cholangiocarcinoma: patterns of spread, the importance of hepatic resection for curative operation, and a presurgical clinical staging system. Ann Surg. 1998;228:385–94.
16. Jarnagin WR, Fong Y, DeMatteo RP, Gonen M, Burke EC, Jessica Bodniewicz BS, Miranda Youssef BA, Klimstra D, Blumgart LH. Staging, resectability, and outcome in 225 patients with hilar cholangiocarcinoma. Ann Surg. 2001;234:507–19.
17. Postlewait LM, Ethun CG, Le N, Pawlik TM, Buettner S, Poultsides G, Tran T, Idrees K, Isom CA, Fields RC, et al. Proposal for a new T-stage classification system for distal cholangiocarcinoma: a 10-institution study from the U.S. Extrahepatic Biliary Malignancy Consortium. HPB (Oxford). 2016;18:793–9.
18. Vauthey J-N, Abdalla EK, Doherty DA, Gertsch P, Fenstermacher MJ, Loyer EM, Lerut J, Materne R, Wang X, Encarnacion A, et al. Body surface area and body weight predict total liver volume in Western adults. Liver Transpl. 2002;8:233–40.
19. Guglielmi A, Ruzzenente A, Conci S, Valdegamberi A, Iacono C. How much remnant is enough in liver resection? Dig Surg. 2012;29:6–17.
20. Narula N, Aloia TA. Portal vein embolization in extended liver resection. Langenbeck's Arch Surg. 2017;402:727–35.
21. Rous P, Larimore LD. Relation of the portal blood to liver maintenance: a demonstration of liver atrophy conditional on compensation. J Exp Med. 1920;31:609–32.
22. Fausto N, Campbell JS, Riehle KJ. Liver regeneration. Hepatology. 2006;43:S45–53.
23. Shindoh J, Truty MJ, Aloia TA, Curley SA, Zimmitti G, Huang SY, Mahvash A, Gupta S, Wallace MJ, Vauthey J-N. Kinetic growth rate after portal vein embolization predicts posthepatectomy outcomes: toward zero liver-related mortality in patients with colorectal liver metastases and small future liver remnant. J Am Coll Surg. 2013;216:201–9.
24. Abulkhir A, Limongelli P, Healey AJ, Damrah O, Tait P, Jackson J, Habib N, Jiao LR. Preoperative portal vein embolization for major liver resection: a meta-analysis. Ann Surg. 2008;1:247.

25. Panzeri F, Crippa S, Castelli P, Aleotti F, Pucci A, Partelli S, Zamboni G, Falconi M. Management of ampullary neoplasms: a tailored approach between endoscopy and surgery. World J Gastroenterol. 2015;21:7970–87.
26. Weber SM, Jarnagin WR, Klimstra D, DeMatteo RP, Fong Y, Blumgart LH. Intrahepatic Cholangiocarcinoma: resectability, recurrence pattern, and outcomes. J Am Coll Surg. 2001;193:384–91.
27. Matsuo K, Rocha FG, Ito K, D'Angelica MI, Allen PJ, Fong Y, DeMatteo RP, Gonen M, Endo I, Jarnagin WR. The blumgart preoperative staging system for hilar cholangiocarcinoma: analysis of resectability and outcomes in 380 patients. J Am Coll Surg. 2012;215:343–55.
28. Ruys AT, Busch OR, Gouma DJ, van Gulik TM. Staging laparoscopy for hilar cholangiocarcinoma: is it still worthwhile? Ann Surg Oncol. 2011;18:2647–53.
29. Reames BN, Ejaz A, Koerkamp BG, Alexandrescu S, Marques HP, Aldrighetti L, Maithel SK, Pulitano C, Bauer TW, Shen F, et al. Impact of major vascular resection on outcomes and survival in patients with intrahepatic cholangiocarcinoma: a multi-institutional analysis. J Surg Oncol. 2017;116:133–9.
30. Levi Sandri GB, Spoletini G, Mascianà G, Colasanti M, Lepiane P, Vennarecci G, D'Andrea V, Ettorre GM. The role of minimally invasive surgery in the treatment of cholangiocarcinoma. Eur J Surg Oncol. 2017;43:1617–21.
31. van Vugt JLA, Gaspersz MP, Coelen RJS, Vugts J, Labeur TA, de Jonge J, Polak WG, Busch ORC, Besselink MG, IJzermans JNM, et al. The prognostic value of portal vein and hepatic artery involvement in patients with perihilar cholangiocarcinoma. HPB. 2018;20:83–92.
32. Hemming AW, Mekeel K, Khanna A, Baquerizo A, Kim RD. Portal Vein Resection in Management of Hilar Cholangiocarcinoma. Journal of the American College of Surgeons. 2011;212:604–13.
33. Maeta T, Ebata T, Hayashi E, Kawahara T, Mizuno S, Matsumoto N, Ohta S, Nagino M, the Nagoya Surgical Oncology Group. Pancreatoduodenectomy with portal vein resection for distal cholangiocarcinoma. Br J Surg. 2017;104:1549–57.
34. Peng C, Zhou D, Meng L, Cao Y, Zhang H, Pan Z, Lin C. The value of combined vein resection in pancreaticoduodenectomy for pancreatic head carcinoma: a meta-analysis. BMC Surg. 2019;19:84.
35. Tseng J, Raut C, Lee J, Pisters P, Vauthey J, Abdalla E, Gomez H, Sun C, Crane C, Wolff R. Pancreaticoduodenectomy with vascular resection: margin status and survival duration. Journal of Gastrointestinal Surgery. 2004;8:935–50.
36. Meyer CG, Penn I, James L. Liver transplantation for cholangiocarcinoma: results in 207 patients. Transplantation. 2000;8:69.
37. Rosen CB. Transplantation versus resection for hilar cholangiocarcinoma: an argument for shifting paradigms for resectable disease in annals of surgery 2018. Ann Surg. 2018;5:267.
38. Ethun CG, Lopez-Aguiar AG, Anderson DJ, Adams AB, Fields RC, Doyle MB, Chapman WC, Krasnick BA, Weber SM, Mezrich JD, et al. Transplantation versus resection for hilar cholangiocarcinoma: an argument for shifting treatment paradigms for resectable disease. Ann Surg. 2018;5:267.
39. Spolverato G, Yakoob MY, Kim Y, Alexandrescu S, Marques HP, Lamelas J, Aldrighetti L, Gamblin TC, Maithel SK, Pulitano C, et al. Impact of complications on long-term survival after resection of intrahepatic cholangiocarcinoma. Cancer. 2015;121:2730–9.
40. Ali SM, Clark CJ, Zaydfudim VM, Que FG, Nagorney DM. Role of Major Vascular Resection in Patients with Intrahepatic Cholangiocarcinoma. Annals of Surgical Oncology. 2013;20:2023–8.
41. Ohtsuka M, Ito H, Kimura F, Shimizu H, Togawa A, Yoshidome H, Shimamura F, Shimizu Y, Miyazaki M. Extended hepatic resection and outcomes in intrahepatic cholangiocarcinoma. Journal of Hepato-Biliary-Pancreatic Surgery. 2003;10:259–64.
42. Allen PJ, Reiner AS, Gonen M, Klimstra DK, Blumgart LH, Brennan MF, D'Angelica M, Dematteo R, Fong Y, Jarnagin WR. Extrahepatic cholangiocarcinoma: a comparison of patients with resected proximal and distal lesions. HPB. 2008;10:341–6.

43. Hasegawa S, Ikai I, Fujii H, Hatano E, Shimahara Y. Surgical Resection of Hilar Cholangiocarcinoma: Analysis of Survival and Postoperative Complications. World Journal of Surgery. 2007;31:1258–65.
44. Nagino M, Kamiya J, Uesaka K, Sano T, Yamamoto H, Hayakawa N, Kanai M, Nimura Y. Complications of Hepatectomy for Hilar Cholangiocarcinoma. World Journal of Surgery. 2001;25:1277–83.
45. Gerhards MF, van Gulik TM, de Wit LT, Obertop H, Gouma DJ. Evaluation of morbidity and mortality after resection for hilar cholangiocarcinoma—a single center experience. Surgery. 2000;127:395–404.
46. Andrianello S, Paiella S, Allegrini V, Ramera M, Pulvirenti A, Malleo G, Salvia R, Bassi C. Pancreaticoduodenectomy for distal cholangiocarcinoma: surgical results, prognostic factors, and long-term follow-up. Langenbeck's Archives of Surgery. 2015;400:623–8.
47. Valle J, Wasan H, Palmer DH, Cunningham D, Anthoney A, Maraveyas A, Madhusudan S, Iveson T, Hughes S, Pereira SP, et al. Cisplatin plus Gemcitabine versus Gemcitabine for Biliary Tract Cancer. N Engl J Med. 2010;362:1273–81.
48. Ebata T, Hirano S, Konishi M, Uesaka K, Tsuchiya Y, Ohtsuka M, Kaneoka Y, Yamamoto M, Ambo Y, Shimizu Y, et al. Randomized clinical trial of adjuvant gemcitabine chemotherapy versus observation in resected bile duct cancer. Br J Surg. 2018;105:192–202.
49. Edeline J, Benabdelghani M, Bertaut A, Watelet J, Hammel P, Joly J-P, Boudjema K, Fartoux L, Bouhier-Leporrier K, Jouve J-L, et al. Gemcitabine and oxaliplatin chemotherapy or surveillance in resected biliary tract cancer (PRODIGE 12-ACCORD 18-UNICANCER GI): a randomized phase III study. J Clin Oncol. 2019;37:658–67.
50. Primrose JN, Fox RP, Palmer DH, Malik HZ, Prasad R, Mirza D, Anthony A, Corrie P, Falk S, Finch-Jones M, et al. Capecitabine compared with observation in resected biliary tract cancer (BILCAP): a randomised, controlled, multicentre, phase 3 study. Lancet Oncol. 2019;20:663–73.
51. Shroff RT, Kennedy EB, Bachini M, Bekaii-Saab T, Crane C, Edeline J, El-Khoueiry A, Feng M, Katz MHG, Primrose J, et al. Adjuvant therapy for resected biliary tract cancer: ASCO clinical practice guideline. J Clin Oncol. 2019;37:1015–27.
52. Ben-Josef E, Guthrie KA, El-Khoueiry AB, Corless CL, Zalupski MM, Lowy AM, Thomas CR, Alberts SR, Dawson LA, Micetich KC, et al. SWOG S0809: A phase II intergroup trial of adjuvant capecitabine and gemcitabine followed by radiotherapy and concurrent capecitabine in extrahepatic cholangiocarcinoma and gallbladder carcinoma. J Clini Oncol. 2014;33:2617–22.
53. Rizvi S, Khan SA, Hallemeier CL, Kelley RK, Gores GJ. Cholangiocarcinoma — evolving concepts and therapeutic strategies. Nat Rev Clin Oncol. 2018;15:95–111.
54. Groot Koerkamp B, Wiggers JK, Allen PJ, Besselink MG, Blumgart LH, Busch ORC, Coelen RJ, D'Angelica MI, DeMatteo RP, Gouma DJ, et al. Recurrence rate and pattern of perihilar cholangiocarcinoma after curative intent resection. J Am Coll Surg. 2015;221:1041–9.
55. Wang C, Pang S, Si-Ma H, Yang N, Zhang H, Fu Y, Yang G. Specific risk factors contributing to early and late recurrences of intrahepatic cholangiocarcinoma after curative resection. World J Surg Oncol. 2019;17:2–2.
56. El-Gendi A, El-Shafei M, El-Gendi S, Shawky A. Laparoscopic Versus Open Hepatic Resection for Solitary Hepatocellular Carcinoma Less Than 5 cm in Cirrhotic Patients: A Randomized Controlled Study. Journal of Laparoendoscopic & Advanced Surgical Techniques. 2017;28:302–10.
57. Fretland ÅA, Dagenborg VJ, Bjørnelv GMW, Kazaryan AM, Kristiansen R, Fagerland MW, Hausken J, Tønnessen TI, Abildgaard A, Barkhatov L, et al. Laparoscopic Versus Open Resection for Colorectal Liver Metastases: The OSLO-COMET Randomized Controlled Trial. Annals of Surgery. 2018:267.
58. Massard C, Michiels S, Ferté C, Le Deley M-C, Lacroix L, Hollebecque A, Verlingue L, Ileana E, Rosellini S, Ammari S, et al. High-throughput genomics and clinical outcome in hard-to-treat advanced cancers: results of the MOSCATO 01 trial. Cancer Discov. 2017;7:586–95.

59. Verlingue L, Malka D, Allorant A, Massard C, Ferté C, Lacroix L, Rouleau E, Auger N, Ngo M, Nicotra C, et al. Precision medicine for patients with advanced biliary tract cancers: an effective strategy within the prospective MOSCATO-01 trial. Eur J Cancer. 2017;87:122–30.
60. Simile MM, Bagella P, Vidili G, Spanu A, Manetti R, Seddaiu MA, Babudieri S, Madeddu G, Serra PA, Altana M, et al. Targeted Therapies in Cholangiocarcinoma: Emerging Evidence from Clinical Trials. Medicina (Kaunas). 2019;55:42.
61. Javle M, Lowery M, Shroff RT, Weiss KH, Springfeld C, Borad MJ, Ramanathan RK, Goyal L, Sadeghi S, Macarulla T, et al. Phase II study of BGJ398 in patients with fgfr-altered advanced cholangiocarcinoma. J Clin Oncol. 2018;36:276–82.
62. Borger DR, Tanabe KK, Fan KC, Lopez HU, Fantin VR, Straley KS, Schenkein DP, Hezel AF, Ancukiewicz M, Liebman HM, et al. Frequent mutation of isocitrate dehydrogenase (IDH)1 and IDH2 in cholangiocarcinoma identified through broad-based tumor genotyping. Oncologist. 2012;17:72–9.
63. Abou-Alfa GK, Macarulla Mercade T, Javle M, Kelley RK, Lubner S, Adeva J, Cleary JM, Catenacci DV, Borad MJ, Bridgewater JA, et al. LBA10_PR - ClarIDHy: A global, phase III, randomized, double-blind study of ivosidenib (IVO) vs placebo in patients with advanced cholangiocarcinoma (CC) with an isocitrate dehydrogenase 1 (IDH1) mutation. Ann Oncol. 2019;30:872–3.

Chapter 15
Liver Transplantation for Cholangiocarcinoma

James R. Butler and Vatche G. Agopian

Abbreviations

CCA	Cholangiocarcinoma
ERCP	Endoscopic retrograde cholangiopancreatography
hCCA	Hilar cholangiocarcinoma
iCCA	Intrahepatic cholangiocarcinoma
LT	Liver transplantation
MELD	Model for end-stage liver disease
PSC	Primary sclerosing cholangitis

Introduction

Biliary tract cancers arise from the biliary epithelium and include cholangiocarcinoma (CCA) and gallbladder carcinoma. The incidence in most developed countries is low, with approximately 9000 new cases in the United States each year. Of all biliary tract cancers, CCA is the most common, with approximately 5000 new cases diagnosed in the United States annually [1]. Although primary sclerosing cholangitis

J. R. Butler
Division of Liver and Pancreas Transplantation, Department of Surgery, University of California, Los Angeles (UCLA), Los Angeles, CA, USA

V. G. Agopian (✉)
Division of Liver and Pancreas Transplantation, Department of Surgery, University of California, Los Angeles (UCLA), Los Angeles, CA, USA

Liver Transplantation and Hepatobiliary Surgery, General Surgery Residency Program, Department of Surgery, David Geffen School of Medicine at UCLA, Ronald Reagan Medical Center, Los Angeles, CA, USA
e-mail: vagopian@mednet.ucla.edu

J. H. Tabibian (ed.), *Diagnosis and Management of Cholangiocarcinoma*,
https://doi.org/10.1007/978-3-030-70936-5_15

(PSC), biliary ductal cysts, parasitic infections, and hepatolithiasis are established risk factors, most patients present without an identifiable underlying cause, thereby obscuring any chance of systematically anticipating this disease. Subsequently, the majority of patients present with unresectable, advanced-stage tumor burden.

CCAs are classified as distal (dCCA), hilar or perihilar (hCCA, i.e., Klatskin's tumor), or intrahepatic (iCCA), depending on their anatomical location – with surgical extirpation being the only curative-intent treatment. However, for the 60–70% of all CCAs which present within 2 cm of the proximal biliary bifurcation (i.e., hCCA), complete margin-negative resection is achieved in only 30–80% of cases following surgical resection [2, 3]. In addition, iCCAs can be large and multifocal and often occur in patients with advanced underlying liver disease and cirrhosis, all of which may limit the ability to perform curative-intent major hepatic resections [4].

Despite recent modest improvements in survival with the use of systemic chemotherapy, immunotherapy, and targeted palliative chemotherapeutic approaches [5–9], median survival without surgery remains a dismal 6–12 months [10, 11]. Even for patients who undergo curative-intent surgical resection, the 5-year survival approaches only 40%, mainly due to negligible 5-year survival rates for the significant proportion of patients in whom a margin-negative resection is not obtained (i.e., R1 resections) [3]. Because achieving negative margins is paramount, liver transplantation (LT) for hCCA and iCCA has emerged as a logical strategy. LT affords complete resection with negative margins even in patients who have locally unresectable disease or insufficient hepatic reserve to support resection.

LT for CCA was first introduced in the 1990s, with underwhelming success. Thomas Starzl's group reported a 5-year survival of 25% in a cohort of 38 patients [12], while Jonas et al. reported the German experience to have a 4-year survival of only 30% and unacceptable morbidity [13] (Table 15.1). However, in these early experiences, there were no stringent patient selection protocols, and utilization of neoadjuvant or adjuvant systemic therapies was highly variable. In fact, the majority of these patients were found to have advanced stage disease, including identification of involved regional lymph nodes and even distant abdominal metastases recognized after total hepatectomy. Not surprisingly, disease-free survival was thus short.

In this chapter, we will review recent data on outcomes of LT for both hCCA and iCCA given the considerable improvements in protocol-driven patient selection and utilization of neoadjuvant and adjuvant therapy.

Hilar Cholangiocarcinoma (hCCA)

Neoadjuvant Therapy

Despite the overall poor results reported in these early studies of LT for hCCA, it was recognized that all 5-year survivors were node-negative at the time of LT. This realization, coupled with the known aggressive natural history of the disease, leads

Table 15.1 Selected series of liver transplantation for hilar cholangiocarcinoma

Author, year	Center	*N*	Patient selection	Neoadjuvant chemoradiotherapy	1-year survival %	5-year survival %	R0%	5-year disease recurrence %
Iwatuski et al., 1998 [12]	Pittsburg, single center	38	None	61%	60	25	81	–
Jonas et al., 1998 [13]	Germany, single center	14	None	0%	56	30 at 3 years	92	57
Sudan et al., 2002 [14]	Nebraska, single center	11	None	100%		33	100	55
Heimbach et al., 2004 [15]	Mayo, single center	28	Mayo	100% Mayo	88	82	–	14
Rea et al., 2005 [24]	Mayo, single center	38	Mayo	100% Mayo	92	82	97	13
Kaiser et al., 2008 [46]	Germany, multi-center	47		0%	61	22	–	–
Rosen et al., 2008 [47]	Mayo, single center	90	Mayo	100% Mayo	90	71	–	–
Darwish et al., 2012 [17]	United States, national	216	Variable	100%	–	53	–	20
Schule et al., 2013 [21]	Germany, single center	16	+LN −LN	0% 0%	–	50 0	100 100	50
Weling et al., 2014 [48]	Michigan, single center	6	Mayo	100%	83	–	100	–
Mantel et al., 2016 [20]	Europe, multinational	105	Mayo (28) Beyond (77)	0% 0%	–	59 21	93 89	46 79
Ethun et al., 2018 [23]	United States, multi center	41	Varied	95%	93	64	90	24
Zabarowski et al., 2020 [49]	Ireland, single center	26	Mayo	100% Mayo	81	55	96	48

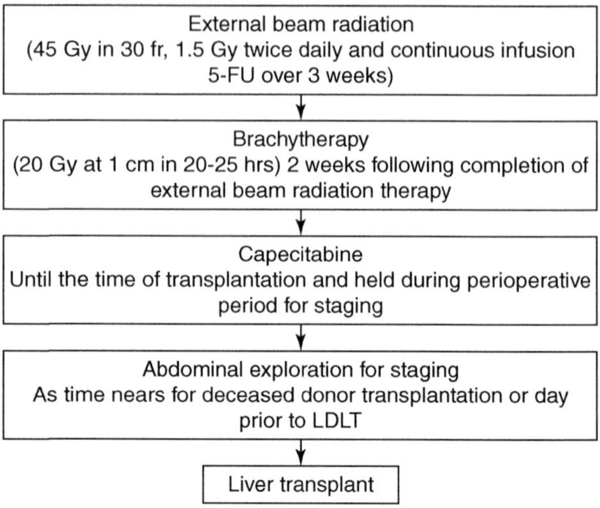

Fig. 15.1 Mayo Clinic neoadjuvant therapy and liver transplantation protocol

physicians at the University of Nebraska to develop the first neoadjuvant chemoradiotherapy protocol to aid in temporizing locally advanced hCCA as bridge to LT [14]. This protocol concept was soon thereafter applied at Mayo Clinic to carefully selected early-stage, unresectable hCCA, yielding unprecedented survival outcomes [15]. In their approach, neoadjuvant external beam radiation was combined with intravenous fluorouracil (5-fluorouracil) sensitization, followed by intraluminal brachytherapy and oral capecitabine while awaiting LT (Fig. 15.1). Their initial results, published in 2000 [16], were updated in 2004 to report an 82% 5-year survival [15]. While there was some criticism regarding the fact that 7/28 (25%) patients had no residual tumor identified in the explant pathology, raising the question of whether these patients truly had hCCA (as opposed to more indolent or precancerous conditions, e.g., PSC), these nonetheless excellent results revived interest in LT for CCA that had been largely abandoned. In fact, numerous contemporary series have reported 5-year survival rates following LT for hCCA that are equivalent to other non-cancer indications for LT utilizing similar neoadjuvant protocols and strict selection criteria (Table 15.1). These uniformly acceptable results have formed the basis for the granting of MELD exception points to prioritize unresectable hCCA patients who meet strict criteria [17].

Patient Selection

Table 15.2 summarizes the inclusion and exclusion criteria as outlined in the initial Mayo Clinic experience. Saliently, this process selects patients with early-stage hCCA which is deemed unresectable or arises within the setting of PSC. Although vascular encasement of hilar vessels is not a contraindication, tumors >3 cm and gallbladder involvement represent contraindications to LT. Prior to LT all patients

Table 15.2 Inclusion and exclusion criteria for Mayo protocol

Inclusion criteria	Exclusion criteria
Diagnosis: Pathologically confirmed hilar cholangiocarcinoma or Malignant appearing stricture + one of the following: Mass at the site of stricture on imaging Serum CA 19-9 > 100 Polysomy on fluorescent in situ hybridization	Intrahepatic cholangiocarcinoma
Radial tumor diameter <3 cm	Prior resection or attempted resection
Absence of intrahepatic or extrahepatic metastases on imaging by cross-sectional imaging and Negative nodal involvement on staging laparotomy	Presence of intrahepatic or extrahepatic metastases
Candidate for LT	History of malignancy within 5 years
Unresectable cancer above the cystic duct	Prior radiation or chemotherapy
Resectable cancer in setting of PSC	Transperitoneal biopsy

undergo a staging abdominal exploration to evaluate for regional lymph node involvement, locally extensive disease, or peritoneal metastases which preclude LT. Although the success of the Mayo Clinic protocol is impressive, it is difficult to assess the relative contribution of neoadjuvant chemoradiotherapy and more rigorous selection practices on the improved outcomes given that they were instituted concurrently. Furthermore, many series utilizing the Mayo Clinic protocol for patient selection report only the post-LT (i.e., per protocol) outcomes and not intent-to-treat analyses, thus limiting the ability to incorporate dynamic changes on the waitlist such as progression versus response to neoadjuvant therapy as potentially useful markers to aid patient selection.

At the tissue level, diagnosis of hCCA can be challenging because intraductal brushing or biopsy is often inconclusive [18]. To address this challenge, the combination of a malignant-appearing stricture on percutaneous transhepatic or endoscopic retrograde cholangiography (ERCP) and *one* of the following additional findings has been deemed sufficient for diagnosis: (1) a mass at the site of stricture by cross-sectional imaging, (2) serum CA 19-9 > 100 U/mL, or (3) polysomy on fluorescent in situ hybridization. Considering this latitude for establishing a diagnosis of hCCA, many patients enter treatment protocols without pretreatment pathologic confirmation of malignancy. However, when studied in multivariate analysis, the absence of pretreatment tissue diagnosis does not inflate 5-year survival except in patients with underlying PSC, where the incidence of benign strictures is much higher [17, 19].

Underscoring the importance of proper patient selection, a recent retrospective analysis of the European Liver Transplant Registry data reported a 5-year overall survival rate of 59% *without* the use of neoadjuvant therapy [20]. In this experience, the authors identified 28 patients of 147 who had undergone LT for hCCA who met strict Mayo Clinic criteria (Table 15.2) but had *not* received neoadjuvant chemoradiotherapy. Given that the results in this small subset of patients were comparable to patients with a pretreatment diagnosis of hCCA who underwent neoadjuvant therapy and subsequent LT, the authors cautiously concluded that patient selection alone may generate improved outcomes following LT for hCCA. Unfortunately, due to a lack of uniformity of neoadjuvant practices in the remaining hCCA patients undergoing LT within this dataset, a comparative analysis to evaluate for a possible benefit of neoadjuvant treatment in addition to strict patient selection could not be performed. Similarly, Schule et al. retrospectively assessed prognostic factors associated with survival in the absence of neoadjuvant therapy. By controlling only for negative lymph node status, they reported an acceptable 5-year survival of 50% *without* multimodal therapy [21]. Considering the 5-year survival in this study was 0% for patients with node-positive disease, this once again raises the question of whether the successful outcomes of the Mayo Clinic protocol are primarily due to its rigorous assessment of nodal involvement as opposed to a benefit of neoadjuvant chemoradiotherapy. As depicted in Table 15.1, patient selection practices and neoadjuvant approaches have varied considerably across studies. Current recommendations to address early hCCA include combination neoadjuvant chemoradiotherapy prior to LT.

Comparing Transplantation with Resection

The rationale of LT in the treatment of unresectable hCCA is intuitive; in fact, outcomes of unresectable patients treated within the Mayo Clinic protocol demonstrate superior 5-year survival to patients undergoing curative-intent resection [22–24]. Foremost, LT offers superior rates of R0 resection despite addressing surgically “unresectable” cohorts (Table 15.1). Even in the most experienced centers, R0 final margin status rates approach only 70% for resection compared to a 90% R0 rate with LT. In addition to superior rates of margin-negative resection following total hepatectomy, LT also appears to confer a lower 90-day mortality than partial hepatectomy for CCA [23, 25]. This fact is likely owed to the complexity of resection required, which often combines extended hepatectomy with bilioenteric anastomosis and vascular reconstruction.

Several nonsurgical factors also affect the disparate outcomes that are reported when comparing surgical resection and LT. A key factor is the variation observed in the proportion of patients that actually make it to surgical resection versus LT. Progression of disease while undergoing neoadjuvant therapy and subsequent “waitlist dropout” while awaiting allograft availability are real issues and may confer a significant positive bias when reporting outcomes in only the patients who make it to LT. Moreover, as wait times for allografts are variable by region and country, waitlist dropout may be variable by geography. Although the practice of granting MELD exception points for this disease, coupled with neoadjuvant therapy, has decreased dropout rates, a significant number of listed hCCA patients still ultimately do not make it to LT, with waitlist dropout reported as high as 23.9% at 12 months [26]. Conversely, resection for hCCA often requires only preoperative biliary drainage, with or without portal vein embolization to support extended hepatectomy. This abbreviated preoperative phase yields less time for aggressive biology to declare itself; subsequently, reported dropout rates for patients undergoing preoperative preparation for non-transplant surgical resection of hCCA are comparably low (less than 20%) [27]. Furthermore, there are no upfront restrictions on making sure lymph node-positive patients do not undergo surgical resection. As such, it is important to appraise any comparison between resection and LT within the context of intent-to-treat analyses.

Interpreting reported differences in outcomes between surgical resection and LT is also challenged by significant cohort heterogeneity between resection and LT patients. To date, this challenge has perhaps been most completely addressed by Ethun et al. describing a retrospective review of LT versus resection in 304 patients from a US multicenter cohort [23], where they report a 5-year overall survival strongly favoring LT over resection for pathologically confirmed hCCA (64% vs 18%, $p = 0.001$). Even after excluding resection cases for patients with variables known to negatively impact survival (e.g., tumors >3 cm and lymph node positivity), the LT group still demonstrated superior 5-year survival compared to surgical resection (54% vs 29% $p = 0.001$). These compelling results have raised the question of whether LT should be considered as preferred therapy even in patients with *resectable* hCCA. This very question is currently under investigation with the European TRANSPHIL study (NCT02232932), an open-label, randomized multicenter trial comparing outcomes for resectable hCCA in patients undergoing either surgical resection or neoadjuvant chemoradiation followed by LT utilizing the Mayo Clinic protocol. The community awaits the results of this study with great anticipation, as they are certain to inform the best curative-intent treatment strategy for patients with this difficult malignancy.

Intrahepatic Cholangiocarcinoma (iCCA)

Intrahepatic cholangiocarcinoma (iCCA) is much less common than hCCA, accounting for under 10% of new cases each year. Similar to HCC, iCCA is strongly associated with underlying cirrhosis and chronic viral hepatitis, and its incidence has been increasing significantly over the past decade [28], which is in part due to the increasing incidence of obesity and the metabolic syndrome [29]. Although iCCA has traditionally been considered a contraindication to LT (Table 15.3), this tenet has recently been challenged due to numerous single-center and retrospective multicenter studies demonstrating acceptable outcomes in well-selected recipients [30]. Similar to hCCA, appropriate patient selection, coupled with neoadjuvant and/or adjuvant protocols, appears to offer an avenue toward favorable post-LT outcomes in this traditionally excluded group of patients.

Table 15.3 Selected series and outcomes of liver transplantation for intrahepatic cholangiocarcinoma

Author, year	Center	*N*	1-year survival %	5-year survival %	Neoadjuvant treatment	5-year disease-free survival %
Shimoda et al., 2001 [50]	Los Angeles, single center	16	62	39 at 3 years	None	35
Robles et al., 2004 [33]	Spain, single center	23	77	42	None	35 at 2 years
Sotiropolus et al., 2008 [51]	Germany, single center	10	70	33	None	–
Vallin et al., 2013 [52]	France, multicenter	10	80	24	None	–
Sapisochin et al., 2014 [53]	Spain, multicenter	27	71	57	None	36
Facciuto et al., 2015 [54]	New York, single center	7	71	57	None	44
Vilchez et al., 2016 [55]	UNOS, national	440	79	47	None	–
Sapisochin et al., 2016 [34]	International, multicenter	15 early[a] 33 advanced[b]	93[a] 79[b]	65[a] 45[b]	None	18[a] 61[b]
Lunsford et al., 2017 [37]	Huston, single center[c]	12	100	83	6-month chemotherapy	50
De Martin et al., 2020 [36]	France, multicenter	49	92	69	Variable	–

[a]Sapisochin et al. found that patients with a single iCCA <2 cm (considered very-early iCCA) had a 5-year survival of 65% after LT and disease recurrence of only 18%. In contrast, patients with advanced disease
[b]Reported a 5-year survival and recurrence rate of 45% and 65%, respectively
[c]Only prospective study on this topic

Initial experiences with LT for iCCA reported very poor survival, mostly attributable to large tumor burden at the time of LT [31, 32]. Subsequently, nearly all published data regarding LT for iCCA is retrospective in nature, with CCA diagnosis identified *after* LT explant tissue analysis. In 2004, Robles et al. retrospectively analyzed a multicenter cohort of 23 patients with iCCA who underwent LT; 5-year survival was 42% [33]. As outlined in Table 15.3, multiple retrospective analyses beginning in 2014 have presented acceptable results for LT in iCCA. The first study to overtly champion the importance of a patient selection strategy to facilitate LT for iCCA was reported by Sapisochin et al. in 2016 [34].

In this multicenter retrospective study, the authors found that patients with a single iCCA <2 cm (considered very-early iCCA) had a 5-year survival of 65% after LT and disease recurrence of only 18%. In contrast, patients with tumors >2 cm reported a 5-year survival and recurrence rate of 45% and 61%, respectively. However, in this subset, it was notable that patients with a known (i.e., non-incidental) iCCA prior to LT had lower tumor recurrence rates and superior actuarial 1-, 3-, and 5-year survival compared to incidentally diagnosed iCCA >2 cm, likely attributable to the fact that 69% of patients with a pre-LT diagnosis received neoadjuvant therapy. Supporting this contention, a UCLA study by Hong et al. of 37 iCCA cases demonstrated that the addition of neoadjuvant and adjuvant therapy with LT significantly reduced recurrence rates for iCCA after LT, with LT recipients receiving both having a 28% recurrence rate compared to 40% for those receiving adjuvant therapy alone and 50% for those receiving neither neoadjuvant nor adjuvant therapy [35]. A multicenter prospective clinical trial is currently underway to validate these retrospective findings, with results expected in 2026 (NCT02878473).

Despite the promise of these selection practices, detection of very-early, <2 cm iCCA in unresectable cirrhotic patients is a challenge. More recently, several groups have also reported their experience with LT with tumors larger than 2 cm with acceptable results. De Martin et al. studied outcomes of 24 patients with iCCA >2 cm and ≤5 cm who underwent LT and reported an overall recurrence rate of 21% and overall survival of 65% at 5 years [36], which represent superior results compared to the multicenter study reported by Sapisochin et al. [34]. A recent prospective study from Lunsford et al. employed LT in patients with *locally advanced* unresectable iCCA, pushing the traditionally acceptable limits by inclusion of iCCA patients with multifocal and large lesions which would be considered beyond the Milan Criteria for HCC [37]. This study enrolled patients with either large (iCCA >5 cm) or multifocal disease (median pre-LT number of four lesions) without vascular invasion, extrahepatic disease, or lymph node involvement. By allowing only iCCA patients demonstrating a sustained response to gemcitabine and cisplatin for a minimum 6 months to receive LT, they were able to achieve 5-year survival of 83% after LT despite large tumor burden identified at explant (median number of seven lesions with median cumulative tumor diameter of 14.2 cm). While the number of patients undergoing LT was quite small ($n = 6$) in this initial report, it provided a strong framework to allow for life-saving LT in highly selected patients with unresectable but not extrahepatic disease.

In summary, LT for iCCA remains controversial, and extrapolating results from retrospective data is challenged by heterogeneity among treatment protocols and small sample sizes. To solidify the practice of LT for iCCA or make an argument for MELD exception, further prospective data will be necessary. Currently available data support consideration of LT either for (1) very-early stage (<2 cm) and intermediate stage (2–5 cm) iCCA diagnosed within the context of chronic liver failure or (2) locally advanced disease in highly selected patients who have demonstrated a sustained tumor response to neoadjuvant treatment.

Perioperative and Technical Considerations

Preoperative Preparation

With the current landscape necessitating neoadjuvant chemoradiotherapy for the majority of patients undergoing LT for CCA, several common sequelae should be anticipated. Radiation therapy confers patients a relatively high rate of duodenal ulceration [38]. As such, it is recommended to employ proton pump inhibitors in these patients during therapy and for a minimum of 1 month afterward. In addition to challenges with tumor cachexia, patients undergoing neoadjuvant chemoradiotherapy are uniquely nutritionally challenged, as radiation therapy often begets gastropathy, gastritis, and gastric dysmotility. The severity of these symptoms may be exacerbated by perioperative narcotics at time of LT. Subsequently, close monitoring for these symptoms preoperatively is important, and surgeons should have a low threshold to employ jejunal feeding access for this at-risk population. Preoperative nutritional optimization has been associated with improved survival in patients undergoing resection for CCA [39]. Although not specifically studied in the context of malignancy, many studies support the benefit of preoperative nutritional optimization to support LT survival as well [40].

Due to the nature of CCA, biliary obstruction and cholangitis are frequent problems encountered in the preoperative course. Despite initial controversy, the use of covered self-expanding metal stents to alleviate these problems does not preclude effective radiotherapy. Such stents are proven to prevent tumor ingrowth but carry a higher rate of migration and cholecystitis [41, 42]. Perhaps most importantly, providers should have low threshold to initiate empiric antibacterial coverage in any patient with suspected acute cholangitis. Prophylactic antibiotics should be considered peri-ERCP and post-procedure according to practice guidelines [43]. As time to repeat ERCP and stent occlusion can be variable, some centers also provide patients with indwelling biliary stents a prescription for antibiotics and instructions to empirically begin treatment at the onset of symptoms indicating worsening biliary obstruction or infection.

Similar to biliary obstruction, cholecystitis often develops in patients awaiting LT for CCA. Its frequent incidence is derivative to tumor obstruction of the cystic duct or complications of biliary stenting. Diagnosis is reliable by ultrasound, as in conventional cases; however, treatment should avoid cholecystectomy as there is a high risk of tumor dissemination [44]. Treatment includes prompt initiation of antibiotics and decompression, with both ERCP and percutaneous stenting as acceptable options.

Operative Considerations

Both deceased donor and living donor LT have been successfully employed to treat CCA. When described, surgical technique for LT follows institutional protocol but favors a bicaval approach when there is caudate involvement. Staging laparotomy described in the Mayo Clinic protocol is performed through a right or bilateral subcostal incision and includes a thorough abdominal exploration, including manual palpation of the hilum. Routine biopsies of nodes overlying the common bile duct as well as the distal hepatic artery at the level of the gastroduodenal artery are performed at this time. Extrahepatic disease or lymph node metastases preclude LT. While this staging laparotomy has initially been described as being performed prior to LT, many centers have now incorporated this staging to be done at the time of an organ offer.

LT performed for hCCA should include very low dissection of the portal structures and routine frozen section of the distal bile duct margin. A positive distal bile duct margin needs to prompt consideration of a pancreaticoduodenectomy to achieve a margin-negative curative intent operation. If a pancreaticoduodenectomy is required, proton pump therapy is recommended for life [45]. Finally, recipients undergoing neoadjuvant intraluminal brachytherapy have been noted to have a higher incidence of vascular complications, particularly hepatic artery thrombosis. Subsequently, routine employment of an infrarenal aortic conduit using donor iliac vessels to supply the donor artery has been described and should be considered.

Conclusion

While LT has been the gold standard treatment for patients with unresectable hepatocellular carcinoma for nearly three decades, a new era of "transplant oncology" has been ushered in with the recognition that LT is also a viable curative therapy for patients with CCA. Given the relative scarcity of available donor liver allografts, rigorous patient selection must be applied to mitigate oncologic risk and ensure meaningful organ utilization (Table 15.4). Although questions exist regarding the

Table 15.4 Data-supported recommendations for LT in hilar vs intrahepatic cholangiocarcinoma

	hCCA	iCCA
Age	<68, absence of comorbidities precluding LT	<65, absence of comorbidities precluding LT
Histologic confirmation	Optional, excluding transperitoneal	Mandatory, often transperitoneal
Size staging	<3 cm	Unresectable <2 cm in setting of chronic liver failure *or* Unresectable >2 cm with sustained response to chemotherapy ± RT
CA 19-9	No upper limit reported	>100 relative contraindication
Multifocality	Contraindication	To be defined
Preoperative lymph node assessment	Mandatory – rule out nodal disease	Mandatory – rule out nodal disease
Neoadjuvant treatment	Chemoradiotherapy	Very early disease – to be defined Advanced disease – recommended as selection tool
Eligibility for MELD exception	Yes	Not currently

application of LT for resectable hCCA and iCCA, diligent patient selection and multimodal neoadjuvant and adjuvant therapy seem to be of paramount importance. With increasing rates of living donor LT, extended criteria organ utilization, and the advances seen within the field of xenotransplantation, the promise of a supply-side fix to organ shortages may further expand opportunities to offer LT as a treatment for CCA.

References

1. Nakeeb A, Pitt HA, Sohn TA, Coleman J, Abrams RA, Piantadosi S, et al. Cholangiocarcinoma. A spectrum of intrahepatic, perihilar, and distal tumors. Ann Surg. 1996;224(4):463–73; discussion 73–5.
2. Jarnagin WR, Fong Y, DeMatteo RP, Gonen M, Burke EC, Bodniewicz BJ, et al. Staging, resectability, and outcome in 225 patients with hilar cholangiocarcinoma. Ann Surg. 2001;234(4):507–17; discussion 17–9.
3. Nagino M, Ebata T, Yokoyama Y, Igami T, Sugawara G, Takahashi Y, et al. Evolution of surgical treatment for perihilar cholangiocarcinoma: a single-center 34-year review of 574 consecutive resections. Ann Surg. 2013;258(1):129–40.
4. Vilana R, Forner A, Bianchi L, Garcia-Criado A, Rimola J, de Lope CR, et al. Intrahepatic peripheral cholangiocarcinoma in cirrhosis patients may display a vascular pattern similar to hepatocellular carcinoma on contrast-enhanced ultrasound. Hepatology. 2010;51(6):2020–9.
5. Ortner ME, Caca K, Berr F, Liebetruth J, Mansmann U, Huster D, et al. Successful photodynamic therapy for nonresectable cholangiocarcinoma: a randomized prospective study. Gastroenterology. 2003;125(5):1355–63.
6. Verderame F, Russo A, Di Leo R, Badalamenti G, Santangelo D, Cicero G, et al. Gemcitabine and oxaliplatin combination chemotherapy in advanced biliary tract cancers. Ann Oncol. 2006;17(Suppl 7):vii68–72.
7. Grendar J, Grendarova P, Sinha R, Dixon E. Neoadjuvant therapy for downstaging of locally advanced hilar cholangiocarcinoma: a systematic review. HPB (Oxford). 2014;16(4):297–303.
8. Abou-Alfa GK, Macarulla T, Javle MM, Kelley RK, Lubner SJ, Adeva J, et al. Ivosidenib in IDH1-mutant, chemotherapy-refractory cholangiocarcinoma (ClarIDHy): a multicentre, randomised, double-blind, placebo-controlled, phase 3 study. Lancet Oncol. 2020;21(6):796–807.
9. Banales JM, Cardinale V, Carpino G, Marzioni M, Andersen JB, Invernizzi P, et al. Expert consensus document: Cholangiocarcinoma: current knowledge and future perspectives consensus statement from the European Network for the Study of Cholangiocarcinoma (ENS-CCA). Nat Rev Gastroenterol Hepatol. 2016;13(5):261–80.
10. Eckel F, Schmid RM. Emerging drugs for biliary cancer. Expert Opin Emerg Drugs. 2007;12(4):571–89.
11. Kelley RK, Bridgewater J, Gores GJ, Zhu AX. Systemic therapies for intrahepatic cholangiocarcinoma. J Hepatol. 2020;72(2):353–63.
12. Iwatsuki S, Todo S, Marsh JW, Madariaga JR, Lee RG, Dvorchik I, et al. Treatment of hilar cholangiocarcinoma (Klatskin tumors) with hepatic resection or transplantation. J Am Coll Surg. 1998;187(4):358–64.
13. Jonas S, Kling N, Guckelberger O, Keck H, Bechstein WO, Neuhaus P. Orthotopic liver transplantation after extended bile duct resection as treatment of hilar cholangiocarcinoma. First long-terms results. Transpl Int. 1998;11(Suppl 1):S206–8.
14. Sudan D, DeRoover A, Chinnakotla S, Fox I, Shaw B Jr, McCashland T, et al. Radiochemotherapy and transplantation allow long-term survival for nonresectable hilar cholangiocarcinoma. Am J Transplant. 2002;2(8):774–9.

15. Heimbach JK, Gores GJ, Haddock MG, Alberts SR, Nyberg SL, Ishitani MB, et al. Liver transplantation for unresectable perihilar cholangiocarcinoma. Semin Liver Dis. 2004;24(2):201–7.
16. De Vreede I, Steers JL, Burch PA, Rosen CB, Gunderson LL, Haddock MG, et al. Prolonged disease-free survival after orthotopic liver transplantation plus adjuvant chemoirradiation for cholangiocarcinoma. Liver Transpl. 2000;6(3):309–16.
17. Rosen CB, Darwish Murad S, Heimbach JK, Nyberg SL, Nagorney DM, Gores GJ. Neoadjuvant therapy and liver transplantation for hilar cholangiocarcinoma: is pretreatment pathological confirmation of diagnosis necessary? J Am Coll Surg. 2012;215(1):31–8; discussion 8–40.
18. Kipp BR, Stadheim LM, Halling SA, Pochron NL, Harmsen S, Nagorney DM, et al. A comparison of routine cytology and fluorescence in situ hybridization for the detection of malignant bile duct strictures. Am J Gastroenterol. 2004;99(9):1675–81.
19. Duignan S, Maguire D, Ravichand CS, Geoghegan J, Hoti E, Fennelly D, et al. Neoadjuvant chemoradiotherapy followed by liver transplantation for unresectable cholangiocarcinoma: a single-centre national experience. HPB (Oxford). 2014;16(1):91–8.
20. Mantel HT, Westerkamp AC, Adam R, Bennet WF, Seehofer D, Settmacher U, et al. Strict selection alone of patients undergoing liver transplantation for hilar cholangiocarcinoma is associated with improved survival. PLoS One. 2016;11(6):e0156127.
21. Schule S, Altendorf-Hofmann A, Utess F, Rauchfuss F, Freesmeyer M, Knosel T, et al. Liver transplantation for hilar cholangiocarcinoma--a single-centre experience. Langenbeck's Arch Surg. 2013;398(1):71–7.
22. Croome KP, Rosen CB, Heimbach JK, Nagorney DM. Is liver transplantation appropriate for patients with potentially resectable de novo hilar cholangiocarcinoma? J Am Coll Surg. 2015;221(1):130–9.
23. Ethun CG, Lopez-Aguiar AG, Anderson DJ, Adams AB, Fields RC, Doyle MB, et al. Transplantation versus resection for hilar cholangiocarcinoma: an argument for shifting treatment paradigms for resectable disease. Ann Surg. 2018;267(5):797–805.
24. Rea DJ, Heimbach JK, Rosen CB, Haddock MG, Alberts SR, Kremers WK, et al. Liver transplantation with neoadjuvant chemoradiation is more effective than resection for hilar cholangiocarcinoma. Ann Surg. 2005;242(3):451–8; discussion 8–61.
25. Matsuo K, Rocha FG, Ito K, D'Angelica MI, Allen PJ, Fong Y, et al. The Blumgart preoperative staging system for hilar cholangiocarcinoma: analysis of resectability and outcomes in 380 patients. J Am Coll Surg. 2012;215(3):343–55.
26. Ziogas IA, Hickman LA, Matsuoka LK, Izzy M, Montenovo MI, Rega SA, et al. Comparison of wait-list mortality between cholangiocarcinoma and hepatocellular carcinoma liver transplant candidates. Liver Transpl. 2020;26:1112–20.
27. Sano T, Shimada K, Sakamoto Y, Yamamoto J, Yamasaki S, Kosuge T. One hundred two consecutive hepatobiliary resections for perihilar cholangiocarcinoma with zero mortality. Ann Surg. 2006;244(2):240–7.
28. Bertuccio P, Malvezzi M, Carioli G, Hashim D, Boffetta P, El-Serag HB, et al. Reply to: “Global trends in mortality from intrahepatic and extrahepatic cholangiocarcinoma”. J Hepatol. 2019;71(6):1262–3.
29. Petrick JL, Thistle JE, Zeleniuch-Jacquotte A, Zhang X, Wactawski-Wende J, Van Dyke AL, et al. Body mass index, diabetes and intrahepatic cholangiocarcinoma risk: the liver cancer pooling project and meta-analysis. Am J Gastroenterol. 2018;113(10):1494–505.
30. Sapisochin G, Javle M, Lerut J, Ohtsuka M, Ghobrial M, Hibi T, et al. Liver transplantation for cholangiocarcinoma and mixed hepatocellular cholangiocarcinoma: working group report from the ILTS transplant oncology consensus conference. Transplantation. 2020;104(6):1125–30.
31. Goldstein RM, Stone M, Tillery GW, Senzer N, Levy M, Husberg BS, et al. Is liver transplantation indicated for cholangiocarcinoma? Am J Surg. 1993;166(6):768–71; discussion 71–2.
32. O’Grady JG, Polson RJ, Rolles K, Calne RY, Williams R. Liver transplantation for malignant disease. Results in 93 consecutive patients. Ann Surg. 1988;207(4):373–9.
33. Robles R, Figueras J, Turrion VS, Margarit C, Moya A, Varo E, et al. Spanish experience in liver transplantation for hilar and peripheral cholangiocarcinoma. Ann Surg. 2004;239(2):265–71.

34. Sapisochin G, Facciuto M, Rubbia-Brandt L, Marti J, Mehta N, Yao FY, et al. Liver transplantation for "very early" intrahepatic cholangiocarcinoma: international retrospective study supporting a prospective assessment. Hepatology. 2016;64(4):1178–88.
35. Hong JC, Jones CM, Duffy JP, Petrowsky H, Farmer DG, French S, et al. Comparative analysis of resection and liver transplantation for intrahepatic and hilar cholangiocarcinoma: a 24-year experience in a single center. Arch Surg. 2011;146(6):683–9.
36. De Martin E, Rayar M, Golse N, Dupeux M, Gelli M, Gnemmi V, et al. Analysis of liver resection versus liver transplantation on outcome of small intrahepatic cholangiocarcinoma and combined hepatocellular-cholangiocarcinoma in the setting of cirrhosis. Liver Transpl. 2020;26(6):785–98.
37. Lunsford KE, Javle M, Heyne K, Shroff RT, Abdel-Wahab R, Gupta N, et al. Liver transplantation for locally advanced intrahepatic cholangiocarcinoma treated with neoadjuvant therapy: a prospective case-series. Lancet Gastroenterol Hepatol. 2018;3(5):337–48.
38. Flickinger JC, Epstein AH, Iwatsuki S, Carr BI, Starzl TE. Radiation therapy for primary carcinoma of the extrahepatic biliary system. An analysis of 63 cases. Cancer. 1991;68(2):289–94.
39. Akgul O, Bagante F, Olsen G, Cloyd JM, Weiss M, Merath K, et al. Preoperative prognostic nutritional index predicts survival of patients with intrahepatic cholangiocarcinoma after curative resection. J Surg Oncol. 2018;118(3):422–30.
40. Sanchez AJ, Aranda-Michel J. Nutrition for the liver transplant patient. Liver Transpl. 2006;12(9):1310–6.
41. Isayama H, Komatsu Y, Tsujino T, Sasahira N, Hirano K, Toda N, et al. A prospective randomised study of "covered" versus "uncovered" diamond stents for the management of distal malignant biliary obstruction. Gut. 2004;53(5):729–34.
42. Jang S, Stevens T, Parsi M, Lopez R, Zuccaro G, Dumot J, et al. Association of covered metallic stents with cholecystitis and stent migration in malignant biliary stricture. Gastrointest Endosc. 2018;87(4):1061–70.
43. ASGE Standards of Practice Committee, Khashab MA, Chithadi KV, Acosta RD, Bruining DH, Chandrasekhara V, et al. Antibiotic prophylaxis for GI endoscopy. Gastrointest Endosc. 2015;81(1):81–9.
44. Razumilava N, Gores GJ. Cholangiocarcinoma. Lancet. 2014;383(9935):2168–79. https://www.thelancet.com/pdfs/journals/lancet/PIIS0140-6736(13)61903-0.pdf.
45. Butler JR, Rogers T, Eckart G, Martens GR, Ceppa EP, House MG, et al. Is antisecretory therapy after pancreatoduodenectomy necessary? Meta-analysis and contemporary practices of pancreatic surgeons. J Gastrointest Surg. 2015;19(4):604–12.
46. Kaiser GM, Sotiropoulos GC, Jauch KW, Lohe F, Hirner A, Kalff JC, et al. Liver transplantation for hilar cholangiocarcinoma: a German survey. Transplant Proc. 2008;40(9):3191–3.
47. Rosen CB, Heimbach JK, Gores GJ. Surgery for cholangiocarcinoma: the role of liver transplantation. HPB (Oxford). 2008;10(3):186–9.
48. Welling TH, Feng M, Wan S, Hwang SY, Volk ML, Lawrence TS, et al. Neoadjuvant stereotactic body radiation therapy, capecitabine, and liver transplantation for unresectable hilar cholangiocarcinoma. Liver Transpl. 2014;20(1):81–8.
49. Zaborowski A, Heneghan HM, Fiore B, Stafford A, Gallagher T, Geoghegan J, et al. Neoadjuvant chemoradiotherapy and liver transplantation for unresectable hilar cholangiocarcinoma: the Irish experience of the Mayo protocol. Transplantation. 2020;104:2097–104.
50. Shimoda M, Farmer DG, Colquhoun SD, Rosove M, Ghobrial RM, Yersiz H, et al. Liver transplantation for cholangiocellular carcinoma: analysis of a single-center experience and review of the literature. Liver Transpl. 2001;7(12):1023–33.
51. Sotiropoulos GC, Kaiser GM, Lang H, Molmenti EP, Beckebaum S, Fouzas I, et al. Liver transplantation as a primary indication for intrahepatic cholangiocarcinoma: a single-center experience. Transplant Proc. 2008;40(9):3194–5.
52. Vallin M, Sturm N, Lamblin G, Guillaud O, Hilleret MN, Hervieu V, et al. Unrecognized intrahepatic cholangiocarcinoma: an analysis of 993 adult cirrhotic liver explants. Clin Transpl. 2013;27(3):403–9.

53. Sapisochin G, Rodriguez de Lope C, Gastaca M, Ortiz de Urbina J, Suarez MA, Santoyo J, et al. "Very early" intrahepatic cholangiocarcinoma in cirrhotic patients: should liver transplantation be reconsidered in these patients? Am J Transplant. 2014;14(3):660–7.
54. Facciuto ME, Singh MK, Lubezky N, Selim MA, Robinson D, Kim-Schluger L, et al. Tumors with intrahepatic bile duct differentiation in cirrhosis: implications on outcomes after liver transplantation. Transplantation. 2015;99(1):151–7.
55. Vilchez V, Shah MB, Daily MF, Pena L, Tzeng CW, Davenport D, et al. Long-term outcome of patients undergoing liver transplantation for mixed hepatocellular carcinoma and cholangiocarcinoma: an analysis of the UNOS database. HPB (Oxford). 2016;18(1):29–34.

Chapter 16
Neoadjuvant and Adjuvant Therapy for Cholangiocarcinoma

Russell C. Kirks and Flavio G. Rocha

Abbreviations

5-FU	5-fluorouracil
ASCO	American Society of Clinical Oncology
ASCOT	Adjuvant S1 for Cholangiocarcinoma Trial
BCAT	Biliary Cancer Adjuvant Trial
BILCAP	Capecitabine compared with observation in resected biliary tract cancer
CCA	Cholangiocarcinoma
dCCA	Distal cholangiocarcinoma
DFS	Disease-free survival
EBRT	External beam radiation therapy
EGFR	Epidermal growth factor receptor
ESPAC	European Study Group for Pancreatic Cancer
FGFR	Fibroblast growth factor receptor
GAP	Gemcitabine, cisplatin, and albumin-bound (nab)-paclitaxel
HAI	Hepatic artery infusion
HARE	Hepatic artery radioembolization
IDH	Isocitrate dehydrogenase
JCOG	Japanese Clinical Oncology Group
LDLT	Living donor liver transplant
NAFLD	Nonalcoholic fatty liver disease
NASH	Nonalcoholic steatohepatitis
NCCN	National Comprehensive Cancer Network
NLR	Neutrophil to lymphocyte ratio
OLT	Orthotopic liver transplantation
OS	Overall survival

R. C. Kirks · F. G. Rocha (✉)
General, Thoracic, and Vascular Surgery, Virginia Mason Medical Center, Seattle, WA, USA
e-mail: Flavio.rocha@virginiamason.org

J. H. Tabibian (ed.), *Diagnosis and Management of Cholangiocarcinoma*,
https://doi.org/10.1007/978-3-030-70936-5_16

pCCA	Perihilar cholangiocarcinoma
PD	Pancreaticoduodenectomy
RFS	Recurrence-free survival
SIRT	Selective internal radiation therapy
SWOG	Southwest Oncology Group
VEGF	Vascular endothelial growth factor

Introduction

Cholangiocarcinoma (CCA) is an epithelial-based tumor arising from the biliary tract which can originate anywhere from the peripheral intrahepatic biliary radicles to the periampullary region. CCA has been historically defined based on the location of disease as intrahepatic CCA (iCCA) arising from the second-order biliary ducts or farther into the livery periphery, perihilar CCA (pCCA) arising from the takeoff of the cystic duct to the main lobar bile ducts, or distal CCA (dCCA) arising from the cystic duct takeoff distally to the ampulla (Chap. 2, Mederos and Girgis) [1]. While the description of site of disease allows for some degree of surgical operative planning for surgically resectable disease, among other potential interventions for resectable or unresectable disease, recent investigations into the molecular characteristics of tumors at different sites suggest that the tumors arising in these respective locations represent distinct disease entities at a biological and molecular level.

The incidence of CCA in the Western world is rising, in large part due to increases in the prevalence of nonalcoholic steatohepatitis (NASH) and nonalcoholic fatty liver disease (NAFLD) as well as changes in the coding and reporting of intrahepatic tumors [1–3]. Long asymptomatic growth periods, the possibility of diagnostic dilemma, and the complex anatomy of the hilum of the liver all contribute to a minority of lesions being resectable at the time of diagnosis [4]. Other factors adding layers of complexity to assessment and therapeutic algorithms in CCA include the presence of portal lymphadenopathy, intrahepatic metastases, multifocal lesions, biliary obstruction, and a background of cirrhosis.

The treatment of CCA underscores the need for a multidisciplinary approach to select from a wide range of therapies. These include endoluminal, surgical, and regional therapies, as well as systemic cytotoxic or molecular targeted agents, with a combination of these being not infrequently used in order to best tailor treatment for an individual patient. Nevertheless, weighing comparatively poor overall survival (OS) rates with chemotherapy alone, the need to consider liver remnant function in certain resections, and the likelihood of residual disease after curative-intent surgical resection, additional disease treatment strategies and therapeutic options have been sought. These include targeted therapies, and, for limited disease in pCCA and iCCA, liver transplantation (Chap. 15, Butler and Agopian). Additional trials continue to better define optimal adjuvant therapeutic strategies in resected disease and treatment regimens that may convert initially advanced disease to surgically resectable disease. In this chapter, we highlight current multidisciplinary CCA treatment focusing on systemic therapies; recent advances in cytotoxic and targeted therapies are discussed along with their roles in patients undergoing curative-intent surgical resection as well as those with locally advanced or metastatic disease.

Prognostic Tools and Factors

While national surgical database outcomes have been used to stratify patients' risks of postoperative complications [5], these databases and online risk calculators have yet to be refined to a level that would allow a confident prediction of disease-specific or cancer-related outcomes. These efforts may be further complicated when considering a disease such as CCA that occurs at different anatomical locations (requiring disparate surgical resections) and our evolving level of understanding of tumor biology and molecular individuality. The use of preoperative prediction tools as compared with postoperative findings such as tumor pathology findings has also been a recent topic of interest in influencing attempts to improve preoperative prediction metrics to include such tools as machine learning [6]. These efforts seek to identify patients at high risk for recurrence, those for whom a neoadjuvant approach may be considered, and the optimal timing for surgery in a multidisciplinary treatment approach.

Multiple clinical preoperative and pathologic tumor analysis factors have been used to form aspects of tumor staging systems as well as to prognosticate upon the biology of disease in CCA as well as the expected chances of disease recurrence. In pCCA and iCCA, the presence of portal lymphadenopathy, surgical margin positivity, multifocal disease or satellite lesions, hilar vascular involvement, and elevated serum tumor markers following biliary decompression have been identified as indicators of more advanced disease and suggest a higher recurrence risk [7–10]. Increased interest in the molecular profiles of CCA as well as understanding of the role of the immune response to tumors has identified easily measured indices that can provide some prognostic information on tumor biology and recurrence risk.

Using preoperative complete blood count with differential, the calculation of neutrophil to lymphocyte ratio (NLR) has been shown to have prognostic validity in resections for other primary and metastatic hepatic tumors [11–13]. A large, multi-institutional, retrospective review confirmed this among a cohort of 991 resected patients with iCCA, finding that elevated NLR was independently associated with worse overall survival. Using a ratio of <5 vs. ≥ 5, patients with elevated NLR had a median survival of 21.9 months compared with 41.7 in the lower NLR group [14]. When adding this score to an established prognostic tool including other standard disease factors such as tumor size, periportal lymphadenopathy, vascular invasion, etc., the overall prognostic ability was improved. Using a high vs. low NLR cutoff of ≥ 3 vs. <3, improvements in 5-year overall survival and recurrence-free survival were also identified in a retrospective single-center US study. A unique subanalysis in this study further demonstrated the improvements in survival in those patients treated with neoadjuvant chemotherapy prior to resection for borderline-resectable or advanced iCCA, showing that those patients treated in a neoadjuvant fashion with NLR <3 had a 95% 5-year OS while those with >3 had an OS of 50% at 5 years [15]. These results include only resected patients and did not include an intention-to-treat analysis; these results must be considered a highly selected surgical group, but the findings of a survival difference based on such an easily measured metric suggest the utility of NLR in patients with iCCA.

Postoperatively, the distribution and maximum number of various types of immune cells have also been studied in patients who underwent resection for iCCA and dCCA. After analyzing a broad review of postoperative factors, Shinke et al. identified significant differences in overall survival, disease-free survival, as well as survival after recurrence based on differences in postoperative peak numbers of neutrophils and eosinophils. Lower peak neutrophil count after resection was associated with improved overall survival at 1, 3, and 5 years (92.0 vs. 80.0%; 66.9% vs. 51.5%; and 49.5% vs. 40.2%; $p = 0.04$) and improved survival 1, 3, and 5 years after recurrence (67.3% vs. 40.0%; 27.7% vs. 10.4%; and 18.5% vs. 0%; $p = 0.03$); a higher peak eosinophil count was also associated with improved OS and survival after recurrence [16]. While these findings are available only following a surgery with a curative intent, they certainly highlight the evolving role and understanding of the immune system and systemic effects occurring in the perioperative period as well as their potential long-term prognostic value. Other biochemical metrics that have been investigated in the postoperative period include measurement of albumin-bilirubin grade and relating this to survival outcomes [17]. It may yet be premature to suggest alterations in therapy decisions or surveillance based on these findings, but such easily followed and measured values such as these could further enrich the comprehensive treatment discussion had with patients who undergo resection for CCA.

Evolving use of online platforms and machine learning technology with image analysis shows promise in determining which patients will benefit most from surgical resection. Developed online risk prediction calculators for iCCA include many conventional prognostic factors such as nodal positivity and R1 resection, factors that can only be determined after resection and pathologic analysis [18]. Using machine learning technology to evaluate preoperative imaging characteristics compared against known survival in a retrospective fashion, algorithms may be developed to determine which patients will benefit from resection as compared with other strategies such as systemic with or without concomitant liver-directed regional therapy [19]. The goal of these new endeavors would certainly be to select patients who will benefit from surgery rather than using surgical specimens to establish prognosis and simultaneously subject low-yield surgical patients to the immunologic challenge of surgery.

For patients presenting with advanced or metastatic disease, prognostic factors and indices focus on expected response to chemotherapy. In addition to assessing a patient's functional status and anatomic disease burden, gauging and communicating the expected response to systemic treatment can enhance an informative and complete discussion of expectation with patients undergoing systemic therapy. Notably, these data concern cytotoxic chemotherapy; while targeted therapy based on tumor molecular profiling may have an evolving role in the treatment of advanced disease, data regarding prognosis with immunotherapy are still being described [20].

Using similar values obtained and mentioned above, several indices use immune cells and nutritional markers to stratify patients' survival on chemotherapy for advanced disease based on immune response as well as inflammatory and nutritional markers [21, 22]. Improved nutritional indices were found to correlate with improved functional status as well as longer overall survival, likely reflecting the effects of cancer-related cachexia, inflammation, and functional reserve in patients presenting with advanced biliary tract malignancy [22]. Notably, these studies focus on patients with a preserved functional status and those who are therefore deemed clinically suitable for palliative chemotherapy for advanced disease which comprises both surgically unresectable and metastatic CCA. Further supporting the idea that CCA may be biologically distinct and behave differently based on site of disease origin (gallbladder, intrahepatic, and distal subtypes), varying prognostic factors for overall survival and progression-free survival times have been described with different prognostic factors based on the different disease sites [23].

Adjuvant Chemotherapy Trials

Due to historically poor survival with surgery alone for CCA as well as the likelihood for margin-positive resections and regional lymphatic metastases, adjuvant chemotherapy has been studied as an integral part of the treatment regimen for patients with surgically resectable disease. The heterogeneity of disease sites in CCA coupled with the typically advanced state of presentation and commensurate minority of patients being unresectable at presentation has limited the early analysis of outcomes to those patients with CCA included with other hepatobiliary and/or pancreatic tumors. Clinical factors and outcomes of completed adjuvant therapy trials are summarized in Table 16.1.

A Japanese study by Takada et al. published in 2002 demonstrated an improvement in survival when adjuvant chemotherapy was administered following curative-intent resection. In this phase III trial, patients undergoing surgery for CCA arising in the extrahepatic bile duct and gallbladder were included for randomization and analysis with patients undergoing resection for pancreatic as well as ampullary tumors. The trial arms were surgery alone compared with surgery followed by 5-fluorouracil (5-FU) and mitomycin C. While the per-protocol analysis resulted in a 5-year OS benefit for patients with resected adenocarcinoma of the gallbladder undergoing adjuvant therapy (36% vs. 14%, $p < 0.0367$), this positive benefit did not extend to all disease sites included in an intention-to-treat analysis [24].

Similarly, dCCA patients were included in the European Study Group for Pancreatic Cancer (ESPAC) 3 trial examining the effect on survival of adjuvant chemotherapy on resected periampullary cancers. As in the Takada trial, dCCA were included in analysis with other periampullary cancers including pancreatic

Table 16.1 Comparison of details from completed adjuvant therapy trials

	SWOG 0809 (United States)	BCAT (Japan)	PRODIGE 12 (France)	BILCAP (United Kingdom)
Design	Single-arm phase II	Randomized phase III	Randomized phase III	Randomized phase III
Treatment	Gem + Cape Followed by Cape + RT	Gem vs. Obs	Gem + Ox vs. Obs	Cape vs. Obs
n	79	225	196	440
Cancer type				
iCCA pCCA Gallbladder dCCA	0 48% 32% 20%	0 48% 0 52	45% 8% 19% 28%	19% 28% 18% 35%
R1 (%)	32	11	15	38
+Lymph node (%)	n/a	35	37	54
End point and summary	2 yr. OS 65%; R0 and R1 OS similar at 35 and 34 months, respectively	OS and RFS similar between treatment and control	RFS similar between treatment and control	Per-protocol analysis shows improved OS in treatment group

Gem gemcitabine, *Cape* capecitabine, *RT* radiotherapy, *Obs* observation, *Ox* oxaliplatin, *Cis* cisplatin, *OS* overall survival, *RFS* recurrence-free survival, *R0* microscopically negative resection margin, *R1* microscopically positive resection margin, *SWOG* Southwest Oncology Group, *BCA* Biliary Cancer Adjuvant Trial

ductal adenocarcinoma and comprised 19% of the 428 patients included in this trial. Patients were randomized to chemotherapy vs. observation with the treatment arm further dividing patients into treatment with 5-FU or gemcitabine. While no difference was noted in survival between the two treatment agents, OS for those patients receiving adjuvant chemotherapy was improved (43.1 vs. 35.2 m) though this did not reach statistical significance ($p > 0.25$) [25].

Completed Adjuvant Therapy Trials

SWOG 0809

A prospective, single-arm phase II published in 2015 by the Southwest Oncology Group (SWOG) investigated survival outcomes for patients with resected extrahepatic (perihilar and distal) CCA and adenocarcinoma of the gallbladder. The treatment regimen of the trial included adjuvant gemcitabine with capecitabine followed by radiotherapy to the resection field (54–59.4 Gy) and surrounding nodal basin (45 Gy) with concurrent capecitabine. Of the 79 patients enrolled in the trial (68% extrahepatic CCA, 32% gallbladder), 86% of patients completed the treatment. In addition to disease site, patients were also stratified in the analysis based on the resection margin; 68% of patients had an R0 margin, while 32% had microscopically positive surgical resection margins. Projected 2-year overall survival in the trial was estimated to be 65%; OS varied slightly in the R0 (67%) and R1 (60%) groups. Two-year disease-free survival was also estimated in the study to be 54%. Using the stratification based upon resection margin status, median overall survival was 34 months for patients with R0 resection and 35 months for patients with R1 resection. Factors limiting the study's results include no outcome stratification based on lymphatic metastases status as well as the absence of an observation arm. The aim of the study, however, was investigational and to establish that treatment could improve historical observation survival findings in addition to the tolerability and feasibility of the regimen [26].

BCAT

The Biliary Cancer Adjuvant Trial (BCAT) was a randomized, phase III, multicenter trial completed in Japan that analyzed the effects of adjuvant gemcitabine chemotherapy on survival following curative-intent resection of CCA. With 225 patients included in final analysis, 117 patients (43.6% pCCA, 56.4% dCCA) were randomized to the treatment arm. While the proportion of lymph node metastases in the treatment arm was similar to other trials, BCAT had the lowest R1 rate among adjuvant trials (9.4% in the treatment arm). Of note, this population underwent a somewhat varied range of surgical interventions including pancreaticoduodenectomy (PD), PD along with partial hepatectomy, and excision of the extrahepatic bile duct with bilioenteric anastomosis. In the treatment arm, 3-year OS was 68.1%, while 5-year OS was 51.7%; this did not differ with 3-year (65.7%) or 5-year (51.6%) OS in the observation arm, suggesting no benefit to adjuvant gemcitabine in this population. Given these findings, the trial was terminated following interim analysis. Further subgroup analysis based on pathologic details did not reveal further prognostic stratification factors [27].

PRODIGE 12-ACCORD 18

The PRODIGE 12-ACCORD 18 was a multicenter, phase III study conducted at 33 French centers that compared treatment with gemcitabine and oxaliplatin versus observation alone in resected biliary tract cancers. The goals of the study were to analyze differences in recurrence-free survival and quality of life. The treatment arm of 95 patients included a somewhat higher percentage of patients with resected iCCA compared with other adjuvant trials including a mixture of CCA disease sites. Analysis of the study results demonstrated no difference in RFS between study and treatment arms (median RFS 30.4 months with treatment, 18.5 months observation). While quality of life was not different between the groups, only 33% of patients in the treatment arm were able to complete the entirety of the planned adjuvant chemotherapy regimen with most stopping treatment due to toxicity [28].

BILCAP

The BILCAP, or capecitabine compared with observation in resected biliary tract cancer, study enrolled 447 over 8 years at 44 hepatobiliary surgery centers across the United Kingdom. Patients randomized between the treatment and observation arms comprised a spectrum of disease sites and were well matched between arms of the trial (treatment: iCCA 19%, pCCA 29%, gallbladder 17%, dCCA 34%). Patients were also stratified for lymph node positivity though routine portal lymphadenectomy was not mandated by trial parameters for patients undergoing partial hepatectomy for iCCA. BILCAP's sensitivity analysis was based upon Takada et al. where 2-year OS was 20% [24]; the goal of the BILCAP trial was to evaluate the ability of the intervention to increase this by 12–32% at 2 years after surgery. To achieve this, the initial trial protocol planned to enroll and randomize 360 patients. On data monitoring committee review after the trial had begun, the target recruitment was increased.

Based on the trial's intention-to-treat analysis, differences in OS and recurrence-free survival outcomes did not reach statistical significance (median OS 51.1 vs. 36.4 months, p 0.097). However when excluding the patients (n = 13) who withdrew from treatment, received no adjuvant chemotherapy drug, or were deemed ineligible to continue, the per-protocol analysis of the treatment arm compared with observation cohort demonstrated a significant improvement in median OS (53 vs. 36 months, p 0.028). Along with these survival results, the demonstrated tolerability of oral capecitabine in this study led the authors to suggest this regimen as a standard of care for resected biliary tract cancer [29].

Ongoing Adjuvant Therapy Trials

While the results of these trials would suggest adjuvant chemotherapy with capecitabine as an efficacious and well-tolerated regimen for patients after curative-intent resection for CCA, additional trials are underway to investigate not only combinations of chemotherapeutic agents but also targeted therapies (Table 16.2). A currently enrolling German phase III trial across several European nations (ACTICCA-1) is seeking to explore the potential survival advantage conferred with gemcitabine and cisplatin as compared with observation alone in patients following curative-intent resection of biliary tract cancer [30]. Building upon results seen in the setting of advanced CCA and the administration of palliative chemotherapy [31], this trial's primary goals are DFS and OS at 24 months.

The Japan Clinical Oncology Group (JCOG) is also conducting a phase III trial to compare survival differences between adjuvant S1 and observation following resection of biliary tract cancer. S1 is an oral fluoropyrimidine agent composed of tegafur,

Table 16.2 Characteristics of ongoing adjuvant therapy trials

	ACTICCA (Germany)	ASCOT (Japan)
Design	Randomized phase 3	Randomized phase 3
Treatment	Gem + Cis vs. Obs	S1 vs. Obs
n	440[a]	440[a]
Cancer type iCCA pCCA Gallbladder dCCA	36%[b]	
End point and summary	Primary outcome will be RFS; OS included as a secondary outcome	Primary outcome will be OS; RFS will be a secondary outcome

Gem gemcitabine, *Cape* capecitabine, *RT* radiotherapy, *Obs* observation, *Cis* cisplatin, *OS* overall survival, *RFS* recurrence-free survival, *R1* microscopically-positive resection margin, *ASCOT* Adjuvant S1 for Cholangiocarcinoma Trial

[a]The ACTICCA and ASCOT trials are currently enrolling. In ACTICCA, the goal enrollment to meet power will be 220 patients per arm with 80 patients per arm having adenocarcinoma of the gallbladder and the other 140 patients having either intrahepatic or hilar/distal (extrahepatic, to include hilum) cholangiocarcinoma. The ASCOT trial will include patients with adenocarcinoma of the ampulla of Vater

[b]By trial design, the ACTICCA trial seeks to enroll and follow 140 patients in the treatment arm, 80 (36%) of whom will receive treatment after resection of muscle-invasive adenocarcinoma of the gallbladder. This is a projected proportion; the trial results are not yet published

5-chloro-2,4-dihydroxypyridine, and potassium oxonate. Previous Japanese clinical trials have demonstrated survival benefit of S1 compared with gemcitabine following resection of pancreatic adenocarcinoma [32] and compared with observation following resection of gastric adenocarcinoma [33]. Further, a phase II trial was also conducted in Japan in which 40 patients were treated with S1 in the setting of advanced and unresected CCA [34]. The Adjuvant S1 for Cholangiocarcinoma Trial (ASCOT) is enrolling treatment-naïve patients treated with curative-intent surgery for CCA at all disease sites and including the ampulla of Vater. The initial sample size was 350 patients but was increased to 440 in 2017 to increase the study's power. The primary outcome will be assessment of overall survival and patients will be stratified by disease site as well as based on the presence of margin positivity and positive surgical margins. Secondary outcomes include recurrence-free survival and the occurrence [35].

Adjuvant Therapy Trials: Conclusion

Difficulty in interpreting the results of these clinical trials in part stems from the heterogeneity of the disease sites/subtypes that were included in analysis; with increasing evidence that tumors at different sites in the biliary tract have disparate mutations and molecular profiles, the inclusion of disparate tumor subtypes in order to facilitate timely accrual into a trial tangentially confuses efforts to interpret the results for any single patient whose tumor is broadly described as "CCA." Ongoing and future clinical trials, potentially aided by international collaborative efforts or registries, may be able to focus in on CCA types by location or even by molecular mutational profile. Currently available results of trials analyzing outcomes of adjuvant therapy must be considered in the context of their examined patient population as well as the examined proportion of each tumor type, the microscopically positive resection margin, and lymph node positivity so as to select a treatment regimen that best fits a patient being considered for adjuvant therapy [36, 37]. As we await results from currently enrolling adjuvant therapy trials in Europe and Japan, current recommendations for adjuvant therapy following curative-intent resection include consideration of the results of the BILCAP and SWOG 0809 trials. Adjuvant chemotherapy with capecitabine and the consideration of chemoradiotherapy in the setting of positive resection margin have been incorporated into American Society of Clinical Oncology (ASCO) Guidelines for resected biliary tract cancers [38].

Neoadjuvant Therapy

The concept of neoadjuvant chemotherapy has been applied to CCA at each of its anatomical sites. The most rigorous neoadjuvant therapy protocols have been applied to pCCA patients enrolled in programs considering orthotopic liver transplantation (OLT) as the surgical intervention. The often advanced nature and large size of iCCA place many patients into a risky category that must consider not only the biology of a tumor detected at a large size but also the size, function, and health of a potential liver remnant after curative-intent surgery. Neoadjuvant therapy prior to hepatectomy for iCCA as part of a comprehensive pre-surgical treatment plan potentially addresses multiple facets of surgical resectability: the administration of systemic therapy allows assessment of disease biology and may decrease the size of the lesion, the extent of hepatic resection may be altered, and liver-directed molding therapies can also be used to increase the size of the future liver remnant. While many studies have assessed the effect of chemotherapy regimens on survival when administered in a palliative intent for advanced CCA, others have focused on the utility of neoadjuvant therapy to downstage a tumor to facilitate surgical resection.

Studies assessing the efficacy of palliative-intent chemotherapy typically consider CCA as "advanced disease" when there is evidence of metastases or when the patients are considered surgically unresectable based on anatomical considerations such as vascular involvement by tumor, intrahepatic metastases, or tumor multifocality. Current (2019) National Comprehensive Cancer Network (NCCN) guidelines for the treatment of iCCA suggest surgical resection for lesions considered able to be resected with R0 margin, while those who are considered unresectable should be treated with palliative chemotherapy, radiotherapy, or other arterial-based local-regional therapies [39]. Unlike in pancreatic cancer, the current version of these guidelines does not specifically note a category of "borderline resectability," leaving clinicians to direct the consideration of neoadjuvant therapy with a goal of surgical resection as part of a multidisciplinary approach.

The currently recommended first-line chemotherapy regimen for advanced iCCA is derived from the ABC-02 trial, a phase III, randomized, multicenter trial conducted in the United Kingdom comparing survival outcomes for patients with advanced CCA; the definition for "advanced" included locally advanced/unresectable disease, recurrent disease after previous resection, and metastatic disease. Extending a previous phase II study in which gemcitabine plus cisplatin was compared with gemcitabine alone in this setting with the finding that the combination of agents improved progression-free survival [31, 40], this study included 410 patients with 204 patients receiving the combination of agents while 206 received gemcitabine alone. This study found that median overall survival (11.7 vs. 8.1 months, $p < 0.0001$) and progression-free survival (8.0 vs. 5.0 months, $p < 0.0001$) were both improved by approximately 3 months in the gemcitabine plus cisplatin group as compared with single-agent gemcitabine. The combination therapy was overall well tolerated; an increase in neutropenia was identified in the gemcitabine plus cisplatin group but did not reach statistical significance [31].

While the ABC-02 trial considers the effects of chemotherapy on survival in the setting of advanced disease or patients who are not considered for surgery regardless of response to therapy, other studies have sought to define a role for converting initially unresectable disease (by unknown biology or extent at detection) to surgical resection. A retrospective review of patients undergoing major resection (n = 32, 30.2% major hepatectomy or n = 72, 69.7% PD) for CCA analyzed outcome and stratified patients based on neoadjuvant chemoradiotherapy (n = 27) versus surgery alone (n = 79). The patients in the neoadjuvant group received three cycles of gemcitabine with 50–60Gy of external beam radiation to the tumor bed and regional nodal basin. The most common indications for surgery were dCCA (n = 72, 69.7%) and pCCA (n = 31, 29.2%). While no difference was found in the incidence of adjuvant therapy, the administration of neoadjuvant therapy was associated with improved 3-year resection-free survival (78.3% vs. 56.8%, p 0.0565); the primary site of disease was not associated with any difference in RFS [41]. While this study's outcomes are limited by its retrospective and non-randomized design, this highlights both the potential difficulty in creating a multi-institutional study for borderline-resectable CCA without an explicit and universal definition of borderline disease and the potential benefit for neoadjuvant therapy.

A French hepatobiliary surgery center has published a single-center experience with downstaging initially unresectable iCCA using systemic therapy [42]. Deemed initially unresectable based on portal lymphadenopathy and vascular invasion, 74 patients underwent a median of 6 cycles of varied chemotherapy regimens, the most common of which was gemcitabine plus oxaliplatin in 44 patients. Four patients in the cohort were treated with selective internal radiation therapy (SIRT) as well as systemic therapy to facilitate resection. Of the 74 patients initially considered unresectable, 39 (52.7%) were considered downstaged to facilitate resection, which was performed. There was no difference in additional hepatic molding procedures such as portal vein embolization or in extended resections between the up-front surgical and neoadjuvant therapy groups.

Even after neoadjuvant therapy, R0 resection was accomplished more frequently in the up-front resectable cohort (59 vs. 31%, $p = 0.004$). Recurrence-free survival and median overall survival did not differ in the groups treated with up-front surgery or surgery after downstaging; there was no difference in the frequency of adjuvant chemotherapy delivery. While this trial is limited by its nonrandomized nature and the diverse treatment regimens delivered in the neoadjuvant cohort, it does demonstrate that neoadjuvant therapy can convert select initially unresectable patients to surgical resectability. The demonstration of no improvement or of disease progression while on therapy also selects patients who would not benefit from an extensive resection. The study's findings did demonstrate overall survival benefit for patients who were able to undergo resection as compared with chemotherapy alone, likely reflecting disease biology as well as the benefits of resection and response to systemic therapy. Median overall survival with up-front surgery was 25.7 months as compared to 24.1 months in the surgery after chemotherapy; without surgery, patients receiving chemotherapy alone had a median OS of 7.8 months. The study's multivariate analysis also demonstrated that, at the time of presentation, standard serum studies such as bilirubin, albumin, and CA 19-9 were not predictive of conversion to resectability, suggesting that additional study is needed to identify reliable markers for predicting response in this patient population [42].

While pooled results of mostly nonrandomized studies suggest the feasibility of delivering neoadjuvant chemoradiotherapy to facilitate improvement in R0 resection rate in pCCA and dCCA [43], the absence of a prospective trial – fueled by the lack of consensus guidelines for borderline disease as well as institutional differences in considerations for borderline resectable disease – limits the strength of recommendations for neoadjuvant treatment in the setting of up-front resectable disease though chemotherapy may be given to test disease biology in patients with iCCA. Basing conclusions on the benefits of neoadjuvant therapy by pathologic stage rather than by disease site may also confound the generalizability of results between disease sites [44], again suggesting that the disease sites may have different prognostic factors separate from their designation as "CCA."

Additional work is proceeding to determine the optimal regimen to be used in a neoadjuvant fashion. Using as a standard previous studies identifying the combination of gemcitabine and cisplatin in the setting of advanced CCA [31], alterations in the systemic chemotherapy for advanced or borderline-resectable CCA are being explored as are varying regional treatments. Building upon experience using the combination of gemcitabine, cisplatin, and albumin-bound (nab)-paclitaxel (GAP) for the treatment of pancreatic adenocarcinoma, this chemotherapy regimen was used in a phase II clinical trial for advanced CCA. This cohort of 60 patients receiving treatment included 63% iCCA, 22% adenocarcinoma of the gallbladder, and 15% extrahepatic CCA; 78% had known metastatic disease, while 22% had locally advanced unresectable disease. Compared with historical controls [31], the median progression-free survival in this cohort was 11.8, while median overall survival was 19.2 months [45]. Given these findings, this treatment regimen has now been advanced to a phase III randomized clinical trial being conducted by the Southwest Oncology Group as trial S1815; the control arm will be current standard-of-care systemic therapy, gemcitabine and cisplatin. The use of regimens such as this in resectable but oncologically high-risk disease (regional lymphadenopathy, multifocal disease, elevated tumor markers, etc.) is also being explored. Given the efficacy of the Mayo/MDACC GAP trial and rapid accrual of S1815, we have begun an exploratory pilot study of neoadjuvant GAP for resectable but oncologically high-risk iCCA (large tumors, major vascular invasion, multifocal disease restricted to same lobe, suspicious or positive portal lymph nodes). It is currently enrolling 34 pts across six high-volume institutions with a primary endpoint of feasibility to deliver the regimen and proceed to resection. Secondary outcomes will be recurrence, survival, and toxicity (personal communication).

Additional Therapies

Radiotherapy for Cholangiocarcinoma

The role of radiotherapy in the treatment of CCA is divided based on the specific treatment indication and patient circumstance. Radiotherapy can be delivered after curative-intent surgery (adjuvant radiotherapy), in a neoadjuvant setting prior to planned OLT for perihilar CCA, as selective internal radiotherapy for local control of a locally advanced liver lesion as well as potentially to induce hypertrophy of a planned future liver remnant, or as local control lesions for which definitive surgical resection is not possible or planned, as also discussed elsewhere in this book (Chap. 17, Hessey and Bridgewater).

Following curative-intent resection, multiple retrospective studies suggest a benefit to adjuvant radiotherapy combined with concurrent chemotherapy. This benefit seems to be highlighted in patients with R1 resection, close margins, or lymph node-positive disease [46, 47]. A more recent meta-analysis including over 1400 patients with dCCA and adenocarcinoma of the gallbladder found 5-year overall survival benefit to adjuvant radiotherapy in patients with positive lymph nodes as well as R1 margins; local recurrence was also reduced in patients who received adjuvant RT. [48]

A US multi-institutional single-arm phase II trial demonstrated safety of a regimen consisting of adjuvant gemcitabine and capecitabine followed by conformal external beam radiation therapy (EBRT) with concurrent capecitabine. This trial included patients with resected perihilar and extrahepatic CCA as well as adenocarcinoma of the gallbladder. While no survival differences were noted between patients with R0 and R1 resection margins, overall survival and local control rates were 68% and 87%, respectively, at 2 years after resection. The regimen was overall well-tolerated [26].

Postoperative radiotherapy or radiotherapy delivered with the goal of local control in the setting of advanced or unresectable disease must consider both local control and toxicity to surrounding structures. Radiotherapy is also typically administered as part of a multidisciplinary protocol for patients with early pCCAs who are deemed eligible for OLT. Publications describing complications in these settings typically highlight the local control afforded contrasted with the described side effects of stereotactic body radiotherapy (SBRT) for locally advanced and unresectable tumors. While local control, described as absence of disease progression in the radiated field, may be attainable, duodenal toxicity hemorrhage, duodenal stenosis, biliary stricture distant from the tumor site, and abdominal pain may result from focused high-dose radiotherapy [49–51]. Patients undergoing RT as part of a treatment algorithm with the possibility of resection must also be surveilled for the development of hepatic or distant metastases [50].

Hepatic artery radioembolization (HARE) or selective internal radiotherapy (SIRT) utilizes the tumor-treating effects of microspheres bonded with radiation-emitting isotopes to treat liver tumors from within their microvascular bed. HARE for iCCA is described for multiple indications including for local-regional therapy to downstage an advanced tumor in conjunction with systemic chemotherapy; to treat tumor while also inducing liver remnant hypertrophy; and to provide local control in a palliative setting when no surgical resection is possible based on tumor extent, liver remnant volume, metastatic disease, or patient factors that preclude curative resection [52].

While many small series demonstrate the feasibility of HARE for unresectable iCCA in a palliative approach, the combined use of HARE with systemic cytotoxic chemotherapy has been studied in a multi-institutional phase II clinical trial after initial results from an institutional study demonstrated local tumor control and the ability to decrease tumor volume and achieve R0 resections in a subset of patients [53]. HARE followed by systemic chemotherapy was used to assess disease biology and potentially enhance the resectability of locally advanced iCCA that was chemotherapy naïve. Response was assessed at 3 months after HARE during which time systemic therapy with gemcitabine and cisplatin was being administered. Over this period, disease control (including failure to progress as well as radiographic response) was 98%. Median overall survival was 22 months in this cohort of 41 patients with 22% of patients found to have disease response to therapy that allowed for surgical resection [54]. In a pooled analysis of studies with varying designs, overall survival following HARE for unresectable iCCA was over 15 months. While this is longer than trials treating patients with definitive chemotherapy for advanced iCCA, many of the trials in this pooled analysis included patients who had been and continued to receive systemic therapy after HARE [55].

Liver Transplantation for Cholangiocarcinoma

OLT has been described for patients with early-stage pCCA and is conducted at a few select centers following rigorous systemic and local-regional radiotherapy followed by surveillance. This procedure is considered for patients meeting strict inclusion criteria: unresectable hilar/perihilar tumor with a diameter of <3 cm and the absence of hepatic or systemic metastases; social history, social support, and patient comorbidity as well as oncologic historical factors required for transplant listing in the setting of end-stage liver disease also apply to patients being considered in OLT for pCCA protocols [56]. The pretransplant therapy consists of hilar radiotherapy with concurrent chemosensitization, brachytherapy, and then a period of chemotherapy during a surveillance period prior to listing for OLT [57]. After meeting these initial inclusion criteria and enjoying favorable response to chemotherapy, patients undergoing OLT for pCCA have been found to have disease-free survival of 65–70% [57, 58].

Centers experienced in OLT for pCCA protocols as well as living donor OLT (LDLT) have published results of LDLT for pCCA. The recipients were treated with similar pretransplant therapy including radiation and chemotherapy. Compared to other LDLT patients, those undergoing LDLT for pCCA developed late vascular anastomotic and bilioenteric anastomotic complications than patients undergoing LDLT for other indications. While the vascular complications did not negatively affect survival in the analysis, residual tumor found in the explanted liver did contribute to inferior survival. Overall survival at 5 years in this cohort of patients was 66.5% [59].

Given the positive outcomes following OLT for pCCA, the feasibility of OLT for iCCA has been investigated as a potential treatment option. An initial retrospective study published in 2014 demonstrated through pooling of results from several European centers a 5-year actuarial survival of 73% in patients with known cirrhosis and what was termed "very early" iCCA; these were defined as tumors less than or equaled to 2 cm in diameter [60]. Of the 29 patients included in the study, 4 had tumors found incidentally in the explanted liver. The study also identified factors associated with tumor recurrence, such as size >2 cm, multinodular tumor, vascular invasion, and poor tumor differentiation. This leads the authors to suggest that patients with known lesions meeting these criteria in a setting of cirrhosis may be able to receive OLT and not be excluded based on the presence of an iCCA.

An international follow-up building upon the 2014 study reaffirmed these findings, this time delineating two groups, "very early" iCCA (tumor $\leq$2 cm) and "advanced" iCCA (any tumor greater than 2 cm in size or multinodular). Those in the "very early" group had a 5-year survival of 65% compared with 45% in the advanced group [61]. Additional selection criteria and description of outcomes of OLT for CCA is discussed further in a separate chapter of this book (Chap. 15, Butler and Agopian).

Hepatic Arterial Infusion Pump Therapy

A recent phase II trial conducted at two high-volume hepatobiliary cancer centers has investigated the use of hepatic arterial infusion (HAI) pump therapy with concurrent systemic chemotherapy for the treatment and potential downstaging of locally advanced and unresectable iCCA. The trial enrolled patients whose disease was considered advanced based on extensive vascular or biliary involvement, multifocal disease, regional lymphadenopathy, or a combination of these findings that would preclude curative surgical therapy with negative (R0) margin; patients with regional nodal disease that could be resected at the time of HAI pump placement were allowed to enroll. In the cohort enrolled at the primary site, 47% of patients had resectable regional nodal disease. With a primary outcome of 80% progression-free survival at 6 months, 42 patients were enrolled at the primary site with 38 of these patients receiving the full treatment regimen of floxuridine via HAI and systemic gemcitabine and oxaliplatin. A confirmatory cohort of 10 patients was enrolled at the second center.

Of the 38 patients receiving therapy at the primary center, 58% achieved radiographic partial response to therapy at 6 months, and 84% of patients had radiographic disease stability at 6 months. Of this cohort of 38 patients, 4 (10.5%) were successfully downstaged by this treatment regimen to the extent that curative surgical resection was pursued. In the entire cohort, median progression-free survival was 11.8 months, while median overall survival was 25 months. There was no survival difference noted between patients with and those without regional lymph node metastases at the time of enrollment.

This trial highlights a potential additional treatment strategy for patients with advanced iCCA without distant metastases in centers with HAI pump experience. Additionally, differences in treatment response were noted based on certain tumor genetic mutations. An important inclusion criterion, the inclusion of patients with resectable regional nodal disease, underscores the ability to attain similar survival outcomes in patients with resectable nodal disease in the setting of aggressive systemic and regional therapy [62].

Targeted Therapy

Evaluation of tumor genomics from the anatomical location subtypes of CCA has demonstrated varying patterns of genetic mutations among tumors occurring at different locations in the biliary tract. While not all of these mutations are currently tied to prognosis, some, such as BAP1 and PBRM1 mutations, are associated with a predilection for bone metastases and worse survival in dCCA [63]. Further study, examining differences in genetic mutations among patients with and without fluke-associated CCA, has demonstrated survival differences [64]. Taken in concert with the immune-related factors associated with prognosis and mentioned previously in this chapter [8, 9, 11], the future treatment of CCA may increasingly integrate the use of targeted molecular therapy along with cytotoxic chemotherapy based on tumor-specific mutational profiles. Previous clinical trials combining cytotoxic

Table 16.3 Prevalence of actionable gene mutations identified in iCCA tumors

Gene mutation	Prevalence
IDH1	30%
ARID1A	23%
BAP1	20%
TP53	20%
FGFR2 (fusion/rearrangement)	14%

Adapted from Lowery et al. [67]
IDH1 isocitrate dehydrogenase 1, *BAP1* ubiquitin carboxyl-terminal hydrolase BAP1, *TP53* tumor protein 53, *FGFR2* fibroblast growth factor receptor 2

chemotherapy with targeted agents have yet to demonstrate significant survival or progression differences in patients with advanced disease [65, 66]. These trials did not, however, have patient-specific targeted therapy based on their tumor's unique mutation profiles.

Tumor molecular profiling studies have identified medication-targetable mutations in multiple genes in iCCA, accounting for the finding of actionable target(s) mutations in approximately 50% of patients [67]. Prevalence of common gene mutations in analyzed iCCA is summarized in Table 16.3.

Multiple clinical trials are currently enrolling to investigate epidermal growth factor receptor (EGFR) inhibitors (regorafenib, apatinib), isocitrate dehydrogenase (IDH) and fibroblast growth factor receptor (FGRF) inhibitors (erdafitinib, ponatinib, niraparib), and checkpoint inhibitors (nivolumab, pembrolizumab, durvalumab) in advanced CCA with or without concurrent cytotoxic chemotherapy [63]. MEK pathway inhibitors, BRAF inhibitors, and vascular endothelial growth factor (VEGF) inhibitors have also been investigated [68–70], among others. A summary of targeted agents along with their corresponding gene mutation is provided in Table 16.4. Additional study is also focusing on using targeted therapies to disrupt the tumor micro-environment to facilitate the delivery of convention cytotoxic therapies into tumors that have been previously chemotherapy-resistant as an additional novel approach to deliver available and indication-approved drugs into intrahepatic tumors [71]. Enrolling and active clinical trials have focused on advanced disease and patients with unresectable tumors; further investigation is underway to establish the roles of targeted therapy following curative-intent resection or in the setting of local or systemic disease recurrence.

Additional interest is beginning to focus on determining the role of targeted therapy agents in the neoadjuvant setting for patients with locally advanced, potentially resectable disease or with oncologically high-risk disease, such as in the presence of a multifocal unilobar tumor, portal lymphadenopathy, or high tumor markers. These patients must be completely staged with cross-sectional imaging, and consideration must be given to peritoneal staging to rule out the presence of occult metastatic disease prior to embarking on therapy with neoadjuvant intent. Further study is needed

Table 16.4 Summary of molecular mutations and targeted therapy agents available or currently enrolling in clinical trials for treatment of CCA

NTRK (gene fusion)	Entrectinib Larotrectinib
FGFR1-3 (fusion/rearrangement)	Pembrolizumab Erdafitinib Ponatinib Infigratinib Ganetespib (hsp90 inhibitor)[a]
IDH1	Ivosedinib
IDH2	Enasidenib
HER2	Trastuzumab emtansine
BRCA mutation	Niraparib
ROS1 kinase fusion protein (including *ALK* fusion)	Ceritinib Entrectinib
KRAS mutation	Selumetinib (*MEK* inhibitor)
BRAF	Vemurafenib
MET/EGFR/MAPK	Tivantinib
VEGFR	Ramucirumab
Checkpoint inhibitor therapy	
PD-1	Pembrolizumab Nivolumab Durvalumab
Anti-CTLA-4 antibodies	Ipilimumab Tremelimumab

NTRK neurotrophic tropomyosin-related kinase, *FGFR* fibroblast growth factor receptor, *IDH* isocitrate dehydrogenase, *HER2* human epidermal growth factor receptor 2, *BRCA* breast cancer gene, *ROS* proto-oncogene tyrosine-protein kinase ROS, *ALK* anaplastic lymphoma kinase, *KRAS* Kirsten rat sarcoma viral oncogene homolog, *EGFR* epidermal growth factor receptor, *MAPK* mitogen-activated protein kinase, *VEGFR* vascular endothelial growth factor receptor, *PD-1* programmed death protein 1, *CTLA-4* cytotoxic T-lymphocyte-associated antigen

[a]Ganetespib is an inhibitor of heat-shock protein 90 (hsp90), a downstream modulator of activity in *FGFR2* mutations

to determine the optimal treatment regimen and if targeted therapy will be given along with or in place of cytotoxic agents. Certainly, tissue biopsy with molecular profiling will be needed in these cases in order to best determine treatment regimens; should they include targeted therapy and cytotoxic chemotherapy, regimens must be tailored to account for drug-specific toxicity profiles. A conceptual algorithm incorporating the evaluation components, decision process for neoadjuvant therapy, and additional considerations such as the use of targeted therapy is provided in Fig.16.1. Cases of this complexity should be thoroughly discussed in multidisciplinary format incorporating medical and surgical oncology as well as interventional gastroenterology and radiology perspectives; when modifiable patient risk factors are identified, additional specialists may be included to augment specific prehabilitation programs.

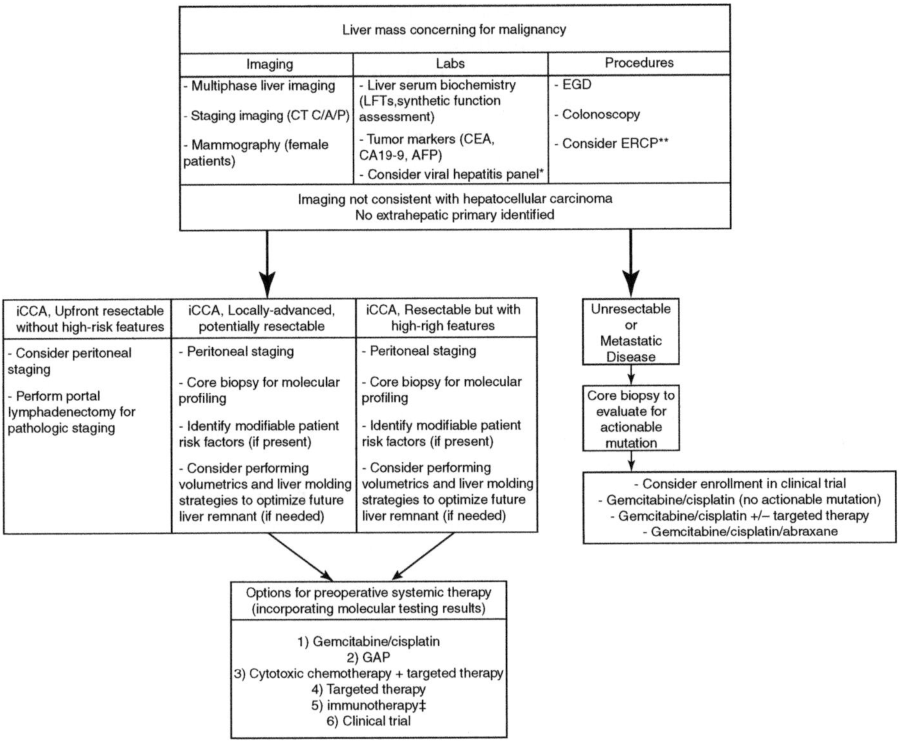

Fig. 16.1 Conceptual treatment flowchart for intrahepatic cholangiocarcinoma incorporating clinical evaluation, staging, and therapeutic options. Abbreviations: CT computed tomography, C/A/P chest/abdomen/pelvis, LFT liver function test, CA19-9 cancer antigen 19-8, AFP α-fetoprotein, EGD esophagogastroduodenoscopy, ERCP endoscopic retrograde cholangiopancreatography, iCCA intrahepatic cholangiocarcinoma, GAP gemcitabine/abraxane/nab-paclitaxel. * Viral hepatitis serology may be considered in patients with known chronic liver disease or in those with concern for exposure to viral hepatitis; ** ERCP may be considered to obtain biopsy if there is a significant intraductal component or for therapeutic purposes should a future liver remnant need to be decompressed prior to initiation of systemic therapy or surgery, when planned; ‡ Immunotherapy is currently indicated for tumors with an identified elevated mutation burden or in cases with identified mismatch repair (MMR) defects

Conclusions

The treatment of CCA has evolved from a strategy based largely upon disease location to one that incorporates tumor- and patient-specific biological considerations. Collaborative efforts and clinical trials are providing data to guide treatment options as well as to identify patient and disease risk factors that suggest when and which patients may benefit from neoadjuvant-intent therapy. For patients with advanced disease, the incorporation of recently developed therapies may lead to improvements over historical survival data derived from trials analyzing palliative therapies. As insights from ongoing trials are gained, the treatment landscape for CCA is likely to continue to evolve to include multidrug regimens, targeted therapies, and regional therapies. The widespread use of molecular profiling of tumors is also expanding our knowledge of this disease process and further argues for an individualized, multidisciplinary approach to care for these patients.

References

1. Rizvi S, Khan SA, Hallemeier CL, et al. Cholangiocarcinoma – evolving concepts and therapeutic strategies. Nat Rev Clin Oncol. 2018;15(2):95–111.
2. Nakeeb A, et al. Cholangiocarcinoma A spectrum of intrahepatic, perihilar, and distal tumors. Ann Surg. 1996;224:463–73.
3. Khan SA, Emadossadaty S, Ladep ND, et al. Rising trends in cholangiocarcinoma: is the ICD classification system misleading us? J Hepatol. 2012;56:848–54.
4. Jarnagin WR, Fong Y, DeMatteo RP, et al. Staging, resectability, and outcome in 225 patients with hilar cholangiocarcinoma. Ann Surg. 2001;234:507–17.
5. https://riskcalculator.facs.org/RiskCalculator/.
6. Moro A, Paredes AZ, Farooq A, et al. Discordance in prediction of prognosis among patients with intrahepatic cholangiocarcinoma: a preoperative vs postoperative perspective. J Surg Oncol. 2019;120(6):946–55.
7. de Jong MC, Nathan H, Sotiropoulos GC, et al. Intrahepatic cholangiocarcinoma: an international multi-institutional analysis of prognostic factors and lymph node assessment. J Clin Oncol. 2011;29:3140–5.
8. Dhanasekaran R, Hemming AW, Zendejas I, et al. Treatment outcomes and prognostic factors of intrahepatic cholangiocarcinoma. Oncol Rep. 2013;29:1259–67.
9. Murakami Y, Uemura K, Sudo T, et al. Prognostic factors after surgical resection for intrahepatic, hilar, and distal cholangiocarcinoma. Ann Surg Oncol. 2011;18:651–8.
10. Guglielmi A, Ruzzenente A, Campagnaro T, et al. Intrahepatic cholangiocarcinoma: prognostic factors after surgical resection. World J Surg. 2009;33:1247–54.
11. Mano Y, Shirabe K, Yamashita Y, et al. Preoperative neutrophil-to-lymphocyte ratio is a predictor of survival after hepatectomy for hepatocellular carcinoma: a retrospective analysis. Ann Surg. 2013;258:301–5.
12. Malik HZ, Prasad KR, Halazun KJ, et al. Preoperative prognostic score for predicting survival after hepatic resection for colorectal liver metastases. Ann Surg. 2007;246:806–14.
13. Halazun KJ, Aldoori A, Malik HZ, et al. Elevated preoperative neutrophil to lymphocyte ratio predicts survival following hepatic resection for colorectal liver metastases. Eur J Surg Oncol. 2008;34:55–60.
14. Buettner S, Spolverato G, Kimbrough CW, et al. The impact of neutrophil-to-lymphocyte ratio and platelet-to-lymphocyte ratio among patients with intrahepatic cholangiocarcinoma. Surgery. 2018;164:411–8.
15. Omichi K, Cloyd JM, Yamashita S, et al. Neutrophil-to-lymphocyte ratio predicts prognosis after neoadjuvant chemotherapy and resection of intrahepatic cholangiocarcinoma. Surgery. 2017;164(2):752–65.
16. Shinke G, Yamada D, Eguchi H, et al. The postoperative peak number of leukocytes after hepatectomy is a significant prognostic factor for cholangiocarcinoma. Mol Clin Oncol. 2019;10(5):531–40.

17. Tsilimigras DI, Hyer JM, Moris D, et al. Prognostic utility of albumin-bilirubin grade for short- and long-term outcomes following hepatic resection for intrahepatic cholangiocarcinoma: a multi-institutional analysis of 706 patients. J Surg Oncol. 2019;120(2):206–13.
18. Sahara K, Tsilimigras DI, Metha R, et al. A novel online prognostic tool to predict long-term survival after liver resection for intrahepatic cholangiocarcinoma: the "metro-ticket" paradigm. J Surg Oncol. 2019;120(2):223–30.
19. Tsilimigras DI, Mehta R, Moris D, et al. A machine-based approach to preoperatively identify patients with the most and least benefit associated with resection for intrahepatic cholangiocarcinoma: an international multi-institutional analysis of 1146 patients. Ann Surg Oncol. 2019. https://doi.org/10.1245/s10434-019-08067-3.
20. Belkouz A, Labeur TA, Dierks J, et al. Prognostic immunohistochemical biomarkers of chemotherapy efficacy in biliary tract cancer: a systematic review and meta-analysis. Crit Rev Oncol Hematol. 2019;141:82–94.
21. Salati M, Caputo F, Cunningham D, et al. The A.L.A.N. score identifies prognostic classes in advanced biliary cancer patients receiving first-line chemotherapy. Eur J Cancer. 2019;117:84–90.
22. Salati M, Filippi R, Vivaldi C, et al. The prognostic nutritional index predicts survival and response to first-line chemotherapy in advanced biliary cancer. Liver Int. 2019. https://doi.org/10.1111/liv.14314.
23. Song BG, Kim HS, Kim K, et al. Prognosis and prognostic factors in patients with advanced biliary tract cancer depending on its anatomical location. Scand J Gastroenterol. 2019;54(6):740–5.
24. Takada T, Amano H, Yasuda H, et al. Is postoperative adjuvant chemotherapy useful for gallbladder carcinoma? A phase III multicenter prospective randomized controlled trial in patients with resected pancreaticobiliary carcinoma. Cancer. 2002;95(8):1685–95.
25. Neoptolemos JP, Moore MJ, Cox TF, et al. Effect of adjuvant chemotherapy with fluorouracil plus folinic acid or gemcitabine vs observation on survival in patients with resected periampullary adenocarcinoma, the ESPAC-3 periampullary cancer randomized trial. JAMA. 2012;308(2):147–56.
26. Ben-Josef E, Guthrie KA, El-Khoueiry AB, et al. SWOG 0809: a phase II intergroup trial of adjuvant capecitabine and gemcitabine followed by radiotherapy and concurrent capecitabine in extrahepatic cholangiocarcinoma and gallbladder carcinoma. J Clin Oncol. 2015;33(24):2617–23.
27. Ebata T, Hirano S, Konishi M, et al. Randomized clinical trial of adjuvant gemcitabine chemotherapy *versus* observation in resected bile duct cancer. Br J Surg. 2018;105:192–202.
28. Edeline J, Benabdelghani M, Bertaut A, et al. Gemcitabine and oxaliplatin chemotherapy or surveillance in resected biliary tract cancer (PRODIGE 12-ACCORD 18-UNICANCER GI): a randomized phase III study. J Clin Oncol. 2019;37(8):658–67.
29. Primrose JN, Fox RP, Palmer DH, et al. Capecitabine compared with observation in resected biliary tract cancer (BILCAP): a randomized, controlled, multicenter, phase 3 study. Lancet Oncol. 2019;20:663–73.
30. Stein A, Arnold D, Bridgewater J, et al. Adjuvant chemotherapy with gemcitabine and cisplatin compared to observation after curative intent resection of cholangiocarcinoma and muscle invasive gallbladder carcinoma (ACTICCA-1 trial) – a randomized, multidisciplinary, multinational phase III trial. BMC Cancer. 2015;15:564.
31. Valle J, Wasan H, Palmer DH, et al. Cisplatin plus gemcitabine versus gemcitabine for biliary tract cancer. N Engl J Med. 2010;362(14):1273–81.
32. Uesaka K, Boku N, Fukutomi A, et al. Adjuvant chemotherapy of S-1 versus gemcitabine for resected pancreatic cancer: a phase 3, open-label, randomised, non-inferiority trial (JASPAC 01). Lancet. 2016;388:248–57.
33. Sakuramoto S, Sasako M, Yamaguchi T, et al. Adjuvant chemotherapy for gastric cancer with S-1, an oral fluoropyrimidine. N Engl J Med. 2007;357:1810–20.

34. Furuse J, Okusaka T, Boku N, et al. S-1 monotherapy as first-line treatment in patients with advanced biliary tract cancer: a multicenter phase II study. Cancer Chemother Pharmacol. 2008;62:849–55.
35. Nakachi K, Konishi M, Ikeda M, et al. A randomized phase III trial of adjuvant S-1 therapy vs. observation alone in resected biliary tract cancer: Japan Clinical Oncology Group Study (JCOG1202, ASCOT). Jpn J Clin Oncol. 2018;48(4):392–5.
36. Horgan AM, Knox JJ. Adjuvant therapy for biliary tract cancers. J Oncol Pract. 2018;14(12):701–8.
37. Cloyd JM, Pawlik TM. Adjuvant therapy for biliary tract cancers: new evidence to resolve old questions. J Clin Oncol. 2018;14(12):723–4.
38. Shroff RT, Kennedy EB, Bachini M, et al. Adjuvant therapy for resected biliary tract cancer: ASCO clinical practice guideline. J Clin Oncol. 2019;37(12):1015–27.
39. National Comprehensive Cancer Network (NCCN). NCCN clinical practice guidelines in oncology. https://www.nccn.org/professionals/physician_gls/default.aspx. Accessed on 26 Feb.
40. Valle JW, Wasan H, Johnson P, et al. Gemcitabine alone or in combination with cisplatin in patients with advanced or metastatic cholangiocarcinomas or other biliary tract tumours: a multicentre randomised phase II study – The UK ABC-01 Study. Br J Cancer. 2009;101(4):621–7.
41. Kobayashi S, Tomokuni A, Gotoh K, et al. A retrospective analysis of the clinical effects of neoadjuvant combination therapy with full-dose gemcitabine and radiation therapy in patients with biliary tract cancer. Eur J Surg Oncol. 2017;43:763–71.
42. Le Roy B, Gelli M, Pittau G, et al. Neoadjuvant chemotherapy for initially unresectable intrahepatic cholangiocarcinoma. Br J Surg. 2018;105:839–47.
43. Frosio F, Mocchegiani F, Conte G, et al. Neoadjuvant therapy in the treatment of hilar cholangiocarcinoma: review of the literature. World J Gastrointest Surg. 2019;11(6):279–86.
44. Yadav S, Xie H, Bin-Riaz I, et al. Neoadjuvant vs. adjuvant chemotherapy for cholangiocarcinoma: a propensity score matched analysis. Eur J Surg Oncol. 2019;45(8):1432–8.
45. Shroff RT, Javle MM, Xiao L, et al. Gemcitabine, cisplatin, and nab-paclitaxel for the treatment of advanced biliary tract cancers a phase 2 clinical trial. JAMA Oncol. 2019;5(6):824–30.
46. Hammad AY, Berger NG, Eastwood D, et al. Is radiotherapy warranted following intrahepatic cholangiocarcinoma resection? The impact of surgical margins and lymph node status on survival. Ann Surg Oncol. 2016;23:912–20.
47. Jia AY, Wu JX, Zhao YT, et al. Intensity-modulated radiotherapy following null-margin resection is associated with improved survival in the treatment of intrahepatic cholangiocarcinoma. J Gastrointest Oncol. 2015;6:126–33.
48. Ren B, Guo Q, Liu L, et al. A meta-analysis of the efficacy of postoperative adjuvant radiotherapy versus no radiotherapy for extrahepatic cholangiocarcinoma and gallbladder carcinoma. Radiat Oncol. 2020;15(1):15.
49. Barney BM, Olivier KR, Miller RC, Haddock MG. Clinical outcomes and toxicity using stereotactic body radiotherapy (SBRT) for advanced cholangiocarcinoma. Radiat Oncol. 2012;7:67.
50. Kozak MM, Toesca DAS, von Eyben R, Pollom EL, Chang DT. Stereotactic body radiation therapy for cholangiocarcinoma: optimizing locoregional control with elective nodal irradiation. Adv Radiat Oncol. 2019;5(1):77–84.
51. Sandler KA, Veruttipong D, Agopian VG, et al. Stereotactic body radiotherapy (SBRT) for locally advanced extrahepatic and intrahepatic cholangiocarcinoma. Adv Radiat Oncol. 2016;1:237–43.
52. Riaz A, Kulik LM, Mulcahy MF, Lewandowski RJ, Salem R. Yttrium-90 radioembolization in the management of liver malignancies. Semin Oncol. 2010;37(2):94–101.
53. Rayar M, Sulpice L, Edeline J, et al. Intra-arterial yttrium-90 radioembolization combined with systemic chemotherapy is a promising method for downstaging unresectable huge intrahepatic cholangiocarcinoma to surgical treatment. Ann Surg Oncol. 2015;22:3102–8.

54. Edeline J, Touchefeu Y, Guiu B, et al. Radioembolization plus chemotherapy for first-line treatment of locally advanced intrahepatic cholangiocarcinoma: a phase two clinical trial. JAMA Oncol. 2019. https://doi.org/10.1001/jamaoncol.2019.3702.
55. Al-Adra DP, Gill RS, Axford SJ, et al. Treatment of unresectable intrahepatic cholangiocarcinoma with yttrium-90 radioembolization: a systematic review and pooled analysis. Eur J Surg Oncol. 2015;41(1):120–7.
56. Rosen CB, Heimbach JK, Gores GJ. Liver transplantation for cholangiocarcinoma. Transpl Int. 2010;23:692–7.
57. Darwish Murad S, et al. Efficacy of neoadjuvant chemoradiation, followed by liver transplantation, for perihilar cholangiocarcinoma at 12 US centers. Gastroenterology. 2012;143:88–98.
58. Zamora-Valdes D, Heimbach JK. Liver transplant for cholangiocarcinoma. Gastroenterol Clin N Am. 2018;47(2):267–80.
59. Tan EK, Rosen CB, Heimbach JK, et al. Living donor liver transplantation for perihilar cholangiocarcinoma: outcomes and complication. J Am Coll Surg. 2020. https://doi.org/10.1016/j.jamcollsurg.2019.12.037.
60. Sapisochin G, Rodriguez de Lope C, Gastaca M, et al. "Very early" intrahepatic cholangiocarcinoma in cirrhotic patients: should liver transplantation be reconsidered in these patients? Am J Transplant. 2014;14:660–7.
61. Sapisochin G, Facciuto M, Rubbia-Brandt L, et al. Liver transplantation for "very early" intrahepatic cholangiocarcinoma: international retrospective study supporting a prospective assessment. Hepatology. 2016;64:1178–88.
62. Cercek A, Boerner T, Tan B, et al. Assessment of hepatic arterial infusion of floxuridine in combination with systemic gemcitabine and oxaliplatin in patients with unresectable intrahepatic cholangiocarcinoma: a phase 2 clinical trial. JAMA Oncol. 2020;6(1):60–7.
63. Saeed A, Park R, Al-Jumayli M, Al-Rajabi R, Weijing S. Biologics, immunotherapy, and future directions in the treatment of advanced cholangiocarcinoma. Clin Colorectal Cancer. 2019;18(2):81–90.
64. Jusakul A, Cutcutache I, Yong CH, et al. Whole-genome and epigenetic landscapes of etiologically-distinct subtypes of cholangiocarcinoma. Cancer Discov. 2017;7:1116–35.
65. Lee J, Park SH, Chang HM, et al. Gemcitabine and oxaliplatin with or without erlotinib in advanced biliary-tract cancer: a multicenter, open-label, randomized, phase 3 study. Lancet Oncol. 2012;13(2):181–8.
66. Malka D, Cervera P, Foulon S, et al. Gemcitabine and oxaliplatin with or without cetuximab in advanced biliary-tract cancer (BINGO): a randomised, open-label, non-comparative phase 2 trial. Lancet Oncol. 2014;15(8):819–28.
67. Lowery MA, Ptashkin R, Joradn E, et al. Comprehensive molecular profiling of intrahepatic and extrahepatic cholangiocarcinomas: potential targets for intervention. Clin Cancer Res. 2018;24:4154–61.
68. El-Khoueiry AB, Rankin CJ, Ben-Josef E, et al. SWOG 0514: a phase II study of sorafenib in patients with unresectable or metastatic gallbladder carcinoma and cholangiocarcinoma. Investig New Drugs. 2012;30:1646–51.
69. Hyman DM, Puzanov I, Subbiah V, et al. Vemurafenib in multiple nonmelanoma cancers with BRAF V600 mutations. N Engl J Med. 2015;373:726–36.
70. Bekaii-Saab T, Phelps MA, Li X, et al. Multi-institutional phase II study of selumetinib in patients with metastatic biliary cancers. J Clin Oncol. 2011;29:2357–63.
71. Yamanaka T, Harimoto N, Yokobori T, et al. Nintedanib inhibits intrahepatic cholangiocarcinoma aggressiveness via suppression of cytokines extracted from activated cancer-associated fibroblasts. Br J Cancer. 2020. https://doi.org/10.1038/s41416-020-0744-7.

Chapter 17
Palliative Chemotherapy and Radiotherapy for Cholangiocarcinoma

Sonya Hessey and John Bridgewater

Abbreviations

BTCs	biliary tract cancers
CI	confidence interval
EBRT	external beam radiotherapy
ECOG	Eastern Cooperative Oncology Group
EGFR	Epidermal growth factor receptor
FOLFIRINOX	5-fluorouracil, leucovorin, oxaliplatin, and irinotecan
5-FU	fluorouracil
GemCis	gemcitabine plus cisplatin
Gem-S1	gemcitabine plus S1
Gy	grey
HR	hazard ratio
ILBT	Intraluminal brachytherapy
MER	merestinib
mFOLFOX	leucovorin, fluorouracil plus oxaliplatin
mGemOx	modified gemcitabine plus oxaliplatin
OS	overall survival
P	p-value
PBT	proton beam therapy
PFS	progression-free survival
PS	performance status
QoL	quality of life

S. Hessey (✉)
Department of Medical Oncology, University College London Hospital, London, UK
e-mail: sonya.hessey2@nhs.net

J. Bridgewater
Department of Medical Oncology, University College London Cancer Institute, London, UK
e-mail: j.bridgewater@ucl.ac.uk

J. H. Tabibian (ed.), *Diagnosis and Management of Cholangiocarcinoma*,
https://doi.org/10.1007/978-3-030-70936-5_17

RAM ramucirumab
SBRT stereotactic body radiotherapy
SEER US Surveillance, Epidemiology, and End Results
SIRT selective internal radiotherapy
VEGF vascular endothelial growth factor

Introduction

Biliary tract cancers (BTCs) are a heterogenous group including cholangiocarcinoma (intrahepatic, hilar, and extrahepatic subtypes), gallbladder carcinoma, and ampullary carcinoma. Their relative rarity leads to BTCs often being pooled in clinical studies in order to achieve sufficient sample sizes. The phase III clinical trials that currently guide practice are no exception; consequently, this chapter describes the management of BTCs. Cholangiocarcinoma-specific data will be emphasized where available.

The majority of BTCs present in an advanced stage of disease owing to late onset or absence of symptoms and aggressive tumour biology. "Advanced" in this context describes distinct disease patterns: locally advanced and metastatic, which are unified by being unresectable at presentation and therefore incurable. The term may also refer to patients who have had surgery but then relapsed with local or metastatic disease or who have had incomplete resection of their disease, although "relapsed" is preferred.

Systemic chemotherapy is the mainstay of management in all of these scenarios. It is administered with palliative intentions: to lessen symptoms, improve quality of life (QoL), and prolong life. Without treatment, the median overall survival (OS) of patients with BTCs is poor, approximately 4 months [1–3].

The first section of this chapter summarizes the evidence that supports the use of chemotherapy as the first-line treatment for advanced BTCs. It also reviews the emerging remit of second-line chemotherapy. Section two of this chapter provides an overview of the evidence for radiotherapy in the management of advanced BTCs, which remains relatively undefined. Figure 17.1 illustrates a summary schematic of the treatment strategy for advanced BTCs as discussed in this chapter.

Palliative Chemotherapy for Advanced BTCs

Two decades ago, it was clear that treatment with systemic chemotherapy improved survival in BTCs compared to best supportive care [1, 3], but evidence favouring one agent over another was sparse. A systematic review published in 2007 identified 104 studies evaluating chemotherapy for advanced BTCs, of which only 3 were randomized controlled trials, each with a small sample size. Their pooled analysis suggested that chemotherapy with gemcitabine alone, fluorouracil alone, or either in combination with a platinum agent yielded the best response rates [4].

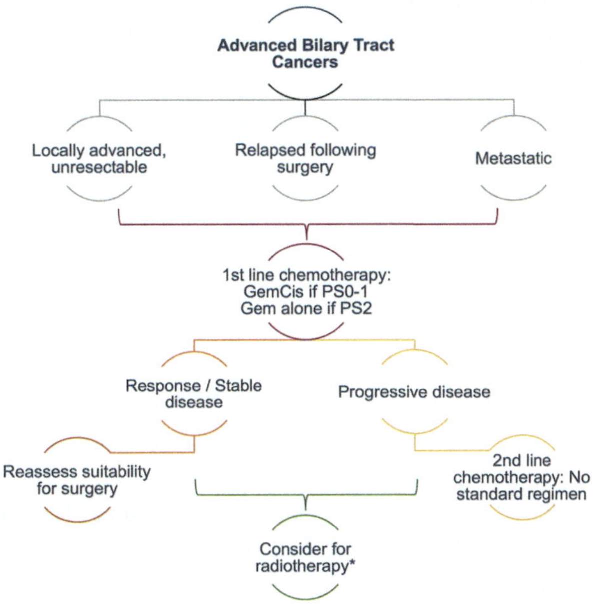

Fig. 17.1 Treatment algorithm for advanced BTCs. Gem gemcitabine, Cis cisplatin. *Low-level evidence: the precise timing, disease setting, and modality of radiotherapy to use remains uncertain

First-Line Systemic Chemotherapy

The Advanced Biliary Tract Cancer (ABC)-02 study was a large, UK-based phase III randomized trial that compared gemcitabine in combination with cisplatin (GemCis) to gemcitabine alone in patients with locally advanced or metastatic BTCs. It was an extension of the ABC-01 phase II randomized trial which demonstrated an improvement in 6-month progression-free survival (PFS) with GemCis over gemcitabine alone [5]. In total, 410 patients were recruited: 242 cholangiocarcinoma (80 intrahepatic, 73 extrahepatic, 57 hilar), 148 gallbladder, and 20 ampullary cancers [6]. As depicted in Fig. 17.2, a statistically significant improvement in median OS was observed with GemCis (11.7 months) compared to gemcitabine alone (8.1 months, hazard ratio [HR] 0.64, 95% confidence interval [CI] 0.52–0.80). The median PFS was also significantly improved in the combination arm (8.0 vs 5.0 months, HR 0.63, 95% CI 0.51–0.77) [6].

At the same time, a parallel study, Biliary Tract (BT) 22 ($n = 83$), was underway in Japan. Using an identical treatment regimen, the BT22 study demonstrated that GemCis improved median OS compared to gemcitabine alone (11.2 vs 7.7 months, respectively, HR 0.69, 95% CI 0.42–1.13) [7]. The outcome data were strikingly consistent to those reported in ABC-02.

To achieve greater statistical power in the evaluation of the treatment effect, the UK and Japanese investigators performed a meta-analysis of the two trials. Confirming prior findings, compared with gemcitabine alone, the GemCis combination was associated with a significant improvement in median PFS and OS [8].

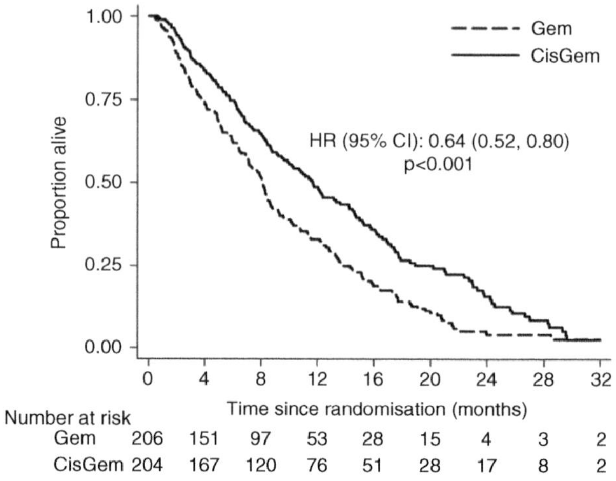

Fig. 17.2 Kaplan–Meier survival curve from the ABC-02 trial demonstrating overall survival in patients with advanced BTCs who received gemcitabine plus cisplatin (solid line) versus gemcitabine alone (dotted line). (Adapted from John Bridgewater's 2009 presentation of the ABC-02 data)

Based on this level 1 evidence, gemcitabine (1000 mg/m^2) and cisplatin (25 mg/m^2), each on days 1 and 8 of a 21-day regimen, became the standard of care for patients with locally advanced, unresectable, or metastatic BTCs [9].

Tolerability

Toxicity

Common adverse effects of GemCis include haematologic toxicity, liver injury, fatigue, nausea, vomiting, alopecia, anorexia, impaired renal function, thromboembolism, and infection. In the ABC-02 trial, there was a non-significant increase in neutropenia in patients treated with GemCis, but the number of infections was similar in the two groups. Liver enzyme levels were more frequently deranged in the gemcitabine alone group (27.1%) compared to the GemCis group (16.7%), likely owing to better disease control in the latter [6].

Quality of Life

The modest survival benefit achieved with GemCis and poor overall prognosis of patients with advanced BTCs warrant careful consideration of the impact of this treatment on QoL. A follow-up study examined the QoL of 324 patients enrolled in the ABC-02 trial before, during, and after their treatment using validated QoL questionnaires. Patients who received GemCis had more favourable scores on scales relating to digestive symptoms, global health, social functioning, appetite loss, financial difficulties, insomnia, and satisfaction with health-care compared to patients who received gemcitabine alone, although statistical significance was not reached. Improved survival outcome was associated with better scores in global health, role functioning, physical functioning, and sexual functioning parameters [10].

Specific Considerations

BTC Subtype

Molecular profiling studies demonstrate significant genetic heterogeneity between BTCs according to their anatomical subtype. Intrahepatic cholangiocarcinoma, in particular, is a distinct entity [11]. Subgroup and post hoc analyses of the ABC trial patients have been performed to investigate the potential differences in response to GemCis chemotherapy between BTC subtypes. No significant difference in PFS or OS was identified between patients with cholangiocarcinoma (all subtypes) and gallbladder or ampullary carcinomas [10].

Among patients who received GemCis, those with intrahepatic cholangiocarcinoma had a longer median OS (15.4 months) compared to all other BTCs (11.7 months, HR 0.72, 95%CI 0.53–0.98, $p = 0.04$). The authors attribute this observation to a difference natural history rather than a better response to palliative chemotherapy [12].

Performance Status

The Eastern Cooperative Oncology Group (ECOG) Scale of Performance Status (PS) is an indicator of a patient's functional level. Ranked on a scale from 0 to 5, PS 0 is fully active, PS 1 is restricted in strenuous activity, PS 2 is ambulatory and self-caring but unable to work, PS 3 is limited ability to self-care, PS 4 is completely disabled, and PS 5 is dead. The ABC-02 trial included patients with PS between 0 and 2. Higher PS was associated with poorer survival in the ABC-02 patients (PS 2, HR: 2.35; 95% CI: 1.68–3.28, $P < 0.001$) [10].

Importantly, patients with a good PS (0–1) appear to derive greater benefit from GemCis combination chemotherapy than patients who are PS 2. A subgroup analysis showed that median OS of patients who were PS 2 was not significantly different between the combination and monotherapy arms (HR 0.88, 95% CI 0.50–1.56) [8]. Hence, it is preferable to consider gemcitabine monotherapy in these patients [9].

Alternative Gemcitabine-Based Regimens

Prior to 2010, when GemCis was established as the first-line standard of care, several chemotherapy regimens were used to treat advanced BTCs. During this time, small, early-phase trials suggested fluoropyrimidines have efficacy against BTCs [4]. This data, as well as the relative comparability of platinum agents, provides rationale for conducting trials evaluating the following combinations.

Gemcitabine Plus S1

S1 is an oral fluoropyrimidine used in gastrointestinal malignancies. FUGA-BT was a Japanese phase III non-inferiority study ($n = 354$) comparing first-line gemcitabine plus S1 (Gem-S1) to the standard of care GemCis for patients with advanced or recurrent BTCs in terms of OS. Gem-S1 was non-inferior to GemCis; median PFS (6.8 vs 5.8 months) and median OS (13.4 vs 15.1 months, respectively, HR 0.945, 90% CI

0.78–1.15, $p = 0.046$ for non-inferiority). There was also no significant difference in the rate of adverse events between the arms (29.9% in Gem-S1, 35.1% in GemCis) [13]. Gem-S1, therefore, is considered an alternative standard of care option. It is predominantly used in Asian countries for patients with advanced or recurrent BTCs.

Gemcitabine Plus Oxaliplatin
Oxaliplatin is an alternative platinum agent to cisplatin which is less ototoxic and less nephrotoxic. Prior to the publication of ABC-02, a single-arm phase II study demonstrated that first-line gemcitabine plus oxaliplatin (GemOx) achieved a median PFS of 3.4 months and median OS of 8.8 months in patients with advanced BTCs [14]. A recent phase III trial conducted in India in patients with advanced gallbladder cancer ($n = 260$) compared first-line modified GemOx (mGemOx) to GemCis. The doses of gemcitabine and oxaliplatin are both lower in the modified regimen compared to the standard GemOx regimen. Median OS was not significantly different between the groups: 9 months in the mGemOx arm and 8.3 months in CisGem arm (HR 0.78, 95% CI 0.60–1.01). Thrombocytopenia and neuropathy were more common in the mGemOx arm, and renal dysfunction was more common in the GemCis arm, in keeping with the known toxicity profiles of the agents [15]. No non-inferiority analysis was performed. This trial did not include any patients with cholangiocarcinoma, limiting its generalizability to management of BTCs in Western countries. Nonetheless, the activity of GemOx is likely to be similar to GemCis; thus GemOx could be considered if a patient was unable to receive cisplatin.

A Fluoropyrimidine Instead of Gemcitabine
Capecitabine is the oral prodrug of the fluoropyrimidine fluorouracil (5-FU). Capecitabine plus oxaliplatin (CapOx) is a well-tolerated combination used in gastric and colorectal malignancies. A phase III non-inferiority trial conducted in South Korea ($n = 222$) investigated the efficacy of CapOx versus GemOx as first-line therapy for advanced BTCs [16]. The median PFS was 5.3 months for the GemOx group and 5.8 months for the CapOx group, meeting their criteria for non-inferiority. There was additionally no difference in OS. While the authors concluded that CapOx is an alternative first-line treatment for advanced BCTs, this has not been widely adopted into our practice.

Adding Targeted Therapies to Chemotherapy

The increased understanding of the molecular basis of BTCs has identified multiple new candidate targeted therapies which are under investigation [11]. To date, the addition of targeted agents to standard of care chemotherapy has not added clinical benefit. While the chapter on targeted therapies will discuss these agents in more depth (Chap. 21, Shroff et al.), the following trials are highlighted because they uphold GemCis as the standard of care.

BINGO was a phase II, open-label trial ($n = 150$) performed in France and Germany that investigated the addition of cetuximab to GemOx for patients with advanced BTCs. Epidermal growth factor receptor (EGFR) signalling regulates biliary epithelial cell growth and proliferation. It is overexpressed in 67–100% of BTCs, hence the rationale for using the EGFR inhibitor cetuximab. The addition of cetuximab to GemOx did not improve PFS or OS. KRAS, BRAF, and EGFR statuses were not associated with patient outcome and did not predict response to treatment [17]. Of note, the median PFS and OS in the GemOx control arm was similar to that achieved by GemCis in ABC-02.

ABC-03 was a phase II trial ($n = 124$) that assessed the effect of adding cediranib to GemCis on PFS in patients with advanced BTCs. Cediranib is a potent oral inhibitor of vascular endothelial growth factor (VEGF) receptors 1, 2, and 3. VEGF is a key regulator of angiogenesis. It is overexpressed in 40–75% of BTCs, and overexpression has been associated with unfavourable clinical phenotypes. There was no significant difference in PFS of patients who received cediranib compared to those who received placebo. Moreover, patients who received cediranib had more grade 3-4 toxicities [18].

A recent phase II placebo-controlled trial ($n = 309$) evaluated the addition of ramucirumab (RAM) or merestinib (MER) to standard of care GemCis chemotherapy. RAM is a VEGF receptor 2 inhibitor and MER inhibits MET, a member of an oncogenic pathway frequently dysregulated in tumours including BTCs. Preliminary results presented in abstract form report that the addition of RAM or MER to GemCis did not improve PFS or OS. Treatment was well tolerated, with safety profiles consistent with known profiles for RAM, MER, and GemCis [19].

The rarity and heterogeneity of BTCs as well as their late presentation and poor prognosis pose challenges to studying targeted therapies in this patient group. Trials that include molecular stratification strategies may help establish the as yet undefined role of targeted therapies in BTC management. For now, combination chemotherapy remains the standard of care.

First-Line Triplet Chemotherapy

The triplet combination of 5-fluorouracil, leucovorin, oxaliplatin, and irinotecan (FOLFIRINOX) was approved as a first-line treatment option for advanced pancreatic cancer after it was shown to significantly improve PFS and OS [20]. BTCs have some histological, biological, and therapeutic similarities to pancreatic cancer, providing rationale for assessing this regimen in patients with BTCs. A single-arm phase II trial evaluating FOLFIRINOX as salvage treatment for patients with progressive disease or excessive toxicity following three or more cycles of GemCis suggests that it can be administered safely in this setting [21]. AMEBICA was a phase II/III randomized trial comparing FOLFIRINOX to GemCis in patients with advanced BTCs that aimed to set a new first-line standard of care [22]. However, the phase II results did not meet the PFS threshold required to proceed to phase III.

Nanoparticle albumin-bound (nab)-paclitaxel used in combination with gemcitabine is an alternative first-line treatment for advanced pancreatic cancer [23].

Following the same logic as with FOLFIRINOX, a phase II open-label single-arm trial ($n = 60$) was set up to evaluate the addition of nab-paclitaxel to GemCis for patients with advanced BTCs. Impressively, the median PFS was 11.8 months (95% CI 6.0–15.6), and median OS was 19.2 months (95% CI 13.2 – not estimable). Most patients completed six cycles and approximately half required a dose reduction. The most common grade 3 or higher adverse event was neutropenia (19 patients, 33%) [24]. Given the extension of PFS and OS observed beyond what is expected from the current standard of care, there is optimism about the planned phase III randomized trial.

Second-Line Systemic Chemotherapy

In contrast, to date there is no established second-line systemic therapy for patients whose disease progresses during or following first-line GemCis combination therapy [9].

In the ABC-02 trial, 15.3% of patient were treated with second-line chemotherapy [6]. In the BT22 trial, 75% of patients received second-line chemotherapy [7]. Despite the difference in the number of patients treated with second-line chemotherapy, the medial OS was similar (11.7 months in ABC-02 and 11.2 months in BT22), raising doubt about the benefit of second-line chemotherapy.

A systematic review of the use of second-line chemotherapy for patients with advanced BTCs published in 2014 captured outcomes of 761 patients from 25 studies. The authors reported that select patients with good performance status might benefit from second-line chemotherapy but concluded that overall there is insufficient evidence to recommend its use [25].

The ABC-06 study is a phase III randomized trial that aims to address this clinical question (NCT 01926236). It compares a combination chemotherapy regimen including leucovorin, fluorouracil, and oxaliplatin (mFOLFOX) with active symptom control to active symptom control alone in patients with advanced BTCs who have progressed on first-line treatment with GemCis. Preliminary results show that patients treated with mFOLFOX had marginally improved median OS (6.2 months) and a clinically meaningful increase in 6- and 12-month OS rates (50.6% and 25.9%) compared to active symptom control (5.2 months, 5.5% and 11.4%, respectively) [26]. Of note, the median OS in the active symptom control arm was better than in previous reports. These findings, when matured, are likely to determine the second-line standard of care for advanced BTCs.

Summary

- GemCis combination chemotherapy improves OS and is the standard of care for patients with unresectable, metastatic, or relapsed BTCs.
- Ongoing studies investigating second-line therapies will continue to build a therapeutic hierarchy for managing advanced BTCs.

- There is no evidence that BTC subtypes should be treated with different chemotherapy regimens, but intrahepatic cholangiocarcinoma represents a distinct disease entity.
- Patients with an ECOG score of PS 2 (or more) do not benefit from combination chemotherapy and should be treated with gemcitabine monotherapy.

Palliative Radiotherapy for Cholangiocarcinoma Management

Nearly one-half of patients with advanced BTCs have disease confined to the liver [12], making loco-regional therapies like radiotherapy attractive options. Additionally, strategies that provide local tumour control have the advantage of avoiding adverse effects of systemic therapy and increasing the treatment options available for patients unfit for systemic therapy. However, owing to a paucity of randomized trial data, there is no standard of care radiotherapy for patients with advanced BTCs.

The current European guidelines state that radiotherapy "may be considered" in patients with localized disease after first-line chemotherapy [9]. Various modalities of radiotherapy have been used to treat advanced BTCs, but high-level evidence supporting one method over another, the timing in relation to chemotherapy or the dose and fractionation of radiation, is scarce. Modalities include external beam radiotherapy (EBRT) using either conventional or conformal treatment planning techniques; brachytherapy with iridium-192; and, more recently, stereotactic body radiotherapy (SBRT). Centres have reported their experiences using these modalities as retrospective series. Data from these series, limited by small sample size and selection bias, emphasize the need for randomized controlled trials to define the role of radiotherapy in the management of BTCs.

Advances in radiotherapy techniques, including intensity-modulated radiotherapy, image-guided radiotherapy, and the use of motion management, enable more focussed treatments to be delivered at higher doses. Such techniques minimize toxicity to the duodenum and adjacent liver tissue, expanding the potential of radiotherapy in managing BTCs. The following section will summarize lessons from historical and contemporary series evaluating radiotherapy techniques in the management of advanced BTCs. It will also introduce the randomized controlled trial that is currently underway.

External Beam Radiotherapy: The Rationale

Several single-centre, retrospective series conducted in the 1980s reported that EBRT might improve survival in patients with unresectable or relapsed BTCs compared to best supportive care [27–29]. More recent series comparing EBRT to best supportive care are, understandably, rare. One such study, conducted in 2008, included patients with unresectable intrahepatic cholangiocarcinoma (n = 84) and compared 35 patients who received EBRT to 49 patients who did not. None of the patients received chemotherapy, and, although not randomized, the groups had comparable baseline characteristics. Treated patients received a median dose of 50 Gy (dose range 30–60 Gy). Median OS was 9.5 months in the treated group and 5.1 months in the untreated group (p = 0.003) [30].

In the early series, patients treated with higher radiation doses consistently achieved higher rates of local disease control and improved OS than patients treated with lower doses [27, 29, 31]. Contemporary studies also report a dose-response relationship [32–34]. One larger retrospective series (n = 79) found that patients with advanced intrahepatic cholangiocarcinoma treated with EBRT who received a >80Gy dose survived longer than those who received <80Gy (73% vs 38% alive at 3 years, respectively) [34]. Although the optimal radiation dose for treating BTCs is not known, this trend has led to modalities that permit safe dose escalation being favoured.

Brachytherapy

Intraluminal brachytherapy (ILBT) is one way to boost the radiation dose. It has the benefit of delivering high radiation doses over a short distance from the radioactive source (iridium-192), thereby sparing the adjacent normal tissues. Access via percutaneous transhepatic biliary drains or endoscopy to the site of disease has facilitated its use in BTC management for decades. Early series suggested that treating advanced BTCs with EBRT combined with ILBT is superior to ERBT alone [35, 36] or ILBT alone [37]. Since then, most retrospective series evaluating radiotherapy for locally advanced BTC have combined EBRT with a ILBT boost. These single-arm series report high 1-year local control rates (50–87%) and median OS rates between 10 and 16 months [38–40].

To compare EBRT to EBRT plus ILBT, the Japanese Radiation Oncology Study Group conducted a large retrospective series and generated a comparison arm using a propensity-score matched-pair analysis. The series included 209 patients with advanced BTCs; 153 received EBRT and 56 received both ILBT and EBRT. The authors concluded that EBRT plus ILBT is associated with improved local control but has no impact on OS compared to EBRT alone. Fifty-seven percent of patients also received chemotherapy, and this was taken into account when generating the matched-pair arm [41].

Despite the number of retrospective series published, their heterogeneity precludes performing a collective analysis of the efficacy of EBRT and ILBT. Poor durability of response following initial good local control is a common trend among the series [32, 42]. This might explain the conflicting and modest impacts on OS. Whether initial local control contributes to a meaningful delay in the development of disease-related symptoms or improvement in QoL is not known.

Chemoradiotherapy

Due to the non-interventional nature of the available evidence, variations in the type and timing of chemotherapy that patients received are too great to draw conclusions about the optimal scheduling of radiotherapy in BTC management. A handful of retrospective series have compared patients treated with chemoradiotherapy to those treated with either chemotherapy or radiotherapy alone.

A retrospective analysis using the US Surveillance, Epidemiology, and End Results (SEER) database evaluated the impact of radiotherapy on survival of elderly patients with inoperable BTCs diagnosed between 1998 and 2011. Of the 2343 patients included, 451 (19%) received radiotherapy within 4 months of diagnosis. In patients who received chemotherapy (n = 1053), treatment with radiotherapy was associated with improved survival (HR 0.82, 95%CI 0.70–0.97, p = 0.02). In patients who did not receive chemotherapy (n = 1290), treatment with radiotherapy was not associated with improved survival (HR 1.09, 95%CI 0.91–1.30, p = 0.34). It is not possible to determine from this data if the addition of radiotherapy to chemotherapy achieves better survival or if patients who received both had more favourable baseline characteristics [43].

Kim et al. published a retrospective series of patients with unresectable intrahepatic cholangiocarcinoma (n = 92) that compared 25 (27.1%) patients who received capecitabine cisplatin (XP) chemotherapy with EBRT and 67 (72.8%) patients who received XP chemotherapy alone. Patients in the chemoradiotherapy group received a mean radiation dose of 44.7 Gy and a mean 5.6 cycles of XP, whereas patients in the chemotherapy group received a mean 4.0 cycles. More patients in the chemoradiotherapy group had a single intrahepatic lesion than those in chemotherapy group (72.0% vs 41.3%, p = 0.007). All other characteristics were balanced. Median PFS (4.3 vs 1.9 months, p = 0.001) and OS (9.3 vs 6.2 months, p = 0.048) were significantly longer in the chemoradiotherapy group than in the chemotherapy group. The disease control rate (56.0% vs 41.5%, p = 0.217) and 1-year survival rates (30.4% vs 22.4%, p = 0.438) did not differ significantly. There was more neutropenia in the chemoradiotherapy group, but otherwise no significant difference in other toxicities [44].

Different results were reported in a phase III trial conducted in France. Patients with unresectable advanced BTCs were randomized to chemoradiotherapy (50Gy with concurrent 5-FU and cisplatin) or combination GemOx chemotherapy. Median PFS and OS were significantly greater in the GemOx arm compared to the chemoradiotherapy arm. Grade 3–4 toxicities were mostly haematological (25% and 23%) and gastrointestinal (6% and 11%), in the GemOx arm and chemoradiotherapy arms, respectively. However, the study closed early after enrolling only 34 patients due to poor recruitment [45].

These conflicting findings provide rationale for performing a randomized trial comparing chemoradiotherapy and/or chemotherapy followed by radiotherapy to standard of care chemotherapy.

Stereotactic Body Radiotherapy

Technical advances in recent years enable more precise delivery of radiation, thereby permitting safer dose escalation. SBRT is one such a technique. SBRT achieves ablative radiation doses with a steep dose gradient and thus reduces toxicity to normal tissues. Fewer fractions are used in SBRT, offering the advantage of a short overall treatment time and ease of sequencing with chemotherapy. SBRT has been applied to primary and metastatic liver lesions and is becoming the predominant method used for BTCs.

At present there is no randomized controlled trial evidence to support using SBRT to treat advanced BTCs. The retrospective studies evaluating SBRT for cholangiocarcinoma management are summarized in Table 17.1. These demonstrate

Table 17.1 Studies evaluating SBRT in patients with advanced BTCs

Author Year Reference	Sample size	Design	No. of patients who had chemotherapy, timing, regimen	Median dose (Gy)/#	1-year local control rate	Median OS (months)	Grade ≥3 toxicities
Tse et al. 2008 [53]	10 ICCA	P	4/10 (40%) All prior 3 GemCap 1 5FU	36/6	65%	15	2 LFT elevation, 2 worsening cirrhosis, 1 late bowel obstruction
Kopek et al. 2010 [48]	29 HCCA 1 ICCA	R	None	45/3	84%	9.6	6 duodenal/ pyloric ulcer, 2 duodenal stenosis
Momm et al. 2010 [50]	13 HCCA	R	6/13 (46%) 2 prior, 4 post Highly variable regimens	47.5/3 or 4	NR	33.5	No severe toxicities
Polistina et al. 2011 [51]	10 HCCA	R	10/10 (100%) All concomitant weekly gemcitabine	30/3	80% at 6 months	35.5	1 duodenal ulcer, 2 duodenal stenosis
Barney et al. 2012[a] [46]	6 ICCA 3 HCCA 1 ECCA	R	8/10 (80%) 4 prior, 4 post Regimens not listed	55/3 or 5	100%	14	1 biliary stenosis, 1 liver failure
Jung et al. 2014[a] [47]	33 ICCA 25 ECCA	R	Not specified	45/3	85%	10	2 gastric/ duodenal ulcer, 1 gastric perforation, 3 biliary infection/ stenosis

Table 17.1 (continued)

Author Year Reference	Sample size	Design	No. of patients who had chemotherapy, timing, regimen	Median dose (Gy)/#	1-year local control rate	Median OS (months)	Grade ≥3 toxicities
Mahadevan et al. 2015[a] [49]	31 ICCA 11 HCCA	R	18/32 (56%) All prior 16 GemCis 2 Gem	30/3	88%	17	2 duodenal ulcer, 1 biliary infection, 1 liver abscess
Sandler et al. 2016[b] [52]	6 ICCA 25 HCCA	R	23/31 (74%) All prior 19 GemCis 2 Gem 1 GemOx 1 CapOx	40/3	78%	15.7	3 duodenal obstruction, 3 duodenal haemorrhage
Tao et al. 2016 [34]	79 ICCA	R	70/79 (87%) prior Most GemCis 50/79 (63%) concurrent Most capecitabine 37/79 (47%) after Most irinotecan	58/3 to 30	81%	30	No severe toxicities

P prospective, *R* retrospective, # fraction, *NR* not reported, *OS* overall survival, *ICCA* intrahepatic cholangiocarcinoma, *HCCA* hilar cholangiocarcinoma, *ECCA* extrahepatic cholangiocarcinoma, *LFT* liver function tests
[a]Study includes patients with post-operative recurrence or residual disease
[b]Study includes patients who proceeded to liver transplantation. *Gem* gemcitabine, *Cap* capecitabine, *Ox* oxaliplatin. Toxicities as per Common Terminology Criteria for Adverse Events

good 1-year local control rates (65–100%), generally superior to those achieved by EBRT [34, 46–53]. Survival outcomes in these series are reasonable, but interpretation is limited by confounding variables such as the natural history of the cholangiocarcinoma subtypes included and additional treatment with chemotherapy.

Although SBRT is well tolerated and associated with fewer adverse effects than EBRT, toxicity remains a recognized limitation of using SBRT to treat hepatobiliary tumours. A phase II trial evaluating SBRT for pancreatic adenocarcinomas following gemcitabine chemotherapy reported severe gastrointestinal toxicity in 13% of patients [54]. Similar rates of toxicities are seen when SBRT is used the treat cholangiocarcinoma (Table 17.1). Rates of toxicity appear to be lower for patients with intrahepatic cholangiocarcinoma, thought to be due to the increased distance between the tumour and structures such as the stomach, duodenum, and jejunum [55, 56].

A 2014 meta-analysis evaluating radiotherapy modalities in primary liver tumours concluded that treating advanced cholangiocarcinoma with SBRT offers promising local control rates and acceptable toxicity, but small patient numbers and a lack of prospective trial data limit the interpretation of its role [55].

Proton Beam Therapy

Proton beam therapy (PBT) is an external beam radiation modality using charged particles. The advantage over conventional radiotherapy is that proton beams have a finite range and therefore no exit dose. This allows normal liver tissue to be spared and permits safe dose escalation [57].

A phase II study evaluated hypofractionated PBT in 43 patients with locally advanced unresectable or recurrent primary liver tumours, 39 of whom had intrahepatic cholangiocarcinoma. The 2-year local control rate was 94%. The median PFS was 8.4 months and median OS was 22.5 months. Three patients (7.7%) had grade 3 toxicity, including liver failure, gastric ulcer, and elevated bilirubin. This median OS surpasses that achieved with standard of care chemotherapy (11.7 months) and approaches that achieved by surgery (27 months). While promising, the interpretation of this OS should take into account the predominance of intrahepatic cholangiocarcinoma patients included and the exclusion patients with extrahepatic disease [58].

A retrospective series of 20 patients with intrahepatic cholangiocarcinoma found similar results, reporting a median OS of 27.5 months among patients with localized disease. Among patients with extrahepatic metastases, however, median OS was 9.6 months [59]. A series of mixed BTCs achieved similarly high local control rates, but the median OS was lower. The most frequent site of first disease progression was out-of-field [60]. Hence, patients with intrahepatic cholangiocarcinoma without extrahepatic metastases are likely to benefit most from PBT and should be the focus of future randomized controlled trials.

The ABC-07 Trial

The variable outcomes in the retrospective studies described demonstrate a clear need for a randomized trial that delineates the role of radiotherapy in the management of BTCs.

The ABC-07 trial is a multi-centre UK-based phase II randomized trial that addresses this need. The study will recruit patients with locally advanced, unresectable intrahepatic or extrahepatic cholangiocarcinoma (excluding gallbladder and ampullary carcinomas). Patients are randomized to receive eight cycles of standard of care GemCis or six cycles of GemCis followed by SBRT. SBRT will be delivered in 5 or 15 fractions depending on tumour size at the time of radiotherapy planning. The primary outcome is the effect of the addition of SBRT to GemCis on PFS. Importantly, secondary outcomes will examine the SBRT toxicity profile, the potential to downstage inoperable disease to operable disease, and the impacts on QoL. This data will offer much needed clarity to the role of radiotherapy in treating advanced BTCs.

Summary

- The currently available published data consists of heterogenous retrospective or single-arm prospective studies, and interpretation of the outcomes is limited by confounding variables (e.g. use of chemotherapy).
- Delivering higher radiation doses confers better outcomes in patients with advanced BTCs.
- Techniques that increase precision and radiation dose (SBRT, PBT) are promising. The role of SBRT will be clarified by the results of the ABC-07 trial.
- Patients with intrahepatic cholangiocarcinoma often have liver-only disease and a favourable prognosis, making them ideal candidates for randomized controlled trials in this area.

References

1. Glimelius B, Hoffman K, Sjoden PO, Jacobsson G, Sellstrom H, Enander LK, et al. Chemotherapy improves survival and quality of life in advanced pancreatic and biliary cancer. Ann Oncol. 1996;7(6):593–600.
2. Park J, Kim MH, Kim KP, Park DH, Moon SH, Song TJ, et al. Natural history and prognostic factors of advanced Cholangiocarcinoma without surgery, chemotherapy, or radiotherapy: a large-scale observational study. Gut Liver. 2009;3(4):298–305.
3. Sharma A, Dwary AD, Mohanti BK, Deo SV, Pal S, Sreenivas V, et al. Best supportive care compared with chemotherapy for unresectable gall bladder cancer: a randomized controlled study. J Clin Oncol. 2010;28(30):4581–6.
4. Eckel F, Schmid RM. Chemotherapy in advanced biliary tract carcinoma: a pooled analysis of clinical trials. Br J Cancer. 2007;96(6):896–902.
5. Valle JW, Wasan H, Johnson P, Jones E, Dixon L, Swindell R, et al. Gemcitabine alone or in combination with cisplatin in patients with advanced or metastatic cholangiocarcinomas or other biliary tract tumours: a multicentre randomised phase II study - The UK ABC-01 Study. Br J Cancer. 2009;101(4):621–7.
6. Valle J, Wasan H, Palmer DH, Cunningham D, Anthoney A, Maraveyas A, et al. Cisplatin plus gemcitabine versus gemcitabine for biliary tract cancer. N Engl J Med. 2010;362(14):1273–81.
7. Okusaka T, Nakachi K, Fukutomi A, Mizuno N, Ohkawa S, Funakoshi A, et al. Gemcitabine alone or in combination with cisplatin in patients with biliary tract cancer: a comparative multicentre study in Japan. Br J Cancer. 2010;103(4):469–74.
8. Valle JW, Furuse J, Jitlal M, Beare S, Mizuno N, Wasan H, et al. Cisplatin and gemcitabine for advanced biliary tract cancer: a meta-analysis of two randomised trials. Ann Oncol. 2014;25(2):391–8.
9. Valle JW, Borbath I, Khan SA, Huguet F, Gruenberger T, Arnold D, et al. Biliary cancer: ESMO clinical practice guidelines for diagnosis, treatment and follow-up. Ann Oncol. 2016;27(suppl 5):v28–37.
10. Bridgewater J, Lopes A, Palmer D, Cunningham D, Anthoney A, Maraveyas A, et al. Quality of life, long-term survivors and long-term outcome from the ABC-02 study. Br J Cancer. 2016;114(9):965–71.
11. Jiao Y, Pawlik TM, Anders RA, Selaru FM, Streppel MM, Lucas DJ, et al. Exome sequencing identifies frequent inactivating mutations in BAP1, ARID1A and PBRM1 in intrahepatic cholangiocarcinomas. Nat Genet. 2013;45(12):1470–3.

12. Lamarca A, Ross P, Wasan HS, Hubner RA, McNamara MG, Lopes A, et al. Advanced intrahepatic Cholangiocarcinoma: Post Hoc analysis of the ABC-01, -02, and -03 clinical trials. J Natl Cancer Inst. 2020;112(2):200–10.
13. Morizane C, Okusaka T, Mizusawa J, Katayama H, Ueno M, Ikeda M, et al. Combination gemcitabine plus S-1 versus gemcitabine plus cisplatin for advanced/recurrent biliary tract cancer: the FUGA-BT (JCOG1113) randomized phase III clinical trial. Ann Oncol. 2019;30(12):1950–8.
14. André T, Reyes-Vidal JM, Fartoux L, Ross P, Leslie M, Rosmorduc O, et al. Gemcitabine and oxaliplatin in advanced biliary tract carcinoma: a phase II study. Br J Cancer. 2008;99(6):862–7.
15. Sharma A, Kalyan Mohanti B, Pal Chaudhary S, Sreenivas V, Kumar Sahoo R, Kumar Shukla N, et al. Modified gemcitabine and oxaliplatin or gemcitabine + cisplatin in unresectable gallbladder cancer: results of a phase III randomised controlled trial. Eur J Cancer. 2019;123:162–70.
16. Kim Seung, Kang Jung, Lee Jeeyun, Lee Hyun, OH SUNG YONG, Jang Joung, et al. Capecitabine Plus Oxaliplatin Versus Gemcitabine Plus Oxaliplatin as First-Line Therapy for Advanced Biliary Tract Cancers: A Multicenter, Open-Label, Randomized, Phase Three, Non-Inferiority Trial. Annals of oncology: official journal of the European Society for Medical Oncology. 2019;30. 10.1093/annonc/mdz058.
17. Malka D, Cervera P, Foulon S, Trarbach T, de la Fouchardiere C, Boucher E, et al. Gemcitabine and oxaliplatin with or without cetuximab in advanced biliary-tract cancer (BINGO): a randomised, open-label, non-comparative phase 2 trial. Lancet Oncol. 2014;15(8):819–28.
18. Valle JW, Wasan H, Lopes A, Backen AC, Palmer DH, Morris K, et al. Cediranib or placebo in combination with cisplatin and gemcitabine chemotherapy for patients with advanced biliary tract cancer (ABC-03): a randomised phase 2 trial. Lancet Oncol. 2015;16(8):967–78.
19. Valle JW, Bai L-Y, Orlova R, Cutsem EV, Alfonso JA, Chen L-T, et al. Ramucirumab (RAM) or merestinib (MER) or placebo (PL) plus gemcitabine (GEM) and cisplatin (CIS) as first-line treatment for advanced or metastatic biliary tract cancer (BTC): a randomized, double-blind, phase II study. J Clin Oncol. 2020;38(4_suppl):477.
20. Conroy T, Hammel P, Hebbar M, Ben Abdelghani M, Wei AC, Raoul JL, et al. FOLFIRINOX or gemcitabine as adjuvant therapy for pancreatic cancer. N Engl J Med. 2018;379(25):2395–406.
21. Belkouz A, de Vos-Geelen J, Mathôt RAA, Eskens FALM, van Gulik TM, van Oijen MGH, et al. Efficacy and safety of FOLFIRINOX as salvage treatment in advanced biliary tract cancer: an open-label, single arm, phase 2 trial. Br J Cancer. 2020;122(5):634–9.
22. Phelip JM, Edeline J, Blanc JF, Barbier E, Michel P, Bourgeois V, et al. Modified FOLFIRINOX versus CisGem first-line chemotherapy for locally advanced non resectable or metastatic biliary tract cancer (AMEBICA)-PRODIGE 38: study protocol for a randomized controlled multicenter phase II/III study. Dig Liver Dis. 2019;51(2):318–20.
23. Von Hoff DD, Ervin T, Arena FP, Chiorean EG, Infante J, Moore M, et al. Increased survival in pancreatic cancer with nab-paclitaxel plus gemcitabine. N Engl J Med. 2013;369(18):1691–703.
24. Shroff RT, Javle MM, Xiao L, Kaseb AO, Varadhachary GR, Wolff RA, et al. Gemcitabine, cisplatin, and nab-paclitaxel for the treatment of advanced biliary tract cancers: a phase 2 clinical trial. JAMA Oncol. 2019;5(6):824–30.
25. Lamarca A, Hubner RA, David Ryder W, Valle JW. Second-line chemotherapy in advanced biliary cancer: a systematic review. Ann Oncol. 2014;25(12):2328–38.
26. Lamarca A, Palmer DH, Wasan HS, Ross PJ, Ma YT, Arora A, et al. ABC-06 | a randomised phase III, multi-centre, open-label study of active symptom control (ASC) alone or ASC with oxaliplatin / 5-FU chemotherapy (ASC+mFOLFOX) for patients (pts) with locally advanced / metastatic biliary tract cancers (ABC) previously-treated with cisplatin/gemcitabine (CisGem) chemotherapy. J Clin Oncol. 2019;37(15_suppl):4003.
27. Alden ME, Mohiuddin M. The impact of radiation dose in combined external beam and intraluminal Ir-192 brachytherapy for bile duct cancer. Int J Radiat Oncol Biol Phys. 1994;28(4):945–51.

28. Gonzalez Gonzalez D, Gerard JP, Maners AW, De la Lande-Guyaux B, Van Dijk-Milatz A, Meerwaldt JH, et al. Results of radiation therapy in carcinoma of the proximal bile duct (Klatskin tumor). Semin Liver Dis. 1990;10(2):131–41.
29. Hayes JK, Sapozink MD, Miller FJ. Definitive radiation therapy in bile duct carcinoma. Int J Radiat Oncol Biol Phys. 1988;15(3):735–44.
30. Chen YX, Zeng ZC, Tang ZY, Fan J, Zhou J, Jiang W, et al. Determining the role of external beam radiotherapy in unresectable intrahepatic cholangiocarcinoma: a retrospective analysis of 84 patients. BMC Cancer. 2010;10:492.
31. Mittal B, Deutsch M, Iwatsuki S. Primary cancers of extrahepatic biliary passages. Int J Radiat Oncol Biol Phys. 1985;11(4):849–54.
32. Ben-David MA, Griffith KA, Abu-Isa E, Lawrence TS, Knol J, Zalupski M, et al. External-beam radiotherapy for localized extrahepatic cholangiocarcinoma. Int J Radiat Oncol Biol Phys. 2006;66(3):772–9.
33. Dawson LA, McGinn CJ, Normolle D, Ten Haken RK, Walker S, Ensminger W, et al. Escalated focal liver radiation and concurrent hepatic artery fluorodeoxyuridine for unresectable intrahepatic malignancies. J Clin Oncol. 2000;18(11):2210–8.
34. Tao R, Krishnan S, Bhosale PR, Javle MM, Aloia TA, Shroff RT, et al. Ablative radiotherapy doses lead to a substantial prolongation of survival in patients with inoperable intrahepatic Cholangiocarcinoma: a retrospective dose response analysis. J Clin Oncol. 2016;34(3):219–26.
35. Fields JN, Emami B. Carcinoma of the extrahepatic biliary system--results of primary and adjuvant radiotherapy. Int J Radiat Oncol Biol Phys. 1987;13(3):331–8.
36. Johnson DW, Safai C, Goffinet DR. Malignant obstructive jaundice: treatment with external-beam and intracavitary radiotherapy. Int J Radiat Oncol Biol Phys. 1985;11(2):411–6.
37. Meyers WC, Jones RS. Internal radiation for bile duct cancer. World J Surg. 1988;12(1): 99–104.
38. Bisello S, Buwenge M, Palloni A, Autorino R, Cellini F, Macchia G, et al. Radiotherapy or chemoradiation in unresectable biliary cancer: a retrospective study. Anticancer Res. 2019;39(6):3095–100.
39. Brunner TB, Schwab D, Meyer T, Sauer R. Chemoradiation may prolong survival of patients with non-bulky unresectable extrahepatic biliary carcinoma. A retrospective analysis. Strahlenther Onkol. 2004;180(12):751–7.
40. Jonczyk M, Collettini F, Schnapauff D, Geisel D, Boning G, Feldhaus F, et al. Cholangiocarcinoma: CT-guided high-dose rate brachytherapy (CT-HDRBT) for limited (<4 cm) and large (>4 cm) tumors. Anticancer Res. 2018;38(10):5843–52.
41. Yoshioka Y, Ogawa K, Oikawa H, Onishi H, Kanesaka N, Tamamoto T, et al. Impact of intraluminal brachytherapy on survival outcome for radiation therapy for unresectable biliary tract cancer: a propensity-score matched-pair analysis. Int J Radiat Oncol Biol Phys. 2014;89(4):822–9.
42. Crane CH, Macdonald KO, Vauthey JN, Yehuda P, Brown T, Curley S, et al. Limitations of conventional doses of chemoradiation for unresectable biliary cancer. Int J Radiat Oncol Biol Phys. 2002;53(4):969–74.
43. Pollom EL, Alagappan M, Park LS, Whittemore AS, Koong AC, Chang DT. Does radiotherapy still have a role in unresected biliary tract cancer? Cancer Med. 2017;6(1):129–41.
44. Kim YI, Park JW, Kim BH, Woo SM, Kim TH, Koh YH, et al. Outcomes of concurrent chemoradiotherapy versus chemotherapy alone for advanced-stage unresectable intrahepatic cholangiocarcinoma. Radiat Oncol. 2013;8:292.
45. Phelip JM, Vendrely V, Rostain F, Subtil F, Jouve JL, Gasmi M, et al. Gemcitabine plus cisplatin versus chemoradiotherapy in locally advanced biliary tract cancer: Federation Francophone de Cancerologie Digestive 9902 phase II randomised study. Eur J Cancer. 2014;50(17):2975–82.
46. Barney BM, Olivier KR, Miller RC, Haddock MG. Clinical outcomes and toxicity using stereotactic body radiotherapy (SBRT) for advanced cholangiocarcinoma. Radiat Oncol. 2012;7:67.

47. Jung DH, Kim MS, Cho CK, Yoo HJ, Jang WI, Seo YS, et al. Outcomes of stereotactic body radiotherapy for unresectable primary or recurrent cholangiocarcinoma. Radiat Oncol J. 2014;32(3):163–9.
48. Kopek N, Holt MI, Hansen AT, Hoyer M. Stereotactic body radiotherapy for unresectable cholangiocarcinoma. Radiother Oncol. 2010;94(1):47–52.
49. Mahadevan A, Dagoglu N, Mancias J, Raven K, Khwaja K, Tseng JF, et al. Stereotactic Body Radiotherapy (SBRT) for intrahepatic and Hilar Cholangiocarcinoma. J Cancer. 2015;6(11):1099–104.
50. Momm F, Schubert E, Henne K, Hodapp N, Frommhold H, Harder J, et al. Stereotactic fractionated radiotherapy for Klatskin tumours. Radiother Oncol. 2010;95(1):99–102.
51. Polistina FA, Guglielmi R, Baiocchi C, Francescon P, Scalchi P, Febbraro A, et al. Chemoradiation treatment with gemcitabine plus stereotactic body radiotherapy for unresectable, non-metastatic, locally advanced hilar cholangiocarcinoma. Results of a five year experience. Radiother Oncol. 2011;99(2):120–3.
52. Sandler KA, Veruttipong D, Agopian VG, Finn RS, Hong JC, Kaldas FM, et al. Stereotactic body radiotherapy (SBRT) for locally advanced extrahepatic and intrahepatic cholangiocarcinoma. Adv Radiat Oncol. 2016;1(4):237–43.
53. Tse RV, Hawkins M, Lockwood G, Kim JJ, Cummings B, Knox J, et al. Phase I study of individualized stereotactic body radiotherapy for hepatocellular carcinoma and intrahepatic cholangiocarcinoma. J Clin Oncol. 2008;26(4):657–64.
54. Herman JM, Chang DT, Goodman KA, Dholakia AS, Raman SP, Hacker-Prietz A, et al. Phase 2 multi-institutional trial evaluating gemcitabine and stereotactic body radiotherapy for patients with locally advanced unresectable pancreatic adenocarcinoma. Cancer. 2015;121(7):1128–37.
55. Aitken KL, Hawkins MA. The role of radiotherapy and chemoradiation in the management of primary liver tumours. Clin Oncol (R Coll Radiol). 2014;26(9):569–80.
56. Kang JK, Kim MS, Cho CK, Yang KM, Yoo HJ, Kim JH, et al. Stereotactic body radiation therapy for inoperable hepatocellular carcinoma as a local salvage treatment after incomplete transarterial chemoembolization. Cancer. 2012;118(21):5424–31.
57. Lee JW, Lee SH. Proton beam therapy as a rising option in treating intrahepatic cholangiocarcinoma. Transl Cancer Res. 2017;6(1):S96–S8.
58. Hong TS, Wo JY, Yeap BY, Ben-Josef E, McDonnell EI, Blaszkowsky LS, et al. Multi-institutional phase II study of high-dose Hypofractionated proton beam therapy in patients with localized, unresectable hepatocellular carcinoma and intrahepatic cholangiocarcinoma. J Clin Oncol. 2016;34(5):460–8.
59. Ohkawa A, Mizumoto M, Ishikawa H, Abei M, Fukuda K, Hashimoto T, et al. Proton beam therapy for unresectable intrahepatic cholangiocarcinoma. J Gastroenterol Hepatol. 2015;30(5):957–63.
60. Makita C, Nakamura T, Takada A, Takayama K, Suzuki M, Ishikawa Y, et al. Clinical outcomes and toxicity of proton beam therapy for advanced cholangiocarcinoma. Radiat Oncol. 2014;9(1):26.

Chapter 18
Interventional Radiology Therapies for Intrahepatic Cholangiocarcinoma

Thomas J. An and Eric Wehrenberg-Klee

Abbreviations

CCA	Cholangiocarcinoma
cTACE	Conventional transarterial chemoembolization
DEB-TACE	Drug-eluting bead transarterial chemoembolization
ECOG	Eastern Cooperative Oncology Group
Gy	Gray
HCC	Hepatocellular carcinoma
iCCA	Intrahepatic cholangiocarcinoma
IR	Interventional radiology
LT	Liver transplantation
MAA	Macro-aggregated albumin
MELD	Model for End-Stage Liver Disease
MWA	Microwave ablation
RECIST	Response Evaluation Criteria in Solid Tumours
RFA	Radiofrequency ablation
TACE	Transarterial chemoembolization
TAE	Bland transarterial embolization
TARE	Transarterial radioembolization

T. J. An
Department of Radiology, Massachusetts General Hospital, Boston, MA, USA

E. Wehrenberg-Klee (✉)
Division of Interventional Radiology, Department of Radiology, Massachusetts General Hospital, Boston, MA, USA
e-mail: EWEHRENBERG-KLEE@PARTNERS.ORG

J. H. Tabibian (ed.), *Diagnosis and Management of Cholangiocarcinoma*,
https://doi.org/10.1007/978-3-030-70936-5_18

Introduction

Cholangiocarcinoma (CCA) is the second most common primary hepatic malignancy after hepatocellular carcinoma. Classification of CCA is typically based on anatomic location, with extrahepatic CCA defined as involving the hilum (i.e., Klatskin tumor) or common bile duct and intrahepatic CCA (iCCA) defined as involving the second-order bile ducts [1]. Over 90% of CCAs are classified as extrahepatic, with the majority of those involving the hilum. The incidence of CCA appears to be increasing over the past several decades in the United States, with a disproportionate increase in particular of iCCA cases [2, 3]. Although many cases of CCA are sporadic, several risk factors for CCA development include chronic viral hepatitis, primary sclerosing cholangitis, and other chronic biliary tract disorders, including parasitic infections such as hepatobiliary flukes [1].

The prognosis for CCA is generally poor, with median 5-year survival of less than 10% [4]. Hepatic resection and liver transplantation (LT) are the only potentially curative options in the treatment of iCCA, with 5-year survival in patients undergoing surgical resection approximately 30% [5]. However, only approximately 30% of patients have resectable disease at the time of diagnosis. In addition, up to half of patients that undergo surgical resection develop recurrent disease, with the most common site of recurrence being within the remnant liver [6]. Most patients are asymptomatic during the initial stages of CCA, which makes early diagnosis and treatment extremely challenging. For patients with unresectable disease, systemic chemotherapy regimens are not very effective, with less than 1-year median overall survival even for standard-of-care chemotherapy with cisplatin and gemcitabine [7].

Interventional radiology (IR) offers several minimally invasive locoregional treatment options for unresectable iCCA and liver-dominant metastatic disease. The minimally invasive nature of interventional radiology procedures makes them well tolerated even in frail patients. Interventional radiology treatment modalities used in this context include thermal ablation, transarterial chemoembolization (TACE), and transarterial radioembolization (TARE). The aim of this chapter is to provide an overview of the different interventional radiology treatments for unresectable iCCA and summarize the available clinical data.

Thermal Ablation

Overview

Percutaneous thermal ablation is a minimally invasive procedure that uses extreme high or low temperatures to cause local tumor necrosis. Due to size constraints of ablation zones, thermal ablation is typically utilized in the setting of small- to medium-sized non-resectable tumors. Percutaneous placement of the ablation probes, which may be performed under CT or ultrasound guidance, makes the procedure well-tolerated even in comorbid patients that are poor surgical candidates. Alternatively, ablation may also be performed concurrently with abdominal surgery through an open incision. Studies comparing percutaneous thermal ablative techniques to surgery for hepatic malignancies have demonstrated decreased morbidity and recovery times compared to open surgical resection [8–10].

Thermal ablation has been used to treat tumors in organs including the liver, kidney, and lung, bone, and soft tissues, which makes it a versatile option for treatment of both iCCA and metastatic disease. The most common ablation techniques include high temperature ablation with microwave ablation (MWA) and radiofrequency ablation (RFA) and low temperature ablation with cryoablation. RFA applies a high-frequency alternating current to tumor cells to generate temperatures up to 100 C and causes local coagulative necrosis. MWA is a more recently developed hyperthermic ablative technique that induces a local electromagnetic field to oscillate water molecules within cells. The resultant kinetic energy results in heating of local tissue to greater than 100 C [11] (Fig. 18.1). MWA can produce larger ablation zones than RFA, as propagation of the RFA ablation zone is limited by current impedance caused by desiccation of tissues. In addition, MWA is less susceptible than RFA to heat-sink effect caused by adjacent vascular structures. With less thermal energy dissipation by flowing blood, probability of tumor-kill is increased with decreased risk of local recurrence [12].

Cryoablation uses extreme low temperatures to cause direct cellular injury and tissue necrosis. The freezing temperatures of cryoablation are generated based on the gas-throttling Joule-Thomson effect, with gas expansion after being forced through a valve resulting in local cooling. During cryoablation, a liquid gas (e.g., argon) flows through the cryoablation probe before rapidly expanding within a chamber at the tip of a probe to generate temperatures down to −160 C in the surrounding tissues. Lethal temperature for tumor cells is typically between −20 and −40 C, with cell death mediated by multiple mechanisms including cell membrane damage by ice crystal formation, vascular injury and thrombosis, and induction of coagulative necrosis [13]. Cryoablation is unique

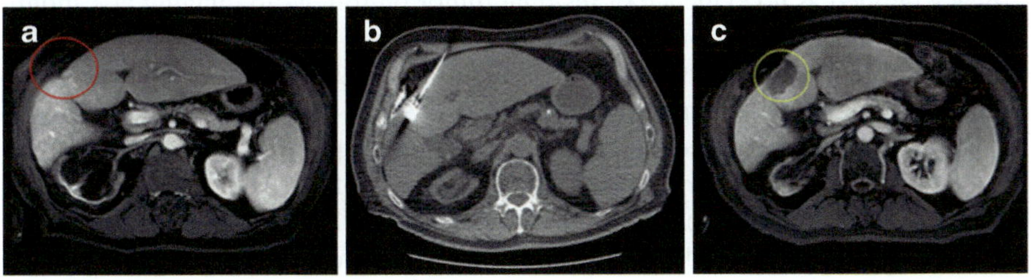

Fig. 18.1 Patient with multifocal intrahepatic cholangiocarcinoma intolerant of chemotherapy. Left hepatic lesions (not shown) were treated with left-lobar Y90 radioembolization. This single right-sided lesion shown on contrast-enhanced MRI (**a**, red circle) was amenable to microwave ablation (**b**). Note high-density hydrodissection (saline with dilute iodinated contrast) to protect peritoneum from thermal injury. One month post-ablation (**c**), contrast-enhanced MRI demonstrates ablation zone with no residual tumor (yellow circle)

among thermal ablation techniques in that it allows for real-time visualization of the cryoablation zone by CT to confirm treatment of the target region.

Novel ablation techniques including irreversible electroporation and high-intensity focused ultrasound have promising initial data regarding safety and efficacy. Irreversible electroporation delivers electrical pulses via percutaneous probes to destabilize cell membranes and induce pore formation to trigger cell death. Histologic studies have demonstrated that irreversible electroporation preserves collagen structures and extracellular matrix within the ablation zone, which makes it an attractive potential option for hepatic tumors in close proximity to vascular structures and bile ducts [14–16]. High-intensity focused ultrasound is an ablative technique that does not require percutaneous probe placement and is performed completely noninvasively. The technique focuses high-intensity ultrasound beams on a small volume of tissue to generate heat and induce coagulative necrosis [17, 18]. Further investigation is necessary to determine the utility of these techniques in the setting of iCCA.

Efficacy and Safety Data

The vast majority of studies on thermal ablation of iCCA have examined the outcomes of hyperthermic ablation with RFA and MWA. Although there is robust outcomes data for cryoablation in the setting of hepatocellular carcinoma and hepatic metastases, additional studies are needed to confirm similar efficacy in the setting of iCCA.

Several retrospective case series have examined the safety and efficacy of radiofrequency ablation in the setting of primary and recurrent CCA. The first case report of radiofrequency ablation for iCCA was published in 2002, which reported technically effective ablation of a single intrahepatic recurrence without evidence of residual disease for 10 months of follow-up [19]. Additional case series on RFA have demonstrated primary efficacy ranging between 70% and 92%, with primary efficacy defined as no evidence of residual tumor on follow-up imaging at 1 month [20–23]. A meta-analysis of radiofrequency ablation in the setting of CCA by Han et al. comprising 84 patients reported median survival time from time of procedure ranging between 20 and 60 months and pooled 1-year, 3-year, and 5-year survival of 82%, 47%, and 24%, respectively. Pooled local tumor progression at 1 month was 21% [24]. Prognostic factors for improved progression-free survival following RFA include fewer treated lesions and smaller tumor size [24, 25].

MWA has demonstrated similar efficacy in the treatment of both primary and recurrent iCCA. A retrospective study by Zhang et al. with 107 patients treated with MWA reported median progression-free survival of 8.9 months and median overall survival of 28 months [26]. An additional retrospective study by Yu et al. demonstrated primary efficacy of 87.5% and overall survival at 6, 12, and 24 months of 79%, 60%, and 60%. Local tumor progression at 4 months was observed in 10.5%

of patients with tumors less than 5 cm and 56% for tumors greater than 5 cm [27]. A study comparing outcomes of MWA and RFA to surgical resection in the setting of recurrent CCA demonstrated no significant difference in disease-free survival or overall survival between the two groups [28]. The incidence of major complications was significantly higher for surgical resection compared to percutaneous ablation (46.9% vs. 3.9%). However, in subgroup analysis of patients with tumors greater than 3 cm, there was greater overall survival in the surgical resection group compared to thermal ablation.

Combination of thermal ablation with additional adjunctive interventional radiology treatments has the potential to further improve efficacy of ablation in the setting of larger tumors. For example, a study by Peng et al. comparing combined RFA with transcatheter arterial chemoembolization (TACE) to RFA alone demonstrated significantly improved overall survival with the combined therapy for lesions greater than 5 cm and in the setting of multiple lesions. Progression-free survival for the combined RFA and TACE at 1, 2, and 3 years was 93%, 83%, and 75% [29]. An additional study by Yang et al. on combined MWA with TACE demonstrated similar improved primary efficacy of 92% without any major complications [30].

Both RFA and MWA are relatively well-tolerated procedures with low rate of complications. A meta-analysis of radiofrequency ablation for CCA reported a major complication rate of 5.9%, which included two cases of liver abscess, biliary stricture, pleural effusion requiring thoracentesis, and pseudoaneurysm formation requiring coiling embolization [24]. Similarly, Zhang et al. reported a low major complication rate of 2.8% among 107 patients that underwent microwave ablation for CCA [26]. In patients that have many medical comorbidities that are poor surgical candidates, thermal ablation is an important potentially curative treatment option to consider.

In addition, thermal ablation combined with immunomodulatory therapies (e.g., checkpoint inhibitors) is an emerging focus in oncology research [31, 32]. Studies have demonstrated that thermal ablation results in a local inflammatory response and stimulation of the immune system [33]. Augmentation of this response with immunotherapy aims to turn exposed tumor antigens into in situ vaccines to trigger a distant antitumor immune response, analogous to the abscopal effect described within the field of radiation oncology. A pilot study by Xie et al. investigated the efficacy of combined anti-CTLA-4 therapy (tremelimumab) and microwave ablation in 20 patients with unresectable biliary tract cancer [34]. Median progression-free survival and overall survival were 3.4 months and 6.0 months, respectively, with an overall response rate of 12.5%. The combined therapy demonstrated an increased global immune response, with peripheral blood flow cytometry showing an approximately threefold increase in activated CD8+ T cells in circulation following treatment. The correlation between the observed immune response and local antitumoral effects requires further investigation. Several additional ongoing clinical trials are currently studying the efficacy of combined thermal ablation with immunotherapy to assess the potential role for this combined therapy in the future of oncology care.

Chemoembolization

Overview

TACE is a minimally invasive endovascular procedure which allows for selective delivery of chemotherapy and embolic material directly to tumor cells in the liver. Originally developed in the 1970s as a treatment for hepatocellular carcinoma, TACE has developed into an important palliative treatment option for unresectable and liver-dominant metastatic iCCA [35, 36].

The liver receives a dual blood supply from both the portal veins and the hepatic arteries. However, hepatic malignancies such as CCA receive the majority of their blood supply from the hepatic arteries [37]. This characteristic allows intra-arterial therapies such as TACE to be effective even for relatively hypovascular malignancies such as CCA. The treatment effect of TACE is mediated by two main mechanisms: concentrated chemotherapy delivery to the tumor and embolic occlusion of hepatic arteries supplying the tumor [38]. Selective delivery of chemotherapy allows a concentrated dose to be administered to the tumor with decreased risk of systemic side effects. Embolization of the hepatic artery has the combined benefit of causing tumor ischemia and increasing retention of chemotherapy within the tumor.

During TACE, the chemotherapy agent is delivered intra-arterially either in combination with lipiodol, an ethiodized oil contrast agent, followed by an embolic agent (e.g., Gelfoam or polyvinyl alcohol) or coated on drug-eluting beads (Fig. 18.2). Administration of chemotherapy in combination with lipiodol and an embolic agent is referred to as conventional TACE (cTACE). The most commonly utilized chemotherapeutic agents utilized during cTACE for CCA include doxorubicin, cisplatin,

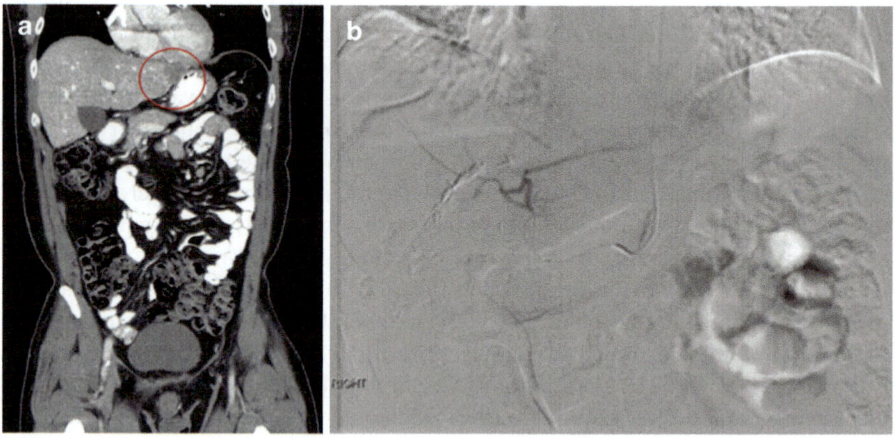

Fig. 18.2 Patient with multifocal intrahepatic cholangiocarcinoma with single lesion in segment II/III not responding to chemotherapy (**a**, red circle). Due to location near stomach and heart, doxorubicin DEB-TACE of this lesion was pursued, with left-hepatic angiogram demonstrating faint tumor blush within segment II (**b**)

gemcitabine, and mitomycin C. Administration of TACE with drug-eluting beads is referred to as DEB-TACE. DEB-TACE, which is typically performed with microbeads measuring between 100 and 300 um in diameter, allows for a sustained release of the chemotherapy from microbeads lodged within the tumor vasculature to maximize the cytotoxic effect [39, 40]. DEB-TACE for CCA is most commonly performed with beads coated with either doxorubicin or irinotecan. Bland transarterial embolization (TAE), which involves embolization of the tumor vasculature without combination with chemotherapy, is another well-recognized approach, and several studies have demonstrated no significant difference in survival benefit compared to cTACE and DEB-TACE in the setting of hepatic malignancies [41, 42].

While TACE may induce local disease control in some patients, it is typically palliative rather than curative. A study by Lee et al. demonstrated residual viable CCA post-TACE in 100% (13/13) of explants following LT. The average percentage tumor necrosis following TACE for patients with CCA was 7.6%, significantly lower than 75.1% tumor necrosis observed for patients with HCC in the same study [43]. Patients with unresectable iCCA routinely undergo multiple TACE treatments in order to control or delay progression of disease. Regular follow-up imaging after TACE is crucial to guide decision-making regarding further treatment with TACE or another therapeutic modality.

Efficacy and Safety Data

Retrospective studies on conventional TACE in the context of unresectable iCCA have demonstrated mean survival between 12 and 21 months post-treatment [35, 44–46]. A retrospective study by Park et al. compared outcomes for 72 patients that underwent cTACE and 83 patients that received supportive therapy alone and demonstrated a significant survival benefit in favor of cTACE of 12.2 months compared to 3.3 months. Another retrospective study by Kiefer et al. with 62 patients showed that cTACE further improves survival when administered sequentially after systemic chemotherapy, with median survival of 28 months with combination therapy relative to 16 months with TACE alone [44]. The treatment benefit of cTACE compared to surgical resection was assessed in a retrospective study by Scheuermann et al., which demonstrated superior median survival for R0 surgical resection compared to cTACE, but no significant difference in median survival for cTACE compared to margin positive resection [47]. Poor prognostic factors for survival in patients undergoing cTACE for iCCA include large tumor size, tumor hypovascularity, Child-Pugh class B, and early tumor progression on imaging following the procedure [45, 48].

DEB-TACE has also been shown to be of value for patients with iCCA. Retrospective studies have demonstrated median survival post-DEB-TACE to be between 12 and 13 months, similar to reported results for cTACE [49, 50]. In a study by Schiffman et al. with 24 patients, DEB-TACE demonstrated improved median overall survival when performed sequentially following systemic chemotherapy (FOLFOX or GEMZAR) compared to systemic chemotherapy alone (17.5 vs. 7.4 months) [49].

Patients that undergo TACE may develop post-embolization syndrome in up to 20–40% of cases, with common symptoms including right upper quadrant pain, nausea, fever, and serum transaminase/bilirubin elevation [51, 52]. These side effects typically self-resolve within 24–48 hours and may require an overnight hospitalization for observation. Major complications from nontarget embolization including gastrointestinal ulceration/perforation, liver abscess, or cholecystitis are rare and occur in less than 2–5% of patients [53, 54].

Most studies on TACE in the setting of iCCA are limited by their retrospective nature and the lack of standardized treatment protocols. Differences in chemotherapeutic agents, embolic agents, and operator experience limit comparison between different types of TACE procedures and other second-line therapeutic options. Based on current evidence, there is no significant difference in overall survival benefit for cTACE compared to DEB-TACE [55, 56]. Future prospective studies are required to better assess the treatment benefit of TACE and evaluate the relative efficacy of DEB-TACE versus cTACE, as well as appropriate combinations with chemotherapy regimens.

Radioembolization

Overview

TARE involves intra-arterial delivery of radioactive microspheres to liver tumors via the hepatic arteries [57]. Similar to TACE, this procedure draws on the concept that hepatic malignancies derive the majority of their blood supply from the hepatic arteries. TARE is performed with Yttrium-90 (^{90}Y)-coated microspheres, which emit high-energy beta radiation with a half-life of approximately 64.2 hours. The Y90-coated microspheres emit high-energy radiation with a mean penetration depth of approximately 2.5 mm, thereby sparing much of the surrounding tissue outside the area of deposition [58, 59]. ^{90}Y radioembolization is also sometimes referred to as selective internal radiation therapy (SIRT) (Fig. 18.3).

There are currently two types of ^{90}Y microspheres available: glass microspheres (TheraSpheres, BTG international) and resin microspheres (SIR-Spheres, Sirtex Medical). Selection of Y90 microsphere type is dependent on operator experience and preference. The two types of microspheres differ in size, with resin microspheres measuring 20–60 um compared to 20–30 um for glass microspheres, and radiation activity, with glass microspheres associated with a higher radiation dose per microsphere compared to resin microspheres. Resin microspheres are FDA approved for treatment of metastatic colorectal cancer to the liver, while glass microspheres are approved with a humanitarian device exception for patients with unresectable hepatocellular carcinoma. However, both are utilized in an investigational and off-label capacity in the context of iCCA.

Although intra-arterial administration of radioactive microspheres allows for high doses of radiation to be delivered selectively to tumors, nontarget delivery

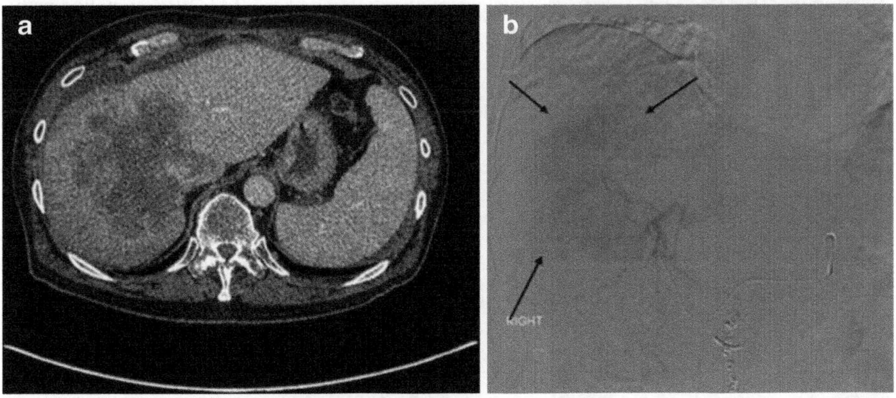

Fig. 18.3 Patient with unresectable liver confined intrahepatic cholangiocarcinoma shown as hypodense mass on axial contrast-enhanced CT (**a**). Patient underwent Y90 radioembolization (**b**). Faint tumor blush can be appreciated on this delayed right hepatic artery angiogram

of the dose has the potential to cause radiation-induced side effects. In order to reduce the risk of nontarget radioembolization, a planning procedure to localize and quantify the anticipated distribution of Y90 microspheres is performed approximately 1–2 weeks prior to the therapy [60]. ^{99m}Technicium-macroaggregated albumin (^{99m}Tc-MAA), a diagnostic radiopharmaceutical that is similar in size to Y90 microspheres, is administered intra-arterially to the hepatic arteries supplying the tumor. SPECT-CT is performed immediately afterward to assess the distribution of particles. The lung shunt fraction, which is the anticipated proportion of the radiation dose delivered to the lungs, is calculated based on the SPECT-CT results to assess the risk for radiation pneumonitis [61] (Fig. 18.4). Progressive dose reduction is typically performed as the lung shunt fraction increases above 10% of the total dose. A radiation dose to the lungs of greater than 30 Gray (Gy) in a single treatment or 50 Gy over a series of treatments is a relative contraindication to TARE [62]. Pre-procedural angiography during 99mTc-MAA administration has the added benefit of characterizing the arterial supply to the tumor and providing an opportunity to coil nontarget arteries that supply the gastrointestinal tract that may arise from hepatic arteries.

Efficacy and Safety Data

TARE has been shown to improve survival in the setting of liver-confined unresectable iCCA relative to historical controls. In several retrospective studies on Y90 TARE for unresectable and limited metastatic disease, medial overall survival from time of procedure ranged between 9.3 and 22 months [63–66]. Factors associated with increased overall survival include higher baseline performance status (ECOG

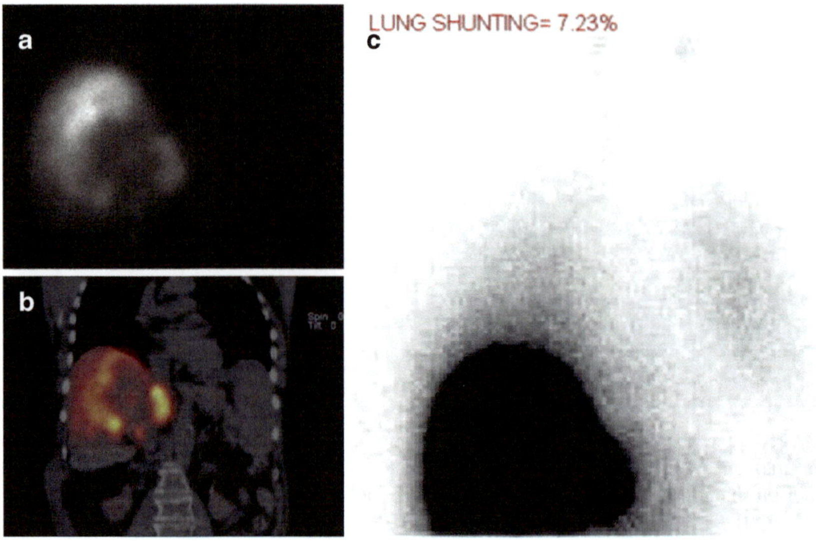

Fig. 18.4 ^{99m}Tc-labeled-MAA scintigraphy was performed in a 68-year-old man with intrahepatic cholangiocarcinoma. (**a**) Single photon emission computed tomography (SPECT) imaging performed by rotating a gamma camera around the patient, which demonstrates high uptake in the expected location of the liver. Region of photopenia in the left lobe of the liver corresponds to an area of central necrosis within a dominant mass. (**b**) SPECT radiotracer uptake superimposed on a low-dose attenuation correction CT demonstrates that the uptake corresponds to the liver without evidence of significant extrahepatic uptake. (**c**) Hepatopulmonary shunt fraction calculated based on planar scintigram demonstrates a lung shunt fraction of 7.23%. The patient was able to undergo successful treatment without radiation dose reduction

0 or 1), tumor burden involving <25% of the liver volume, tumor response to treatment (i.e., partial response or stable disease), and higher radiation dose delivered [64, 66]. Decreased overall survival was associated with increased INR, bilirubin, CA 19–9, ALT, and MELD score post-treatment [67]. A prospective multicenter observational study on the safety and efficacy of TARE for unresectable or limited metastatic, chemotherapy refractory iCCA by White et al. demonstrated overall survival of 8.7 months and progression-free survival of 2.8 months at a median follow-up of 13.9 months [68]. Overall, survival outcomes for TARE are comparable to alternative intra-arterial therapies including cTACE and DEB-TACE. However, there are no randomized clinical trials directly comparing efficacy of TARE, TACE, and other second-line therapies for iCCA. A meta-analysis by Boehm et al. comparing outcomes from TARE and TACE demonstrated slightly higher median overall survival for TARE compared to TACE (13.9 +/− 4.4 months vs. 12.4 +/− 1.5 months). The response to therapy demonstrated in the meta-analysis (complete or partial response) was higher for TARE compared to TACE (27.4 +/− 10% vs. 17.3 +/− 11.5%) [56].

Treatment with TARE also has the potential benefit of downstaging patients with borderline unresectable tumors into surgical candidates. In a study by Mouli et al.,

46 patients with unresectable iCCA were treated with a total of 92 total TARE treatments. Among the 46 patients, 5 (11%) had disease response that allowed them to be converted to resectable status and undergo curative R0 resection [69]. Another phase II clinical trial combining first-line chemotherapy and TARE for unresectable disease demonstrated an overall response rate of 39% by RECIST criteria and allowed 22% of patients to be downstaged to surgically resectable status [70]. The survival benefit of downstaging tumors for surgical resection was demonstrated in a retrospective study by Bourien et al., in which 19% of the patients were downstaged to surgical resection and had a subsequent median overall survival of 51.9 months, which was significantly higher than 16.4 months for patients treated with TARE alone [64].

TARE is well tolerated in the majority of patients and is typically performed as an outpatient procedure. Following the procedure, patients may develop post-radioembolization syndrome in up to 20–40% of cases, which includes fatigue, nausea, malaise, and right upper quadrant pain. The symptoms of post-radioembolization syndrome are typically less severe than post-embolization syndrome observed following TACE and rarely require hospitalization. Side effects related to nontarget deposition of radioactive microspheres including gastrointestinal ulceration, radiation pneumonitis, and liver dysfunction are relatively rare [71, 72].

Conclusion

Most patients with iCCA are diagnosed at an advanced stage and have a poor prognosis. Although surgical resection and LT are potentially curative treatment options, only a minority of patients have resectable disease at the time of diagnosis. In patients with unresectable and liver-confined or liver-dominant metastatic disease, locoregional therapies performed by interventional radiology offer effective palliative options. Thermal ablation and arterially directed therapies such as TACE and TARE have demonstrated survival benefit in retrospective studies comparable or even favorable to standard-of-care systemic chemotherapy. In addition, interventional radiology procedures are minimally invasive with lower risk for complications compared to surgical resection.

Robust clinical data on the efficacy of interventional radiology procedures for iCCA is limited by the rarity of the disease, lack of standardized treatment protocols, and retrospective nature of the majority of published studies. In addition, the technology within the field of interventional radiology evolves rapidly, with new devices and equipment being utilized every few years. Updated prospective trials will be necessary to accurately assess the efficacy of interventional radiology procedures and develop evidence-based indications and guidelines.

Overall, interventional radiology treatments such as thermal ablation and arterially directed therapies should be considered important components of the treatment arsenal for unresectable iCCA. In the setting of liver-confined or liver-dominant disease, these therapies can be used in combination with or as an alternative to systemic chemotherapy.

References

1. Rizvi S, Gores GJ. Pathogenesis, diagnosis, and management of cholangiocarcinoma. Gastroenterology. 2013;145(6):1215–29. https://doi.org/10.1053/j.gastro.2013.10.013.
2. Bergquist A, von Seth E. Epidemiology of cholangiocarcinoma. Best Pract Res Clin Gastroenterol. 2015;29(2):221–32. https://doi.org/10.1016/j.bpg.2015.02.003.
3. Saha SK, Zhu AX, Fuchs CS, Brooks GA. Forty-year trends in cholangiocarcinoma incidence in the U.S.: intrahepatic disease on the rise. Oncologist. 2016;21(5):594–9. https://doi.org/10.1634/theoncologist.2015-0446.
4. Shaib Y, El-Serag H. The epidemiology of cholangiocarcinoma. Semin Liver Dis. 2004;24(02):115–25. https://doi.org/10.1055/s-2004-828889.
5. Mavros MN, Economopoulos KP, Alexiou VG, Pawlik TM. Treatment and prognosis for patients with intrahepatic cholangiocarcinoma. JAMA Surg. 2014;149(6):565. https://doi.org/10.1001/jamasurg.2013.5137.
6. Hyder O, Hatzaras I, Sotiropoulos GC, et al. Recurrence after operative management of intrahepatic cholangiocarcinoma. Surgery. 2013;153(6):811–8. https://doi.org/10.1016/j.surg.2012.12.005.
7. Valle J, Wasan H, Palmer DH, et al. Cisplatin plus gemcitabine versus gemcitabine for biliary tract cancer. N Engl J Med. 2010;362(14):1273–81. https://doi.org/10.1056/NEJMoa0908721.
8. Meijerink MR, Puijk RS, van Tilborg AAJM, et al. Radiofrequency and microwave ablation compared to systemic chemotherapy and to partial hepatectomy in the treatment of colorectal liver metastases: a systematic review and meta-analysis. Cardiovasc Intervent Radiol. 2018;41(8):1189–204. https://doi.org/10.1007/s00270-018-1959-3.
9. Yazici P, Akyuz M, Yigitbas H, et al. A comparison of perioperative outcomes in elderly patients with malignant liver tumors undergoing laparoscopic liver resection versus radiofrequency ablation. Surg Endosc. 2017;31(3):1269–74. https://doi.org/10.1007/s00464-016-5105-5.
10. Fang Y, Chen W, Liang X, et al. Comparison of long-term effectiveness and complications of radiofrequency ablation with hepatectomy for small hepatocellular carcinoma. J Gastroenterol Hepatol. 2014;29(1):193–200. https://doi.org/10.1111/jgh.12441.
11. Lubner MG, Brace CL, Hinshaw JL, Lee FT. Microwave tumor ablation: mechanism of action, clinical results, and devices. J Vasc Interv Radiol. 2010;21(8):S192–203. https://doi.org/10.1016/j.jvir.2010.04.007.
12. Brace CL. Radiofrequency and microwave ablation of the liver, lung, kidney, and bone: what are the differences? Curr Probl Diagn Radiol. 2009;38(3):135–43. https://doi.org/10.1067/J.CPRADIOL.2007.10.001.
13. Baust JG, Gage AA, Bjerklund Johansen TE, Baust JM. Mechanisms of cryoablation: clinical consequences on malignant tumors. Cryobiology. 2014;68(1):1–11. https://doi.org/10.1016/j.cryobiol.2013.11.001.
14. Wagstaff PG, Buijs M, van den Bos W, et al. Irreversible electroporation: state of the art. Onco Targets Ther. 2016;9:2437–46. https://doi.org/10.2147/OTT.S88086.
15. Martin RCG, Kwon D, Chalikonda S, et al. Treatment of 200 locally advanced (stage III) pancreatic adenocarcinoma patients with irreversible electroporation. Ann Surg. 2015;262(3):486–94. https://doi.org/10.1097/SLA.0000000000001441.
16. Davalos RV, Mir LM, Rubinsky B. Tissue ablation with irreversible electroporation. Ann Biomed Eng. 2005;33(2):223–31. https://doi.org/10.1007/s10439-005-8981-8.
17. van den Bijgaart RJE, Eikelenboom DC, Hoogenboom M, Fütterer JJ, den Brok MH, Adema GJ. Thermal and mechanical high-intensity focused ultrasound: perspectives on tumor ablation, immune effects and combination strategies. Cancer Immunol Immunother. 2017;66(2):247–58. https://doi.org/10.1007/s00262-016-1891-9.
18. Orsi F, Zhang L, Arnone P, et al. High-intensity focused ultrasound ablation: effective and safe therapy for solid tumors in difficult locations. Am J Roentgenol. 2010;195(3):W245–52. https://doi.org/10.2214/AJR.09.3321.

19. Slakey DP. Radiofrequency ablation of recurrent cholangiocarcinoma. Am Surg. 2002;68(4):395–7. http://www.ncbi.nlm.nih.gov/pubmed/11952256. Accessed 1 Mar 2020
20. Butros SR, Shenoy-Bhangle A, Mueller PR, Arellano RS. Radiofrequency ablation of intrahepatic cholangiocarcinoma: feasibility, local tumor control, and long-term outcome. Clin Imaging. 2014;38(4):490–4. https://doi.org/10.1016/j.clinimag.2014.01.013.
21. Haidu M, Dobrozemsky G, Schullian P, et al. Stereotactic radiofrequency ablation of unresectable intrahepatic cholangiocarcinomas: a retrospective study. Cardiovasc Intervent Radiol. 2012;35(5):1074–82. https://doi.org/10.1007/s00270-011-0288-6.
22. Kim JH, Won HJ, Shin YM, Kim K-A, Kim PN. Radiofrequency ablation for the treatment of primary intrahepatic cholangiocarcinoma. Am J Roentgenol. 2011;196(2):W205–9. https://doi.org/10.2214/AJR.10.4937.
23. Giorgio A, Calisti G, DE Stefano G, et al. Radiofrequency ablation for intrahepatic cholangiocarcinoma: retrospective analysis of a single centre experience. Anticancer Res. 2011; 31(12):4575–80. http://www.ncbi.nlm.nih.gov/pubmed/22199333. Accessed 1 Mar 2020
24. Han K, Ko HK, Kim KW, Won HJ, Shin YM, Kim PN. Radiofrequency ablation in the treatment of unresectable intrahepatic cholangiocarcinoma: systematic review and meta-analysis. J Vasc Interv Radiol. 2015;26(7):943–8. https://doi.org/10.1016/j.jvir.2015.02.024.
25. Xu H-X, Wang Y, Lu M-D, Liu L-N. Percutaneous ultrasound-guided thermal ablation for intrahepatic cholangiocarcinoma. Br J Radiol. 2012;85(1016):1078–84. https://doi.org/10.1259/bjr/24563774.
26. Zhang K, Yu J, Yu X, et al. Clinical and survival outcomes of percutaneous microwave ablation for intrahepatic cholangiocarcinoma. Int J Hyperth. 2018;34(3):292–7. https://doi.org/10.1080/02656736.2017.1327678.
27. Yu M-A, Liang P, Yu X-L, et al. Sonography-guided percutaneous microwave ablation of intrahepatic primary cholangiocarcinoma. Eur J Radiol. 2011;80(2):548–52. https://doi.org/10.1016/j.ejrad.2011.01.014.
28. Zhang S-J, Hu P, Wang N, et al. Thermal ablation versus repeated hepatic resection for recurrent intrahepatic cholangiocarcinoma. Ann Surg Oncol. 2013;20(11):3596–602. https://doi.org/10.1245/s10434-013-3035-1.
29. Peng Z-W, Chen M-S, Liang H-H, et al. A case-control study comparing percutaneous radiofrequency ablation alone or combined with transcatheter arterial chemoembolization for hepatocellular carcinoma. Eur J Surg Oncol. 2010;36(3):257–63. https://doi.org/10.1016/j.ejso.2009.07.007.
30. Yang G, Zhao Q, Qian S, et al. Percutaneous microwave ablation combined with simultaneous transarterial chemoembolization for the treatment of advanced intrahepatic cholangiocarcinoma. Onco Targets Ther. 2015;8:1245. https://doi.org/10.2147/OTT.S84764.
31. Mehta A, Oklu R, Sheth RA. Thermal ablative therapies and immune checkpoint modulation: can locoregional approaches effect a systemic response? Gastroenterol Res Pract. 2016;2016:1–11. https://doi.org/10.1155/2016/9251375.
32. Slovak R, Ludwig JM, Gettinger SN, Herbst RS, Kim HS. Immuno-thermal ablations – boosting the anticancer immune response. J Immunother Cancer. 2017;5(1):78. https://doi.org/10.1186/s40425-017-0284-8.
33. Chu KF, Dupuy DE. Thermal ablation of tumours: biological mechanisms and advances in therapy. Nat Rev Cancer. 2014;14(3):199–208. https://doi.org/10.1038/nrc3672.
34. Xie C, Duffy AG, Mabry-Hrones D, et al. Tremelimumab in combination with microwave ablation in patients with refractory biliary tract cancer. Hepatology. 2019;69(5) https://doi.org/10.1002/HEP.30482.
35. Herber S, Otto G, Schneider J, et al. Transarterial chemoembolization (TACE) for inoperable intrahepatic cholangiocarcinoma. Cardiovasc Intervent Radiol. 2007;30(6):1156–65. https://doi.org/10.1007/s00270-007-9032-7.
36. Zechlinski JJ, Rilling WS. Transarterial therapies for the treatment of intrahepatic cholangiocarcinoma. Semin Intervent Radiol. 2013;30(1):21–7. https://doi.org/10.1055/s-0033-1333650.

37. Breedis C, Young G. The blood supply of neoplasms in the liver. Am J Pathol. 1954;30(5):969–77. http://www.ncbi.nlm.nih.gov/pubmed/13197542. Accessed 16 Feb 2020
38. Gonsalves CF, Brown DB. Chemoembolization of hepatic malignancy. Abdom Imaging. 2009;34(5):557–65. https://doi.org/10.1007/s00261-008-9446-y.
39. Lencioni R, Petruzzi P, Crocetti L. Chemoembolization of hepatocellular carcinoma. Semin Intervent Radiol. 2013;30(1):3–11. https://doi.org/10.1055/s-0033-1333648.
40. Lencioni R, de Baere T, Burrel M, et al. Transcatheter treatment of hepatocellular carcinoma with doxorubicin-loaded DC bead (DEBDOX): technical recommendations. Cardiovasc Intervent Radiol. 2012;35(5):980–5. https://doi.org/10.1007/s00270-011-0287-7.
41. Marelli L, Stigliano R, Triantos C, et al. Transarterial therapy for hepatocellular carcinoma: which technique is more effective? A systematic review of cohort and randomized studies. Cardiovasc Intervent Radiol. 2007;30(1):6–25. https://doi.org/10.1007/s00270-006-0062-3.
42. Pleguezuelo M, Marelli L, Misseri M, et al. TACE versus TAE as therapy for hepatocellular carcinoma. Expert Rev Anticancer Ther. 2008;8(10):1623–41. https://doi.org/10.1586/14737140.8.10.1623.
43. Lee DD, Croome KP, Musto KR, et al. Liver transplantation for intrahepatic cholangiocarcinoma. Liver Transpl. 2018;24(5):634–44. https://doi.org/10.1002/lt.25052.
44. Kiefer MV, Albert M, McNally M, et al. Chemoembolization of intrahepatic cholangiocarcinoma with cisplatinum, doxorubicin, mitomycin C, ethiodol, and polyvinyl alcohol. Cancer. 2011;117(7):1498–505. https://doi.org/10.1002/cncr.25625.
45. Vogl TJ, Naguib NNN, Nour-Eldin N-EA, et al. Transarterial chemoembolization in the treatment of patients with unresectable cholangiocarcinoma: results and prognostic factors governing treatment success. Int J Cancer. 2012;131(3):733–40. https://doi.org/10.1002/ijc.26407.
46. Burger I, Hong K, Schulick R, et al. Transcatheter arterial chemoembolization in unresectable cholangiocarcinoma: initial experience in a single institution. J Vasc Interv Radiol. 2005;16(3):353–61. https://doi.org/10.1097/01.RVI.0000143768.60751.78.
47. Scheuermann U, Kaths JM, Heise M, et al. Comparison of resection and transarterial chemoembolisation in the treatment of advanced intrahepatic cholangiocarcinoma – a single-center experience. Eur J Surg Oncol. 2013;39(6):593–600. https://doi.org/10.1016/j.ejso.2013.03.010.
48. Kim JH, Yoon H-K, Sung K-B, et al. Transcatheter arterial chemoembolization or chemoinfusion for unresectable intrahepatic cholangiocarcinoma. Cancer. 2008;113(7):1614–22. https://doi.org/10.1002/cncr.23787.
49. Schiffman SC, Metzger T, Dubel G, et al. Precision hepatic arterial Irinotecan therapy in the treatment of unresectable intrahepatic cholangiocellular carcinoma: optimal tolerance and prolonged overall survival. Ann Surg Oncol. 2011;18(2):431–8. https://doi.org/10.1245/s10434-010-1333-4.
50. Aliberti C, Benea G, Tilli M, Fiorentini G. Chemoembolization (TACE) of unresectable intrahepatic cholangiocarcinoma with slow-release doxorubicin-eluting beads: preliminary results. Cardiovasc Intervent Radiol. 2008;31(5):883–8. https://doi.org/10.1007/s00270-008-9336-2.
51. Pomoni M, Malagari K, Moschouris H, et al. Post embolization syndrome in doxorubicin eluting chemoembolization with DC bead. Hepato-Gastroenterology. 2011;59(115):820–5. https://doi.org/10.5754/hge11347.
52. Lencioni R, de Baere T, Soulen MC, Rilling WS, Geschwind J-FH. Lipiodol transarterial chemoembolization for hepatocellular carcinoma: a systematic review of efficacy and safety data. Hepatology. 2016;64(1):106–16. https://doi.org/10.1002/hep.28453.
53. Tu J, Jia Z, Ying X, et al. The incidence and outcome of major complication following conventional TAE/TACE for hepatocellular carcinoma. Medicine (Baltimore). 2016;95(49):e5606. https://doi.org/10.1097/MD.0000000000005606.
54. Clark TWI. Complications of hepatic chemoembolization. Semin Intervent Radiol. 2006;23(2):119–25. https://doi.org/10.1055/s-2006-941442.
55. Kuhlmann JB, Euringer W, Spangenberg HC, et al. Treatment of unresectable cholangiocarcinoma. Eur J Gastroenterol Hepatol. 2012;24(4):1. https://doi.org/10.1097/MEG.0b013e3283502241.

56. Boehm LM, Jayakrishnan TT, Miura JT, et al. Comparative effectiveness of hepatic artery based therapies for unresectable intrahepatic cholangiocarcinoma. J Surg Oncol. 2015;111(2):213–20. https://doi.org/10.1002/jso.23781.
57. Tong AKT, Kao YH, Too CW, Chin KFW, Ng DCE, Chow PKH. Yttrium-90 hepatic radioembolization: clinical review and current techniques in interventional radiology and personalized dosimetry. Br J Radiol. 2016;89(1062):20150943. https://doi.org/10.1259/bjr.20150943.
58. Kennedy A, Nag S, Salem R, et al. Recommendations for radioembolization of hepatic malignancies using yttrium-90 microsphere brachytherapy: a consensus panel report from the radioembolization brachytherapy oncology consortium. Int J Radiat Oncol. 2007;68(1):13–23. https://doi.org/10.1016/j.ijrobp.2006.11.060.
59. Lewandowski RJ, Geschwind J-F, Liapi E, Salem R. Transcatheter intraarterial therapies: rationale and overview. Radiology. 2011;259(3):641–57. https://doi.org/10.1148/radiol.11081489.
60. Leung WT, Lau WY, Ho SK, et al. Measuring lung shunting in hepatocellular carcinoma with intrahepatic-arterial technetium-99m macroaggregated albumin. J Nucl Med. 1994;35(1):70–3. http://www.ncbi.nlm.nih.gov/pubmed/8271063. Accessed 20 Feb 2020
61. Leung TW, Lau WY, Ho SK, et al. Radiation pneumonitis after selective internal radiation treatment with intraarterial 90yttrium-microspheres for inoperable hepatic tumors. Int J Radiat Oncol Biol Phys. 1995;33(4):919–24. https://doi.org/10.1016/0360-3016(95)00039-3.
62. Ho S, Lau WY, Leung TWT, Johnson PJ. Internal radiation therapy for patients with primary or metastatic hepatic cancer. Cancer. 1998;83(9):1894–907. https://doi.org/10.1002/(SICI)1097-0142(19981101)83:9<1894::AID-CNCR4>3.0.CO;2-O.
63. Rafi S, Piduru SM, El-Rayes B, et al. Yttrium-90 radioembolization for unresectable standard-chemorefractory intrahepatic cholangiocarcinoma: survival, efficacy, and safety study. Cardiovasc Intervent Radiol. 2013;36(2):440–8. https://doi.org/10.1007/s00270-012-0463-4.
64. Bourien H, Palard X, Rolland Y, et al. Yttrium-90 glass microspheres radioembolization (RE) for biliary tract cancer: a large single-center experience. Eur J Nucl Med Mol Imaging. 2019;46(3):669–76. https://doi.org/10.1007/s00259-018-4199-5.
65. Saxena A, Bester L, Chua TC, Chu FC, Morris DL. Yttrium-90 radiotherapy for unresectable intrahepatic cholangiocarcinoma: a preliminary assessment of this novel treatment option. Ann Surg Oncol. 2010;17(2):484–91. https://doi.org/10.1245/s10434-009-0777-x.
66. Hoffmann R-T, Paprottka PM, Schön A, et al. Transarterial hepatic yttrium-90 radioembolization in patients with unresectable intrahepatic cholangiocarcinoma: factors associated with prolonged survival. Cardiovasc Intervent Radiol. 2012;35(1):105–16. https://doi.org/10.1007/s00270-011-0142-x.
67. Gangi A, Shah J, Hatfield N, et al. Intrahepatic cholangiocarcinoma treated with transarterial yttrium-90 glass microsphere radioembolization: results of a single institution retrospective study. J Vasc Interv Radiol. 2018;29(8):1101–8. https://doi.org/10.1016/j.jvir.2018.04.001.
68. White J, Carolan-Rees G, Dale M, et al. Yttrium-90 transarterial radioembolization for chemotherapy-refractory intrahepatic cholangiocarcinoma: a prospective, observational study. J Vasc Interv Radiol. 2019;30(8):1185–92. https://doi.org/10.1016/j.jvir.2019.03.018.
69. Mouli S, Memon K, Baker T, et al. Yttrium-90 radioembolization for intrahepatic cholangiocarcinoma: safety, response, and survival analysis. J Vasc Interv Radiol. 2013;24(8):1227–34. https://doi.org/10.1016/j.jvir.2013.02.031.
70. Edeline J, Touchefeu Y, Guiu B, et al. Radioembolization plus chemotherapy for first-line treatment of locally advanced intrahepatic cholangiocarcinoma. JAMA Oncol. 2020;6(1):51. https://doi.org/10.1001/jamaoncol.2019.3702.
71. Riaz A, Awais R, Salem R. Side effects of yttrium-90 radioembolization. Front Oncol. 2014;4:198. https://doi.org/10.3389/fonc.2014.00198.
72. Sangro B, Iñarrairaegui M, Bilbao JI. Radioembolization for hepatocellular carcinoma. J Hepatol. 2012;56(2):464–73. https://doi.org/10.1016/j.jhep.2011.07.012.

Chapter 19
Established and Emerging Biomarkers for Prediction, Early Detection, and Prognostication of Cholangiocarcinoma

Andrés García-Sampedro, Pilar Acedo, and Stephen P. Pereira

Abbreviations

BBD	benign biliary disorders
CCA	cholangiocarcinoma
CT	computed tomography
CTCs	circulating tumour cells
eCCA	extrahepatic cholangiocarcinoma
ERCP	endoscopic retrograde cholangiopancreatography
EUS	endoscopic ultrasonography
EVs	extracellular vesicles
HCC	hepatocellular carcinoma
iCCA	intrahepatic cholangiocarcinoma
MRI	magnetic resonance imaging
pCCA	perihilar cholangiocarcinoma
PSC	primary sclerosing cholangitis
PTC	percutaneous transhepatic cholangiography
UC	ulcerative colitis
VOCs	volatile organic compounds

A. García-Sampedro · P. Acedo · S. P. Pereira (✉)
Institute for Liver & Digestive Health, University College London, Royal Free Hospital Campus, London, UK
e-mail: andres.sampedro.17@ucl.ac.uk; p.nunez@ucl.ac.uk; stephen.pereira@ucl.ac.uk

J. H. Tabibian (ed.), *Diagnosis and Management of Cholangiocarcinoma*,
https://doi.org/10.1007/978-3-030-70936-5_19

Introduction

The term "biomarker" in clinical care refers to biomolecules produced by different cell populations in the human body that have been strongly linked with a particular disease or disorder [1, 2]. The detection and quantification of these molecules have become particularly useful to diagnose diseases at an early stage as well as to select the best therapeutic option for personalised medicine. Similarly, some biomarkers can also predict patient prognosis and risk of disease relapse [2, 3]. For clinical use, an ideal biomarker should be highly specific and sensitive for a disease, being able to differentiate the disease from other biologically related conditions (specificity) and detect the disease when low levels of the biomolecule of interest are present (sensitivity) [4, 5].

In the case of CCA, early diagnosis remains an area of critical need, as presently 65% of patients are diagnosed with an advanced stage of the disease when treatment options are very limited [6]. The frequently late diagnosis of CCA is mainly due to the non-specific symptoms and clinical manifestations of CCA, which are common to other biliary obstructive conditions [7, 8]. In contrast, the 35% of the cases diagnosed at early stages have potentially curative options, such as surgical resection or liver transplantation [9].

The diagnosis of CCA is based largely on non-invasive imaging, which may include contrast-enhanced computed tomography (CT) and magnetic resonance imaging (MRI). Endoscopic ultrasonography (EUS), endoscopic retrograde cholangiopancreatography (ERCP), and percutaneous transhepatic cholangiography (PTC) have additional roles in tissue acquisition and stenting of biliary strictures, with a very small risk of peritoneal seeding reported with PTC- and EUS-guided biopsy [10]. Serum biomarkers for diagnosis lack sensitivity and specificity [5, 6, 11], and there are currently no biomarkers established to predict patient outcome for the different disease sites: extrahepatic CCA (eCCA), intrahepatic CCA (iCCA), and perihilar CCA (pCCA) [11].

In this chapter we will review current biomarkers used in the clinical setting for the detection of CCA as well as novel strategies still under development for early diagnosis, surveillance, and prognostication and grouped according to tissue source (see Fig. 19.1).

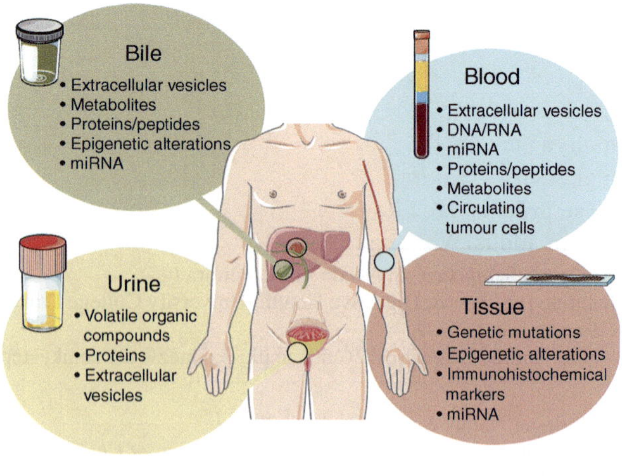

Fig. 19.1 Emerging biomarkers for the detection and prognostication of CCA according to tissue source. (This figure was created using images from Servier Medical Art Commons Attribution 3.0 Unported License (http://smart.servier.com). Servier Medical Art by Servier is licensed under a Creative Commons Attribution 3.0 Unported License)

Established Serum Biomarkers

The most commonly used serum biomarkers for the detection of CCA are carbohydrate antigen 19-9 (CA19-9) and carcinoembryonic antigen (CEA). However, they have low sensitivity and specificity and are not adequate for early diagnosis [3, 7].

CA19-9

CA19-9 is a sialylated Lewis blood group antigen reported for the first time in colorectal cancer cells [12]. Synthesis of this biomolecule is directly linked to the activity of its two precursor enzymes known as fucosyltransferases 2 and 3 (FUT2 and FUT3). Patient genotype regarding these enzymes affects the overall amount of CA19-9 liberated into the bloodstream, and it is estimated that 10% of the population have inactive FUT3, thus being CA19-9 antigen negative (even in the presence of tissue-proven CCA) [13].

The sensitivity and specificity of CA19-9 for CCA vary among studies and patient cohorts analysed but are estimated to be around 50–80% and 40–70%, respectively [14]. Its low specificity arises from the fact that this marker is also detected in the serum of patients with other malignancies, such as pancreatic cancer, colorectal cancer, and hepatocellular carcinoma (HCC), as well as in benign inflammatory conditions including acute cholangitis, pancreatitis, choledocholithiasis, hepatitis, and cirrhosis [15, 16]. Levels of CA19-9 greater than 100 U/mL, in the absence of cholangitis, tend to indicate the presence of malignancy in the biliary tree [14, 15, 17]. Lastly, levels of CA19-9 are also elevated in some respiratory conditions such as bronchiectasis, pulmonary fibrosis, and emphysema. For these reasons, it is estimated that around 10% of patients with elevated CA19-9 levels do not have any cancer of the biliary tree but instead some kind of benign disease [19].

CEA

CEA is a group of 12 glycoproteins involved in cell adhesion that was linked to malignancy for the first time in colorectal cancer specimens [20]. Generally, levels higher than 5 ng/mL are considered abnormal in clinical practice [21]. Levels of these proteins are elevated during foetal development, but their expression is minimal in adults. Although CEA represents a reliable biomarker for colorectal cancer, it is only elevated in 30% of patients with CCA. Like CA19-9, CEA may also be elevated in other conditions such as pancreatic cancer, colorectal cancer, cirrhosis, hepatitis, cholangitis, and inflammatory bowel disease [22]. Thus, detection of CEA in patients with suspected CCA may indicate a different primary malignancy metastatic to the hepatobiliary system.

CA-125

The carbohydrate antigen 125, also known as mucin 16, is a large cell surface protein encoded by the MUC16 gene generally found in the epithelia of the endometrium, ovaries, bronchi, and cornea [23]. It is elevated in about 65% of CCA patients (normal upper limit of 37 U/mL) but also in pancreatic, colon, ovarian, breast, and lung cancers as well as in benign hepatobiliary conditions like cirrhosis [18, 24]. As with CEA, this serum biomarker is generally only tested when another primary malignancy is suspected.

Emerging Biomarkers

Blood Biomarkers

Among all the non-invasive sources of biomarkers, blood is easily and routinely collected and is rich in biomolecules. Therefore, the majority of published and ongoing research studies have sought to identify more specific and sensitive blood biomarkers for CCA or to combine several biomarkers into a panel to improve their performance (see Table 19.1).

Extracellular Vesicles

Extracellular vesicles (EVs) have emerged as a promising source of biomarkers. EVs consist of a heterogeneous population of lipid bilayer spheres containing different biomolecules such as proteins, nucleic acids (DNA and RNA), lipids, and other metabolites [25]. Cells use these biomolecules for intercellular communication and, in the context of disease, to modulate pathological pathways [26]. EVs have been found in all body fluids including blood [27], urine [28], bile [29], saliva [30], and ascites [31].

Based on their diameter (30 nm–2 μm), EVs have been classified into two main groups: (i) small EVs or exosomes (30–100 nm in diameter) and (ii) large EVs or microvesicles (>100 nm) [27]. Small EVs constitute the most studied group. They have their origin in vesicles derived from the endomembranous system, which accumulate to form multivesicular bodies and merge with the plasma membrane releasing the exosomes to the extracellular space. In contrast, large EVs bud directly from the cell membrane of the parental cell [32, 33].

The amount, content, and surface markers of EVs have proven to reflect the biological features and staging of different types of cancer, including CCA [35]. In one study performed by Arbelaiz et al., the total amount and protein content of EVs isolated from patients with CCA, primary sclerosing cholangitis (PSC), HCC, and healthy individuals were compared [36]. HCC patients had the highest EV density

Table 19.1 Emerging biomarkers for CCA detection in blood

Biomarker	Source	Comparison	SEN (%)	SPE (%)	AUC	References
Protein-containing EVs						
AMPN	Serum	CCA vs healthy	90.7	65.6	0.878	[36]
VNN1	Serum	CCA vs healthy	72.1	87.5	0.876	[36]
PIGR	Serum	CCA vs healthy	83.7	71.8	0.844	[36]
FIBG	Serum	CCA vs PSC	88.4	63.3	0.796	[36]
A1AG1	Serum	CCA vs PSC	76.7	70.0	0.794	[36]
S100A8	Serum	CCA vs PSC	69.8	66.6	0.759	[36]
FCN2	Serum	Early-stage CCA (I-II) vs PSC	100.0	80.9	0.956	[36]
ITIH4	Serum	Early-stage CCA (I-II) vs PSC	91.7	80.9	0.881	[36]
FIBG	Serum	Early-stage CCA (I-II) vs PSC	91.7	80.9	0.881	[36]
RNA-containing EVs						
RFFL	Serum	CCA vs [PSC+UC+healthy]	100.0	100.0	1.00	[37]
ZNF266	Serum	CCA vs [PSC+UC+healthy]	91.7	91.3	0.976	[37]
OR4F3	Serum	CCA vs [PSC+UC+healthy]	100.0	87.1	0.960	[37]
miR-551B	Serum	CCA vs [PSC+UC+healthy]	83.3	87.0	0.909	[37]
PMS2L4	Serum	CCA vs [PSC+UC+healthy]	91.7	87.0	0.880	[37]
LOC643955	Serum	CCA vs [PSC+UC+healthy]	83.3	87.0	0.873	[37]
EV surface markers						
AnnexinV^{+} EpCAM^{+} AS6PR1^{+}	Serum	CCA vs liver disorders	65.8	47.0	0.621	[38]
microRNA markers						
miR-21	Serum	CCA vs healthy	–	–	0.910	[44]
miR-21	Plasma	CCA vs healthy	–	–	0.940	[44]
miR-26a	Serum	CCA vs healthy	84.8	81.8	0.900	[46]
miR-150	Plasma	iCCA vs healthy	80.6	58.1	0.791	[47]
miR-192	Serum	CCA vs healthy	74.0	72.0	0.809	[48]
miR-106a	Serum	CCA vs healthy	81.6	85.0	0.890	[49]
miR-222 miR-483-5p	Serum	CCA vs PSC-derived CCA	–	–	0.770	[50]
miR-126	Serum	CCA vs PSC	68.0	93.0	0.870	[51]
miR-1281	Serum	CCA vs PSC	55.0	90.0	0.830	[51]
miR-30b	Serum	CCA vs PSC	52.0	88.0	0.780	[51]
miR-122	Serum	CCA vs PSC	32.0	90.0	0.650	[51]
Protein biomarkers						
OPN	Serum	CCA vs healthy	88.0	100.0	0.964	[56]

(continued)

Table 19.1 (continued)

Biomarker	Source	Comparison	SEN (%)	SPE (%)	AUC	References
IL-6	Serum	CCA vs healthy	73.0	92.0	0.875	[61]
TGF-β1	Serum	CCA vs healthy	71.1	68.9	0.668	[63]
TGF-β1	Serum	CCA vs BBD	68.0	71.1	0.644	[63]
CYFRA 21-1	Serum	iCCA vs BBD	75.6	96.2	0.879	[66]
CYFRA 21-1 PKM2 MUC5AC GGT	Serum	CCA vs PSC	81.8	90.0	0.903	[68]
MMP-7	Serum	CCA vs BBD	75.0	78.0	0.730	[73]
S100A6	Serum	CCA vs healthy	86.0	91.0	0.909	[74]
DKK1	Serum	CCA vs healthy	76.0	100.0	0.872	[75]
SSP411	Serum	CCA vs BBD	90.0	83.0	0.913	[76]
AFP	Serum	iCCA vs HCC	91.1	–	–	[80]
AFP CA-242	Serum	iCCA vs HCC	93.4	89.7	–	[80]
Metabolites						
TSA	Serum	CCA vs [BBD+healthy]	71.9	81.4	0.856	[82]
TSA	Serum	CCA vs HCC	82.6	83.1	0.885	[83]
TSA	Serum	CCA vs [chronic hepatitis + cirrhosis + healthy]	82.6	86.0	0.964	[83]
21-deoxycortisol Bilirubin LysoPC (14:0) LysoPC (15:0)	Serum	CCA vs healthy	98.5	99.2	0.993	[84]

SEN sensitivity, *SPE* specificity, *AUC* area under (ROC) curve, *Ref* reference, *EV* extracellular vesicles, *CCA* cholangiocarcinoma, *PSC* primary sclerosing cholangitis, *UC* ulcerative colitis, *iCCA* intrahepatic cholangiocarcinoma, *BBD* benign biliary disorders, *HCC* hepatocellular cholangiocarcinoma

in serum compared to the other groups. A range of different proteins were suggested as potential biomarkers to distinguish CCA from the other groups. Among these proteins, AMPN (aminopeptidase N), VNN1 (pantetheinase), and PIGR (polymeric immunoglobulin receptor) showed the highest diagnostic values when comparing CCA patients to healthy controls (AUC 0.878, 0.876, and 0.844, respectively), whereas FIBG (fibrinogen gamma chain), A1AG1 (alpha-1-acid glycoprotein), and protein S100A8 (AUC 0.796, 0.794, and 0.759, respectively) were the most promising candidates to differentiate PSC from CCA. Lastly, the proteins FCN2 (ficolin 2), ITIH4 (inter-alpha-trypsin inhibitor heavy chain 4), and FIBG (AUC 0.956, 0.881 and 0.881, respectively) showed promise for the differential diagnosis of early-stage CCA (stages I–II) and PSC.

Transcriptomic analysis of EV content revealed messenger RNA (mRNA) and different non-coding RNA molecules (such as microRNAs [miRs], long non-coding RNAs, and small nucleolar RNAs) with potential for CCA diagnosis. In a recent study by Lapitz et al., the serum EV content of CCA patients was compared with benign biliary conditions like PSC and ulcerative colitis (UC) as well as with healthy individuals [37]. A total of 1932 transcripts were differentially expressed in the CCA group compared to the other 3 subgroups combined into a single group, with RFFL (E3 ubiquitin-protein ligase rififylin), ZNF266 (zinc finger protein 266), and OR4F3 (olfactory receptor family 4 subfamily F member 3) being the mRNAs with the highest diagnostic potential (AUC 1.00, 0.976, and 0.960, respectively). The best-performing non-coding RNAs were miR-551B, PMS2L4, and LOC643955 (AUC 0.909, 0.880, and 0.873, respectively).

The fact that large EVs bud from the plasma membrane of the parental cell is particularly interesting because some of the surface markers will remain on the vesicle lipid bilayer and mirror the pathobiological cues of the disease. For instance, tumour-associated microparticles (taMPs) carrying markers such as Annexin V, EpCAM (epithelial cellular adhesion molecule), and ASGPR1 (asialoglycoprotein receptor 1) allowed the differentiation of patients with liver malignancies (including CCA and HCC) from patients bearing non-liver cancers and cirrhosis, with 65.8% sensitivity but only 47% specificity. These taMPs decreased significantly at 7 days after curative resection, demonstrating their potential prognostic value [38, 39].

Nucleic Acid Biomarkers

Similar to EVs, cell-free nucleic acids are released by healthy and cancer cells into different body fluids such as blood, urine, or bile [3, 34]. In terms of circulating DNA, some of the most commonly mutated genes in CCA, including KRAS, NRAS, BRAF, and PIK3CA, were first screened in tumour tissue by multiplex PCR and then in DNA isolated from matched plasma samples from patients. The mutation pattern of the tumour was conserved in plasma suggesting the suitability of the technique for cancer detection [40].

Another group of nucleic acid biomarkers are circulating RNAs, with some studies suggesting their diagnostic value in CCA [41, 42]. Among them, miR-21, a small transcript with important roles in development, inflammation, and cancer invasion [43], was the most commonly upregulated miR in CCA, and in one study, it differentiated iCCA patients from healthy individuals with an AUC 0.91 in serum and 0.94 in plasma [44]. However, it was also upregulated in the blood of patients with other cancers such as HCC, limiting its specificity [45]. Patients with CCA have also shown increased levels of miR-26a [46], miR-150 [47], and miR-192 [48] and decreased levels of miR-106a [49].

Interestingly, a comparison of the differential expression of miRs in the blood of PSC-derived CCA patients (n = 7) and CCA alone patients (n = 63) showed increased levels of miR-222 and miR-483-5p in the latter group, achieving an AUC of 0.770 when combined [50]. Another study reported a panel of five miRs in serum (miR-126, -1281, -26a, -30b, and -122) with an individual maximum AUC of 0.870, though a combination of the different miRs in a logistic regression model did not significantly improve their diagnostic accuracy [51]. However, further studies with larger cohorts are needed to validate these findings.

One of the strongest features that makes cell-free nucleic acids good candidate biomarkers for CCA is their ability to reflect the very heterogeneous pattern of mutations of these tumours. In addition, they can be easily isolated from blood, amplified, and detected by well-established targeted techniques such as qRT-PCR and microarray or by untargeted techniques such as whole genome sequencing (WGS) or whole transcriptome sequencing (also known as total RNA sequencing, RNA-Seq) [52, 53]. Although the above-mentioned publications support the potential of nucleic acid biomarkers for the early detection of CCA and patient stratification, further studies are still needed to validate these findings.

Proteins and Peptides

Proteins are generally more stable and abundant in blood than nucleic acids. In recent years, many studies have taken a proteomic approach aiming at identifying a protein signature for CCA [19].

Osteopontin (OPN) is a potential novel biomarker for CCA. This glycoprotein is involved in normal physiological processes like bone biomineralisation and in pathological conditions such as chronic inflammation [54] and tumour formation [55]. Serum levels of OPN have been reported to be elevated in patients with CCA compared to PSC and healthy controls, with an AUC of 0.964. Persistently high levels post-tumour resection were associated with poor postoperative survival, highlighting its potential role as a prognostic biomarker [56].

Interleukin-6 (IL-6) is an inflammatory cytokine secreted by cholangiocytes upon inflammatory stimuli [57, 58, 59]. In CCA, the cancerous cells also produce this protein, which upregulates Bcl-2, an antiapoptotic cytosolic protein, promoting tumour growth [60]. Serum levels of IL-6 had a 73% sensitivity and 92% specificity (AUC 0.875) for distinguishing CCA patients from healthy controls [61]. Additionally, the concentration of IL-6 in blood decreased after tumour resection. Of note, IL-6 was also elevated in patients with other liver cancers like HCC [62]. Similarly, the cytokine transforming growth factor-β1 (TGF-β1), associated with cell invasion and microenvironment modification, was also found to be elevated in patients with CCA compared to healthy individuals (AUC 0.668) and to other inflammatory conditions (AUC 0.644) [63].

Another proposed CCA biomarker is the soluble fragment of cytokeratin-19, i.e. CYFRA 21-1 [64]. This marker has been studied in other cancers, e.g. lung cancer [65], and in one study it distinguished CCA from other benign biliary conditions with 75.6% sensitivity and 96.2% specificity [66]. CYFRA 21-1 levels have also been reported to correlate with tumour stage and patient prognosis, with a 3-year survival rate of 76% in patients with low levels of CYFRA 21-1 compared with only 25% in patients with high concentrations [67]. One study from our group by Cuenco et al. reported that a panel of serum protein biomarkers, which included CYFRA21-1, PKM2 (pyruvate kinase M2), MUC5AC (mucin 5AC), and GGT (gamma-glutamyltransferase), was able to differentiate CCA from PSC alone with 81.8% sensitivity and 90.0% specificity (AUC 0.903) [68].

Matrix metalloproteinases 7 and 9 (MMP-7 and MMP-9) are two enzymes responsible for the degradation and remodelling of the extracellular matrix in processes of tissue repair, embryonic development, and angiogenesis [69]. They also play an important role in tumour formation, and as such, increased levels of these proteins in blood have been linked to tumour presence [70–72]. Increased serum levels of MMP-7 in CCA patients compared with individuals with benign biliary conditions showed an AUC of 0.730, but MMP-9 did not reliably differentiate between the two groups [73].

Several other proteins for CCA detection have been described. For example, serum S100A6, a calcium-binding protein, had an AUC of 0.909 when comparing CCA to healthy controls [74], while Dickkopf-related protein 1 (DKK1) had an AUC of 0.872 in iCCA versus healthy controls [75]. Spermatogenesis-associated protein 20 (SSP411) showed an AUC of 0.913 in CCA versus benign biliary disorders and healthy controls [76]. A specific glycoprotein known as KL-6, a type of MUC1, has also showed potential when comparing blood levels of CCA patients to healthy individuals, HCC patients, and metastatic liver cancer patients [77]. Serum alpha fetoprotein (AFP) showed good results differentiating HCC from CCA patients, but low specificity [78]. However, when combining AFP with carbohydrate antigen 242 (CA-242), a potential marker of pancreatic cancer [79], the overall sensitivity and specificity increased to 93.4% and 89.7%, respectively [80]. Larger studies are needed to validate these findings.

Serum Metabolites

In addition to the previously mentioned biochemical groups, small molecules have also been reported to be altered in the blood of patients with CCA. Sialic acid (TSA) is a neurotransmitter which has been linked to different cancers including brain tumours, leukaemia, melanoma, and also CCA [81]. In one study by Wongkham et al., the total amount of TSA in CCA patients compared with individuals with benign biliary conditions (including cholangitis, cirrhosis, and gallstones, among others) had an AUC of 0.670, which increased to 0.856 when compared to healthy controls alone [82]. In another study, Kongtawelert et al. compared TSA levels in blood of CCA versus HCC patients (AUC 0.885) and CCA versus cirrhosis and chronic hepatitis patients (AUC 0.964) [83].

Liang et al. performed a metabolomic analysis of the serum of CCA patients and compared it with healthy individuals. During the initial discovery phase, 75 differentially expressed metabolites were found between groups. After the validation phase in 225 CCA and 101 healthy serum samples, the 4 markers that showed the best diagnostic performance were 21-deoxycortisol (under-expressed in CCA), bilirubin (over-expressed), lysophosphatidylcholine 14:0 (lysoPC (14:0), under-expressed), and lysophosphatidylcholine (lysoPC (15:0), over-expressed). The calculated AUCs were 0.918, 0.922, 0.954, and 0.927, respectively, which increased to 0.993 when the four metabolites were combined [84]. Further validation studies of these metabolites are expected.

Circulating Tumour Cells

Circulating tumour cells (CTCs) represent a potential tool for the detection of CCA and have been reported in other cancers including HCC [85], pancreatic cancer [86], and colorectal carcinoma [87]. CTCs have also been studied as a cause of metastasis and tumour relapse, opening the possibility of their use as prognostic biomarkers [88]. To date, the only FDA-approved system for cancer detection is the CellSearch® system, which selects CTCs positive for DAPI, CK-8/18 (hepatocyte antigens), and CK-19 (cholangiocytes antigen) and negative for CD45 staining (leukocyte antigen). However, in one study, only 25% of patients with CCA showed elevated CTC levels [89].

The accuracy of CTCs as prognostic biomarkers has not yet been well-studied in CCA, and only a few studies have reported small subgroups of CCA patients within their cohorts of patients with hepatobiliary disorders. One study isolated CTCs from the blood of CCA patients and showed a high variability in mutations on exon 12 of KRAS gene [88]. Others have reported that CTCs could play an important role in tumour metastasis through their interaction with different T-cell populations in the circulation [86].

Bile Biomarkers

Bile is a complex mix of biomolecules synthesised by the liver and used in the process of digestion. Its major components include bile acids, phospholipids, cholesterol, urea, bilirubin and a variety of hormones and digestive enzymes. In recent years, bile has gained attention as a source of potential novel biomarkers for biliary disorders like CCA [89, 90]. Different groups have used approaches based on omics to identify alterations in the concentration and composition of these organic molecules.

Bile Metabolites

Metabolomic studies performed by several groups have identified alterations in the composition of bile in CCA patients [91]. Bile acids, phospholipids, and cholesterol have shown the biggest differences between disease groups, highlighting their promising diagnostic potential.

Bile acids are steroid acids synthesised from cholesterol by hepatocytes. They regulate levels of cholesterol in the body, assist in fat absorption, and allow phospholipid transport. Analyses of the total content of bile acids in CCA patients have shown a reduction in secondary bile acids, such as deoxycholic and lithocholic acids, compared to patients with biliary tract stones and healthy individuals [92]. A decrease in glycine- and taurine-conjugated bile acids, phospholipids, and cholesterol was also observed in CCA patients compared to benign controls [93]. However, when comparing bile from CCA and PSC patients, the levels of glycine-conjugated acids and phosphatidylcholines were significantly increased in the cancer group [94]. In another study, magnetic resonance spectroscopy of bile had an 88.9% sensitivity and an 87.1% specificity in distinguishing CCA from non-PSC benign biliary conditions [95].

Proteins and Peptides

Analysis of the bile proteome has also been widely explored to identify proteins abnormally expressed in CCA patients. In this context, biliary levels of insulin-like growth factor 1 (IGF-1), also called somatomedin C, a hormone synthesised in the liver with important roles in growth and development, was increased in eCCA patients compared with those with pancreatic cancer or non-malignant disorders (AUC 1.00) [96]. Lipocalin-2 (LCN2), a secreted protein responsible for the transport of some hydrophobic substances, was found elevated in the bile of 30 CCA patients compared to 36 gallstone patients, with a sensitivity of 87% and an AUC of 0.81 [97].

Minichromosome maintenance (MCM) proteins are a family of proteins conserved in all eukaryotic cells due to their role in DNA replication [98] which have been explored as markers of proliferation and cancer progression [99]. Specifically, MCM-7 has been linked to the activation of oncogenes in CCA [100]. In a study conducted in our laboratory by Ayaru et al., biliary MCM-5 as a marker of pancreatobiliary malignancy (including CCA) had a sensitivity of 66% compared to 20% for biliary brush cytology (AUC 0.800) [101].

The ratio of pancreatic elastase (PE) and amylase in bile could be another possible marker of CCA. Low levels of amylase may be associated with complete biliary obstruction caused by a tumour. Patients with CCA had an increased PE/amylase ratio compared with gallstone patients, with a sensitivity of 82% and a specificity of 89% (AUC 0.877) [102].

Lastly, increased biliary levels of Mac-2-binding protein (Mac-2BP), a cell-adhesive protein of the extracellular matrix found upregulated in many cancers, showed promising values for the differential diagnosis of CCA from patients with benign biliary disorders including PSC. The study reported an AUC of 0.700 that increased to 0.750 when Mac-2BP levels were combined with biliary levels of CA19-9 [103].

Extracellular Vesicles

EVs in bile have also been studied for the differential diagnosis of CCA. The total amount of EVs in bile in CCA patients was compared to patients with non-malignant bile duct stenoses. Cancer patients showed an increased total amount of EVs (4.00×10^{15} compared to 1.26×10^{14} nanoparticles/L), being able to differentiate malignant from non-malignant patients with 100% sensitivity and 100% specificity (AUC 1.00) [104]. Another study compared the transcriptomic content of

EVs in patients with the same conditions and found a panel of five miRs (miR-191, miR-486-3p, miR-1274b, miR-16, miR-484) able to differentiate CCA with 67% sensitivity and 96% specificity [105].

Genetic Biomarkers

Circulating RNAs have also been reported in bile. In one study by Plieskatt et al., the content of miRs in bile was compared between patients with malignant and benign biliary tract conditions like choledocholithiasis. miR-9 and miR-145 showed the highest diagnostic accuracy (AUC 0.975 in both cases) to differentiate between the two groups [106]. A different research group found that the expression of miR-150-5p was decreased in the bile of CCA patients compared to healthy individuals [47]. In terms of their ability to differentiate PSC-derived CCA from benign PSC, four miRs were identified (miR-412, miR-640, miR-1537, and miR-3189) showing AUC ranging from 0.78 to 0.81. The combination of biliary miR-1537 and CA19-9 levels had an AUC of 0.91 [51].

Changes in DNA methylation in CCA bile samples have been studied by a few groups. Shin et al. described a biomarker panel based on the altered methylation pattern of five genes involved in tumour growth, invasion, migration, and differentiation (CCND2, CDH13, GRIN2B, RUNX3, and TWIST1). The combination was able to differentiate eCCA from a control group of patients with benign disorders like cholecystitis and cholangitis with 83.3% sensitivity and 100% specificity [107]. Thus, the detection of DNA methylation alterations could be a powerful diagnostic strategy for patients with CCA, but further studies are needed to consolidate these data.

Serotonin

Serotonin is a neurotransmitter which also plays an important role in liver regeneration and is overexpressed in CCA [108]. Alpini et al. reported increased levels of TPH-1, an enzyme involved in the route of serotonin synthesis, in 48 tumour biopsies of CCA patients compared to healthy liver tissue. Decreased levels of enzymes responsible for serotonin degradation, such as monoamine oxidase A, were also observed. Finally, increased levels of serotonin were found in the bile of CCA patients but not in patients with intrahepatic stones [109].

Urine Biomarkers

Urine has been shown to be a useful non-invasive source of biomarkers for different cancers, including bladder [110], kidney [111], liver [112], and pancreas [113], with advantages of ease of access and low proteome complexity compared to blood [114]. However, its applicability to biliary tract cancers has been only recently explored.

Volatile Organic Compounds

Urine is a body fluid rich in a variety of volatile organic compounds (VOCs) that have been screened for markers that may differentiate CCA from benign biliary conditions. Navaneethan et al. used selected-ion flow-tube mass spectrometry (SIFT-MS) to measure the concentration of VOCs in urine. Results showed that a combination of ethane and 1-octene levels distinguished CCA from PSC patients with an 80% sensitivity and 100% specificity (AUC 0.900). In addition, by comparing the concentration of 2-propanol and acetonitrile, the authors reported an efficient tool for separating CCA cases from a mixed group of PSC and other benign biliary conditions (AUC 0.862) [115].

Proteomic Profile

The total urinary proteome of 41 patients bearing different biliary conditions including CCA, PSC, and other benign disorders has also been analysed with the aim of finding a singular proteomic signature able to detect and differentiate malignancies. Around 5600 different peptides were selected from the samples with a frequency higher than 20%. Out of these, 43 peptides were chosen as potential biomarkers of CCA showing AUC ranging from 0.630 to 0.890 [116]. Some of these peptides were assigned to well-known proteins such as collagen α-1 and α-2 (extracellular matrix components), osteopontin, uromodulin (an inhibitor of calcium crystallisation in renal fluids), and the antigen CD99 (involved in transmembrane transport). The panel of identified distinct markers was then validated in a different cohort of 123 patients that included CCA, PSC, and other benign biliary disorders, proving efficiency in discriminating CCA cases with a sensitivity of 83% and a specificity of 79% (AUC 0.870) [117].

Extracellular Vesicles

EVs have also been sourced from urine showing particularly good potential when their transcriptomic content was analysed. In a comparative study of the RNA content of EVs from CCA ($n = 23$), PSC ($n = 5$), UC ($n = 12$), and healthy individuals ($n = 5$), a total number of 27,319 transcripts were identified, out of which 1470 were unique in CCA samples. Messenger RNAs INO80D, MAP6D1, and RRAGD (AUC 1.00 for all) and non-coding RNAs HCG4, MIR200C, and LOC100134868 (AUC 0.930, 0.904, and 0.896, respectively) were the best candidate markers for the differential diagnosis of CCA versus healthy individuals. CLIP3, VCAM1, and TRIM33 messenger RNAs (AUC 0.965 for all) were able to differentiate CCA versus PSC; whereas MT1F, GPX3, and LDHA (AUC 0.915, 0.897, 0.894, respectively) were selected to distinguish CCA from a control group that combined PSC, UC, and healthy patients [37].

Histological Markers

Biopsy confirmation is often required for the clinical diagnosis of CCA [10]. In this regard, biomarkers analysed in resected tissue may provide complementary information for patient stratification, prognosis, and personalised therapies.

Genomic Markers

Considering the high heterogeneity of mutations between the different subtypes of CCA tumours, finding key and specific altered genes can inform treatment options and predict patient outcome after tumour resection [118]. Mutations in DNA repair and cell growth genes (such as TP53 and KRAS, respectively) have been linked to worse patient prognosis than mutations in metabolic genes like IDH-1 and IDH-2 (encoding the enzymes isocitrate dehydrogenases 1 and 2) [7, 119–122]. The fibroblast growth factor receptor 2 gene (FGFR2) has been frequently reported mutated in iCCA patients and not in other liver cancers, suggesting the diagnostic potential of this genetic marker [118]. However, studies involving larger patient cohorts are required to validate these markers.

CCA tissue samples have also been used to identify novel biomarkers based on epigenetic alterations. A study conducted by Andresen and co-workers identified a four-gene panel (CDO1, CNRIP1, SEPT9, VIM) using tissue from brush cytologies. The panel showed a sensitivity of 85% and a specificity of 98% (AUC 0.944) in discriminating CCA from PSC patients [123]. Similarly, and although less investigated, other genes have also shown abnormal methylation patterns in CCA such as MLH1, DCLK1, CDO1, ZSCAN18, and ZNF331. These genes play key roles in DNA repair, stemness, and tumour growth and invasion [124, 125]. To date, the characterisation of the CCA methylome is still limited. A summary of the main steps towards the implementation of a novel biomarker is represented in Fig. 19.2.

Transcriptomic Markers

Whole transcriptome sequencing of resected tumour tissue has allowed researchers to better understand the biology and behaviour of CCA. In an integrative molecular analysis that combined gene expression levels, single-nucleotide polymorphisms (SNPs), and immunohistochemical markers of 153 patients, two subtypes of iCCA were found. In the so-called inflammatory type, an overexpression of inflammation-related genes (such as different cytokines and STAT3) was reported, whereas in the 'proliferation type', an activation of oncogenes (KRAS, MAPKs, and MET) was observed and linked to worse patient outcome [126].

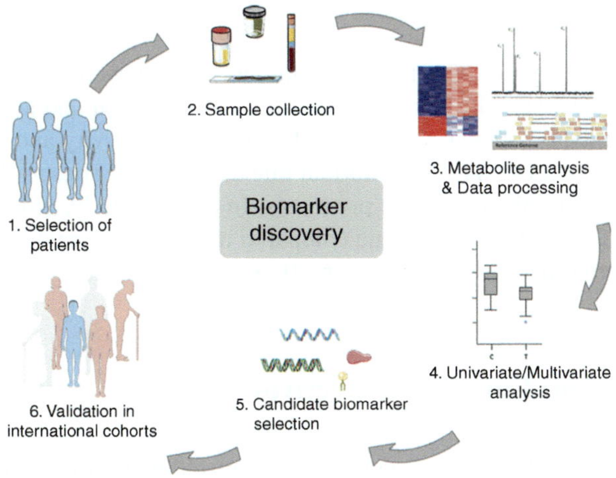

Fig. 19.2 Steps to cancer biomarker discovery. The process starts with the selection of a cohort of patients for biomarker discovery. Samples (blood, bile, urine, tissue) are screened for potential altered biomolecules. Levels of these molecules are then compared between cancer and control groups, and statistical differences and diagnostic potential are calculated. Only a few biomolecules (or a combination) get selected for further validation in larger cohorts. (This figure was created using images from Servier Medical Art Commons Attribution 3.0 Unported License (http://smart.servier.com). Servier Medical Art by Servier is licensed under a Creative Commons Attribution 3.0 Unported License)

A different study examining the recurrence-free interval after resection of CCA and gallbladder cancer linked the overexpression of CTL4 (cytotoxic T-lymphocyte-associated protein 4) and FOXP3 (marker of naturally occurring regulatory T cells) to patients with no CCA recurrence up to 18 months after resection [127]. Recently, the expression of IL-33 in tumour tissue was also associated with better prognosis in both iCCA and pCCA patients [128].

Immunohistochemical Markers

A number of prognostic markers for CCA have been identified using histological tumour samples. In one of the largest meta-studies to date, the histological signature of 4126 CCA patients was compared, identifying 77 potential prognostic biomarkers. Some of these markers were fascin (an actin bundling protein), the epithelial growth factor receptor (EGFR), mucins 1 and 4 (MUC1/4), and p27 (a tumour suppressor protein able to block the proliferation of cancer cells). Over-expression of these five proteins was linked to increased patient survival [129]. Similarly, Suzuki et al. reported that increased expression of the pyruvate kinase type M2 (PKM2) in tumour tissue may enhance tumour cell invasion and promote lymph node metastasis in iCCA cases [130].

micro-RNA

Microarray profiling of CCA resected tumours has allowed the identification of small RNA molecules with the potential for CCA detection and staging [39]. The best characterised is miR-21, which has shown 95% sensitivity and 100% specificity in the detection of CCA versus normal bile duct and liver tissue [131, 132]. This miR has also been linked to worse prognosis. In another study, miR-21 had similar expression in CCA and PDAC tissue compared to normal surrounding tissue, while a panel of seven other miRs were differently expressed [133].

Conclusion and Future Perspectives

CCA remains a deadly disease due in part to the lack of accurate non-invasive diagnostic tests, especially for early-stage disease. The identification and validation of specific markers could not only help discriminate which patients could undergo tumour resection, the only available curative option to date, but also predict the risk of recurrence after surgery. A great number of biomarkers including genetic material (DNA/RNA), circulating proteins, extracellular vesicles, bile acids, and metabolites, among others, have been identified in blood, bile, urine, and tumour tissue of CCA patients. However, in order to be translated to the clinical setting, the diagnostic and prognostic potential of these biological entities need to be validated in large international cohorts and compared with appropriate disease control groups.

References

1. Ongen Z. What do biomarkers mark? Anatol J Cardiol. 2016;16(2):75.
2. Diamandis EP. Towards identification of true cancer biomarkers. BMC Med. 2014;12(1):156.
3. Srivastava A, Creek DJ. Discovery and validation of clinical biomarkers of cancer: a review combining metabolomics and proteomics. Proteomics. 2019;19(10):e1700448.
4. Henry NL, Hayes DF. Cancer biomarkers. Mol Oncol. 2012;6(2):140–6.
5. Macias RIR, et al. The search for novel diagnostic and prognostic biomarkers in cholangiocarcinoma. Biochim Biophys Acta Mol basis Dis. 2018;1864(4 Pt B):1468–77.
6. Banales JM, et al. Expert consensus document: Cholangiocarcinoma: current knowledge and future perspectives consensus statement from the European Network for the Study of Cholangiocarcinoma (ENS-CCA). Nat Rev Gastroenterol Hepatol. 2016;13(5):261–80.
7. Marin JJG, et al. Chemoresistance and chemosensitization in cholangiocarcinoma. Biochim Biophys Acta Mol basis Dis. 2018;1864(4 Pt B):1444–53.
8. Banales JM, et al. Cholangiocarcinoma 2020: the next horizon in mechanisms and management. Nat Rev Gastroenterol Hepatol. 2020;17:557.
9. Rizvi S, Khan SA, Hallemeier CL, Kelley RK, Gores GJ. Cholangiocarcinoma - evolving concepts and therapeutic strategies. Nat Rev Clin Oncol. 2018;15(2):95–111.
10. Eloubeidi MA, et al. Endoscopic ultrasound-guided fine needle aspiration biopsy of suspected cholangiocarcinoma. Clin Gastroenterol Hepatol. 2004;2(3):209–13.

11. Macias RIR, et al. Diagnostic and prognostic biomarkers in cholangiocarcinoma. Liver Int. 2019;39(Suppl 1):108–22.
12. Malaguarnera G, Paladina I, Giordano M, Malaguarnera M, Bertino G, Berretta M. Serum markers of intrahepatic cholangiocarcinoma. Dis Markers. 2013;34(4):219–28.
13. Wannhoff A, et al. FUT2 and FUT3 genotype determines CA19-9 cut-off values for detection of cholangiocarcinoma in patients with primary sclerosing cholangitis. J Hepatol. 2013;59(6):1278–84.
14. Khan SA, et al. Guidelines for the diagnosis and treatment of cholangiocarcinoma: an update. Gut. 2012;61(12):1657–69.
15. Wadsworth CA, Lim A, Taylor-Robinson SD, Khan SA. The risk factors and diagnosis of cholangiocarcinoma. Hepatol Int. 2013;7(2):377–93.
16. Dumonceau J-M, Delhaye M, Charette N, Farina A. Challenging biliary strictures: pathophysiological features, differential diagnosis, diagnostic algorithms, and new clinically relevant biomarkers - part 1. Ther Adv Gastroenterol. 2020;13:1756284820927292.
17. Levy C, Lymp J, Angulo P, Gores GJ, Larusso N, Lindor KD. The value of serum CA 19-9 in predicting cholangiocarcinomas in patients with primary sclerosing cholangitis. Dig Dis Sci. 2005;50(9):1734–40.
18. He X-D, et al. The risk of carcinogenesis in congenital choledochal cyst patients: an analysis of 214 cases. Ann Hepatol. 2014;13(6):819–26.
19. Galli C, Basso D, Plebani M. CA 19-9: handle with care. Clin Chem Lab Med. 2013;51(7):1369–83.
20. Beauchemin N, Arabzadeh A. Carcinoembryonic antigen-related cell adhesion molecules (CEACAMs) in cancer progression and metastasis. Cancer Metastasis Rev. 2013; 32(3–4):643–71.
21. Fang T, Wang H, Wang Y, Lin X, Cui Y, Wang Z. Clinical significance of preoperative serum CEA, CA125, and CA19-9 levels in predicting the Resectability of Cholangiocarcinoma. Dis Markers. 2019;2019:6016931.
22. Rule AH, Goleski-Reilly C, Sachar DB, Vandevoorde J, Janowitz HD. Circulating carcinoembryonic antigen (CEA): relationship to clinical status of patients with inflammatory bowel disease. Gut. 1973;14(11):880–4.
23. Felder M, et al. MUC16 (CA125): tumor biomarker to cancer therapy, a work in progress. Mol Cancer. 2014;13:129.
24. Moss EL, Hollingworth J, Reynolds TM. The role of CA125 in clinical practice. J Clin Pathol. 2005;58(3):308–12.
25. Lapitz A, et al. Extracellular vesicles in hepatobiliary malignancies. Front Immunol. 2018;9:2270.
26. Yanez-Mo M, et al. Biological properties of extracellular vesicles and their physiological functions. J Extracell Vesicles. 2015;4:27066.
27. Caby M-P, Lankar D, Vincendeau-Scherrer C, Raposo G, Bonnerot C. Exosomal-like vesicles are present in human blood plasma. Int Immunol. 2005;17(7):879–87.
28. Pisitkun T, Shen R-F, Knepper MA. Identification and proteomic profiling of exosomes in human urine. Proc Natl Acad Sci U S A. 2004;101(36):13368 LP–13373.
29. Masyuk AI, et al. Biliary exosomes influence cholangiocyte regulatory mechanisms and proliferation through interaction with primary cilia. Am J Physiol Gastrointest Liver Physiol. 2010;299(4):G990–9.
30. Ogawa Y, et al. Proteomic analysis of two types of exosomes in human whole saliva. Biol Pharm Bull. 2011;34(1):13–23.
31. Li X, Wang X. The emerging roles and therapeutic potential of exosomes in epithelial ovarian cancer. Mol Cancer. 2017;16(1):92.
32. Hirsova P, et al. Extracellular vesicles in liver pathobiology: small particles with big impact. Hepatology. 2016;64(6):2219–33.
33. Gonzalez E, Falcon-Perez JM. Cell-derived extracellular vesicles as a platform to identify low-invasive disease biomarkers. Expert Rev Mol Diagn. 2015;15(7):907–23.

34. Raposo G, Stoorvogel W. Extracellular vesicles: exosomes, microvesicles, and friends. J Cell Biol. 2013;200(4):373–83.
35. Xie F, Feng S, Yang H, Mao Y. Extracellular vesicles in hepatocellular cancer and cholangiocarcinoma. Ann Transl Med. 2019;7(5):86.
36. Arbelaiz A, et al. Serum extracellular vesicles contain protein biomarkers for primary sclerosing cholangitis and cholangiocarcinoma. Hepatology. 2017;66(4):1125–43.
37. Lapitz A, et al. Patients with Cholangiocarcinoma present specific RNA profiles in serum and urine extracellular vesicles mirroring the tumor expression: novel liquid biopsy biomarkers for disease diagnosis. Cell. 2020;9(3):721.
38. Julich-Haertel H, et al. Cancer-associated circulating large extracellular vesicles in cholangiocarcinoma and hepatocellular carcinoma. J Hepatol. 2017;67(2):282–92.
39. Olaizola P, et al. MicroRNAs and extracellular vesicles in cholangiopathies. Biochim Biophys Acta Mol basis Dis. 2018;1864(4 Pt B):1293–307.
40. Andersen RF, Jakobsen A. Screening for circulating RAS/RAF mutations by multiplex digital PCR. Clin Chim Acta. 2016;458:138–43.
41. Liang Z, Liu X, Zhang Q, Wang C, Zhao Y. Diagnostic value of microRNAs as biomarkers for cholangiocarcinoma. Dig Liver Dis. 2016;48(10):1227–32.
42. Zhou J, Liu Z, Yang S, Li X. Identification of microRNAs as biomarkers for cholangiocarcinoma detection: a diagnostic meta-analysis. Clin Res Hepatol Gastroenterol. 2017;41(2): 156–62.
43. Kumarswamy R, Volkmann I, Thum T. Regulation and function of miRNA-21 in health and disease. RNA Biol. 2011;8(5):706–13.
44. Correa-Gallego C, et al. Circulating plasma levels of MicroRNA-21 and MicroRNA-221 are potential diagnostic markers for primary intrahepatic Cholangiocarcinoma. PLoS One. 2016;11(9):e0163699.
45. Huang C-S, et al. Increased expression of miR-21 predicts poor prognosis in patients with hepatocellular carcinoma. Int J Clin Exp Pathol. 2015;8(6):7234–8.
46. Wang L-J, et al. Serum miR-26a as a diagnostic and prognostic biomarker in cholangiocarcinoma. Oncotarget. 2015;6(21):18631–40.
47. Wu X, et al. Profiling of downregulated blood-circulating miR-150-5p as a novel tumor marker for cholangiocarcinoma. Tumour Biol. 2016;37(11):15019–29.
48. Silakit R, et al. Circulating miR-192 in liver fluke-associated cholangiocarcinoma patients: a prospective prognostic indicator. J Hepatobiliary Pancreat Sci. 2014;21(12):864–72.
49. Cheng Q, et al. Circulating miR-106a is a novel prognostic and lymph node metastasis Indicator for Cholangiocarcinoma. Sci Rep. 2015;5(1):16103.
50. Bernuzzi F, et al. Serum microRNAs as novel biomarkers for primary sclerosing cholangitis and cholangiocarcinoma. Clin Exp Immunol. 2016;185(1):61–71.
51. Voigtlander T, et al. MicroRNAs in serum and bile of patients with primary sclerosing cholangitis and/or Cholangiocarcinoma. PLoS One. 2015;10(10):e0139305.
52. Elazezy M, Joosse SA. Techniques of using circulating tumor DNA as a liquid biopsy component in cancer management. Comput Struct Biotechnol J. 2018;16:370–8.
53. Glenn TC. Field guide to next-generation DNA sequencers. Mol Ecol Resour. 2011;11(5):759–69.
54. Giachelli CM, Steitz S. Osteopontin: a versatile regulator of inflammation and biomineralization. Matrix Biol. 2000;19(7):615–22.
55. Wai PY, Kuo PC. Osteopontin: regulation in tumor metastasis. Cancer Metastasis Rev. 2008;27(1):103–18.
56. Loosen SH, et al. Elevated levels of circulating osteopontin are associated with a poor survival after resection of cholangiocarcinoma. J Hepatol. 2017;67(4):749–57.
57. O'Hara SP, Splinter PL, Trussoni CE, Gajdos GB, Lineswala PN, LaRusso NF. Cholangiocyte N-Ras protein mediates lipopolysaccharide-induced interleukin 6 secretion and proliferation. J Biol Chem. 2011;286(35):30352–60.

58. Tabibian JH, O'Hara SP, Splinter PL, Trussoni CE, LaRusso NF. Cholangiocyte senescence by way of N-ras activation is a characteristic of primary sclerosing cholangitis. Hepatology. 2014;59(6):2263–75.
59. Tabibian JH, Trussoni CE, O'Hara SP, Splinter PL, Heimbach JK, LaRusso NF. Characterization of cultured cholangiocytes isolated from livers of patients with primary sclerosing cholangitis. Lab Investig. 2014;94(10):1126–33.
60. Kumari N, Dwarakanath BS, Das A, Bhatt AN. Role of interleukin-6 in cancer progression and therapeutic resistance. Tumour Biol. 2016;37(9):11553–72.
61. Cheon YK, et al. Diagnostic utility of interleukin-6 (IL-6) for primary bile duct cancer and changes in serum IL-6 levels following photodynamic therapy. Am J Gastroenterol. 2007;102(10):2164–70.
62. Wang C-Q, et al. Interleukin-6 enhances cancer stemness and promotes metastasis of hepatocellular carcinoma via up-regulating osteopontin expression. Am J Cancer Res. 2016;6(9):1873–89.
63. Kimawaha P, Jusakul A, Junsawang P, Loilome W, Khuntikeo N, Techasen A. Circulating TGF-β1 as the potential epithelial mesenchymal transition-biomarker for diagnosis of cholangiocarcinoma. J Gastrointest Oncol. 2020;11(2):304–18.
64. Chapman MH, et al. Circulating CYFRA 21-1 is a specific diagnostic and prognostic biomarker in biliary tract cancer. J Clin Exp Hepatol. 2011;1(1):6–12.
65. Edelman MJ, et al. CYFRA 21-1 as a prognostic and predictive marker in advanced non-small-cell lung cancer in a prospective trial: CALGB 150304. J Thorac Oncol. 2012;7(4):649–54.
66. Huang L, et al. Serum CYFRA 21-1 in biliary tract cancers: a reliable biomarker for gallbladder carcinoma and intrahepatic Cholangiocarcinoma. Dig Dis Sci. 2015;60(5):1273–83.
67. Uenishi T, et al. Serum cytokeratin 19 fragment (CYFRA21-1) as a prognostic factor in intrahepatic cholangiocarcinoma. Ann Surg Oncol. 2008;15(2):583–9.
68. Cuenco J, et al. Identification of a serum biomarker panel for the differential diagnosis of cholangiocarcinoma and primary sclerosing cholangitis. Oncotarget. 2018;9(25):17430–42.
69. Vairaktaris E, et al. High gene expression of matrix metalloproteinase-7 is associated with early stages of oral cancer. Anticancer Res. 2007;27(4B):2493–8.
70. Štrbac D, Goričar K, Dolžan V, Kovač V. Evaluation of matrix metalloproteinase 9 serum concentration as a biomarker in malignant mesothelioma. Dis Markers. 2019;2019:1242964.
71. Nanda DP, Sil H, Moulik S, Biswas J, Mandal SS, Chatterjee A. Matrix metalloproteinase-9 as a potential tumor marker in breast cancer. J Environ Pathol Toxicol Oncol. 2013;32(2):115–29.
72. Lawicki S, Glazewska EK, Sobolewska M, Bedkowska GE, Szmitkowski M. Plasma levels and diagnostic utility of macrophage Colony-stimulating factor, matrix Metalloproteinase-9, and tissue inhibitor of Metalloproteinases-1 as new biomarkers of breast cancer. Ann Lab Med. 2016;36(3):223–9.
73. Leelawat K, Sakchinabut S, Narong S, Wannaprasert J. Detection of serum MMP-7 and MMP-9 in cholangiocarcinoma patients: evaluation of diagnostic accuracy. BMC Gastroenterol. 2009;9:30.
74. Onsurathum S, et al. Proteomics detection of S100A6 in tumor tissue interstitial fluid and evaluation of its potential as a biomarker of cholangiocarcinoma. Tumour Biol. 2018;40(4):1010428318767195.
75. Shi R-Y, et al. High expression of Dickkopf-related protein 1 is related to lymphatic metastasis and indicates poor prognosis in intrahepatic cholangiocarcinoma patients after surgery. Cancer. 2013;119(5):993–1003.
76. Shen J, et al. Comparative proteomic profiling of human bile reveals SSP411 as a novel biomarker of cholangiocarcinoma. PLoS One. 2012;7(10):e47476–6.
77. Xu H, et al. Elevation of serum KL-6 mucin levels in patients with cholangiocarcinoma. Hepato-Gastroenterology. 2008;55(88):2000–4.
78. Li Y, et al. Application of joint detection of AFP, CA19-9, CA125 and CEA in identification and diagnosis of Cholangiocarcinoma. Asian Pac J Cancer Prev. 2015;16(8):3451–5.

79. Zhang Y, Yang J, Li H, Wu Y, Zhang H, Chen W. Tumor markers CA19-9, CA242 and CEA in the diagnosis of pancreatic cancer: a meta-analysis. Int J Clin Exp Med. 2015;8(7):11683–91.
80. Tao L-Y, Cai L, He X-D, Liu W, Qu Q. Comparison of serum tumor markers for intrahepatic cholangiocarcinoma and hepatocellular carcinoma. Am Surg. 2010;76(11):1210–3.
81. Wongkham S, et al. Clinical significance of serum total sialic acid in cholangiocarcinoma. Clin Chim Acta. 2003;327(1–2):139–47.
82. Wongkham S, Boonla C, Kongkham S, Wongkham C, Bhudhisawasdi V, Sripa B. Serum total sialic acid in cholangiocarcinoma patients: an ROC curve analysis. Clin Biochem. 2001;34(7):537–41.
83. Kongtawelert P, Tangkijvanich P, Ong-Chai S, Poovorawan Y. Role of serum total sialic acid in differentiating cholangiocarcinoma from hepatocellular carcinoma. World J Gastroenterol. 2003;9(10):2178–81.
84. Liang Q, Liu H, Zhang T, Jiang Y, Xing H, Zhang H. Serum metabolomics uncovering specific metabolite signatures of intra- and extrahepatic cholangiocarcinoma. Mol BioSyst. 2016;12(2):334–40.
85. Sun Y-F, et al. Circulating stem cell-like epithelial cell adhesion molecule-positive tumor cells indicate poor prognosis of hepatocellular carcinoma after curative resection. Hepatology. 2013;57(4):1458–68.
86. Arnoletti JP, et al. Pancreatic and bile duct cancer circulating tumor cells (CTC) form immune-resistant multi-cell type clusters in the portal venous circulation. Cancer Biol Ther. 2018;19(10):887–97.
87. Tan CRC, Zhou L, El-Deiry WS. Circulating tumor cells versus circulating tumor DNA in colorectal cancer: Pros and Cons. Curr Colorectal Cancer Rep. 2016;12(3):151–61.
88. Arnoletti JP, et al. Portal venous blood circulation supports immunosuppressive environment and pancreatic cancer circulating tumor cell activation. Pancreas. 2017;46(1):116–23.
89. Al Ustwani O, Iancu D, Yacoub R, Iyer R. Detection of circulating tumor cells in cancers of biliary origin. J Gastrointest Oncol. 2012;3(2):97–104.
90. Intuyod K, Armartmuntree N, Jusakul A, Sakonsinsiri C, Thanan R, Pinlaor S. Current omics-based biomarkers for cholangiocarcinoma. Expert Rev Mol Diagn. 2019;19(11):997–1005.
91. Son KH, Ahn CB, Kim HJ, Kim JS. Quantitative proteomic analysis of bile in extrahepatic cholangiocarcinoma patients. J Cancer. 2020;11(14):4073–80.
92. Park JY, Park BK, Ko JS, Bang S, Song SY, Chung JB. Bile acid analysis in biliary tract cancer. Yonsei Med J. 2006;47(6):817–25.
93. Nagana Gowda GA, Shanaiah N, Cooper A, Maluccio M, Raftery D. Bile acids conjugation in human bile is not random: new insights from (1)H-NMR spectroscopy at 800 MHz. Lipids. 2009;44(6):527–35.
94. Sharif AW, et al. Metabolic profiling of bile in cholangiocarcinoma using in vitro magnetic resonance spectroscopy. HPB (Oxford). 2010;12(6):396–402.
95. Albiin N, et al. Detection of cholangiocarcinoma with magnetic resonance spectroscopy of bile in patients with and without primary sclerosing cholangitis. Acta Radiol. 2008;49(8):855–62.
96. Alvaro D, et al. Serum and biliary insulin-like growth factor I and vascular endothelial growth factor in determining the cause of obstructive cholestasis. Ann Intern Med. 2007;147(7):451–9.
97. Chiang K-C, et al. Lipocalin 2 (LCN2) is a promising target for cholangiocarcinoma treatment and bile LCN2 level is a potential cholangiocarcinoma diagnostic marker. Sci Rep. 2016;6:36138.
98. Tye BK. MCM proteins in DNA replication. Annu Rev Biochem. 1999;68:649–86.
99. Ren B, et al. MCM7 amplification and overexpression are associated with prostate cancer progression. Oncogene. 2006;25(7):1090–8.
100. Kim D-W, et al. Transcriptional induction of minichromosome maintenance protein 7 (Mcm7) in human cholangiocarcinoma cells treated with Clonorchis sinensis excretory-secretory products. Mol Biochem Parasitol. 2010;173(1):10–6.

101. Ayaru L, et al. Diagnosis of pancreaticobiliary malignancy by detection of minichromosome maintenance protein 5 in bile aspirates. Br J Cancer. 2008;98(9):1548–54.
102. Chen C-Y, Tsai W-L, Wu H-C, Syu M-J, Wu C-C, Shiesh S-C. Diagnostic role of biliary pancreatic elastase for cholangiocarcinoma in patients with cholestasis. Clin Chim Acta. 2008;390(1–2):82–9.
103. Koopmann J, et al. Mac-2-binding protein is a diagnostic marker for biliary tract carcinoma. Cancer. 2004;101(7):1609–15.
104. Severino V, et al. Extracellular vesicles in bile as markers of malignant biliary Stenoses. Gastroenterology. 2017;153(2):495–504.e8.
105. Li L, et al. Human bile contains microRNA-laden extracellular vesicles that can be used for cholangiocarcinoma diagnosis. Hepatology. 2014;60(3):896–907.
106. Plieskatt J, et al. A microRNA profile associated with Opisthorchis viverrini-induced cholangiocarcinoma in tissue and plasma. BMC Cancer. 2015;15:309.
107. Shin S-H, et al. Bile-based detection of extrahepatic cholangiocarcinoma with quantitative DNA methylation markers and its high sensitivity. J Mol Diagn. 2012;14(3):256–63.
108. Lesurtel M, et al. Platelet-derived serotonin mediates liver regeneration. Science. 2006;312(5770):104–7.
109. Alpini G, et al. Serotonin metabolism is dysregulated in cholangiocarcinoma, which has implications for tumor growth. Cancer Res. 2008;68(22):9184–93.
110. Smith ZL, Guzzo TJ. Urinary markers for bladder cancer. F1000Prime Rep. 2013;5:21.
111. Morrissey JJ, London AN, Luo J, Kharasch ED. Urinary biomarkers for the early diagnosis of kidney cancer. Mayo Clin Proc. 2010;85(5):413–21.
112. Cartlidge CR, U Abellona MR, Alkhatib AMA, Taylor-Robinson SD. The utility of biomarkers in hepatocellular carcinoma: review of urine-based (1)H-NMR studies - what the clinician needs to know. Int J Gen Med. 2017;10:431–42.
113. Radon TP, et al. Identification of a three-biomarker panel in urine for early detection of pancreatic adenocarcinoma. Clin Cancer Res. 2015;21(15):3512–21.
114. Jing J, Gao Y. Urine biomarkers in the early stages of diseases: current status and perspective. Discov Med. 2018;25(136):57–65.
115. Navaneethan U, et al. Volatile organic compounds in urine for noninvasive diagnosis of malignant biliary strictures: a pilot study. Dig Dis Sci. 2015;60(7):2150–7.
116. Metzger J, et al. Urine proteomic analysis differentiates cholangiocarcinoma from primary sclerosing cholangitis and other benign biliary disorders. Gut. 2013;62(1):122–30.
117. Voigtländer T, et al. Bile and urine peptide marker profiles: access keys to molecular pathways and biological processes in cholangiocarcinoma. J Biomed Sci. 2020;27(1):13.
118. Borad MJ, et al. Integrated genomic characterization reveals novel, therapeutically relevant drug targets in FGFR and EGFR pathways in sporadic intrahepatic cholangiocarcinoma. PLoS Genet. 2014;10(2):e1004135.
119. Zou S, et al. Mutational landscape of intrahepatic cholangiocarcinoma. Nat Commun. 2014;5:5696.
120. Wang P, et al. Mutations in isocitrate dehydrogenase 1 and 2 occur frequently in intrahepatic cholangiocarcinomas and share hypermethylation targets with glioblastomas. Oncogene. 2013;32(25):3091–100.
121. Nakamura H, et al. Genomic spectra of biliary tract cancer. Nat Genet. 2015;47(9):1003–10.
122. Nepal C, et al. Genomic perturbations reveal distinct regulatory networks in intrahepatic cholangiocarcinoma. Hepatology. 2018;68(3):949–63.
123. Andresen K, et al. Four DNA methylation biomarkers in biliary brush samples accurately identify the presence of cholangiocarcinoma. Hepatology. 2015;61(5):1651–9.
124. Limpaiboon T, et al. Promoter hypermethylation is a major event of hMLH1 gene inactivation in liver fluke related cholangiocarcinoma. Cancer Lett. 2005;217(2):213–9.
125. Vedeld HM, et al. The novel colorectal cancer biomarkers CDO1, ZSCAN18 and ZNF331 are frequently methylated across gastrointestinal cancers. Int J Cancer. 2015;136(4):844–53.

126. Sia D, et al. Integrative molecular analysis of intrahepatic cholangiocarcinoma reveals 2 classes that have different outcomes. Gastroenterology. 2013;144(4):829–40.
127. Ghidini M, et al. Characterisation of the immune-related transcriptome in resected biliary tract cancers. Eur J Cancer. 2017;86:158–65.
128. Sawada R, et al. Interleukin-33 overexpression reflects less aggressive tumour features in large-duct type cholangiocarcinomas. Histopathology. 2018;73(2):259–72.
129. Ruys AT, Groot Koerkamp B, Wiggers JK, Klumpen H-J, ten Kate FJ, van Gulik TM. Prognostic biomarkers in patients with resected cholangiocarcinoma: a systematic review and meta-analysis. Ann Surg Oncol. 2014;21(2):487–500.
130. Suzuki H, et al. Relationship between 18-F-fluoro-deoxy-D-glucose uptake and expression of glucose transporter 1 and pyruvate kinase M2 in intrahepatic cholangiocarcinoma. Dig Liver Dis. 2015;47(7):590–6.
131. Selaru FM, et al. MicroRNA-21 is overexpressed in human cholangiocarcinoma and regulates programmed cell death 4 and tissue inhibitor of metalloproteinase 3. Hepatology. 2009;49(5):1595–601.
132. He Q, et al. Ars2 is overexpressed in human cholangiocarcinomas and its depletion increases PTEN and PDCD4 by decreasing microRNA-21. Mol Carcinog. 2013;52(4):286–96.
133. Collins AL, et al. A differential microRNA profile distinguishes cholangiocarcinoma from pancreatic adenocarcinoma. Ann Surg Oncol. 2014;21(1):133–8.

Chapter 20
Cholangiocarcinoma Surveillance in Primary Sclerosing Cholangitis and IgG4-Related Sclerosing Cholangitis

Ahmad Hassan Ali and Elizabeth J. Carey

Abbreviations

AIH	Autoimmune hepatitis
CA 19–9	Carbohydrate antigen 19–9
CCA	Cholangiocarcinoma
CT	Computed tomography
FISH	Fluorescence in situ hybridization
GWAS	Genome-wide association studies
HBCa	Hepatobiliary cancers
HPB	Hepatopancreatobiliary cancers
IBD	Inflammatory bowel disease
IgG4-RD	Immunoglobulin G4-related disease
IgG4-SC	Immunoglobulin G4-related sclerosing cholangitis
MRCP	Magnetic resonance cholangiopancreatography
MRI	Magnetic resonance imaging
PSC	Primary sclerosing cholangitis
UC	Ulcerative colitis
UDCA	Ursodeoxycholic acid
US	Ultrasound

A. H. Ali (✉)
Division of Gastroenterology and Hepatology, Mayo Clinic Rochester, Rochester, MN, USA

Department of Internal Medicine, Texas Tech University Health Sciences Center, Amarillo, TX, USA
e-mail: ali.ahmad@mayo.edu; ahmad.ali@ttuhsc.edu

E. J. Carey
Division of Gastroenterology and Hepatology, Mayo Clinic Arizona, Phoenix, AZ, USA

J. H. Tabibian (ed.), *Diagnosis and Management of Cholangiocarcinoma*,
https://doi.org/10.1007/978-3-030-70936-5_20

Introduction

Cholangiocarcinoma (CCA) represents a diverse group of biliary tract malignancies comprising nearly 3% of all gastrointestinal tract cancers [1]. CCA is classically subdivided into three anatomical groups: intrahepatic, perihilar, and distal CCA. The incidence of CCA shows variable geographical distribution, ranging between 0.3 and 85 per 100,000 individuals [2]; similarly, risk factors for CCA vary by geographic region (Chap. 5). In the Western world, primary sclerosing cholangitis (PSC) is the most important risk factor for CCA. Although not yet recognized as standard of care, experts recommend surveillance for CCA in PSC patients [3]. Immunoglobulin G4-related sclerosing cholangitis (IgG4-SC) has been recently described as the biliary manifestation of IgG4-related disease (IgG4-RD). A few recent studies have reported CCA as an outcome in IgG4-SC patients; however, the role of CCA surveillance in IgG4-SC patients is less clear.

In this chapter, we focus on the role of surveillance for CCA in PSC and the evidence supporting it. We also discuss the association between CCA and IgG4-SC as well as closely related topics.

Primary Sclerosing Cholangitis

Background

Primary sclerosing cholangitis (PSC) is a progressive fibroinflammatory disease of the bile ducts that ultimately leads to cirrhosis and its consequent complications [4]. PSC is often associated with inflammatory bowel disease (IBD), especially ulcerative colitis (UC), with a reported IBD prevalence of 70–80% in PSC patients [5]. The etiopathogenesis of PSC remains enigmatic. However, with ongoing research and advanced technologies, such as genome-wide association studies (GWAS), the complex relationship between human genes, the environment, and PSC has begun to unravel [6–13]. Further, the gut microbiome concept, originally introduced in the 1980s, has become increasingly recognized as a key player in the pathophysiology of PSC and IBD [14–18].

PSC is a very heterogeneous disease in several ways: it affects men and women; children and adults; individuals of different ethnic and racial backgrounds; and small and large bile ducts and occurs with (diagnosed before, contemporaneously, or after) or without IBD [19]. In addition, PSC can coexist (i.e., “overlap”) with autoimmune hepatitis (AIH), a phenomenon observed more commonly in children (~33%) compared to adults (~6.6%) [20, 21].

Risk of Malignancy in Primary Sclerosing Cholangitis

The risk of malignancy in PSC patients has been firmly established [22, 23]. In fact, PSC has been designated as a "premalignant condition" by experts [24]. Several observational studies have reported a substantial increased risk for hepatobiliary (HBCa) and colorectal cancers in PSC patients compared to the general population [23, 25–30]. Among all, CCA is considered the most dreaded malignant complication of PSC. According to the largest, population-based study to date, CCA has been reported to be the most common cause of liver-related death in PSC patients [31]. The risk of CCA has been reported to be more than 1000-fold greater in PSC compared to the general population [32]. The lifetime risk of CCA in PSC is estimated to be 7–13% [33]. Due to the increased proportion of patients with asymptomatic disease, PSC and CCA are often simultaneously diagnosed. In a recent multicenter, international study, nearly 30% of all CCA cases were diagnosed within the first year of PSC diagnosis [21].

CCA is one of the most aggressive tumors of the biliary tract, with a reported median survival in all anatomical types (intrahepatic, perihilar, and distal CCA) without surgery ranging between 5 and 12 months [34]. Unfortunately, many CCA patients (~28%) present with advanced-stage CCA, which disqualifies them from curative treatment [34]. Collectively, these data highlight the notoriety of CCA in the setting of PSC.

Diagnosis of Cholangiocarcinoma in Primary Sclerosing Cholangitis

In the setting of PSC, CCA diagnosis is based on the finding of a mass or dominant biliary stricture on cross-sectional imaging and/or endoscopic retrograde cholangiopancreatography (ERCP), often associated with serum carbohydrate antigen 19–9 (CA 19–9) elevation, and confirmed by positive biliary cytology and/or fluorescence in situ hybridization (FISH) polysomy. The diagnosis of CCA, especially in the context of PSC, is often extremely difficult and requires a multidisciplinary approach. Further details regarding the diagnosis of CCA and associated challenges are discussed elsewhere in this book (Chaps. 6, 7, 8, 9, and 10).

Therapies for Primary Sclerosing Cholangitis and Associated Cholangiocarcinoma

Detailed discussion of therapies for PSC, including novel ones, is beyond the scope of this chapter. In brief, however, it should be noted that no medical or surgical therapy has been conclusively proven to halt disease progression or prevent CCA in

PSC. Ursodeoxycholic acid (UDCA) has been extensively investigated, but randomized trials did not show clinical benefits in PSC [35, 36]. Details regarding treatment options for CCA complicating PSC are discussed elsewhere in this book (Chaps. 10, 12, 14, 15, 16, 17, 18, and 21).

Cancer Surveillance in Primary Sclerosing Cholangitis

Overview Regarding Surveillance

The term "surveillance" stems from the French compound word *surveiller* (*sur-*, "over"; *veiller*, "to watch"), meaning "to watch over" or "to oversee." In the medical field, surveillance implies continued and close monitoring for an anticipated event in an at-risk population, with the overall goal of improving outcomes. Prior to applying a surveillance strategy, there are key elements that need to be considered:

(a) Identification of the target population to be under surveillance.
(b) Identification of what needs to be surveilled for.
(c) Identification of the surveillance tools and their availability and costs.
(d) Data collection from the population under surveillance.
(e) Treatment of the condition surveilled for should be effective, available, and standard.
(f) The surveillance and treatment should be cost-effective and improve the survival of the target population.

The leading societies recommend surveillance for gallbladder cancer (abdominal imaging on an annual basis) and colorectal cancer (screening colonoscopy every 1–2 years) in PSC patients as well as surveillance for hepatocellular carcinoma in the subset of PSC patients with cirrhosis [37–40]. However, surveillance for CCA has been relatively controversial, in large part due to a paucity of data demonstrating overall benefit. Prospective studies designed to examine the clinical benefit of surveillance for CCA in PSC are lacking. Nevertheless, experts have advocated for surveillance for CCA in PSC [3, 26, 41, 42], and supportive data have recently emerged in this regard, as discussed below.

Evidence Supporting the Implementation of CCA Surveillance in PSC

In 1995, a surveillance program for HBCa in PSC patients launched at the Mayo Clinic Rochester. Surveillance for CCA consisted of annual imaging with abdominal ultrasound (US), computed tomography (CT), or magnetic resonance imaging (MRI)/cholangiopancreatography (MRCP) plus serum CA 19–9. Not all patients and their providers participated in this surveillance program; as a result, there were two groups of PSC patients based on surveillance status (surveillance vs. no-surveillance groups). Using the extensive PSC database at Mayo Clinic, a retrospective study was conducted to examine the role of surveillance for HBCa, including CCA, in PSC patients seen between 1995 and 2015 [43]. PSC patients were included if they had at least 1 year of clinical follow-up and were categorized according to their surveillance status. HBCa-related adverse event was defined as HBCa recurrence or HBCa-related death. The primary endpoints were HBCa recurrence, HBCa-related death, and overall survival. A total of 830 PSC patients met the inclusion criteria (40 in the surveillance group and 39 in the no-surveillance group), with a cumulative follow-up of 712 and 283 person-years pre- and post-HBCa diagnosis, respectively [43]. During the follow-up, a total of 79 patients developed HBCa; 56 patients were diagnosed with CCA. Overall, PSC patients in the surveillance group had a better 5-year overall survival (68% vs. 20%) and a lower 5-year probability of experiencing an HBCa-related adverse event (32% vs. 75%) compared to PSC patients in the no-surveillance group.

CCA groups were then analyzed separately based on tumor location; 37 PSC patients developed extrahepatic CCA, and 19 PSC patients developed intrahepatic CCA. Regarding the PSC patients who developed extrahepatic CCA, 14 were in the surveillance group and 23 were in the no-surveillance groups [43]. Upon subgroup statistical analysis of those who developed extrahepatic CCA, those in the surveillance group were more likely to present without lymph node metastases (93% vs. 50%) and without extrahepatic metastases (100% vs. 68%) and were more likely to receive liver transplantation as a treatment for CCA (93% vs. 45%) compared to those in the no-surveillance group [43]. More importantly, the 5-year probability of an extrahepatic CCA-related adverse event (i.e., recurrence or cancer-related death) was lower in the surveillance vs. the no-surveillance group (14% vs. 64%, respectively). Regarding the PSC patients who developed intrahepatic CCA (n = 19), 6 were in the surveillance group, and 13 were in the no-surveillance group [43]. Upon subgroup analysis of those who developed intrahepatic CCA, there was a tendency toward presenting without intrahepatic metastases (67% vs. 38%) and a tendency toward a higher rate of undergoing surgical resection of the tumor (50% vs. 31%) in the surveillance group compared to the no-surveillance group. Further, there was a tendency toward higher 5-year intrahepatic CCA-related survival (21% vs. 8%) and a tendency toward longer survival (median time from intrahepatic CCA diagnosis until death) in the surveillance compared to the no-surveillance group (24.5 months vs. 7.5 months, respectively) [43].

Combining all PSC patients who developed CCA (n = 56), 20 patients were in the surveillance group and 36 were in the no-surveillance group. The 5-year probability of experiencing a CCA-related adverse event (i.e., recurrence or cancer-related death) was lower in the surveillance vs. the no-surveillance group (29% vs. 75%, respectively) [43]. It is important to point out the limitations of this study, the main ones being its retrospective design and the relatively low number of events of interest (i.e., development of HBCa).

In a recent large UK nationwide study that included 2588 PSC-IBD patients identified over a 10-year period, a total of 334 patients developed hepatopancreatobiliary cancer (HPB), of whom 164 patients developed CCA [44]. The group reported greater than twofold risk reduction in HPB-related death. After excluding all CCA cases that were diagnosed within the first year of PSC diagnosis (n = 111/164), there was no difference in post-CCA survival between the surveillance and no-surveillance groups [44]. It is unclear why there was no difference in the post-CCA survival between the surveillance and the no-surveillance group in the UK study. One possible explanation is that the number of PSC-IBD patients who underwent annual imaging surveillance and developed CCA was too small ($n = 7$) to detect a statistically significantly difference in the post-CCA between surveillance and the no-surveillance group [44].

There is continued debate on the optimal strategy for CCA surveillance in PSC. Some experts in the field recommend abdominal US with CA 19–9 every 6–12 months [27, 45]. A recent statement by expert radiologists and hepatologists of the International PSC Study Group provided quality standards for the use of MRI/MRCP as a screening tool for CCA in PSC patients [46]. In a recent study at our institution, clinical, biochemical, cholangiographic, and imaging data on 226 adult patients with large-duct PSC cared for at the three Mayo Clinic sites (Rochester, Florida, and Arizona), of whom 120 patients developed perihilar CCA, were examined [47]. All patients underwent US and MRI/MRCP within 3 months of each other. Patients with CCA were required to have their imaging studies within 3 months of CCA diagnosis, and those without CCA were required to have a minimum follow-up of 2 years after imaging to mitigate the possibility of an occult CCA. Imaging studies were re-reviewed by radiologists who were blinded to the patients' clinical and biochemical data [47]. There were several important findings in this study. MRI was found to have a significantly better diagnostic performance in detecting early-stage perihilar CCA compared to US (area under curve: 0.87 vs. 0.70, respectively) [47]. In addition, the absence of symptoms at the time of CCA diagnosis was associated with better 5-year overall survival (82% vs. 46%, respectively), better 5-year progression-free survival among those listed for liver transplantation as curative treatment for perihilar CCA (77% vs. 37%, respectively), and better 5-year recurrence-free survival following liver transplantation (89% vs. 65%, respectively) compared to those who had symptoms at the time of CCA diagnosis [47]. Furthermore, individuals who were asymptomatic at the time of CCA diagnosis and had their cancer detected by MRI only were found to have a better 5-year overall survival (100% vs. 33%, respectively) and a better 5-year progression-free survival among those listed for liver transplantation as curative treatment for perihilar CCA (88% vs. 33%, respectively) compared to those who were asymptomatic at the time of CCA diagnosis and had their cancer detected by US [47]. These findings (a) show that MRI/MRCP is superior to US in detecting perihilar CCA at an early stage, which translates into improved survival, and (b) confirm our earlier observation that surveillance for hepatobiliary cancers in PSC is associated with improved outcomes [43].

Take-Home Points Regarding CCA Surveillance in PSC

Routine surveillance for CCA in PSC is rational and prudent. There are no prospective studies comparing between the diagnostic accuracy of US, CT, and MRI abdomen with contrast and MRCP. A common practice in many high-volume institutions is surveillance with MRI abdomen with contrast and MRCP with or without CA 19–9 on an annual basis [48, 49]. We recommend beginning surveillance for CCA in PSC patients (MRI/MRCP or US with CA 19–9 annually; Fig. 20.1) as soon as the diagnosis of PSC is established, regardless of the stage of PSC. This is because 8%

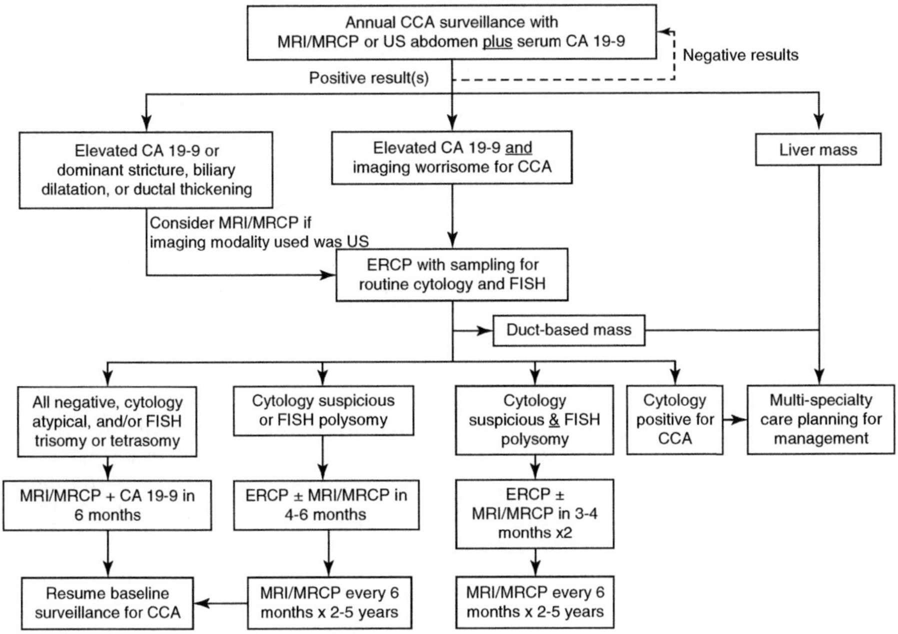

Fig. 20.1 Proposed algorithm for CCA surveillance in patients with PSC. *Abbreviations*: CA 19–9 carbohydrate antigen 19–9, CCA cholangiocarcinoma, ERCP endoscopic retrograde cholangiopancreatography, EUS endoscopic ultrasound, FISH fluorescence in situ hybridization, MRI magnetic resonance imaging, MRCP magnetic resonance cholangiopancreatography, US ultrasound

of all CCA cases in the aforementioned study had early histological stage PSC at the time of CCA diagnosis [43], validating earlier observations [21]. The American Gastroenterology Association recently introduced surveillance for HBCa, including CCA, in the updated PSC clinical practice guidelines [50]. Further, the Italian Association for the Study of the Liver (AISF) in collaboration with the International Liver Cancer Association (ILCA) recently recommended implementing surveillance for CCA in patients with PSC every 6–12 months using cross-sectional imaging of the liver/bile ducts (US, MRI/MRCP, or CT) combined with serum CA 19–9 [51].

Immunoglobulin G4-Related Sclerosing Cholangitis

Background

Immunoglobulin G4-related sclerosing cholangitis (IgG4-SC) is relapsing-remitting, autoimmune disease of the biliary tract characterized cholangiographically by biliary strictures (intrahepatic, extrahepatic, or both) and histopathologically by infiltration of the biliary tree with IgG4-positive plasma cells and often serologically by elevated IgG4 levels [52, 53]. It is a rare disease, mostly affecting men who are 50 years of age or older [54]. It is often associated with autoimmune pancreatitis, which is the pancreatic manifestation of IgG4-related disease (IgG4-RD). IgG4-SC can mimic malignancy, presenting as a dominant stricture, soft tissue enhancement, or even a biliary mass [55]. Thus, akin to PSC, differentiating between IgG4-SC and CCA can be challenging, often exposing the patients to unnecessary procedures and surgeries. By extension, distinguishing IgG4-SC from PSC can also be challenging, as discussed elsewhere [56, 57].

Therapies for Immunoglobulin G4-Related Sclerosing Cholangitis

Immunosuppressive therapy is the mainstay treatment for patients with IgG4-SC. Nearly 90% of IgG4-SC patients respond to steroids. However, relapse is quite common, often requiring re-administration of steroids or initiation of steroid-sparing agents or B cell depletion therapy [58, 59]. A detailed description of steroids and other immunosuppressive regimens is beyond the scope of this chapter but has been recently discussed elsewhere [58, 60].

Risk of Malignancy in Immunoglobulin G4-Related Sclerosing Cholangitis

IgG4-SC is a newly described entity of IgG4-RD; hence, the epidemiology of IgG4-SC has not been well studied. Studies have reported an overall increased risk of malignancy in IgG4-RD patients, ranging between 5.4% and 21.5% [61–68]. The incidence and lifetime risk of CCA in IgG4-SC are not well defined due to the rarity of the disease but appear to be increased compared to the general population. In the largest outcomes study to date including 527 Japanese patients with IgG4-SC, CCA was reported in only 0.4% of the cohort [69]. A higher prevalence of CCA was reported in Western cohorts, 3.2% in a British cohort [70], and 10% in a German cohort [71].

In a recently published report on the largest IgG4-SC cohort in North America, 3 of the 89 IgG4-SC patients developed CCA during a median follow-up of 5.7 years [72]. Based on these data, compared to the average nationwide in the United States, the incidence of CCA was found to be nearly 130 times greater in the IgG4-SC group [72].

Surveillance for Cholangiocarcinoma in Immunoglobulin G4-Related Sclerosing Cholangitis

To date, there is no consensus on surveillance for CCA in IgG4-SC patients. Although still debatable, based on limited data and expert opinion, surveillance for CCA as a part of IgG4-SC management is reasonable (Fig. 20.2).

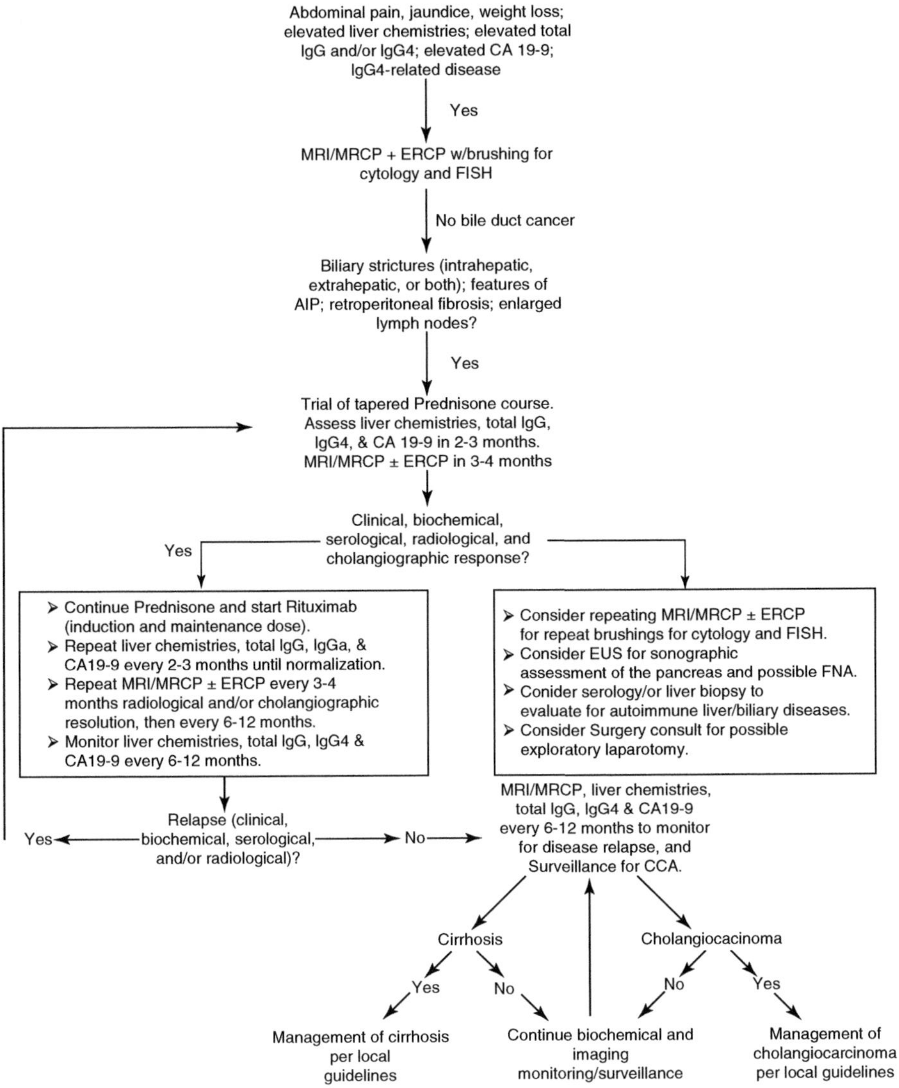

Fig. 20.2 Proposal for CCA surveillance in patients with IgG4-SC. *Abbreviations*: AIP autoimmune pancreatitis, CA 19–9 carbohydrate antigen 19–9, CCA cholangiocarcinoma, ERCP endoscopic retrograde cholangiopancreatography, EUS endoscopic ultrasound, FISH fluorescence in situ hybridization, IgG immunoglobulin, IgG4 immunoglobulin G4, MRI magnetic resonance imaging, MRCP magnetic resonance cholangiopancreatography

Future Directions

There are several key questions and issues regarding surveillance for CCA in PSC and IgG4-SC. Which PSC and IgG4-SC patients benefit most from CCA surveillance? What modalities and biomarkers are most effective for surveillance? Is surveillance cost-effective? In PSC patients, should surveillance be only for those who have persistently abnormal liver chemistries? In IgG4-SC patients, what is the risk of CCA, and what is the optimal surveillance interval? It is our hope that advanced technology, such as GWAS and multi-omics approaches using combined data from genomics, proteomics, methylomics, transcriptomics, and metabolomics, might identify alterations contributing to the development of malignancy in PSC patients and thus optimize surveillance strategies in PSC and IgG4-SC patients.

Conclusions

CCA is the most feared complication of PSC. Early diagnosis of CCA is crucial for optimal outcomes. Surveillance for CCA in PSC has historically been controversial, though recent data and guidelines now support it [43, 50]. The approach in many high-volume centers is annual MRI/MRCP coupled with serum CA 19–9, though better and more tailored approaches are expected. Surveillance for CCA in PSC patients should begin as soon as the diagnosis of PSC is established, irrespective of the stage of PSC. With regard to IgG4-SC, the risk of CCA is less defined, and there is no consensus regarding the need for surveillance. Larger studies are required to better examine the risk of CCA in IgG4-SC patients, though available data demonstrate that it is significantly increased, thus suggesting a role for surveillance.

Acknowledgments The first author of this chapter would like to dedicate this work to his lovely wife, Hala, and their children Zaina, Maryam, Malek, Yousuf, and Abdulrahman.

References

1. Rizvi S, Khan SA, Hallemeier CL, Kelley RK, Gores GJ. Cholangiocarcinoma — evolving concepts and therapeutic strategies. Nat Rev Clin Oncol. 2018;15(2):95–111.
2. Khan SA, Tavolari S, Brandi G. Cholangiocarcinoma: epidemiology and risk factors. Liver Int. 2019;39(S1):19–31.
3. Razumilava N, Gores GJ. Surveillance for cholangiocarcinoma in patients with primary sclerosing cholangitis: effective and justified? Clin Liver Dis (Hoboken). 2016;8(2):43–7.
4. Dyson JK, Beuers U, Jones DEJ, Lohse AW, Hudson M. Primary sclerosing cholangitis. Lancet. 2018;391(10139):2547–59.
5. Palmela C, Peerani F, Castaneda D, Torres J, Itzkowitz SH. Inflammatory bowel disease and primary sclerosing cholangitis: a review of the phenotype and associated specific features. Gut Liver. 2018;12(1):17–29.
6. Alberts R, de Vries EMG, Goode EC, Jiang X, Sampaziotis F, Rombouts K, et al. Genetic association analysis identifies variants associated with disease progression in primary sclerosing cholangitis. Gut. 2018;67(8):1517–24.
7. Ji SG, Juran BD, Mucha S, Folseraas T, Jostins L, Melum E, et al. Genome-wide association study of primary sclerosing cholangitis identifies new risk loci and quantifies the genetic relationship with inflammatory bowel disease. Nat Genet. 2017;49(2):269–73.

8. Ellinghaus D, Jostins L, Spain SL, Cortes A, Bethune J, Han B, et al. Analysis of five chronic inflammatory diseases identifies 27 new associations and highlights disease-specific patterns at shared loci. Nat Genet. 2016;48(5):510–8.
9. Liu JZ, Hov JR, Folseraas T, Ellinghaus E, Rushbrook SM, Doncheva NT, et al. Dense genotyping of immune-related disease regions identifies nine new risk loci for primary sclerosing cholangitis. Nat Genet. 2013;45(6):670–5.
10. Ellinghaus D, Folseraas T, Holm K, Ellinghaus E, Melum E, Balschun T, et al. Genome-wide association analysis in primary sclerosing cholangitis and ulcerative colitis identifies risk loci at GPR35 and TCF4. Hepatology. 2013;58(3):1074–83.
11. Folseraas T, Melum E, Rausch P, Juran BD, Ellinghaus E, Shiryaev A, et al. Extended analysis of a genome-wide association study in primary sclerosing cholangitis detects multiple novel risk loci. J Hepatol. 2012;57(2):366–75.
12. Melum E, Franke A, Schramm C, Weismuller TJ, Gotthardt DN, Offner FA, et al. Genome-wide association analysis in primary sclerosing cholangitis identifies two non-HLA susceptibility loci. Nat Genet. 2011;43(1):17–9.
13. Karlsen TH, Franke A, Melum E, Kaser A, Hov JR, Balschun T, et al. Genome-wide association analysis in primary sclerosing cholangitis. Gastroenterology. 2010;138(3):1102–11.
14. Ali AH, Carey EJ, Lindor KD. The microbiome and primary sclerosing cholangitis. Semin Liver Dis. 2016;36(4):340–8.
15. Damman JL, Rodriguez EA, Ali AH, Buness CW, Cox KL, Carey EJ, et al. Review article: the evidence that vancomycin is a therapeutic option for primary sclerosing cholangitis. Aliment Pharmacol Ther. 2018;47(7):886–95.
16. Nakamoto N, Sasaki N, Aoki R, Miyamoto K, Suda W, Teratani T, et al. Gut pathobionts underlie intestinal barrier dysfunction and liver T helper 17 cell immune response in primary sclerosing cholangitis. Nat Microbiol. 2019;4(3):492–503.
17. Dean G, Hanauer S, Levitsky J. The role of the intestine in the pathogenesis of primary sclerosing cholangitis: evidence and therapeutic implications. Hepatology. 2020;72(3):1127–38.
18. Shah A, Macdonald GA, Morrison M, Holtmann G. Targeting the gut microbiome as a treatment for primary sclerosing cholangitis: a conceptional framework. Am J Gastroenterol. 2020;115(6):814–22.
19. Lazaridis KN, LaRusso NF. Primary sclerosing cholangitis. N Engl J Med. 2016;375(25):2501–2.
20. Deneau MR, El-Matary W, Valentino PL, Abdou R, Alqoaer K, Amin M, et al. The natural history of primary sclerosing cholangitis in 781 children: a multicenter, international collaboration. Hepatology. 2017;66(2):518–27.
21. Weismuller TJ, Trivedi PJ, Bergquist A, Imam M, Lenzen H, Ponsioen CY, et al. Patient age, sex, and inflammatory bowel disease phenotype associate with course of primary sclerosing cholangitis. Gastroenterology. 2017;152(8):1975–84. e8
22. Grimsrud MM, Folseraas T. Pathogenesis, diagnosis and treatment of premalignant and malignant stages of cholangiocarcinoma in primary sclerosing cholangitis. Liver Int. 2019; 39(12):2230–7.
23. Fung BM, Lindor KD, Tabibian JH. Cancer risk in primary sclerosing cholangitis: epidemiology, prevention, and surveillance strategies. World J Gastroenterol. 2019;25(6):659–71.
24. Rizvi S, Eaton JE, Gores GJ. Primary sclerosing cholangitis as a premalignant biliary tract disease: surveillance and management. Clin Gastroenterol Hepatol. 2015;13(12):2152–65.
25. Karlsen TH, Schrumpf E, Boberg KM. Gallbladder polyps in primary sclerosing cholangitis: not so benign. Curr Opin Gastroenterol. 2008;24(3):395–9.
26. Folseraas T, Boberg KM. Cancer risk and surveillance in primary sclerosing cholangitis. Clin Liver Dis. 2016;20(1):79–98.
27. Chascsa DM, Lindor KD. Cancer risk, screening and surveillance in primary sclerosing cholangitis. Minerva Gastroenterol Dietol. 2019;65(3):214–28.
28. Broome U, Bergquist A. Primary sclerosing cholangitis, inflammatory bowel disease, and colon cancer. Semin Liver Dis. 2006;26(1):31–41.

29. de Valle MB, Björnsson E, Lindkvist B. Mortality and cancer risk related to primary sclerosing cholangitis in a Swedish population-based cohort. Liver Int. 2012;32(3):441–8.
30. Torabi Sagvand B, Edwards K, Shen B. Frequency, risk factors, and outcome of gallbladder polyps in patients with primary sclerosing cholangitis: a case-control study. Hepatol Commun. 2018;2(12):1440–5.
31. Boonstra K, Weersma RK, van Erpecum KJ, Rauws EA, Spanier BW, Poen AC, et al. Population-based epidemiology, malignancy risk, and outcome of primary sclerosing cholangitis. Hepatology. 2013;58(6):2045–55.
32. Burak K, Angulo P, Pasha TM, Egan K, Petz J, Lindor KD. Incidence and risk factors for cholangiocarcinoma in primary sclerosing cholangitis. Am J Gastroenterol. 2004;99(3):523–6.
33. Tabibian JH, Ali AH, Lindor KD. Primary sclerosing cholangitis, part 2: cancer risk, prevention, and surveillance. Gastroenterol Hepatol (N Y). 2018;14(7):427–32.
34. Waseem D, Tushar P. Intrahepatic, perihilar and distal cholangiocarcinoma: management and outcomes. Ann Hepatol. 2017;16(1):133–9.
35. Olsson R, Boberg KM, de Muckadell OS, Lindgren S, Hultcrantz R, Folvik G, et al. High-dose ursodeoxycholic acid in primary sclerosing cholangitis: a 5-year multicenter, randomized, controlled study. Gastroenterology. 2005;129(5):1464–72.
36. Lindor KD, Kowdley KV, Luketic VA, Harrison ME, McCashland T, Befeler AS, et al. High-dose ursodeoxycholic acid for the treatment of primary sclerosing cholangitis. Hepatology. 2009;50(3):808–14.
37. Chapman R, Fevery J, Kalloo A, Nagorney DM, Boberg KM, Shneider B, et al. Diagnosis and management of primary sclerosing cholangitis. Hepatology. 2010;51(2):660–78.
38. Chapman MH, Thorburn D, Hirschfield GM, Webster GGJ, Rushbrook SM, Alexander G, et al. British Society of Gastroenterology and UK-PSC guidelines for the diagnosis and management of primary sclerosing cholangitis. Gut. 2019;68(8):1356–78.
39. Lindor KD, Kowdley KV, Harrison ME, American College of G. ACG clinical guideline: primary sclerosing cholangitis. Am J Gastroenterol. 2015;110(5):646–59. quiz 60
40. European Association for the Study of the L. EASL clinical practice guidelines: management of cholestatic liver diseases. J Hepatol. 2009;51(2):237–67.
41. Boyd S, Mustonen H, Tenca A, Jokelainen K, Arola J, Farkkila MA. Surveillance of primary sclerosing cholangitis with ERC and brush cytology: risk factors for cholangiocarcinoma. Scand J Gastroenterol. 2017;52(2):242–9.
42. Razumilava N, Gores GJ, Lindor KD. Cancer surveillance in patients with primary sclerosing cholangitis. Hepatology. 2011;54(5):1842–52.
43. Ali AH, Tabibian JH, Nasser-Ghodsi N, Lennon RJ, DeLeon T, Borad MJ, et al. Surveillance for hepatobiliary cancers in patients with primary sclerosing cholangitis. Hepatology. 2018;67(6):2338–51.
44. Trivedi PJ, Crothers H, Mytton J, Bosch S, Iqbal T, Ferguson J, et al. Effects of primary sclerosing cholangitis on risks of cancer and death in people with inflammatory bowel disease, based on sex, race, and age. Gastroenterology. 2020;159(3):915–28.
45. Charatcharoenwitthaya P, Enders FB, Halling KC, Lindor KD. Utility of serum tumor markers, imaging, and biliary cytology for detecting cholangiocarcinoma in primary sclerosing cholangitis. Hepatology. 2008;48(4):1106–17.
46. Schramm C, Eaton J, Ringe KI, Venkatesh S, Yamamura J. IPSCSG MRIwgot. Recommendations on the use of magnetic resonance imaging in PSC-A position statement from the International PSC Study Group. Hepatology. 2017;66(5):1675–88.
47. Eaton JE, Welle CL, Bakhshi Z, Sheedy SP, Idilman IS, Gores GJ, et al. Early cholangiocarcinoma detection with magnetic resonance imaging versus ultrasound in primary sclerosing cholangitis. Hepatology. 2020; (in press)
48. Zenouzi R, Welle CL, Venkatesh SK, Schramm C, Eaton JE. Magnetic resonance imaging in primary sclerosing cholangitis-current state and future directions. Semin Liver Dis. 2019;39(3):369–80.

49. Zenouzi R, Liwinski T, Yamamura J, Weiler-Normann C, Sebode M, Keller S, et al. Follow-up magnetic resonance imaging/3D-magnetic resonance cholangiopancreatography in patients with primary sclerosing cholangitis: challenging for experts to interpret. Aliment Pharmacol Ther. 2018;48(2):169–78.
50. Bowlus CL, Lim JK, Lindor KD. AGA clinical practice update on surveillance for hepatobiliary cancers in patients with primary sclerosing cholangitis: expert review. Clin Gastroenterol Hepatol. 2019;17(12):2416–22.
51. Alvaro D, Hassan C, Cardinale V, Carpino G, Fabris L, Gringeri E, et al. Italian clinical practice guidelines on cholangiocarcinoma – part I: classification, diagnosis and staging. Dig Liver Dis. 2020;52(11):1282–93.
52. Stone JH, Zen Y, Deshpande V. IgG4-related disease. N Engl J Med. 2012;366(6):539–51.
53. Okazaki K, Uchida K, Koyabu M, Miyoshi H, Ikeura T, Takaoka M. IgG4 cholangiopathy: current concept, diagnosis, and pathogenesis. J Hepatol. 2014;61(3):690–5.
54. Tanaka A, Mori M, Kubota K, Naitoh I, Nakazawa T, Takikawa H, et al. Epidemiological features of immunoglobulin G4-related sclerosing cholangitis in Japan. J Hepatobiliary Pancreat Sci. 2020;
55. Tanaka A. IgG4-related sclerosing cholangitis and primary sclerosing cholangitis. Gut Liver. 2019;13(3):300–7.
56. Doorenspleet ME, Hubers LM, Culver EL, Maillette de Buy Wenniger LJ, Klarenbeek PL, Chapman RW, et al. Immunoglobulin G4(+) B-cell receptor clones distinguish immunoglobulin G 4-related disease from primary sclerosing cholangitis and biliary/pancreatic malignancies. Hepatology. 2016;64(2):501–7.
57. Tabibian JH, Lindor KD. Distinguishing immunoglobulin G4-related disease from its pancreatobiliary mimics: are we there now? Hepatology. 2016;64(2):340–3.
58. Miyabe K, Zen Y, Cornell LD, Rajagopalan G, Chowdhary VR, Roberts LR, et al. Gastrointestinal and extra-intestinal manifestations of IgG4-related disease. Gastroenterology. 2018;155(4):990–1003. e1
59. Majumder S, Mohapatra S, Lennon RJ, Piovezani Ramos G, Postier N, Gleeson FC, et al. Rituximab maintenance therapy reduces rate of relapse of pancreaticobiliary immunoglobulin G4-related disease. Clin Gastroenterol Hepatol. 2018;16(12):1947–53.
60. Hart PA, Topazian MD, Witzig TE, Clain JE, Gleeson FC, Klebig RR, et al. Treatment of relapsing autoimmune pancreatitis with immunomodulators and rituximab: the Mayo Clinic experience. Gut. 2013;62(11):1607–15.
61. Ahn SS, Song JJ, Park YB, Lee SW. Malignancies in Korean patients with immunoglobulin G4-related disease. Int J Rheum Dis. 2017;20(8):1028–35.
62. Asano J, Watanabe T, Oguchi T, Kanai K, Maruyama M, Ito T, et al. Association between immunoglobulin G4-related disease and malignancy within 12 years after diagnosis: an analysis after long term follow up. J Rheumatol. 2015;42(11):2135–42.
63. Detlefsen S, Mortensen MB, Pless TK, Cribe AS, de Muckadell OB. Laparoscopic and percutaneous core needle biopsy plays a central role for the diagnosis of autoimmune pancreatitis in a single-center study from Denmark. Pancreas. 2015;44(6):845–58.
64. Hart PA, Kamisawa T, Brugge WR, Chung JB, Culver EL, Czako L, et al. Long-term outcomes of autoimmune pancreatitis: a multicentre, international analysis. Gut. 2013;62(12):1771–6.
65. Schneider A, Michaely H, Ruckert F, Weiss C, Strobel P, Belle S, et al. Diagnosing autoimmune pancreatitis with the unifying-autoimmune-pancreatitis-criteria. Pancreatology. 2017;17(3):381–94.
66. Schneider A, Michaely H, Weiss C, Hirth M, Ruckert F, Wilhelm TJ, et al. Prevalence and incidence of autoimmune pancreatitis in the population living in the southwest of Germany. Digestion. 2017;96(4):187–98.
67. Wallace ZS, Wallace CJ, Lu N, Choi HK, Stone JH. Association of IgG4-related disease with history of malignancy. Arthritis Rheumatol. 2016;68(9):2283–9.
68. Yamamoto M, Takahashi H, Tabeya T, Suzuki C, Naishiro Y, Ishigami K, et al. Risk of malignancies in IgG4-related disease. Mod Rheumatol. 2012;22(3):414–8.

69. Tanaka A, Tazuma S, Okazaki K, Nakazawa T, Inui K, Chiba T, et al. Clinical features, response to treatment, and outcomes of IgG4-related sclerosing cholangitis. Clin Gastroenterol Hepatol. 2017;15(6):920–6. e3
70. Huggett MT, Culver EL, Kumar M, Hurst JM, Rodriguez-Justo M, Chapman MH, et al. Type 1 autoimmune pancreatitis and IgG4-related sclerosing cholangitis is associated with extrapancreatic organ failure, malignancy, and mortality in a prospective UK cohort. Am J Gastroenterol. 2014;109(10):1675–83.
71. Buechter M, Manka P, Heinemann FM, Lindemann M, Juntermanns B, Canbay A, et al. Outcome and genetic factors in IgG4-associated autoimmune pancreatitis and cholangitis: a single center experience. Gastroenterol Res Pract. 2017;2017:6126707.
72. Ali AH, Bi Y, Machicado JD, Garg S, Lennon RJ, Zhang L, et al. The long-term outcomes of patients with immunoglobulin G4-related sclerosing cholangitis: the Mayo Clinic experience. J Gastroenterol. 2020;55(11):1087–97.

Chapter 21
Novel Targeted Therapies in Clinical Use and on the Horizon for Cholangiocarcinoma

Nishant V. Munugala, Amisha Singh, and Rachna T. Shroff

Abbreviations

2-HG	2-hydroxyglutarate
BTC	Biliary tract cancer
CCA	Cholangiocarcinoma
CGP	Capture-based genomic profiling
cPRS	complete partial remission
ctDNA	circulating tumor DNA
DSBs	Double-stranded DNA breaks
FGFR	Fibroblast growth factor receptor
Gem-cis	Gemcitabine-cisplatin
Her2	Human epidermal growth factor receptor
HR	Hazard ratio
iCCA	intrahepatic cholangiocarcinoma
IDH	Isocitrate dehydrogenase gene
IVO	Ivosidenib
MMR	Mismatch repair
MSI	Microsatellite instability
NGS	Next-generation sequencing
ORR	Objective response rate
OS	Overall survival
PARP	Poly-ADP-ribose polymerase
PBO	Placebo
PD-1	Program cell death protein 1

N. V. Munugala · A. Singh
Internal Medicine, University of Arizona, Tucson, AZ, USA

R. T. Shroff (✉)
Hematology/Oncology, University of Arizona Cancer Center, Tucson, AZ, USA
e-mail: rshroff@email.arizona.edu

J. H. Tabibian (ed.), *Diagnosis and Management of Cholangiocarcinoma*,
https://doi.org/10.1007/978-3-030-70936-5_21

PD-L1	Program cell death protein 1 ligand
PFS	Progression-free survival
RPSFT	Rank preserving structural failure time
TKI	Tyrosine kinase inhibitor

Introduction

Since 2010, the standard of care in treating all advanced, inoperable biliary tract cancers has been combination gemcitabine and cisplatin (gem-cis). Valle et al. demonstrated in the phase 3, randomized ABC-02 trial, a median overall survival (OS) of 11.7 months with this combination compared to 8.1 months with single-agent gemcitabine in patients with unresectable, recurrent, or metastatic biliary tract cancers, including cholangiocarcinoma (CCA). The rate of tumor control among patients in the cisplatin-gemcitabine group was significantly increased (81.4% vs 71.8%, $P = 0.049$) [1]. Additionally, these benefits were seen without the addition of substantial toxicity, establishing gem-cis as the standard of care for all biliary tract cancers.

Until recently, the treatment for advanced biliary tract cancers in the second-line setting has been relatively less clear. Data informing treatment in the second-line setting had been lacking, with no prospective, phase 3 studies performed until 2019. Rogers et al. were the first to explore this matter, performing a single institution retrospective study between 2009 and 2012 to evaluate progression-free survival (PFS) in patients with advanced CCA who were started on second-line systemic treatment. Fifty-six patients were included in the analysis, with 95% having intrahepatic CCA [2]. Second-line treatment regimens were classified into four groups—gemcitabine plus platinum (19.6%), gemcitabine plus fluoropyrimidine (28.6%), other FU combination (37.5%), and others (14.3%). Median PFS was 2.7 months (95% CI, 2.3–3.8 months) with a median OS of 13.8 months (95% CI, 12–19.3 months) and a disease control rate of 50% [2]. Despite a potential survival benefit with second-line systemic therapy, no significant difference in survival was identified between the four treatment groups [2].

Delving deeper, Lamarca et al. conducted a systemic review evaluating the quality of evidence supporting the use of second-line chemotherapy for patients with advanced biliary tract cancers. The study evaluated OS, response rate (RR), toxicity, and quality of life. Twenty-five studies were included in the analysis—14 phase 2 clinical trials, 9 retrospective analyses, and 2 case reports with data collected from 761 patients [3]. The mean OS was 7.2 months [95% confidence interval (CI) 6.2–8.2] [3]. The mean PFS, RR, and disease control rate were 3.2 months (95% CI 2.7–3.7), 7.7% (95% CI 4.6–10.9), and 49.5% (95% CI 41.4–57.7), respectively [3]. Despite the low standards in terms of outcomes (OS, PFS) of second-line chemotherapy in advanced biliary tract cancers, the data suggests select patients, particularly those with adequate performance status, may benefit from treatment.

The largest cohort of patients with advanced biliary tract cancers failing first-line therapy was studied in a multicentered trial across three US academic medical centers that evaluated treatment practice and outcomes for second-line chemotherapy [4]. Institutional registries were reviewed from April 2010 to March 2015, and 198 patients were identified (intrahepatic CCA 61.1%, extrahepatic CCA 14.1%, and 24.8% gallbladder carcinoma) [4]. The median overall survival from initiation of second-line therapy (OS2) was 11 months (95% confidence interval [CI], 8.8–13.1 months). The median OS2 for patients with intrahepatic CCA was 13.4 months (95% CI, 10.7–17.8 months), which was longer than that for patients with extrahepatic CCA (6.8 months; 95% CI, 5–10.6 months) or gallbladder carcinoma (9.4 months; 95% CI, 7.2–12.3 months; $p = 0.018$) [4]. Survival was longer than expected compared to prior studies, likely reflecting more favorable tumor biology among patients who were able to receive second-line therapy after the progression of disease on first-line chemotherapy [3, 4]. The median time to second-line treatment failure was 2.2 months (95% CI, 1.8–2.7 months), and it was similar across tumor locations ($p = 0.60$), highlighting the limited efficacy of standard second-line regimens [4]. The study noted more than half of the patients went on to receive additional lines of treatment, further underlining the need for new efficacious therapies.

Early Progress in Systemic Therapies

Despite the seeming lack of therapies in the treatment of CCA, several recent studies have shown signs of progress. In the recently concluded ABC-06 trial, 162 patients with advanced biliary tract cancers who failed treatment with gem-cis were randomized 1:1 (March 2014 to Jan 2018) into two arms—treatment with active symptom control (ASC) or ASC plus folinic acid, fluorouracil, and oxaliplatin (mFOLFOX) [5]. Initial results revealed a survival benefit with ASC + FOLFOX arm with an adjusted HR of 0.69 (95% CI 0.50–0.97; $p = 0.031$; ASC + mFOLFOX vs ASC) [5]. Median OS and OS rate (%) at 6 months and 12 months, respectively, were 5.3 months, 35.5%, and 11.4% for the ASC arm and 6.2 months, 50.6%, and 25.9% for the ASC + mFOLFOX arm, respectively [5]. The survival seen in the ASC arm was greater than assumed, while ASC + mFOLFOX improved OS after progression with gem-cis treatment with a clinically meaningful increase in 6-month and 12-month OS rate [5]. Though awaiting final results, initial data from this trial is suggestive of ASC + mFOLFOX becoming the standard of care in the second-line setting for advanced biliary tract cancers (NCT01926236).

A step forward in systemic therapies came in a phase 2 clinical trial evaluating the association between PFS and the addition of nanoparticle albumin-bound (nab)-paclitaxel to gem-cis [6]. Existing preclinical data suggest nab-paclitaxel enhances gemcitabine delivery in pancreatic tumors, raising the possibility of similar effects in biliary tract cancers [6]. This open-label, single-arm, phase 2 clinical trial was conducted at the University of Texas MD Anderson Cancer Center and the Mayo

Clinic in Phoenix, Arizona. A total of 62 patients with advanced biliary tract cancers were enrolled between April 2015 and April 2017. Of 60 patients who started treatment, the mean (SD) age was 58.4 (11.0) years, 38 (63%) had intrahepatic CCA, 9 (15%) had extrahepatic CCA, 13 (22%) had gallbladder cancer, 47 (78%) had metastatic disease, and 13 (22%) had locally advanced disease [5]. Dose adjustments were made due to adverse hematologic events among the first 32 patients enrolled, resulting in the remaining 28 patients having dose-reduced regimens. Median PFS in 58 patients was 11.8 (95% CI, 6.0 to 15.6) months. The median overall survival was 19.2 months in 57 patients (95% CI, 13.2 months to not estimable) [6]. Treatment response data were available for 51 patients, and the partial RR was 45%, with a disease control rate of 84%. Grade 3 or higher adverse events occurred in 58% of patients, and 9 patients (16%) withdrew owing to adverse events [5]. Post hoc analyses showed that treatment efficacy was not significantly associated with starting dose, tumor type, or disease status and that tolerability was improved with reduced vs high-dose treatment [6]. Additionally, with treatment, 12 patients were converted from unresectable to resectable disease allowing surgical intervention; 2 of these patients subsequently achieved a pathologic complete response [6]. This study demonstrated that the addition of nab-paclitaxel to gem-cis notably prolonged median PFS when compared to the historical control of gem-cis alone [1, 6]. These findings are being tested in a phase 3 randomized clinical trial (S1815 Study, NCT03768414).

Despite some encouraging progress in systemic therapies, the reality is the 5-year survival for CCA remains poor at 5–10% [1, 6]. There is a dire need for improved treatment options for patients with CCA in both the first-line and second-line settings, particularly given the known toxicity profile of geme-cis [6]. Part of the challenge is that CCA has varying molecular etiologies and is clinically heterogeneous, differing in presentation and complexities depending on the location of the tumor and underlying hepatobiliary disease. This has made development of universal treatments challenging, raising the question if targeted therapies will yield more promising results.

Importance of Molecular Profiling

Next-Generation Sequencing in Cholangiocarcinoma

Next-generation sequencing (NGS) refers to several different modern sequencing technologies that allow for sequencing of DNA and RNA much more quickly and inexpensively than the previously used Sanger sequencing method [7]. It has expanded in the last decades with significant improvements in reliability, gene sequencing, analyses, and data interpretation that has played a key role advancing the study of genomics and molecular biology. Improved efficacy and affordability have further made the use of NGS feasible in modern clinical practice with applications ranging from mutation detection in inherited cancer syndromes, detection of spliceogenic variants, cancer somatic mutation analysis, pharmacogenetics, and liquid biopsy [7]. NGS has been central in advancing understanding of cancer biology with the identification of genetic variances contributing to tumor growth, development and metastasis, driver genes, driver mutations, and passenger mutations [7]. Furthermore, NGS has opened doors in the clinical realm via improved patient classification, prognostication, targeted treatments, drug resistance, and pharmacogenetics. Recent advances in the understanding of the pathogenesis of CCA are linked to molecular insights provided by NGS.

Jusakul et al. were among the first to begin to explore the molecular and epigenomic landscape in CCA. In this study, a cohort of nearly 500 CCA specimens from distinct geographical regions was analyzed with NGS at the whole genome level [8]. Four distinct etiological clusters were recognized, defined by differences in gene expression, mutations, copy number changes, and epigenetic changes. The specific mutations noted were ERBB2 amplification, TP53 mutations, levels of PD-1/PD-L2 expression, IDH1/2 and BAP1 epigenetic mutations, and FGFR/PRKA-related gene rearrangements [8]. The relevance of classifying CCAs by these driver genes, noncoding promoter mutations, and structural variants is that each subtype exhibited distinct molecular and clinicopathologic features. Molecular profiling of these CCAs provided insight beyond the anatomical location of the tumor. Additionally, CCAs in different anatomical locations did not differ in their survival trends, while CCAs stratified by molecular clusters showed significant differences in survival [8]. This highlights how distinct cancer subtypes in the same organ may arise through varying oncogenic processes. Given this, NGS offers the potential to identify disease subsets with differing prognostic and therapeutic implications, while further informing the development of targeted therapies.

The concept of developing targeted therapies based on a CCA molecular profile has prompted the search for these actionable mutations (Table 21.1). Emerging data from NGS analyses have identified two such mutations holding considerable promise, the *FGFR2* fusion and *IDH1* and *IDH2* mutations, which are the two most common genetic alterations seen in intrahepatic CCA [9].

Isocitrate Dehydrogenase (IDH1/IDH2) Mutations

Mutations in the isocitrate dehydrogenase genes (*IDH1* and *IDH2*) were first discovered using NGS, and collaborative efforts to characterize *IDH* mutations have shown these mutations are higher in intrahepatic CCA (iCCA) than extrahepatic CCA [9]. *IDH* mutations are seen in about 20–25% of iCCA [8, 9]. However, the prognostic significance of *IDH* mutations remains unclear.

IDH1 and IDH2 are metabolic enzymes that normally function as components of the tricarboxylic acid cycle, catalyzing the interconversion of isocitrate and alpha-ketoglutarate. The mutant IDH loses its normal enzymatic activity and instead produces increased amounts of the oncometabolite 2-hydroxyglutarate(2-HG) [9]. 2-HG can competitively inhibit dioxygenases, which play a role in DNA

Table 21.1 Actionable mutations in cholangiocarcinoma

Actionable mutation	Prevalence	Targeted therapies	Mechanism of action
IDH 1 and IDH 2 mutation	20–25% of iCCA	Ivosidenib	Blocks the function of mutant IDH1 or IDH2, which reduces the levels of oncometabolite 2-HG
FGFR2 fusion	15–20% of iCCA	Infigratinib, TAS-120, pemigatinib[a]	Inhibits the constitutively active FGFR signaling that promotes cell proliferation and inhibits apoptosis
KRAS	7–24% in iCCA	AMG510[b]	Binds to the cysteine residue in KRAS G12C mutations, holding the protein in its inactive form
B-raf	3–5% of CCA	Vemurafenib, dabrafenib[c]	Selectively inhibits the mutated BRAF V600E kinase that leads to reduced signaling through the aberrant mitogen-activated protein kinase (MAPK) pathway
BRCA1, BRCA2, and PARP inhibition	Unknown	Niraparib, olaparib	Inhibits the role of PARP-1 and PARP-2 in DNA repair. By blocking PARP enzymatic activity and increasing the formation of PARP-DNA complexes, these inhibitors induce DNA damage and cell death
Her2/neu	9–20% of CCA	Varlitinib, lapatinib, pertuzumab, trastuzumab	Varlitinib and lapatinib selectively and reversibly bind to both EGFR (ErbB-1) and Her2/neu (ErbB-2) and prevent their phosphorylation and activation, which may result in inhibition of the associated signal transduction pathways, inhibition of cellular proliferation and cell death

[a]*Pemigatinib is currently the only FDA-approved drug for CCA*
[b]*AMG510 is only for the KRAS G12C mutation which is rare in CCA*
[c]*Given in combination with MEK inhibitors*

demethylation. Increased amounts of 2-HG can be detected both in the tumor and blood [9]. Furthermore, *IDH* and *KRAS* mutations can cooperate to drive the expansion of the liver, progenitor cells, development of premalignant biliary lesions, and progression to metastatic iCCA [9].

Highly specific IDH inhibitors have been developed. These inhibitors block the function of mutant IDH1 or IDH2, which reduces the levels of oncometabolite 2-HG [10]. One such inhibitor, ivosidenib (IVO), an oral, reversible inhibitor of mutant IDH1 (mIDH1) was well tolerated among patients with advanced solid tumors with *IDH1* mutations in a phase 1 I trial (NCT02073994). IVO is currently approved in the USA for the treatment of mIDH1 acute myeloid leukemia in newly diagnosed patients ineligible for intensive chemotherapy and patients with relapsed or refractory disease. Seventy-three patients with mIDH1-CCA were enrolled in the study and received IVO [10]. These patients had a median of two prior treatments (range 1–5), pointing to a refractory study population. The median PFS was 3.8 months (95% CI 3.6–7.3), 6-month PFS was 40.1% (28.4–51.6), and 12-month PFS was 21.8% (12.3–33.0) [10]. Median OS was 13.8 months (95% CI 11.1–29.3);

however, data were censored for 48 patients (66%) [10]. No dose-limiting toxicities were reported, and maximum tolerated dose was not reached [10]. Given these encouraging results, 500 mg daily dose of IVO was selected for expansion in a phase 3 trial [10].

The ClarIDHy study, is the phase 3 clinical trial that evaluated IVO versus placebo (PBO) in patients with previously treated nonresectable or metastatic mIDH1-CCA. As of January 2019, 185 pts. were randomized to IVO (n = 124) or PBO (n = 61) [11]. Crossover from PBO group to IVO was permitted when progressive disease was documented. Initial results are promising, showing PFS 2.7 vs 1.4 months (IVO vs PBO). PFS rates at 6 and 12 months were 32.0% and 21.9% in IVO arm. On the other hand, no PBO patients were progression-free for ≥6 months at data cutoff [11]. The primary endpoint was PFS, with IVO showing clear benefit with a hazard ratio = 0.37 (95% CI 0.25, 0.54; $p < 0.001$) [11]. IVO's efficacy was seen across all subgroups. Intention to treat analysis showed median OS was 10.8 mo for IVO compared to 9.7 months for PBO (HR = 0.69; one-sided $p = 0.06$) with 57% of PBO patients crossed over to IVO [10]. The rank preserving structural failure time (RPSFT)-adjusted median OS was 6 months for PBO (HR = 0.46; $p = 0.0008$) [11]. Grade ≥ 3 adverse events reported in 46% IVO vs 36% PBO, and there were no treatment-related deaths. This study demonstrated significant improvement in PFS with IVO and a favorable OS trend compared to PBO [11]. This is the first pivotal study demonstrating the clinical benefit of targeting mIDH1 in patients with advanced mutant IDH1 CCA.

Other clinical trials testing IDH1 and IDH2 inhibitors are ongoing (NCT02746081, NCT02273739, NCT02381886, NCT02481154) [9]. The promise of targeting IDH1 and IDH2 with these targeted therapies raises questions on how these treatments should be used—as first-line therapy in certain populations or whether these inhibitors should be combined with chemotherapy or other treatment modalities. Additionally, the utility of these inhibitors in the adjuvant and neoadjuvant settings will need to be explored. Regardless, the potential of these inhibitors offers optimism for improved therapies and a direction for future drug development.

Fibroblast Growth Factor Receptor 2 (FGFR2) Fusions

The second touted actionable mutation in CCA is the fibroblast growth factor receptor 2 (FGFR2) fusion. This genetic phenotype is seen in about 15–20% of iCCA [9]. Genome-wide structural analyses first showed recurrent translocation events involving the *FGFR2* locus [9]. The mechanism by which *FGFR2* fusions drive oncogenesis has yet to be fully elucidated. However, it is thought that genetic alterations of FGFR can alter FGFR kinase activity and result in constitutively active FGFR signaling that promotes cell proliferation and inhibits apoptosis [12]. Jain et al. reported on clinical characteristics and treatment outcomes of biliary tract cancers with *FGFR* genetic alterations in a retrospective analysis and found this subtype to be associated with an indolent disease course and prolonged survival. It was additionally noted this subtype affected a disproportionate number of young women [12]. Since the initial discovery of recurrent *FGFR2* fusions being present in multiple tumor types and particularly in iCCA, it has become the focus of developing targeted therapies.

The earliest reported data of selective FGFR inhibition in CCA is with oral agent BGJ398. BGJ398 is an orally bioavailable, selective pan-FGFR kinase inhibitor that has shown preliminary clinical activity against tumors with FGFR alterations [13]. A multicenter, open-label, phase 2 study (NCT02150967) evaluated BGJ398 antitumor activity in patients age $\geq$ 18 years with advanced or metastatic CCA containing FGFR2 fusions or other FGFR alterations whose disease progressed on prior therapy [13]. Sixty-one patients (median age, 57 years) with FGFR2 fusion ($n = 48$), mutation ($n = 8$), or amplification ($n = 3$) participated. At the prespecified data cutoff (June 30, 2016), 50 patients had discontinued treatment. All responsive tumors contained FGFR2 fusions. The overall RR was 14.8% (18.8% in FGFR2 fusions population), disease control rate was 75.4% (83.3% FGFR2 fusions population), and estimated median PFS was 5.8 months (95% CI, 4.3 to 7.6 months) [13]. BGJ398 is a first-in-class FGFR kinase inhibitor with a manageable toxicity profile, showing meaningful clinical activity against refractory CCA containing FGFR2 fusions. This promising antitumor activity supports continued development of BGJ398 in this patient population and further suggests FGFR inhibitor therapy as a viable therapeutic option in advanced biliary tract malignancies. The PROOF trial is currently ongoing, evaluating the efficacy of BGJ398 vs gem-cis in first-line treatment of patients with unresectable locally advanced or metastatic CCA with FGFR2 fusions or translocations (NCT03773302). It is a multicenter, open-label, randomized, controlled phase 3 clinical trial aiming to enroll 384 patients [14]. Patients will be randomized 2:1 to infigratinib versus standard of care, with the ability for patients who are unresponsive to gem-cis to cross over and receive infigratinib [14]. In January 2020, infigratinib (BGJ398) received fast-track and orphan drug designations by the FDA, highlighting the optimism surrounding the drug's potential to treat CCA in this select patient population [14].

TAS-120 is another irreversible FGFR inhibitor showing promise in clinical trials. A phase 1 study of TAS-120 (8–24 mg QD) in adult patients with advanced solid tumors (NCT02052778) found the maximum tolerated dose to be 20 mg QD [15]. Meric-Bernstam et al. specifically analyzed patients with CCA enrolled in this study. 45 patients with CCA (intrahepatic $n = 41$) with FGF/FGFR aberrations were treated at 16 ($n = 24$), 20 ($n = 14$), and 24 mg ($n = 7$) QD (median age 53 y [range 29–73]). Of note, 76% of the patients were female. 28 patients (62%) had tumor FGFR2 gene fusions, while 17 (38%) had other FGF/FGFR aberrations [15]. All patients received prior systemic therapy, 28.9% with reversible FGFR inhibitor, revealing a highly refractory patient population with prior FGFR inhibitor exposure. Of the 28 pts. with FGFR2 gene fusions, 20 (71%) experienced tumor shrinkage, and 7 achieved confirmed partial responses [13]. The objective RR was 25%. 15 of 28 (54%) patients had stable disease as best response [15]. The disease control rate was 79%. Of the 17 patients with other FGF/FGFR aberrations, 3 had cPRs (all had FGFR2 rearrangements; 1 also had FGFR2 amplification). Median treatment time was 7.4 months. Of the 13 patients with prior FGFR inhibitor treatment, 4 (3 with

FGFR2 gene fusions, 1 with FGFR2 amplification) had cPRs [15]. Grade ≥ 3 treatment-related adverse events were reported in 23 of 45 (51%) patients, with the most common being hyperphosphatemia (22%) [15]. TAS-120 showed notable clinical activity with manageable toxicities in patients with CCA and FGFR2 fusions. The drug further showed efficacy in patients who had progressed on prior FGFR inhibitors. A phase 2 study testing TAS-120 in patients with FGFR2 gene fusions is ongoing. Interim analysis as of May 2020 reported data for 67 patients with a minimum of 6 months of follow-up and found the ORR was 37.3% (1 CR = 1.5%; 24 PR = 35.8%) [16]. Median duration of response was 8.31 months. The most common treatment-related adverse events (all grades, grade 3) at the time of analysis were hyperphosphatemia (80.6%; 26.9%), diarrhea (37.3%; 0%), and dry mouth (32.8%; 0%) [16]. There were no grade 4 treatment-related adverse events. This initial analysis is encouraging that TAS-120 may have clinically meaningful benefit in patients with refractory iCCA with FGFR2 gene fusions.

Pemigatinib is an orally bioavailable inhibitor of FGFR 1, 2, and 3 currently being investigated. The Fight-202 trial is a phase 2, open-label, single-arm, multicenter study evaluating the efficacy of pemigatinib in patients with advanced or surgically unresectable CCA with FGFR2 translocation who have failed at least one previous treatment (NCT02924376). Patients were enrolled in three cohorts—those with FGFR2 translocations (A), those with other FGF/FGFR genetic alterations (B), or those with neither (C) [17]. Each cohort received pemigatinib 13.5 mg daily on a 21-day cycle until disease progression or intolerable toxicity. Interim data presented in September 2019 showed an objective RR of 35.5% in cohort A [17]. Median duration of response in this group was 7.5 months. No response was seen in cohort B or C. Median PFS was 6.9 months in cohort A compared with 2.1 months in cohort B and 1.7 months in cohort C [18]. This data supports FGFR inhibition being a meaningful treatment for this subset of patients with CCA. Based on the data from FIGHT-202, a phase 3 study of pemigatinib versus gem-cis chemotherapy in first-line treatment of patients with unresectable or metastatic CCA with FGFR2 rearrangements is underway (NCT03656536). As of April 2020, pemigatinib became the first FDA-approved targeted therapy for treatment of adults with previously treated, unresectable locally advanced or metastatic CCA with a fibroblast growth factor receptor 2 *(FGFR2)* fusion or other rearrangement [18].

Other selective FGFR inhibitors including Debio-1347(Debiopharm, NCT01948297), are currently being evaluated in early phase trials in patients with advanced solid tumors, including iCCA [9]. A third nonselective TKI, ARQ-087 (ArQule, NCT01752920), has shown some encouraging antitumor activity in advanced iCCA with FGFR2 fusion as well [9]. Overall, the preliminary data for FGFR inhibitors in advanced ICC provides some optimism. However, some debate exists regarding if these trends in survival can be attributed to these targeted therapies or to the natural history of FGFR phenotype, given its favorable survival profile. Looking to the future, questions remain whether these drugs can evolve into frontline therapies or if they should be used with chemotherapy or other forms of therapy.

Mechanisms of Resistance

Initial clinical trials of targeted therapies in CCA, though encouraging, have also raised concerns of drug resistance [9]. Mechanisms of resistance are not fully understood at this time, and adequately addressing resistance will likely determine the durability of these targeted therapies.

A mechanism for acquired resistance to IDH inhibitors, known as isoform switching, was first detailed in four clinical cases [19]. Harding et al. describe a selective pressure of inhibiting mutant IDH activity in one subcellular compartment, which in turn provides a growth advantage for malignant subclones with unchecked mutant IDH activity in another subcellular compartment. In other words, by "isoform switching" from mutant IDH1 to mutant IDH2 or vice versa, IDH-mutant cancers can develop resistance to isoform-selective IDH inhibitors and restore the production of oncometabolite 2-HG, ultimately promoting tumor progression [19]. The frequency of mutant IDH isoform switching as a mechanism of resistance to IDH inhibition remains uncertain.

Development of acquired resistance to FGFR kinase inhibitors has been even more prevalent, threatening the durability of benefit. The emergence of secondary FGFR2 kinase domain mutations has been observed in patients in the BGJ398 clinical trials [13]. Furthermore, Goyal et al. reported that the irreversible FGFR inhibitor TAS-120 demonstrated efficacy in four patients with *FGFR*2 fusion-positive iCCA who developed resistance to BGJ398 or Debio-1347. After examining serial biopsies, circulating tumor DNA, and patient-derived iCCA cells, it was found that TAS-120 was active against multiple FGFR2 mutations which conferred resistance to BGJ398 or Debio-1347 [20]. Functional assessment and modeling of the clonal outgrowth of individual resistance mutations from polyclonal cell pools mirrored the resistance profiles observed clinically for each inhibitor [20]. These findings suggest that strategic sequencing of FGFR inhibitors, guided by serial biopsy and ctDNA analysis, may prolong the duration of benefit from FGFR inhibition in patients with *FGFR2* fusion-positive iCCA. Moving forward, therapeutic strategies to prevent or overcome resistance will be pivotal to sustained success of these developing targeted therapies.

Smaller Targets in Cholangiocarcinoma

KRAS

The KRAS proto-oncogene encodes for a small GTPase that participates in several cell signaling pathways, including the MAPK-ERK pathway which regulates cell differentiation and proliferation. Mutations can disable the GTPase activity of KRAS, keeping it constitutively active in a GTP-bound state. This leads to continuous activation of downstream signal transduction pathways that drive tumor growth, remodeling, and migration [21].

The reported prevalence of KRAS mutations in intrahepatic CCA varies considerably between studies from 7% to 24% [22–25]. Although the reported frequency of KRAS mutations is variable, there is some data to suggest that testing for KRAS mutations may carry prognostic value. Robertson et al. conducted DNA extraction and pyrosequencing of 54 iCCA cases and found that four cases carried KRAS mutations. The reported median overall survival was 13.5 months for KRAS mutant cases, compared to 37.3 months for wild-type cases, suggesting a worse prognosis for KRAS mutant cases. KRAS mutant cases were also associated with higher tumor stage and greater likelihood of lymph node involvement at time of resection [23]. Javle et al. reported similar findings from a multicenter study using hybrid capture-based comprehensive genomic profiling (CGP) of 412 intrahepatic CCA samples. KRAS mutations were observed in 22% of iCCA samples, and among the 224 iCCA cases analyzed, KRAS-mutated tumors were associated with poorer overall survival ($P = 0.048$) in comparison with KRAS wild-type tumors [26]. Although these studies suggest that KRAS mutations may carry prognostic significance, target specific treatments for this pathway are still in the early stages of development. The Amgen pharmaceutical company has introduced an irreversible KRAS p.G12C inhibitor (AMG510) which is being tested in phase 1/2 trials (NCT03600883). However, the G12C mutation has not been commonly reported in CCA, and as such AMG510 may have limited practical significance in treating CCA.

B-raf

The B-raf proto-oncogene encodes a serine-threonine protein kinase which engages the MAPK/ERK proliferation signaling pathway. Activating mutations in B-raf, such as BRAF V600E, lead to continuous activation of its downstream signaling molecules, resulting in cell cycle progression [27]. The nucleotide sequence of the raf gene was first determined from murine sarcoma virus 3611 (MSV-3611) in 1983 [28, 29]. Raf or "rapidly accelerated fibrosarcoma" was discovered after MSV-3611 was shown to enhance fibrosarcoma induction in mice. Two years later, the C-raf-1 gene was cloned from human cells, and shortly afterward, the A-raf and B-raf isoforms were discovered.

The B-raf gene gained attention in 2002 when researchers identified B-raf somatic missense mutations in 66% of malignant melanomas [30]. The BRAF V600E mutation accounted for 80% of these mutations, providing a promising new therapeutic target. BRAF inhibitors, dabrafenib and vemurafenib, have shown dramatic results in BRAF V600E-mutated metastatic melanoma and, therefore, might be effective treatments for BRAF-mutated CCA. However, in CCA, B-raf mutations occur at a low frequency (3–5%) compared to the frequency of these mutations in melanoma [22, 24, 31]. There are limited studies that evaluate the efficacy of vemurafenib in BRAF-mutated CCA cases. In a phase 2 basket study of vemurafenib in BRAF V600E-mutated non-melanoma cancers, one patient from a cohort of eight patients with CCA achieved a durable partial response of over 1 year [32]. ROAR, a phase 2 trial investigating combination therapy with B-raf and MEK inhibition (dabrafenib and trametinib) in subjects with BRAF V600E-mutated rare cancers, is ongoing (NCT02034110). Preliminary data for the ROAR trial was presented at the 2019 Gastrointestinal Cancers Symposium [33]. Of the 33 biliary tract cancer patients enrolled in the study, 30 patients harbored BRAF V600E mutations. The objective RR was 41% (13/32; 95% CI, 24–59%), with 6 of 13 responses ongoing at data cutoff, and 7 of 13 (54%) patients with a duration of response ≥6 months. The median PFS was 7.2 months (95% CI, 4.6–10.1 months), and median overall survival was 11.3 months (95% CI, 7.3–17.6 months).

BRCA1 and BRCA2: PPAR Inhibition

The BRCA1 and BRCA2 tumor-suppressor genes encode proteins that repair double-stranded DNA breaks (DSBs) by homologous recombination. BRCA1/2-mutated cells are unable to carry out homologous recombination and perform DNA repair by alternative error-prone mechanisms, making them more prone to genomic instability [34]. One approach to targeting BRCA-mutated tumors is by inhibiting both BRCA and poly-ADP-ribose polymerase (PARP) proteins. Normally, PARP enzymes repair single-stranded DNA breaks via base excision repair. In PARP-deficient cells, single-stranded DNA breaks remain unrepaired and, when encountered by a replication fork, evolve into double-stranded breaks. BRCA-mutated cells are unable to repair these DSBs and overcome the collapsed replication fork [35]. In this way, PARP inhibition can exploit the inherent vulnerability of BRCA-mutated tumors as well as other DNA repair deficient cells.

In a retrospective analysis of patients with BRCA-mutated CCA (n = 18), one of four patients who received PARP inhibitors had a sustained disease response with a PFS duration of 42.6 months [36]. However, given the limited number of patients in this study, more research is needed to establish the success of PARP inhibition in BRCA-mutated CCA. A phase 2 trial of PARP inhibitor, niraparib, is underway at the University of Florida (NCT03207347). A basket phase 2 trial of PARP inhibitor, olaparib, is also ongoing and will include patients with metastatic solid tumors harboring IDH1 or IDH2 mutations (NCT03212274).

Her2/neu

The Her2/neu gene was initially discovered when a series of neuroglioblastomas from carcinogen treated rats were found to have the same oncogene [37]. The Her2/neu gene encodes for the Her2 (human epidermal growth factor receptor 2) protein, a transmembrane receptor with tyrosine kinase activity which lies upstream of multiple signal transduction pathways that drive tumorigenesis. Overexpression of Her2 has long been used as a predictive marker in breast and gastric cancers. However, the prevalence of Her2 overexpression in biliary tract cancers was previously understudied.

In 2017, a systematic review and meta-analysis of 40 studies (including 3839 patients in total) by Galdy et al. demonstrated that extrahepatic biliary tumors have higher Her2 overexpression compared to intrahepatic CCA: 19.9% (95% CI, 12.8–27.1%) vs 4.8% (95% CI, 0–14.5%), respectively [38]. In addition to the low prevalence of Her2 mutations in intrahepatic CCA, previous phase 2 trials of lapatinib, a dual inhibitor of EGFR and Her2/neu, have shown poor results [39]. A phase 2 study of lapatinib in 17 patients with advanced biliary tract cancer reported a median PFS duration of 1.8 months with a zero percent RR. A similar phase 2 study of lapatinib in nine biliary tract cancer patients reported zero responses and a median PFS of 2.6 months [39, 40]. In comparison to lapatinib, monoclonal antibodies such as trastuzumab might be better alternatives for Her2 overexpressing biliary tract cancers. Varlitinib, a small molecule Her 1/2/4 inhibitor, is also being investigated in a phase 2/3 study in combination with capecitabine as second-line treatment for unselected advanced biliary tract cancers [41]. Preliminary results from an ongoing clinical trial (NCT02091141) has shown that pertuzumab plus trastuzumab has activity in *Her2*-mutated biliary tract cancers, further supporting *Her2* as a potential therapeutic target for these cancers. Additionally, data from a phase 1 study showed single-agent ZW25, a bispecific antibody, induced antitumor activity in heavily pretreated patients with a variety of *Her2*-expressing cancers, including CCA [42]. Phase 2 clinical trials are currently underway testing ZW25 in breast, gastric, and other *Her2*-expressing cancers.

Role of Immunotherapy in Cholangiocarcinoma

As immunotherapy gains popularity as a treatment option for cancers such as melanoma and colorectal cancer, studies investigating the role of immunotherapy in CCA are also emerging. Immunotherapies such as programmed cell death protein 1 (PD-1) inhibitors enable tumor recognition by blocking the PD-1 and PD-L1 (programmed cell death protein 1 ligand) interaction that allows tumor cells to evade T-cell recognition. The presence of mismatch repair (MMR) deficiency further enhances tumor recognition since MMR deficiency results in a high mutation burden with subsequent creation of neoantigens and microsatellite instability. Consequently, tumors with MMR deficiency have been shown to be especially sensitive to PD-1 inhibitors such as pembrolizumab [43]. With regard to the prevalence of MMR deficiency in CCA, Goyal et al. report a 9% rate of MMR protein loss, with only 4.5% patients being microsatellite instability (MSI)-high [44].

The phase 1b KEYNOTE-028 trial evaluated 24 patients with biliary tract cancers, all of whom were PD-L1-positive but negative for MSI-H. The reported overall RR to pembrolizumab was 13.0% (3/23, all partial response; 95% CI, 2.8–33.6%), and median duration of response was not reached (range, 21.5 to 29.4+ mo). Median OS and PFS were 6.2 mo (95% CI, 3.8–10.3) and 1.8 mo (95% CI, 1.4–3.7), respectively [45]. In the larger KEYNOTE-158 phase 2 basket trial, 104 patients were enrolled in the biliary tract cancer cohort and treated with pembrolizumab; 58% were PD-L1-positive and none harbored MSI-H. The overall RR was 5.8% (6/104, all partial response; 95% CI, 2.1–12.1%), and median duration of response was not reached (range, 6.2 to 23.2+ mo). Results from these trials, especially the low overall RR in the larger KEYNOTE-158 trial, suggest that pembrolizumab is not an effective single-agent treatment option for CCA. Although there is no existing literature for immunotherapy combination regimens in CCA, combination therapy with atezolizumab and cobimetinib is being studied in the treatment of metastatic colorectal cancer. Results from a phase 3, randomized controlled trial with 363 metastatic colorectal cancer patients showed a median OS of 8.8 months (95% CI, 7.00–10.61) with atezolizumab plus cobimetinib, compared to 7.1 months (95% CI, 6.05–10.05) with atezolizumab, and 8.5 months (95% CI, 6.41–10.71) with regorafenib [46]. Although these results do not demonstrate that immunotherapy combinations are superior, this trial presents the possibilities for studying immunotherapy combinations. The first randomized trial of immunotherapy in BTC was the phase 2 trial of atezolizumab plus cobimetinib in metastatic, unresectable CCA in 2017. 86 patients were enrolled in 23 centers across the USA (NCT03201458). Results were notable for a median PFS of 3.65 months (cobimetinib + atezolizumab) vs 1.87 months (atezolizumab monotherapy) ($p = 0.027$) [47]. OS data was still pending at the time of analysis. Treatment was well tolerated in both groups as grade 3–4 treatment-related adverse events were similar in both arms, and there were no treatment-related deaths [47]. Ultimately, the combination of atezolizumab + cobimetinib significantly prolonged PFS as compared to atezolizumab monotherapy in BTC without significant toxicity, warranting further investigation in treatment of biliary tract cancers.

A single-center, prospective cohort study, conducted between May 2018 and February 2019 in Korea, evaluated the efficacy and safety of pembrolizumab in patients who were positive for programmed death ligand-1 (PD-L1) and progressed on first-line gemcitabine plus cisplatin. A total of 40 patients were enrolled, and pembrolizumab 200 mg was administered intravenously every 3 weeks. The objective response rate was 10% and 12.5% by Response Evaluation Criteria in Solid Tumor (RECIST) v1.1 and immune-modified RECIST (imRECIST), and median duration of response was 6.3 months [48]. The median PFS and OS were 1.5 months (95% confidence interval [CI], 0.0 to 3.0) and 4.3 months (95% CI, 3.5 to 5.1), respectively, and objective response per imRECIST was significantly associated with PFS ($p < 0.001$) and OS ($p = 0.001$) [48]. The data presented in this study suggests pembrolizumab having modest antitumor activity in heavily pretreated PD-L1-positive BTC patients, with a durable response seen in patients who showed objective response.

In a recent phase 2 trial, Kim et al. investigated the efficacy of nivolumab, a PD-1 inhibitor in refractory biliary tract cancers. 54 patients were enrolled in this multicenter study between October 2016 and December 2018 [49]. Of these patients, 46 were examined for objective response via radiologic imaging. Investigator-assessed objective responses (all partial responses) were observed in 10 (22%) of 46 patients.

Additionally, it was noted 17 (37%) patients had stable disease, yielding DCR of 59%. Of note, all responses were observed in patients with mismatch repair protein-proficient tumors. Among all 54 patients, median PFS was 3.68 months, and median OS was 14.24 months [49]. Patients with PD-L1-positive tumors had significantly prolonged PFS (median = 10.4 vs 2.3 months, HR = 0.23, $P < 0.001$) and nonsignificantly prolonged overall survival (median = not reached vs 10.8 months, $P = 0.19$) vs patients with PD-L1-negative tumors [49]. This study found nivolumab was well tolerated and showed modest efficacy and durable response with patients with refractory BTC. The median OS of 14.24 months was impressive given the refractory patient population. Additionally, the ORR of 22% was a strikingly higher ORR than what has been previously reported with other checkpoint inhibitors, such as pembrolizumab. However, it is important to note centrally reviewed ORR was lower at 11% and more in line with previously published results. Interestingly, although all the patients were noted to be mismatch repair-proficient, there appeared to be a correlation between PD-L1 positivity and response. Moving forward, further studies to both verify these findings and to evaluate biomarkers for improved treatment selection are needed.

One such ongoing study is a randomized, multi-institutional, phase 2 study investigating the role of combinational immunotherapy, using nivolumab with chemotherapy (gemcitabine/cisplatin) or as dual immunotherapy (nivolumab and ipilimumab) in patients with advanced BTC (NCT03101566). The primary objective is to evaluate the PFS rate at 6 months. Secondary objectives include evaluation of ORR, median PFS and OS, and safety. Exploratory objectives include identification of biomarker predictors of response and mechanisms of resistance through serial biopsies and blood collection, including sequential whole exome/transcriptomic analysis and immune cell analysis of tissue and blood [50]. Patient accrual was completed as of January 2020 and final data analysis is pending. These results will not only provide information regarding efficacy of nivolumab in combination with gem-cis and ipilimumab but may also elucidate the role of NGS data in guiding treatment selection for patients.

Conclusion: Future Directions of Targeted Therapy

Since gem-cis combination therapy was established as first-line therapy in the treatment of advanced biliary tract cancers in 2010, advances in systemic options extending to standard clinical practice have been minimal. NGS has started to elucidate the pathogenesis of CCA at a molecular level, bringing hope of identifying actionable mutations for the development of targeted therapies. The notion of a "one size fits all" for the treatment of CCA is likely outdated, given the varying etiologies and heterogeneity of the disease. Looking to the future, NGS should become central to clinical and therapeutic decision-making, and there is clear need to sequence all patients with CCA. IDH1 inhibitor IVO showed considerable promise in the ClarIDHy study, and FGFR inhibitors BGJ398 and TAS-120 have also shown meaningful activity in phase 2 clinical trials. Marking a big step for targeted therapies, pemigatinib became the first FDA-approved therapy for CCA patients with *FGFR2* fusions, as of April 2020. It is not unrealistic to expect more of these targeted therapies to enter the front line of care in coming years.

Although other molecular targets, such as B-raf and BRCA mutations, occur at lower frequencies in CCA, many of these targets are actionable with approved therapies in other cancer types. Therefore, further investigation is needed to evaluate the efficacy of targeting these mutations in CCA. One approach to increasing these investigations is through basket trials, which allow for evaluation of rare tumor subsets with shared controls. Introducing more basket trials should provide researchers with more opportunities for studying infrequent mutations in rare cancers such as CCA.

While immunotherapy has shown promising results for malignancies such as melanoma and colorectal cancer, results for pembrolizumab treatment in CCA have been mixed. Kang et al. reported modest efficacy of pembrolizumab in PD-L1-positive patients, but the applicability of this study remains unknown given all patients were enrolled were Asian. Additionally, the results of Kim et al. study are intriguing given reported ORR 22%, which was notably higher than prior studies, namely, the large KEYNOTE-158 study. The data was certainly suggestive of durable response in patients who responded to nivolumab. However, it is important to note no molecular profiling data was reported in patients to this study. Looking to the future, the possibilities of using immunotherapy combinations in treating CCA remain ripe for further investigation, particularly with trials incorporating NGS information.

Challenges remain despite the optimism surrounding targeted therapies, particularly regarding how targeted therapies will be used—whether in combination with systemic therapies or other treatment modalities. Additionally, as noted in clinical trials, issues with resistance to IDH and FGFR inhibitors and durability of treatment will need to be explored further and appropriately addressed. Furthermore, it is clear not all CCAs are created equal; however, how to stratify CCA remains a mystery. Despite the unknowns that remain in the treatment of CCA, targeted therapies have provided a hope of a future in which patients with this disease will have improved survival.

References

1. Valle J, Wasan H, Palmer D, Cunningham D, Anthoney A, Maraveyas A, et al. Cisplatin plus Gemcitabine versus Gemcitabine for Biliary Tract Cancer. N Engl J Med. 2010;362(14):1273–81.
2. Rogers J, Law L, Nguyen D, Qiao W, Javle M, Kaseb A, et al. Second-line systemic treatment for advanced cholangiocarcinoma. J Clin Oncol. 2014;32(3_suppl):371.
3. Lamarca A, Hubner R, David Ryder W, Valle J. Second-line chemotherapy in advanced biliary cancer: a systematic review. Ann Oncol. 2014;25(12):2328–38.
4. Lowery M, Goff L, Keenan B, Jordan E, Wang R, Bocobo A, et al. Second-line chemotherapy in advanced biliary cancers: a retrospective, multicenter analysis of outcomes. Cancer. 2019;125(24):4426–34.

5. Lamarca A, Palmer D, Wasan H, Ross P, Ma Y, Arora A, et al. ABC-06 I A randomised phase III, multi-centre, open-label study of active symptom control (ASC) alone or ASC with oxaliplatin / 5-FU chemotherapy (ASC+mFOLFOX) for patients (pts) with locally advanced / metastatic biliary tract cancers (ABC) previously-treated with cisplatin/gemcitabine (CisGem) chemotherapy. J Clin Oncol. 2019;37(15_suppl):4003.
6. Shroff R, Javle M, Xiao L, Kaseb A, Varadhachary G, Wolff R, et al. Gemcitabine, Cisplatin, and nab-Paclitaxel for the treatment of advanced biliary tract cancers. JAMA Oncol. 2019;5(6):824.
7. Kamps R, Brandão R, Bosch B, Paulussen A, Xanthoulea S, Blok M, et al. Next-generation sequencing in oncology: genetic diagnosis, risk prediction and cancer classification. Int J Mol Sci. 2017;18(2):308.
8. Jusakul A, Cutcutache I, Yong C, Lim J, Huang M, Padmanabhan N, et al. Whole-genome and epigenomic landscapes of etiologically distinct subtypes of cholangiocarcinoma. Cancer Discov. 2017;7(10):1116–35.
9. Valle J, Lamarca A, Goyal L, Barriuso J, Zhu A. New horizons for precision medicine in biliary tract cancers. Cancer Discov. 2017;7(9):943–62.
10. Lowery M, Burris H, Janku F, Shroff R, Cleary J, Azad N, et al. Safety and activity of ivosidenib in patients with IDH1-mutant advanced cholangiocarcinoma: a phase 1 study. Lancet Gastroenterol Hepatol. 2019;4(9):711–20.
11. Abou-Alfa, Ghassan K, et al. Ivosidenib in IDH1-Mutant, Chemotherapy-Refractory Cholangiocarcinoma (ClarIDHy): a multicentre, randomised, double-blind, placebo-controlled, phase 3 study. Lancet Oncol. 2020;21(6):796–807. https://doi.org/10.1016/s1470-2045(20)30157-1.
12. Jain A, Borad M, Kelley R, Wang Y, Abdel-Wahab R, Meric-Bernstam F, et al. Cholangiocarcinoma with FGFR genetic aberrations: a unique clinical phenotype. JCO Precis Oncol. 2018;2:1–12.
13. Javle M, Lowery M, Shroff R, Weiss K, Springfeld C, Borad M, et al. Phase II study of BGJ398 in patients with FGFR-altered advanced cholangiocarcinoma. J Clin Oncol. 2018;36(3):276–82.
14. BridgeBio. BridgeBio Pharma's QED therapeutics receives fast track designation for infigratinib in adults with first-line advanced or metastatic cholangiocarcinoma and orphan drug designation for infigratinib for treatment of cholangiocarcinoma. 2020.
15. Meric-Bernstam F, Arkenau H, Tran B, Bahleda R, Kelley R, Hierro C, et al. Efficacy of TAS-120, an irreversible fibroblast growth factor receptor (FGFR) inhibitor, in cholangiocarcinoma patients with FGFR pathway alterations who were previously treated with chemotherapy and other FGFR inhibitors. Ann Oncol. 2018;29:v100.
16. Taiho Oncology. (2020). Presentation of data for futibatinib in advanced INTRAHEPATIC Cholangiocarcinoma at 2020 ASCO meeting [Press release]. Retrieved 2020, from https://www.biospace.com/article/releases/taiho-oncology-announces-presentation-of-data-for-futibatinib-in-advanced-intrahepatic-cholangiocarcinoma-at-2020-asco-meeting/.
17. Vogel A, Sahai V, Hollebecque A, et al. FIGHT-202: a phase 2 study of pemigatinib in patients (pts) with previously treated locally advanced or metastatic cholangiocarcinoma (CCA). Presented at: 2019 ESMO Congress; September 27–October 1, 2019; Barcelona, Spain. Abstract LBA40.
18. Jermias S. FDA approves orphan drug pemigatinib for rare bile duct cancer cholangiocarcinoma. AJMC. April 2020.
19. Harding J, Lowery M, Shih A, Schvartzman J, Hou S, Famulare C, et al. Isoform switching as a mechanism of acquired resistance to mutant isocitrate dehydrogenase inhibition. Cancer Discov. 2018;8(12):1540–7.
20. Goyal L, Shi L, Liu L, Fece de la Cruz F, Lennerz J, Raghavan S, et al. TAS-120 overcomes resistance to ATP-competitive FGFR inhibitors in patients with FGFR2 fusion–positive intrahepatic cholangiocarcinoma. Cancer Discov. 2019;9(8):1064–79.
21. Eser S, Schnieke A, Schneider G, Saur D. Oncogenic KRAS signalling in pancreatic cancer. Br J Cancer. 2014;111(5):817–22. https://doi.org/10.1038/bjc.2014.215.

22. Churi CR, Shroff R, Wang Y, Rashid A, Kang HC, Weatherly J, Zuo M, Zinner R, Hong D, Meric-Bernstam F, Janku F, Crane CH, Mishra L, Vauthey JN, Wolff RA, Mills G, Javle M. Mutation profiling in cholangiocarcinoma: prognostic and therapeutic implications. PLoS One. 2014;9(12):e115383. https://doi.org/10.1371/journal.pone.0115383.
23. Robertson S, Hyder O, Dodson R, Nayar SK, Poling J, Beierl K, Eshleman JR, Lin MT, Pawlik TM, Anders RA. The frequency of KRAS and BRAF mutations in intrahepatic cholangiocarcinomas and their correlation with clinical outcome. Hum Pathol. 2013;44(12):2768–73. https://doi.org/10.1016/j.humpath.2013.07.026.
24. Zhu AX, Borger DR, Kim Y, Cosgrove D, Ejaz A, Alexandrescu S, Groeschl RT, Deshpande V, Lindberg JM, Ferrone C, Sempoux C, Yau T, Poon R, Popescu I, Bauer TW, Gamblin TC, Gigot JF, Anders RA, Pawlik TM. Genomic profiling of intrahepatic cholangiocarcinoma: refining prognosis and identifying therapeutic targets. Ann Surg Oncol. 2014;21(12):3827–34. https://doi.org/10.1245/s10434-014-3828-x.
25. Ross JS, Wang K, Gay L, Al-Rohil R, Rand JV, Jones DM, Lee HJ, Sheehan CE, Otto GA, Palmer G, Yelensky R, Lipson D, Morosini D, Hawryluk M, Catenacci DV, Miller VA, Churi C, Ali S, Stephens PJ. New routes to targeted therapy of intrahepatic cholangiocarcinomas revealed by next-generation sequencing. Oncologist. 2014;19(3):235–42. https://doi.org/10.1634/theoncologist.2013-0352.
26. Javle M, Bekaii-Saab T, Jain A, Wang Y, Kelley RK, Wang K, Kang HC, Catenacci D, Ali S, Krishnan S, Ahn D, Bocobo AG, Zuo M, Kaseb A, Miller V, Stephens PJ, Meric-Bernstam F, Shroff R, Ross J. Biliary cancer: utility of next-generation sequencing for clinical management. Cancer. 2016;122(24):3838–47. https://doi.org/10.1002/cncr.30254.
27. Wan PT, Garnett MJ, Roe SM, Lee S, Niculescu-Duvaz D, Good VM, Jones CM, Marshall CJ, Springer CJ, Barford D, Marais R. Mechanism of activation of the RAF-ERK signaling pathway by oncogenic mutations of B-RAF. Cell. 2004;116(6):855–67. https://doi.org/10.1016/s0092-8674(04)00215-6.
28. Mark GE, Rapp UR. Primary structure of v-raf: relatedness to the src family of oncogenes. Science. 1984;224(4646):285–9. https://doi.org/10.1126/science.6324342.
29. Zebisch A, Troppmair J. Back to the roots: the remarkable RAF oncogene story. Cell Mol Life Sci. 2006;63(11):1314–30. https://doi.org/10.1007/s00018-006-6005-y.
30. Davies H, Bignell GR, Cox C, Stephens P, Edkins S, Clegg S, Teague J, Woffendin H, Garnett MJ, Bottomley W, Davis N, Dicks E, Ewing R, Floyd Y, Gray K, Hall S, Hawes R, Hughes J, Kosmidou V, Menzies A, Mould C, Parker A, Stevens C, Watt S, Hooper S, Wilson R, Jayatilake H, Gusterson BA, Cooper C, Shipley J, Hargrave D, Pritchard-Jones K, Maitland N, Chenevix-Trench G, Riggins GJ, Bigner DD, Palmieri G, Cossu A, Flanagan A, Nicholson A, Ho JW, Leung SY, Yuen ST, Weber BL, Seigler HF, Darrow TL, Paterson H, Marais R, Marshall CJ, Wooster R, Stratton MR, Futreal PA. Mutations of the BRAF gene in human cancer. Nature. 2002;417(6892):949–54. https://doi.org/10.1038/nature00766.
31. Goeppert B, Frauenschuh L, Renner M, Roessler S, Stenzinger A, Klauschen F, Warth A, Vogel MN, Mehrabi A, Hafezi M, Boehmer K, von Deimling A, Schirmacher P, Weichert W, Capper D. BRAF V600E-specific immunohistochemistry reveals low mutation rates in biliary tract cancer and restriction to intrahepatic cholangiocarcinoma. Mod Pathol. 2014;27(7):1028–34. https://doi.org/10.1038/modpathol.2013.206.
32. Hyman DM, Puzanov I, Subbiah V, Faris JE, Chau I, Blay JY, Wolf J, Raje NS, Diamond EL, Hollebecque A, Gervais R, Elez-Fernandez ME, Italiano A, Hofheinz RD, Hidalgo M, Chan E, Schuler M, Lasserre SF, Makrutzki M, Sirzen F, Veronese ML, Tabernero J, Baselga J. Vemurafenib in Multiple Nonmelanoma cancers with BRAF V600 mutations. N Engl J Med. 2015;373(8):726–36. https://doi.org/10.1056/NEJMoa1502309.
33. Wainberg ZA, Lassen UN, Elez E, Italiano A, Curigliano G, Braud FGD, Prager G, Greil R, Stein A, Fasolo A, Schellens JHM, Wen PY, Boran AD, Burgess P, Gasal E, Ilankumaran P, Subbiah V. Efficacy and safety of dabrafenib (D) and trametinib (T) in patients (pts) with BRAF V600E–mutated biliary tract cancer (BTC): a cohort of the ROAR basket trial. J Clin Oncol. 2019;37(4_suppl):187. https://doi.org/10.1200/JCO.2019.37.4_suppl.187.

34. Gudmundsdottir K, Ashworth A. The roles of BRCA1 and BRCA2 and associated proteins in the maintenance of genomic stability. Oncogene. 2006;25(43):5864–74. https://doi.org/10.1038/sj.onc.1209874.
35. Bryant HE, Schultz N, Thomas HD, Parker KM, Flower D, Lopez E, Kyle S, Meuth M, Curtin NJ, Helleday T. Specific killing of BRCA2-deficient tumours with inhibitors of poly(ADP-ribose) polymerase. Nature. 2005;434(7035):913–7. https://doi.org/10.1038/nature03443.
36. Golan T, Raitses-Gurevich M, Kelley RK, Bocobo AG, Borgida A, Shroff RT, Holter S, Gallinger S, Ahn DH, Aderka D, Apurva J, Bekaii-Saab T, Friedman E, Javle M. Overall survival and clinical characteristics of BRCA-associated cholangiocarcinoma: a multicenter retrospective study. Oncologist. 2017;22(7):804–10. https://doi.org/10.1634/theoncologist.2016-0415.
37. Schechter AL, Stern DF, Vaidyanathan L, Decker SJ, Drebin JA, Greene MI, Weinberg RA. The neu oncogene: an erb-B-related gene encoding a 185,000-Mr tumour antigen. Nature. 1984;312(5994):513–6. https://doi.org/10.1038/312513a0.
38. Galdy S, Lamarca A, McNamara MG, Hubner RA, Cella CA, Fazio N, Valle JW. HER2/HER3 pathway in biliary tract malignancies; systematic review and meta-analysis: a potential therapeutic target? Cancer Metastasis Rev. 2017;36(1):141–57. https://doi.org/10.1007/s10555-016-9645-x.
39. Ramanathan RK, Belani CP, Singh DA, Tanaka M, Lenz HJ, Yen Y, Kindler HL, Iqbal S, Longmate J, Mack PC, Lurje G, Gandour-Edwards R, Dancey J, Gandara DR. A phase II study of lapatinib in patients with advanced biliary tree and hepatocellular cancer. Cancer Chemother Pharmacol. 2009;64(4):777–83. https://doi.org/10.1007/s00280-009-0927-7.
40. Peck J, Wei L, Zalupski M, O'Neil B, Villalona Calero M, Bekaii-Saab T. HER2/neu may not be an interesting target in biliary cancers: results of an early phase II study with lapatinib. Oncology. 2012;82(3):175–9. https://doi.org/10.1159/000336488.
41. Javle MM, Oh D-Y, Ikeda M, Qin S, Yong W-P, Chao Y, McIntyre N, Hsieh C-Y, Chow L, Chang A, McHale M, Lindmark B. TREETOPP: A phase 2/3 study of varlitinib plus capecitabine versus placebo plus capecitabine as second-line treatment in patients with advanced or metastatic biliary tract cancers (BTCs). J Clin Oncol. 2018;36(15_suppl):TPS4143. https://doi.org/10.1200/JCO.2018.36.15_suppl.TPS4143.
42. Meric-Bernstam F, Beeram M, Mayordomo JI, Hanna DL, Ajani JA, Murphy MAB, et al. Single agent activity of ZW25, a HER2-targeted bispecific antibody, in heavily pretreated HER2-expressing cancers. J Clin Oncol. 2018;36(15_suppl):2500.
43. Le DT, Uram JN, Wang H, Bartlett BR, Kemberling H, Eyring AD, Skora AD, Luber BS, Azad NS, Laheru D, Biedrzycki B, Donehower RC, Zaheer A, Fisher GA, Crocenzi TS, Lee JJ, Duffy SM, Goldberg RM, de la Chapelle A, Koshiji M, Bhaijee F, Huebner T, Hruban RH, Wood LD, Cuka N, Pardoll DM, Papadopoulos N, Kinzler KW, Zhou S, Cornish TC, Taube JM, Anders RA, Eshleman JR, Vogelstein B, Diaz LA Jr. PD-1 blockade in tumors with mismatch-repair deficiency. N Engl J Med. 2015;372(26):2509–20. https://doi.org/10.1056/NEJMoa1500596.
44. Goyal L, Deshpande V, Chung DC, Groeschl RT, Gamblin TC, Zhu AX. Mismatch repair protein loss and microsatellite instability in cholangiocarcinoma. J Clin Oncol. 2014;32(3_suppl):237. https://doi.org/10.1200/jco.2014.32.3_suppl.237.
45. Bang Y-J, Ueno M, Malka D, Chung HC, Nagrial A, Kelley RK, Piha-Paul SA, Ros W, Italiano A, Nakagawa K, Rugo HS, Braud FGD, Varga AI, Hansen AR, Gao C, Krishnan S, Norwood K, Doi T. Pembrolizumab (pembro) for advanced biliary adenocarcinoma: results from the KEYNOTE-028 (KN028) and KEYNOTE-158 (KN158) basket studies. J Clin Oncol. 2019;37(15_suppl):4079. https://doi.org/10.1200/JCO.2019.37.15_suppl.4079.
46. Eng C, Kim TW, Bendell J, Argiles G, Tebbutt NC, Di Bartolomeo M, Falcone A, Fakih M, Kozloff M, Segal NH, Sobrero A, Yan Y, Chang I, Uyei A, Roberts L, Ciardiello F. Atezolizumab with or without cobimetinib versus regorafenib in previously treated metastatic colorectal cancer (IMblaze370): a multicentre, open-label, phase 3, randomised, controlled trial. Lancet Oncol. 2019;20(6):849–61. https://doi.org/10.1016/s1470-2045(19)30027-0.

47. CHOLANGIOCARCINOMA: PD-L1 + MEK inhibition improved PFS versus PD-L1 alone in the second/third line setting. (AACR 2020). In CHOLANGIOCARCINOMA: PD-L1 + MEK inhibition improved PFS versus PD-L1 alone in the second/third line setting.
48. Kang J, Jeong JH, Hwang H, Lee SS, Park DH, Oh DW, et al. Efficacy and safety of pembrolizumab in patients with refractory advanced biliary tract cancer: tumor proportion score as a potential biomarker for response. Cancer Res Treat. 2020;52(2):594–603. https://doi.org/10.4143/crt.2019.493.
49. Kim RD, Chung V, Alese OB, El-Rayes BF, Li D, Al-Toubah TE, et al. A phase 2 multi-institutional study of nivolumab for patients with advanced refractory biliary tract cancer. JAMA Oncol. 2020;6(6):888. https://doi.org/10.1001/jamaoncol.2020.0930.
50. Sahai V, Griffith KA, Zalupski M. A multicenter randomized phase II study of nivolumab in combination with gemcitabine/cisplatin or ipilimumab as first-line therapy for patients with advanced unresectable biliary tract cancer. J Clin Oncol. 2018;36(4_suppl):TPS541. https://doi.org/10.1200/jco.2018.36.4_suppl.tps541.

Part III
Experimental and Translational Facets of Cholangiocarcinoma

Chapter 22
In Vitro and In Vivo Model Systems of Cholangiocarcinoma

Giovanni Brandi and Simona Tavolari

Abbreviations

2D	Two-dimensional
3D	Three-dimensional
CCA	Cholangiocarcinoma
CCl_4	Carbon tetrachloride
DEN	Diethylnitrosamine
eCCA	extrahepatic cholangiocarcinoma
ECM	Extracellular matrix
GEMM	Genetically engineered mouse model
HCC	Hepatocellular carcinoma
HTVI	Hydrodynamic tail vein injection
iCCA	intrahepatic cholangiocarcinoma
LMBDL	Left and median bile duct
NICD	Notch intracellular domain
PDX	Patient-derived xenograft
ROS	Reactive oxygen species
SB	Sleeping Beauty
TAA	Thioacetamide

G. Brandi (✉)
Department of Experimental, Diagnostic and Specialty Medicine, S. Orsola-Malpighi University Hospital, Bologna, Italy
e-mail: giovanni.brandi@unibo.it

S. Tavolari
Division of Medical Oncology, IRCSS, Azienda Ospedaliero-Universitaria of Bologna, Bologna, Italy

Center for Applied Biomedical Research, S.Orsola-Malpighi University Hospital, Bologna, Italy
e-mail: simona.tavolari@unibo.it

J. H. Tabibian (ed.), *Diagnosis and Management of Cholangiocarcinoma*,
https://doi.org/10.1007/978-3-030-70936-5_22

Introduction

Cholangiocarcinoma (CCA) encompasses a group of malignancies that may emerge at different anatomic sites along the intrahepatic (iCCA) and extrahepatic (eCCA) biliary tree. Recent studies have revealed that the molecular landscape of CCA is heterogeneous and segregates with the anatomical location and underlying risk factors [1]. The highly dismal prognosis of CCA, along with the rising global incidence, highlights the critical need for new therapeutic strategies for this disease. In an effort to address this challenge, the development of preclinical models allowing high-throughput experimental approaches to quickly gain insight into biological processes and effectiveness of therapies have becomes a paramount in understanding CCA carcinogenesis, progression, and therapeutic strategies. To date, two-dimensional (2D) and three-dimensional (3D) cell culture as well as animal models have been employed for the study of liver physiology, disease pathogenesis, and treatment. In CCA, the lack of a uniform phenotype and molecular signature makes more challenging the development of preclinical models that accurately represent the phenotypic and genetic complexity that characterizes this disease. Despite this drawback, the spectrum of currently available in vitro and in vivo models of CCA (Fig. 22.1) offers an unprecedented opportunity to elucidate the molecular mechanisms underlying cholangiocarcinogenesis as well as to develop more efficacious treatment options for this disease.

This chapter summarizes the current knowledge and understanding of the preclinical in vitro and in vivo models of CCA, critically underlining their translational usefulness as well as their limitations.

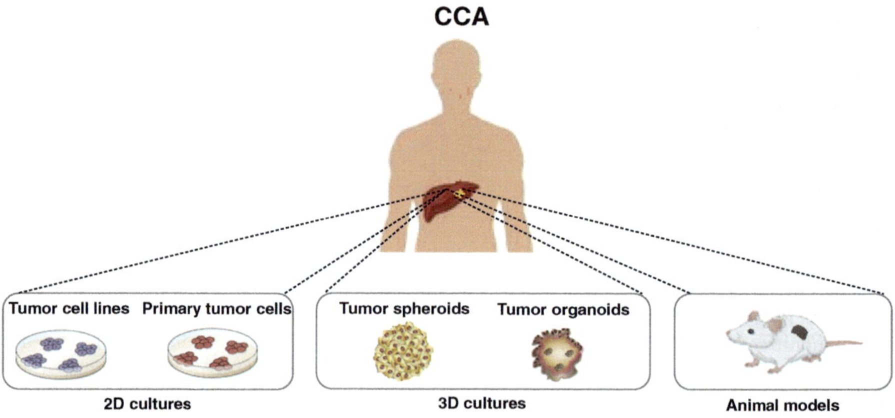

Fig. 22.1 Current preclinical models available for CCA

CCA In Vitro Culture Systems

Two-Dimensional (2D) Cell Cultures

Much of our understanding on the biological mechanisms underlying tumor cellular functions, such as proliferation, migration, invasion, and differentiation, has been garnered from studies of two-dimensional (2D) cell cultures. For this purpose, the use of tumor cell lines is essential. Cell line models have the advantage of guaranteeing a large amount of material, allowing high reproducibility and highly controlled experimental conditions; moreover, these models are relatively simple to use and manage [2]. The first well-characterized CCA cell line was established in 1985 from a specimen of an iCCA patient's autopsy; this cell line was known as HChol-Y1 [3]. Since then, different CCA cell lines have been established and characterized. Currently available CCA cell lines are derived from iCCA, eCCA, perihilar CCA (i.e., Klatskin tumor), and CCA metastases (Table 22.1). Of these, iCCA and eCCA represent approximately 39% and 37%, respectively, of the primary sites from which CCA cell lines have been isolated; cell lines of Klatskin tumor account only for 5% of all CCA cell lines, while the remaining 19% are derived from CCA metastases [35]. Molecular characterization has revealed a heterogeneous pattern of protein expression among these cell lines, akin to the molecular heterogeneity of CCA [36].

Table 22.1 Current established cell lines for iCCA, eCCA, and Klatskin CCA

iCCA	eCCA	Klatsin CCA
HChol-Y1 [3]	Sk-ChA-1 [7, 20]	HBDC [33]
Oz [4]	EGI-1 [7]	SNU-1196 [16]
HuH-28 [5]	MEC [21]	KKU-100 [34]
HuCC-T1 [6, 7]	KMBC + BDC [7, 22]	
SG231 [8, 9]	BDC [23, 24]	
HuCCA-1 [10]	TFK-1 [7, 25]	
KMC-1 [11]	OCUCh-LM1 [26]	
CC-SW-1 + CC-LP-1 [12]	ICBD-1 [27]	
KMCH-2 [13]	TK [28]	
ETK1 [14]	SCK + JCK + Cho-CK+ Choi-CK [29]	
RBA+ SSP-25 [15]	SNU-245 [16]	
SNU-1079 [16]	TGBC-47 [30]	
HKGZ-CC [17]	TBCN6 [31]	
NCC-CC1 + NCC-CC3–1 + NCC-CC3–2+ NCC-CC4–1 [18]	RMCCA-1 [32]	
HCCC-9810 [19]	NCC-BD1 + NCC-BD2 [18]	

Depending on the cell line, expression of receptors (EGFR, HGFR, IGF1R IGF2R, VEGFR1, VEGFR2), intermediate filaments (keratin, vimentin), antigens (HLA-1), or secreted proteins such as tumor markers CA-19-9, CEA, AFP, and CA125 have been observed [3, 7, 14, 20, 28, 31, 32, 34, 37]. Currently the establishment of a CCA cell line can be achieved with a success rate of approximately 10% [35]. This unsatisfactory result is mainly related to the stringent selection by 2D culture, to possible fungal or bacterial contamination and also to frequent fibroblast overgrowth in the culture plate [35]. Moreover, the time from sampling to processing has a critical role in success rate, as cells are prone to undergoing necrosis in a nonphysiological environment.

Despite cell lines representing an important tool for functional studies to better understand the molecular pathogenesis of CCA, they have several important limitations. First, the homogeneity of cell line populations cannot sufficiently represent the complex molecular and phenotypic heterogeneity of CCA [36]. Second, the high number of passages in monolayer systems makes these models prone to genetic drift that may alter the tumor genome over time; therefore, their genetic profile, as well as their gene expression pattern, may significantly differ from that of patient tumor tissue [38–40]. Furthermore, 2D systems fail to faithfully capture the physiological behavior of cells in vivo, as they lack realistic cell-cell and cell-matrix interactions [41]. Indeed, in vivo, cells exist embedded within a complex environment containing multiple extracellular matrix (ECM) components, mixed cell populations that interact with each other, and a medley of cell-secreted factors [42]. This is particularly true in the context of CCA, whose highly malignant behavior relies on a tight interplay between tumor cells and tumor microenvironment, including stromal, endothelial, and immune cells [43]. The suboptimal clinical translational value of cell lines may be responsible for the failure of many compounds in clinical trials and has encouraged researchers to explore new ways of cancer modelling. Accordingly, primary cultures from patient-derived tumor samples have been established in recent years [44, 45]. These preclinical models better (though still only partially) reproduce the natural in situ tumor microenvironment, maintaining the cross talk between malignant and healthy components [2]. In addition, conversely to immortalized tumor cell lines, primary cultures also may preserve cancer subpopulations, including cancer cells with stem-like phenotypes. This is of particular relevance, as cancer stem cells are known to play an important role in drug resistance [46]. However, primary cultures from patient tissue are very laborious and less efficient. In particular, in highly desmoplastic tumors such as CCA, the overgrowth of stromal cells may significantly reduce establishment efficiency [16]. Moreover, primary cultures have to be used shortly after isolation in order to retain most of the patient tumor features [47]. Another important caveat of these models is that they can be established only from surgically resected specimens; therefore, their applicability is limited only to patients who have undergone tumor resection.

Three-Dimensional (3D) Cell Cultures

Many cell types, when isolated from tissues and placed into 2D cell culture, become progressively flatter, divide aberrantly, and lose their differentiated phenotype. Interestingly, most of these cells can maintain their physiological form and function when cultured in a 3D system [42]. This observation has led to the notion that the dimension in which cells are cultured in vitro (2D or 3D) is a crucial determinant of cell fate and that while culturing cells in 2D monolayer may drive abnormal cell function or dedifferentiation, 3D cultures are able to better reproduce a more physiological state. This aspect should particularly be kept in mind when culturing tumor cells in vitro. Indeed, tumors are dynamic cell systems where malignant and healthy cell populations of the stroma are in continuous coevolution, supported by an extracellular 3D matrix that is constantly remodelled [42]. The complexity of this interaction cannot be faithfully reproduced in 2D monolayer models.

To overcome these drawbacks, 3D cell cultures models that more realistically mimic the pathophysiological features of the tumor niche have been developed. Tumor spheroids are in vitro aggregates of tumor cells grown in suspension or embedded in a 3D matrix; despite their establishment being more expensive and time-consuming compared to 2D cell cultures, they are widely used as in vitro experimental models on the basis of their advantages [41]. Indeed, they can mimic the growth characteristics of in vivo solid tumors, including cell-cell and cell-matrix interactions between tumor cells and the microenvironment, which collectively lead to tumor genetic and adaptive changes [41]. Moreover, as it occurs in vivo, tumor cells in spheroids are exposed to concentration gradients of signalling effector molecules, nutrients, and waste products; conversely, in 2D monolayers, cells are exposed to a uniform concentration of factors due to direct contact with the culture medium [48]. In terms of therapeutic applications, this may, in part, explain the failure of 2D cell culture systems to recapitulate drug screening outcomes as seen in vivo [49].

When performing experiments with spheroids, tumor size represents an important variable. Indeed, spheroids ranging from 200 to 500 μm diameter are sufficiently large to develop gradients of oxygen, nutrients, and catabolites [50]; conversely, spheroids not reaching a diameter of approximately 200 μm can reproduce cell-cell and cell-matrix interactions but are not large enough to recapitulate oxygen gradients with hypoxic regions or proliferation gradients [50]. On the other hand, above a critical size of 400–600 μm diameter, tumor spheroids typically develop a necrotic core, similar to what observed in poorly vascularized tumors [50]. Currently, spheroids have been established from both CCA cancer cell lines and primary cultures. The pattern of protein expression in two cell lines arising from a differentiated (Mz-ChA-1) and undifferentiated (SK-ChA-1) eCCA and undergoing spheroid formation has been recently investigated [51]. Compared to 2D cultures, ECC spheroids displayed a decrease in E-cadherin and vimentin expression and an increased expression of several enzymes involved in glycolysis, hypoxia signalling, protein ubiquitination pathway, NADH repair, and superoxide radical degradation [51]. These effects are likely to increase cell growth rate and redifferentiation of cholangiocytes in the 3D aggregation form, which is therefore likely to associate with more invasive behavior in vivo. In another recent study, CCA spheroids were established from SG231, HuCC-T1, CC-LP1, and primary human iCCA-derived (CCA4) cell lines [52]. Characterization of these CCA spheroids revealed that they were highly enriched for cancer stem cells; moreover, a core of 30 common dysregulated genes was identified in all CCA spheroid types. In particular, an increased expression of key genes involved in pluripotency and self-renewal, drug resistance and survival, as well as stem-like surface markers was reported; in addition, an overexpression of the hepatic oncogenic drivers CDKN1A, BCL2L1, CTNNB1, IGF2, ITGB1, and LEF1 was found [52]. Intriguingly, these CCA spheroids engrafted in 100% of transplanted mice, showing a sustained tumorigenic potential through diverse xenograft generations [52].

A more recent promising culture system to bridge the gap between 2D cultures and in vivo mouse/human models is represented by organoids, an innovative 3D model established from resected specimens and core needle biopsies [53]. A comprehensive discussion about the development of CCA organoids is discussed elsewhere in this book (Chap. 23, *Mertens et al.*).

CCA in Vivo Models

Preclinical in vivo CCA models are an intermediate step of experimentation between 2D/3D cell cultures and human clinical trials, thus representing a valuable tool to gain new insights into the pathophysiology of these diseases as well as to investigate the efficacy of therapies. Compared to in vitro systems, in vivo models of CCA may more closely mimic the complex interplay between tumor and stromal cells [54]. To date a repertoire of different murine models for CCA (including neoplastic transformation of biliary cells, CCA progression, and metastasis) have been developed, including carcinogen-based, genetic, xenograft, and syngeneic models (Fig. 22.2).

Carcinogen-Based Murine Models

With carcinogen-based models, CCA development is induced by the administration of a chemical carcinogen, typically diethylnitrosamine (DEN), furan, thioacetamide (TAA), or carbon tetrachloride (CCl_4). These carcinogens are able to induce a genotoxic effect by affecting the DNA structure or by promoting tumor development by expansion of preneoplastic cells. The main advantage of carcinogen-based murine CCA models is that tumor development is closely associated with chronic liver injury, thus mimicking human disease [55].

Diethylnitrosamine (DEN) promotes carcinogenesis inducing DNA methylation [56]. DEN administration in mice results in formation of multifocal biliary cystic

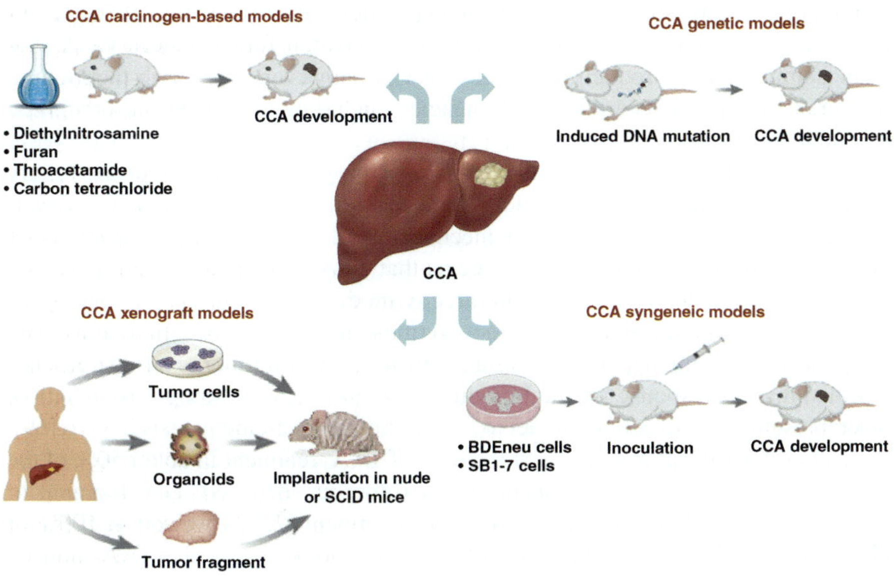

Fig. 22.2 Current in vivo models available for CCA

lesions and may induce CCA development when administered in combination with pentachlorophenol [57, 58]. However, the formation of both CCA and hepatocellular carcinoma (HCC) in this model limits its applicability for the study of iCCA. In another murine model, DEN administration was combined with cholestasis induced by surgical ligation of the left and median bile duct (LMBDL) [59]. This combination was found to result in CCA formation in 50% of the animals by week 28, whereas none of the animals undergoing LMBDL alone or DEN administration alone developed CCA [59]. The main advantages of this model are the higher tumor incidence and the shorter duration to tumor development compared to other similar models, but it requires significant technical skills.

Furan is a heterocyclic compound whose carcinogenic effects are related to the ability to induce oxidative stress, thus generating DNA mutations in target cells [60]. Furan-induced CCA is one of the most commonly used animal models of liver cancer. In rats, chronic administration of furan at a high dose of 8 mg/kg for 15 months was able to promote CCA development in 98% of animals [61]. At higher doses (15–60 mg/kg/per day), furan administration induced a rapid development of cholangiofibrosis (i.e., fibrosis of the bile ducts) after 2–3 weeks of treatment; cholangiofibrosis in the caudate liver lobe with the development of dysplastic glands persisted also after 6 weeks from treatment [62], thus mimicking the natural progression from chronic bile duct lesions inducing cholangiofibrosis to subsequent CCA development. Molecular analysis have shown that in rat liver furan may affect the expression of several genes involved in cell proliferation, apoptosis, and DNA repair; moreover changes in miRNA expression profile and DNA methylation have been reported, suggesting that genetic and epigenetic alterations may also contribute to furan-induced iCCA carcinogenesis [63]. Overall furan-induced CCA provides a simple and reproducible model of iCCA. However, it is worth mentioning that furan can also induce other malignancies, including malignant mesothelioma and mononuclear cell leukemia [64].

TAA is a potent hepatotoxin able to induce a progressive damage of the biliary epithelium that, starting from a typical dysplasia, ultimately results in iCCA development [65]. Though the molecular mechanisms of TAA-induced carcinogenesis have not yet been fully elucidated, it seems that TAA may induce reactive oxygen species (ROS) production, which can directly modify amine groups on membrane proteins or phospholipids and interfere with ribosomal activity [66]. In rodents TAA is capable of inducing hepatic fibrosis and cirrhosis [67, 68]; moreover it stimulates an inflammatory response on the bile ducts and an intense desmoplastic reaction, thus representing an excellent model to assess cholangiocarcinogenesis in vivo [69]. Typically biliary dysplasia occurs at 9 weeks of TAA treatment in about 50% of the rats, and after 12–16 weeks, cancerous microfoci are detected. Development of mass-forming iCCA lesions occurs at longer treatment (22–24 weeks) in 100% of all treated animals [65]. Notably, the molecular phenotype observed in TAA-induced CCA shares traits with the human disease, including ErbB2 and c-Met overexpression and upregulation of c-Kit, estrogen receptor, EGFR, and mucin 1 [65, 69, 70]. The main advantages of this model are its feasibility and reproducibility, as no surgical intervention is required; however, this model has been standardized only in rats.

CCl_4 is a potent hepatotoxin that induces membrane lipid peroxidation and ROS production [71]. When administered in mice, a pronounced toxic effect on the biliary epithelium, resulting in widespread bile duct injury and necrosis, is observed [72]. Experiments conducted on $p53^{+/+}$, $p53^{+/-}$, and $p53^{-/-}$ mice treated with CCl_4 have shown that mass-forming iCCA occurred in 54% of $p53^{-/-}$ mice, while only in 18% of $p53^{+/-}$ mice [72]. Notably, the neoplastic lesions were embedded in a highly desmoplastic stroma, thus well reproducing what occurs in human disease [73]. Loss of p53 seems a prerequisite for CCA development in this in vivo model. It is indeed conceivable that loss of p53 tumor suppressor activity may cooperate with biliary injury, inflammation, and fibrosis induced by CCl_4. The main limitations of this model are the time span for tumor development, which may be longer than 50 weeks, and the limited number of mice that ultimately develop CCA.

Genetically Engineered Mouse Models

Currently, genetically engineered mouse models (GEMMs) represent the most sophisticated animal model for the study of human cancer. In these models, tumor develops in an immunocompetent host with the appropriate tumor microenvironment and under tight control of specific genetic modifications, faithfully reproducing most of the histopathological and molecular features of human cancer [74]. To date, different GEMMs harboring some of the most frequent molecular alterations of human CCA have been developed. The main advantage of these models is that tumors arise through different stages of cholangiocarcinogenesis, in some cases also including the formation of preneoplastic lesions. However, it should be noted that in GEMMs, CCA develops in the absence of chronic tissue injury, and in most cases tumor latency is relatively long; in addition, the generation of GEMMs is technically challenging, time-consuming, and expensive.

The first GEMM of CCA was established by combined disruption of SMAD4 and PTEN tumor suppressor genes using Cre-loxP recombination [75]. In this model, mice harboring a conditional knockout allele for SMAD4 and PTEN genes were crossed with mice carrying a Cre-recombinase gene under the control of albumin promoter *(Alb-Cre)*. In the resulting *Alb-Cre*/$SMAD4^{flox/flox}$/$PTEN^{flox/flox}$ model, mice typically display bile duct hyperplasia within 2–3 months, multiple tumor foci within 4–5 months, and iCCA between 4 and 7 months of age. Once established, tumor progressively increases in size, resulting in animal death before 10 months of age. Therefore, this model reproduces the sequential progression from bile duct hyperplasia-dysplasia-carcinoma in situ to invasive iCCA, as frequently seen in humans. From a molecular point of view, tumors show increased ERK and AKT phosphorylation and cyclin D1 overexpression [75]. Some important limitations of the *Alb-Cre*/$SMAD4^{flox/flox}$/$PTEN^{flox/flox}$ model are that, unlike human CCA, the tumors arise in the absence of chronic liver injury and inflammation, and metastases do not develop. Additionally, it is worth recognizing that it might not represent a pure iCCA model, as in the majority of mice, liver-specific disruption of PTEN results in HCC development at 74–78 weeks of age [76].

Using the same *Alb-Cre* approach, a GEMM carrying the $KRAS^{G12D}$ mutation and TP53 deletion was established [77]. This model was developed by intercrossing *Alb-Cre* mutants with $KRAS^{G12D}$ mice with or without TP53 deletion. Among the resulting genotypes (*Alb-Cre*/$KRAS^{G12D}$, *Alb-Cre*/$KRAS^{G12D}$/$p53^{L/L}$ and *Alb-Cre*/$KRAS^{G12D}$/$p53^{L/+}$), only mice with homozygous p53 deletion (*Alb-Cre*/$KRAS^{G12D}$/$p53^{L/L}$) developed tumors at 9 weeks of age. Of these, 83% histologically resembled iCCA, while the remaining 17% displayed a mixed HCC/iCCA or HCC phenotype. Molecular characterization of iCCA tumors showed the activation of the MAPK and PI3K/ AKT pathways, similar to a subset of human CCA [78]. In line with the human disease, iCCAs were characterized by an extensive collagen deposition and displayed adjacent organ invasion or distant metastasis. Notably, the presence of preneoplastic biliary lesions closely resembling intraductal papillary neoplasms of the bile duct highlights the ability of this model to recapitulate the multistage histopathologic progression of human CCA. Nevertheless, this model does not reproduce the background of chronic liver injury and the inflammatory microenvironment typical of human CCA. Moreover, as also observed in *Alb-Cre*/$SMAD4^{flox/flox}$/$PTEN^{flox/flox}$ model, it does not exclusively develop iCCA, as 17% of the liver tumors are consistent with mixed HCC/iCCA or HCC.

Another CCA GEMM established using the Cre-loxP system was developed by combining $KRAS^{G12D}$ mutation with PTEN deletion [79]. *Alb-Cre*/$KRAS^{G12D}$/$PTEN^{flox/flox}$ mice developed macroscopic CCA-like nodules at 7 weeks of age, preceded by biliary hyperplasia at 4 weeks and by bile duct dysplasia at 5 weeks. Mouse death occurred after 46 days, making this CCA GEMM one of the fastest described to date using the *Alb-Cre* strain. Histologically, the tumors displayed variable grading and were accompanied by an abundant desmoplastic stroma closely resembling well-differentiated iCCA; however, no evidence of metastatic disease was observed. Notably, while *Alb-Cre*/KRAS^{G12D}/PTEN$^{flox/flox}$ mice exclusively developed iCCA, *Alb-Cre*/KRAS^{G12D}/PTEN$^{f+/+}$ developed hepatocellular dysplasia but no iCCA, suggesting that PTEN may play a pivotal role in hepatotumorigenesis. The main advantages of this model are the relatively short time required for tumor development without the need for highly technical skills.

Several other GEMMS have been described based on observations in human CCA. For instance, IDH1 and IDH2 gain of function occurs in approximately 20–25% of human CCAs [80] and has been reported to block progenitor cell differentiation toward hepatocyte lineage by downregulation of hepatocyte nuclear factor-4α expression due to aberrant production of 2-hydroxyglutarate (2-HG) onco-metabolite [81]. Intercrossing a transgenic IDH2$^{LSL-R172K}$ mouse strain with KRAS$^{SLSL-G12D}$ and *Alb-Cre* mice led to the generation of *Alb-Cre*/ IDH2$^{LSL-R172K}$/ KRAS$^{SLSL-G12D}$ animals showing multifocal liver masses consistent with iCCA from 33 to 58 weeks of age [81]. Notably, precancerous lesions, as well as splenic invasion and peritoneal metastases at later time, were observed, thus recapitulating the multistage progression of human CCA [81].

Notch signalling is known to be involved in biliary tree development during embryogenesis [82], and aberrant activation of this pathway occurs during CCA carcinogenesis [83]. Basing on these findings, a CCA GEMM with constitutive Notch expression in liver tissue has been developed by crossing transgenic mice with tissue-specific overexpression of the intracellular domain of Notch 1 (NICD) (Rosa26Notch1C) with *Alb-Cre* mice [83]. When NICD was expressed under the regulation of *Alb-Cre,* epithelial cells with features of hepatocytes and cholangiocyte differentiation were observed in liver of mice at 7 months of age, whereas initial features of malignant transformations by the age of 8 months; notably, xenotransplantation of these altered cells into immunodeficient mice resulted in formation of tumors with histopathologic features of human iCCAs, including a desmoplastic stroma and CK7 and CK17 expression [83].

Another CCA GEMM, reproducing liver mitochondrial dysfunction, has been developed by Yuan et al. [84]. Mitochondrial dysfunction is indeed known to lead to increased ROS levels, inflammation, and severe liver injury, a condition often linked to CCA development. In order to reproduce hepatic mitochondrial dysfunction, mice with liver-specific *Hspd1* deletion (*AlbCre;Hspd1*$^{flox/flox}$) were generated by crossing *Hspd1*$^{flox/flox}$ mice with *Alb-Cre* strain. Though cholangiocellular lesions resembling human biliary intraepithelial neoplasia were observed at 8 weeks of age, these animals died prior to iCCA development due to severe liver injury. However, transplantation of liver tissues was found to give rise to tumors showing histological features of CCA [84]. Despite this model not allowing long-term experiments due to the premature death of mice, it provides a unique opportunity to study the role of the microenvironment in the context of chronic liver injury promoting CCA development.

Overall the abovementioned GEMMs are representative only for iCCA. In 2017 the first eCCA GEMM, namely, $KRAS^{LSL\text{-}G12D}/Tgfbr2^{flox/flox}/Cdh1^{flox/flox};Ck19\text{-}Cre^{ERT}$, was established [85]. These mice, after 4 weeks of tamoxifen administration, developed moderately differentiated adenocarcinomas resembling human Klatskin CCA/eCCA; peribiliary glands, located within the walls of the extrahepatic bile ducts, have been shown to be the site of malignant transformation. An important caveat of this model is the concomitant development of lung cancer, resulting in mouse death, thus limiting its applicability for survival studies.

Transposon-Based Models

Transposons are nonviral gene delivery vectors able to stably integrate into the genome of target cells by specific recombinase-mediated mechanisms, enabling persistent expression of genes of interest. Sleeping Beauty (SB) transposon-based systems represent a sophisticated technology for genetic manipulation [86]. The first transposon-based CCA model was developed combining lobar bile duct ligation in C57BL/6 mice with injection into the biliary tree of SB transposons with active AKT and YAP, followed by intraperitoneal injection of recombinant IL-33 for 3 days [87]. Ten weeks later tumors were observed in 72% of mice receiving SB transposons plus IL-33 as compared to only 20% of mice receiving SB transposons alone, suggesting a pivotal tumorigenic role of IL-33 in this model [87]. Morphologic and phenotypic analysis of these tumors showed hyperplasia, SOX9 expression, and abundant α-SMA positive myofibroblasts. Overall this represents a time-efficient in vivo CCA model recapitulating many features of the human disease, including a desmoplastic stroma and alterations in signalling pathways involved in CCA development. However, SB transposon-based models require high technical skills.

Combination delivery of SB transposon systems with hydrodynamic tail vein injection (HTVI) may better allow for stable integration of transgenes in target tissues [88]. In HTVI, controlled hydrodynamic pressure in capillaries increases the permeability of endothelial and parenchymal cells, thus allowing DNA uptake in target cells by the transient opening of membrane pores [89]. In the liver, DNA is efficiently delivered only to 10% of cells by HTVI; therefore, this model may mimic the human setting, where normal and transformed cells coexist. In addition, in HTVI models, tumors develop in 1–2 months, thus providing an efficient in vivo tool for accelerating experimental procedures. The main drawbacks of these models are that tumors develop in the absence of an inflammatory microenvironment, thus limiting their applicability to studies of tumor-stroma interaction; moreover, they represent a good model for the early stages of carcinogenesis, but not for progression and metastasis [89].

The first transposon-based system in combination with HTVI was developed by the exogenous expression of $NRAS^{G12V}$ oncogene in $Arf^{-/-}$ mice [90]. Despite the advantageous early onset of liver tumors (4–6 weeks), both HCC and iCCA developed in this model, limiting its application for CCA studies. Similarly, HTVI of $NRAS^{G12V}$ and of a constitutively active AKT (myrAKT) failed to induce only iCCA, as HCC also occurred in mice at 3–4 weeks after injection [91].

In another study, stable overexpression of the intracellular domain of Notch1 receptor (NICD) in the liver of mice by HTVI resulted in development of CCA-like lesions in 100% of animals at 20 weeks after injection [92]; similar lesions were observed after 3.5 weeks when NICD plasmid was injected with an AKT plasmid by HTVI. Such lesions replaced most of the liver parenchyma by 5 weeks following injection and were associated with strong mitotic activity and tissue invasion [92]. Notably, concomitant delivery of these oncogenic pathways exclusively resulted in iCCA formation at 8 weeks postinjection [93].

A similar HTVI model investigated the effect of yes-associated protein (YAP) and AKT overexpression on liver carcinogenesis [94, 95]. In the said model, YAP/AKT mice developed iCCA by 3 weeks postinjection, whereas death occurred by 5.5–7.5 weeks. As expected, tumors expressed active AKT, mTOR, and downstream targets of the PI3K-AKTmTOR pathway; high levels of pyruvate kinaseM1/M2, hexokinase ½, and survivin were also observed [95]. In another transposon-based HTVI model, an active-mutant form of YAP (S127A) was simultaneously delivered with PIK3CA (H1047R) into mice liver, resulting in liver tumor formation approximately by 12–13 weeks postinjection. However, in this model tumor lesions resembled HCC (40%), iCCA (10%), and mixed HCC/iCCA (50%) [96].

A combination of two of the most common genetic events in human CCA has been studied by the overexpression of a NICD plasmid in $KRA^{SLSL\text{-}G12D}$ mice, showing development of cholangiocellular tumors closely resembling human iCCA at 8 weeks postinjection [97]. Notably, no HCC or mixed HCC/iCCA lesions occurred in K-Ras/NICD mice. Thus, this model represents an ideal preclinical tool to study KRAS-driven iCCA development in vivo and to evaluate the therapeutic potential of drugs targeting the Ras pathway for iCCA treatment.

In a further pioneer study, HTVI was combined with the CRISPR-Cas9 approach to establish iCCA [98]. CRISPR-Cas9 technology provides an efficient tool to generate functional knockout of cancer-related genes or to recreate oncogenic driver mutations [99]. In this iCCA model, HTVI of single guide RNAs targeting TP53 and PTEN resulted in tumors of biliary differentiation 3 months after injection into wild-type FVB mice, faithfully reproducing the liver lesions observed in adeno-Cre-activated/$TP53^{flox/flox}$/$PTEN^{flox/flox}$ mice [98].

Alternatives to HTVI for Targeted Gene Delivery

An alternative technique to HTVI for efficient liver gene delivery is represented by electroporation, where plasmids are injected into the liver parenchyma by an electric pulse. In this context, a recent study showed that while delivery of Myc and $NRAS^{G12V}$ (or Myc and AKT1) by HTVI technology gives rise to multifocal liver tumors with HCC-like histology, their delivery by electroporation gives rise to combined HCC-iCCA tumors, highlighting the pivotal role of surrounding hepatic microenvironment in determining the phenotypic differentiation of liver tumors [100]. Therefore both HTVI and liver electroporation approaches failed to induce only iCCA development.

To bypass this limitation, a novel model of direct intrabiliary injection coupled with lobar bile duct ligation has been recently described [87]. In this model, introduction of AKT and YAP transgenes into biliary cells led to iCCA development in 20% of mice 10 weeks after in vivo transfection [87]. However, tumor formation was not restricted to the intrahepatic biliary tree but also to the extrahepatic, suggesting that this model, although technically challenging, may be suitable also for eCCA development.

Xenograft Models

The main limitation of carcinogen-based and genetically engineered CCA models is the slow tumor growth. To overcome this issue, CCA xenograft models have been established by implantation of tumor cells subcutaneously (heterotopic xenograft) or into the liver (orthotopic xenograft) of athymic nude or severe combined immunodeficient mice. Tumor xenografts have the advantage of closely resembling the molecular alterations occurring in human tumors. However, these models generally reflect an advanced stage of the disease, being therefore unsuitable to study the early stages of CCA tumorigenesis [55]; moreover, the host is immuno-compromised, and a species mismatch between the human tumor and the murine host microenvironment typically occurs.

The most common xenograft model is a heterotopic graft, where human tumor cells are subcutaneously implanted into the flank of immunodeficient or nude mice. To date, xenograft models have been developed employing different CCA cell lines, including the QBC939 and Sk-ChA-1 eCCA cells, as well as the HuCC-T1 and CC-LP-1 iCCA cells, with a tumor formation success rate of nearly 100% [55, 101].

More recently, a heterotopic xenograft mouse model using CCA organoids has been developed [102]. Interestingly, organoid xenografts from patients with metastatic CCA reproduce the same metastatic profile in mice; moreover, this model maintains the same mutational profile after long-term culturing and has a high engraftment rate, with 100% of mice developing tumors [53, 102]. However, xenograft models using cancer cell lines have some important limitations. The first is that they do not reflect the complex phenotypic and molecular heterogeneity of the tumor of origin. Indeed, most tumors contain highly heterogeneous subpopulations of cancer cells, resulting from genomic instability that increases the complexity of the cancer phenotype by the simultaneous alterations in several oncogenes and tumor suppressors [103]. Moreover, xenograft models using cancer cell lines do not reproduce the tumor microenvironment (fibroblasts, vessel cells, and immune cells), whose interaction with tumor cells is a critical factor for tumor behavior and response to treatments.

To overcome these limitations, there has been an increasing interest in patient-derived xenograft (PDX) development as a more advanced preclinical in vivo cancer model. In this model, a tumor specimen is directly implanted into immunodeficient mice either by subcutaneous injection or by direct injection into target organs. PDXs are able to retain the histological features, molecular characteristics, and intratumoral heterogeneity of human cancer, thus providing a faithful representation of individual tumor phenotype and genotype [104]. Typically, the first generation of mice receiving the patient's tumor fragment is commonly denoted as F0. When the tumor reaches 1 cm3 size, it is reimplanted into another recipient mice; each generation thereafter is denoted as F1, F2, F3, and Fn [104]. Recently, two heterotopic PDX models have been established in CCA. The first has been generated from an Italian patient with iCCA. This PDX model harbors a KRAS mutation, and the fourth generation of PDXs was found to share the same biliary epithelial markers, tissue architecture, and genetic aberrations of the native tumor [105]. The second PDX model has been established from a metastatic lung nodule of an iCCA patient; this PDX model, designated LIV31, endogenously expresses the fusion protein FGFR2-CCDC6 [106]. Overall the creation of PDX models is expensive and time-consuming, with a long engraftment period and a rate of efficacy variable among cancer types [104]; in particular, successfully engraftment is low for CCA, as reported in previous studies [105, 107, 108]. However, a recent study showed that in CCA PDX models failing primary engraftment, secondary engraftment of cryopreserved patient tissues resulted in a high success rate (70%) of secondary PDX generation [109].

An important caveat of heterotopic tumor xenografts is the considerable difference between the microenvironment of the subcutaneous tissue where tumors are implanted and the microenvironment wherein the primary tumor originates and disseminates. Conversely, in orthotopic xenograft models, tumor cells are implanted into the organ of origin. The organ-specific microenvironment induces tumor growth and dissemination similar to that observed in the original tumor. In addition, as drug responsiveness is dependent on tumor location, orthotopic models more faithfully reproduce human pharmacodynamics, thus providing a more accurate model to predict clinical therapeutic outcomes [55]. Intrahepatic orthotopic xenografts can be established by injecting human cancer cells through the mouse portal or splenic vein or directly into the liver parenchyma. Though intrasplenic injection is technically easier and at lower risk of perioperative complications compared to intraportal injection, tumor cells generally engraft not only in the liver, but also in the spleen [110]. Recently, spheroids from cancer stem cells of human CCA primary cell cultures have been injected into the liver of normal and cirrhotic NOD/SCID mice; notably, after 4 weeks, only cirrhotic mice developed several intrahepatic tumor masses [111]. Unfortunately, the generation of orthotopic xenograft models is time-consuming, and the assessment of tumor growth and metastatic dissemination is complex, relying on imaging techniques and/or on the sacrifice of the experimental animal [112].

Syngeneic Models

Syngeneic tumor models allow for the use of immunocompetent recipient animals, as transplanted cells derive from a donor strain that belongs to the same species. This model overcomes many of the immunologic and stromal limitations of other xenograft models; however, murine and rat tumors are not able to fully recapitulate the complex biological and molecular heterogeneity of human tumors [55].

The first syngeneic CCA model was established by inoculation of BDEneu tumor rat cholangiocytes into the bile ducts of Fisher 344 rats [113]. Following transplantation, BDEneu cells generated macroscopic, moderately differentiated, iCCA nodules; clinically, rats developed severe biliary obstruction, with increased serum bilirubin levels and peritoneal metastases. Similar features of tumor growth and metastatic dissemination were also obtained by inoculating BDEneu cells under the capsule of the left hepatic lobe in rats previously having undergone bile duct ligation [113]. In these models, CCA development was rapidly achieved and faithfully reproduced, with clinicopathological, cellular, and molecular features of human advanced CCA; in particular, this rodent model recapitulates the high desmoplastic reaction typical of human CCA [54]. However, this model requires abdominal manipulation and consequent surgical risks for animals; moreover, it does not reproduce de novo CCA development, since tumors arise following implantation of malignant cells.

More recently, a syngeneic mouse model has been described. In this model seven malignant mouse cell lines (SB1–7) were established from tumor nodules derived from a genetic transposon-based CCA model [87]. These cell lines have been implanted into the medial lobe of mouse liver; the resulting tumors showed histopathologic characteristics of human CCA including desmoplasia, malignant glands, and CK-19 expression [114]. This model has the potential to be a valuable tool to increase our knowledge of CCA tumor-stroma interactions, pathogenesis, and therapeutics.

Conclusions

The recent advances of high-throughput techniques such as next-generation sequencing and other omics approaches have provided an unprecedented opportunity to broaden our understanding of the molecular mechanisms driving CCA development, progression, and metastasis, leading to an extremely large body of data that need to be properly interpreted and translated into clinical practice. To address this issue, several in vitro and in vivo models recapitulating many of the molecular alterations of human CCA have been developed in the last years, providing new insights regarding the potential role of such alterations in this disease. Nonetheless, the possibility to translate into clinical practice the results obtained with these models still remains limited, as they are not able to fully recapitulate the extreme phenotypic and molecular heterogeneity of CCA. This observation implies that existing and future in vitro and in vivo models should be devoted to addressing more specific and clinically relevant issues in CCA. In this context, the development of models mimicking specific molecular features of human CCA would serve as preclinical platforms to address important questions of cholangiocarcinogenesis as well as to develop novel, more personalized, and effective treatments against this aggressive malignancy.

References

1. Khan SA, Tavolari S, Brandi G. Cholangiocarcinoma: epidemiology and risk factors. Liver Int. 2019;39(Suppl 1):19–31. https://doi.org/10.1111/liv.14095.
2. Miserocchi G, Mercatali L, Liverani C, De Vita A, Spadazzi C, Pieri F, Bongiovanni A, Recine F, Amadori D, Ibrahim T. Management and potentialities of primary cancer cultures in preclinical and translational studies. J Transl Med. 2017;15(1):229. https://doi.org/10.1186/s12967-017-1328-z.
3. Yamaguchi N, Morioka H, Ohkura H, Hirohashi S, Kawai K. Establishment and characterization of the human cholangiocarcinoma cell line HChol-Y1 in a serum-free, chemically defined medium. J Natl Cancer Inst. 1985;75(1):29–35.
4. Homma S, Nagamori S, Fujise K, Yamazaki K, Hasumura S, Sujino H, Matsuura T, Shimizu K, Kameda H, Takaki K. Human bile duct carcinoma cell line producing abundant mucin in vitro. Gastroenterol Jpn. 1987;22(4):474–9. https://doi.org/10.1007/bf02773816.
5. Kusaka Y, Tokiwa T, Sato J. Establishment and characterization of a cell line from a human cholangiocellular carcinoma. Res Exp Med (Berl). 1988;188(5):367–75. https://doi.org/10.1007/bf01851205.
6. Miyagiwa M, Ichida T, Tokiwa T, Sato J, Sasaki H. A new human cholangiocellular carcinoma cell line (HuCC-T1) producing carbohydrate antigen 19/9 in serum-free medium. In Vitro Cell Dev Biol. 1989;25(6):503–10. https://doi.org/10.1007/bf02623562.
7. Andresen K, Boberg KM, Vedeld HM, Honne H, Hektoen M, Wadsworth CA, Clausen OP, Karlsen TH, Foss A, Mathisen O, Schrumpf E, Lothe RA, Lind GE. Novel target genes and a valid biomarker panel identified for cholangiocarcinoma. Epigenetics. 2012;7(11):1249–57. https://doi.org/10.4161/epi.22191.
8. Storto PD, Saidman SL, Demetris AJ, Letessier E, Whiteside TL, Gollin SM. Chromosomal breakpoints in cholangiocarcinoma cell lines. Genes Chromosomes Cancer. 1990;2(4):300–10. https://doi.org/10.1002/gcc.2870020408.
9. Yokomuro S, Tsuji H, Lunz JG 3rd, Sakamoto T, Ezure T, Murase N, Demetris AJ. Growth control of human biliary epithelial cells by interleukin 6, hepatocyte growth factor, transforming growth factor beta1, and activin A: comparison of a cholangiocarcinoma cell line with primary cultures of non-neoplastic biliary epithelial cells. Hepatology. 2000;32(1):26–35. https://doi.org/10.1053/jhep.2000.8535.
10. Sirisinha S, Tengchaisri T, Boonpucknavig S, Prempracha N, Ratanarapee S, Pausawasdi A. Establishment and characterization of a cholangiocarcinoma cell line from a Thai patient with intrahepatic bile duct cancer. Asian Pac J Allergy Immunol. 1991;9(2):153–7.
11. Iemura A, Maruiwa M, Yano H, Kojiro M. A new human cholangiocellular carcinoma cell line (KMC-1). J Hepatol. 1992;15(3):288–98. https://doi.org/10.1016/0168-8278(92)90058-w.
12. Shimizu Y, Demetris AJ, Gollin SM, Storto PD, Bedford HM, Altarac S, Iwatsuki S, Herberman RB, Whiteside TL. Two new human cholangiocarcinoma cell lines and their cytogenetics and responses to growth factors, hormones, cytokines or immunologic effector cells. Int J Cancer. 1992;52(2):252–60. https://doi.org/10.1002/ijc.2910520217.

13. Yano H, Iemura A, Haramaki M, Momosaki S, Ogasawara S, Higaki K, Kojiro M. A human combined hepatocellular and cholangiocarcinoma cell line (KMCH-2) that shows the features of hepatocellular carcinoma or cholangiocarcinoma under different growth conditions. J Hepatol. 1996;24(4):413–22. https://doi.org/10.1016/s0168-8278(96)80161-9.
14. Enjoji M, Nakashima M, Honda M, Sakai H, Nawata H. Hepatocytic phenotypes induced in sarcomatous cholangiocarcinoma cells treated with 5-azacytidine. Hepatology. 1997;26(2):288–94. https://doi.org/10.1002/hep.510260206.
15. Enjoji M, Sakai H, Nawata H, Kajiyama K, Tsuneyoshi M. Sarcomatous and adenocarcinoma cell lines from the same nodule of cholangiocarcinoma. In Vitro Cell Dev Biol Anim. 1997;33(9):681–3. https://doi.org/10.1007/s11626-997-0125-z.
16. Ku JL, Yoon KA, Kim IJ, Kim WH, Jang JY, Suh KS, Kim SW, Park YH, Hwang JH, Yoon YB, Park JG. Establishment and characterisation of six human biliary tract cancer cell lines. Br J Cancer. 2002;87(2):187–93. https://doi.org/10.1038/sj.bjc.6600440.
17. Ma S, Hu L, Huang XH, Cao LQ, Chan KW, Wang Q, Guan XY. Establishment and characterization of a human cholangiocarcinoma cell line. Oncol Rep. 2007;18(5):1195–200.
18. Ojima H, Yoshikawa D, Ino Y, Shimizu H, Miyamoto M, Kokubu A, Hiraoka N, Morofuji N, Kondo T, Onaya H, Okusaka T, Shimada K, Sakamoto Y, Esaki M, Nara S, Kosuge T, Hirohashi S, Kanai Y, Shibata T. Establishment of six new human biliary tract carcinoma cell lines and identification of MAGEH1 as a candidate biomarker for predicting the efficacy of gemcitabine treatment. Cancer Sci. 2010;101(4):882–8. https://doi.org/10.1111/j.1349-7006.2009.01462.x.
19. Liu J, Han G, Liu H, Qin C. Suppression of cholangiocarcinoma cell growth by human umbilical cord mesenchymal stem cells: a possible role of Wnt and Akt signaling. PLoS One. 2013;8(4):e62844. https://doi.org/10.1371/journal.pone.0062844.
20. Knuth A, Gabbert H, Dippold W, Klein O, Sachsse W, Bitter-Suermann D, Prellwitz W, Meyer zum Buschenfelde KH. Biliary adenocarcinoma. Characterisation of three new human tumor cell lines. J Hepatol. 1985;1(6):579–96. https://doi.org/10.1016/s0168-8278(85)80002-7.
21. Yoshida K, Tomizawa H, Ota T, Nagashima T, Kikuchi H, Watanabe H, Hashizaki K, Yonaha A. Establishment and characterization of human cholangiocarcinoma, MEC, producing carbohydrate antigen 19-9. Hum Cell. 1990;3(4):346–51.
22. Yano H, Maruiwa M, Iemura A, Mizoguchi A, Kojiro M. Establishment and characterization of a new human extrahepatic bile duct carcinoma cell line (KMBC). Cancer. 1992;69(7):1664–73. https://doi.org/10.1002/1097-0142(19920401)69:7<1664::aid-cncr2820690705>3.0.co;2-p.
23. Purdum PP 3rd, Ulissi A, Hylemon PB, Shiffman ML, Moore EW. Cultured human gallbladder epithelia. Methods and partial characterization of a carcinoma-derived model. Lab Investig. 1993;68(3):345–53.
24. Oertel M, Schastak SI, Tannapfel A, Hermann R, Sack U, Mossner J, Berr F. Novel bacteriochlorine for high tissue-penetration: photodynamic properties in human biliary tract cancer cells in vitro and in a mouse tumor model. J Photochem Photobiol B. 2003;71(1–3):1–10. https://doi.org/10.1016/s1011-1344(03)00091-5.
25. Saijyo S, Kudo T, Suzuki M, Katayose Y, Shinoda M, Muto T, Fukuhara K, Suzuki T, Matsuno S. Establishment of a new extrahepatic bile duct carcinoma cell line, TFK-1. Tohoku J Exp Med. 1995;177(1):61–71. https://doi.org/10.1620/tjem.177.61.
26. Yamada N, Chung YS, Arimoto Y, Sawada T, Seki S, Sowa M. Establishment of a new human extrahepatic bile duct carcinoma cell line (OCUCh-LM1) and experimental liver metastatic model. Br J Cancer. 1995;71(3):543–8. https://doi.org/10.1038/bjc.1995.107.
27. Takiyama I, Terashima M, Ikeda K, Kawamura H, Kashiwaba M, Tamura G, Suto T, Nakashima F, Sasaki R, Saito K. Establishment and characterization of a new human extrahepatic bile duct carcinoma cell line (ICBD-1). Oncol Rep. 1998;5(2):463–7. https://doi.org/10.3892/or.5.2.463.
28. Watanabe M, Chigusa M, Takahashi H, Nakamura J, Tanaka H, Ohno T. High level of CA19-9, CA50, and CEA-producible human cholangiocarcinoma cell line changes in the

secretion ratios in vitro or in vivo. In Vitro Cell Dev Biol Anim. 2000;36(2):104–9. https://doi.org/10.1290/1071-2690(2000)036<0104:HLOCCA>2.0.CO;2.
29. Kim DG, Park SY, You KR, Lee GB, Kim H, Moon WS, Chun YH, Park SH. Establishment and characterization of chromosomal aberrations in human cholangiocarcinoma cell lines by cross-species color banding. Genes Chromosomes Cancer. 2001;30(1):48–56. https://doi.org/10.1002/1098-2264(2000)9999:9999<::aid-gcc1053>3.0.co;2-p.
30. Emura F, Kamma H, Ghosh M, Koike N, Kawamoto T, Saijo K, Ohno T, Ohkohchi N, Todoroki T. Establishment and characterization of novel xenograft models of human biliary tract carcinomas. Int J Oncol. 2003;23(5):1293–300.
31. Ghosh M, Koike N, Tsunoda S, Hirano T, Kaul S, Kashiwagi H, Kawamoto T, Ohkohchi N, Saijo K, Ohno T, Miwa M, Todoroki T. Characterization and genetic analysis in the newly established human bile duct cancer cell lines. Int J Oncol. 2005;26(2):449–56.
32. Rattanasinganchan P, Leelawat K, Treepongkaruna SA, Tocharoentanaphol C, Subwongcharoen S, Suthiphongchai T, Tohtong R. Establishment and characterization of a cholangiocarcinoma cell line (RMCCA-1) from a Thai patient. World J Gastroenterol. 2006;12(40):6500–6. https://doi.org/10.3748/wjg.v12.i40.6500.
33. Jiao W, Yakushiji H, Kitajima Y, Ogawa A, Miyazaki K. Establishment and characterization of human hilar bile duct carcinoma cell line and cell strain. J Hepato-Biliary-Pancreat Surg. 2000;7(4):417–25. https://doi.org/10.1007/s005340070038.
34. Sripa B, Leungwattanawanit S, Nitta T, Wongkham C, Bhudhisawasdi V, Puapairoj A, Sripa C, Miwa M. Establishment and characterization of an opisthorchiasis-associated cholangiocarcinoma cell line (KKU-100). World J Gastroenterol. 2005;11(22):3392–7. https://doi.org/10.3748/wjg.v11.i22.3392.
35. Zach S, Birgin E, Rückert F. Primary Cholangiocellular carcinoma cell lines. J Stem Cell Res Transplant. 2015;2(1):1013.
36. Brandi G, Farioli A, Astolfi A, Biasco G, Tavolari S. Genetic heterogeneity in cholangiocarcinoma: a major challenge for targeted therapies. Oncotarget. 2015;6(17):14744–53. https://doi.org/10.18632/oncotarget.4539.
37. Xu L, Hausmann M, Dietmaier W, Kellermeier S, Pesch T, Stieber-Gunckel M, Lippert E, Klebl F, Rogler G. Expression of growth factor receptors and targeting of EGFR in cholangiocarcinoma cell lines. BMC Cancer. 2010;10:302. https://doi.org/10.1186/1471-2407-10-302.
38. Domcke S, Sinha R, Levine DA, Sander C, Schultz N. Evaluating cell lines as tumor models by comparison of genomic profiles. Nat Commun. 2013;4:2126. https://doi.org/10.1038/ncomms3126.
39. Ertel A, Verghese A, Byers SW, Ochs M, Tozeren A. Pathway-specific differences between tumor cell lines and normal and tumor tissue cells. Mol Cancer. 2006;5(1):55. https://doi.org/10.1186/1476-4598-5-55.
40. Gillet JP, Calcagno AM, Varma S, Marino M, Green LJ, Vora MI, Patel C, Orina JN, Eliseeva TA, Singal V, Padmanabhan R, Davidson B, Ganapathi R, Sood AK, Rueda BR, Ambudkar SV, Gottesman MM. Redefining the relevance of established cancer cell lines to the study of mechanisms of clinical anti-cancer drug resistance. Proc Natl Acad Sci U S A. 2011;108(46):18708–13. https://doi.org/10.1073/pnas.111184010.
41. Nath S, Devi GR. Three-dimensional culture systems in cancer research: focus on tumor spheroid model. Pharmacol Ther. 2016;163:94–108. https://doi.org/10.1016/j.pharmthera.2016.03.013.
42. Baker BM, Chen CS. Deconstructing the third dimension: how 3D culture microenvironments alter cellular cues. J Cell Sci. 2012;125(Pt 13):3015–24. https://doi.org/10.1242/jcs.079509.
43. Raggi C, Invernizzi P, Andersen JB. Impact of microenvironment and stem-like plasticity in cholangiocarcinoma: molecular networks and biological concepts. J Hepatol. 2015;62(1):198–207. https://doi.org/10.1016/j.jhep.2014.09.007.
44. Massani M, Stecca T, Fabris L, Caratozzolo E, Ruffolo C, Furlanetto A, Morton S, Cadamuro M, Strazzabosco M, Bassi N. Isolation and characterization of biliary epithelial and stromal

cells from resected human cholangiocarcinoma: a novel in vitro model to study tumor-stroma interactions. Oncol Rep. 2013;30(3):1143–8. https://doi.org/10.3892/or.2013.2568.
45. Fraveto A, Cardinale V, Bragazzi MC, Giuliante F, De Rose AM, Grazi GL, Napoletano C, Semeraro R, Lustri AM, Costantini D, Nevi L, Di Matteo S, Renzi A, Carpino G, Gaudio E, Alvaro D. Sensitivity of human intrahepatic cholangiocarcinoma subtypes to chemotherapeutics and molecular targeted agents: a study on primary cell cultures. PLoS One. 2015;10(11):e0142124. https://doi.org/10.1371/journal.pone.0142124.
46. Shibue T, Weinberg RA. EMT, CSCs, and drug resistance: the mechanistic link and clinical implications. Nat Rev Clin Oncol. 2017;14(10):611–29. https://doi.org/10.1038/nrclinonc.2017.44.
47. Cree IA, Glaysher S, Harvey AL. Efficacy of anti-cancer agents in cell lines versus human primary tumor tissue. Curr Opin Pharmacol. 2010;10(4):375–9. https://doi.org/10.1016/j.coph.2010.05.001.
48. Prior N, Inacio P, Huch M. Liver organoids: from basic research to therapeutic applications. Gut. 2019;68(12):2228–37. https://doi.org/10.1136/gutjnl-2019-319256.
49. Weaver VM, Lelievre S, Lakins JN, Chrenek MA, Jones JC, Giancotti F, Werb Z, Bissell MJ. beta4 integrin-dependent formation of polarized three-dimensional architecture confers resistance to apoptosis in normal and malignant mammary epithelium. Cancer Cell. 2002;2(3):205–16. https://doi.org/10.1016/s1535-6108(02)00125-3.
50. Hirschhaeuser F, Menne H, Dittfeld C, West J, Mueller-Klieser W, Kunz-Schughart LA. Multicellular tumor spheroids: an underestimated tool is catching up again. J Biotechnol. 2010;148(1):3–15. https://doi.org/10.1016/j.jbiotec.2010.01.012.
51. Mischiati C, Ura B, Roncoroni L, Elli L, Cervellati C, Squerzanti M, Conte D, Doneda L, Polverino de Laureto P, de Franceschi G, Calza R, Barrero CA, Merali S, Ferrari C, Bergamini CM, Agostinelli E. Changes in protein expression in two cholangiocarcinoma cell lines undergoing formation of multicellular tumor spheroids in vitro. PLoS One. 2015;10(3):e0118906. https://doi.org/10.1371/journal.pone.0118906.
52. Raggi C, Correnti M, Sica A, Andersen JB, Cardinale V, Alvaro D, Chiorino G, Forti E, Glaser S, Alpini G, Destro A, Sozio F, Di Tommaso L, Roncalli M, Banales JM, Coulouarn C, Bujanda L, Torzilli G, Invernizzi P. Cholangiocarcinoma stem-like subset shapes tumor-initiating niche by educating associated macrophages. J Hepatol. 2017;66(1):102–15. https://doi.org/10.1016/j.jhep.2016.08.012.
53. Broutier L, Mastrogiovanni G, Verstegen MM, Francies HE, Gavarro LM, Bradshaw CR, Allen GE, Arnes-Benito R, Sidorova O, Gaspersz MP, Georgakopoulos N, Koo BK, Dietmann S, Davies SE, Praseedom RK, Lieshout R, JNM IJ, Wigmore SJ, Saeb-Parsy K, Garnett MJ, van der Laan LJ, Huch M. Human primary liver cancer-derived organoid cultures for disease modeling and drug screening. Nat Med. 2017;23(12):1424–35. https://doi.org/10.1038/nm.4438.
54. Brivio S, Cadamuro M, Strazzabosco M, Fabris L. Tumor reactive stroma in cholangiocarcinoma: the fuel behind cancer aggressiveness. World J Hepatol. 2017;9(9):455–68. https://doi.org/10.4254/wjh.v9.i9.455.
55. De Minicis S, Kisseleva T, Francis H, Baroni GS, Benedetti A, Brenner D, Alvaro D, Alpini G, Marzioni M. Liver carcinogenesis: rodent models of hepatocarcinoma and cholangiocarcinoma. Dig Liver Dis. 2013;45(6):450–9. https://doi.org/10.1016/j.dld.2012.10.008.
56. Heindryckx F, Colle I, Van Vlierberghe H. Experimental mouse models for hepatocellular carcinoma research. Int J Exp Pathol. 2009;90(4):367–86. https://doi.org/10.1111/j.1365-2613.2009.00656.x.
57. Umemura T, Kai S, Hasegawa R, Kanki K, Kitamura Y, Nishikawa A, Hirose M. Prevention of dual promoting effects of pentachlorophenol, an environmental pollutant, on diethylnitrosamine-induced hepato- and cholangiocarcinogenesis in mice by green tea infusion. Carcinogenesis. 2003;24(6):1105–9. https://doi.org/10.1093/carcin/bgg053.
58. Umemura T, Kodama Y, Kanki K, Iatropoulos MJ, Nishikawa A, Hirose M, Williams GM. Pentachlorophenol (but not phenobarbital) promotes intrahepatic biliary cysts induced

by diethylnitrosamine to cholangio cystic neoplasms in B6C3F1 mice possibly due to oxidative stress. Toxicol Pathol. 2003;31(1):10–3. https://doi.org/10.1080/01926230390173806.
59. Yang H, Li TW, Peng J, Tang X, Ko KS, Xia M, Aller MA. A mouse model of cholestasis-associated cholangiocarcinoma and transcription factors involved in progression. Gastroenterology. 2011;141(1):378–88, 388 e371-374. https://doi.org/10.1053/j.gastro.2011.03.044.
60. Hickling KC, Hitchcock JM, Oreffo V, Mally A, Hammond TG, Evans JG, Chipman JK. Evidence of oxidative stress and associated DNA damage, increased proliferative drive, and altered gene expression in rat liver produced by the cholangiocarcinogenic agent furan. Toxicol Pathol. 2010;38(2):230–43. https://doi.org/10.1177/0192623309357946.
61. Maronpot RR, Giles HD, Dykes DJ, Irwin RD. Furan-induced hepatic cholangiocarcinomas in Fischer 344 rats. Toxicol Pathol. 1991;19(4 Pt 2):561–70. https://doi.org/10.1177/019262339101900401.
62. Elmore LW, Sirica AE. Phenotypic characterization of metaplastic intestinal glands and ductular hepatocytes in cholangiofibrotic lesions rapidly induced in the caudate liver lobe of rats treated with furan. Cancer Res. 1991;51(20):5752–9.
63. Chen T, Williams TD, Mally A, Hamberger C, Mirbahai L, Hickling K, Chipman JK. Gene expression and epigenetic changes by furan in rat liver. Toxicology. 2012;292(2–3):63–70. https://doi.org/10.1016/j.tox.2011.10.020.
64. Von Tungeln LS, Walker NJ, Olson GR, Mendoza MC, Felton RP, Thorn BT, Marques MM, Pogribny IP, Doerge DR, Beland FA. Low dose assessment of the carcinogenicity of furan in male F344/N Nctr rats in a 2-year gavage study. Food Chem Toxicol. 2017;99:170–81. https://doi.org/10.1016/j.fct.2016.11.015.
65. Yeh CN, Maitra A, Lee KF, Jan YY, Chen MF. Thioacetamide-induced intestinal-type cholangiocarcinoma in rat: an animal model recapitulating the multi-stage progression of human cholangiocarcinoma. Carcinogenesis. 2004;25(4):631–6. https://doi.org/10.1093/carcin/bgh037.
66. Hajovsky H, Hu G, Koen Y, Sarma D, Cui W, Moore DS, Staudinger JL, Hanzlik RP. Metabolism and toxicity of thioacetamide and thioacetamide S-oxide in rat hepatocytes. Chem Res Toxicol. 2012;25(9):1955–63. https://doi.org/10.1021/tx3002719.
67. Yang MC, Chang CP, Lei HY. Induction of liver fibrosis in a murine hepatoma model by thioacetamide is associated with enhanced tumor growth and suppressed antitumor immunity. Lab Investig. 2010;90:1782–93.
68. Al-Bader A, Mathew TC, Abul H, Al-Sayer H, Singal PK, Dashti HM. Cholangiocarcinoma and liver cirrhosis in relation to changes due to thioacetamide. Mol Cell Biochem. 2000;208(1–2):1–10. https://doi.org/10.1023/a:1007082515548.
69. Marzioni M, Torrice A, Saccomanno S, Rychlicki C, Agostinelli L, Pierantonelli I, Rhonnstad P, Trozzi L, Apelqvist T, Gentile R, Candelaresi C, Fava G, Semeraro R, Benedetti A, Gaudio E, Franchitto A, Onori P, De Minicis S, Carpino G, Kallin E, Alvaro D, Nilsson S. An oestrogen receptor beta-selective agonist exerts anti-neoplastic effects in experimental intrahepatic cholangiocarcinoma. Dig Liver Dis. 2012;44(2):134–42. https://doi.org/10.1016/j.dld.2011.06.014.
70. Mansuroglu T, Ramadori P, Dudas J, Malik I, Hammerich K, Fuzesi L, Ramadori G. Expression of stem cell factor and its receptor c-Kit during the development of intrahepatic cholangiocarcinoma. Lab Investig. 2009;89(5):562–74. https://doi.org/10.1038/labinvest.2009.15.
71. Eastmond DA. Evaluating genotoxicity data to identify a mode of action and its application in estimating cancer risk at low doses: a case study involving carbon tetrachloride. Environ Mol Mutagen. 2008;49(2):132–41. https://doi.org/10.1002/em.20368.
72. Farazi PA, Zeisberg M, Glickman J, Zhang Y, Kalluri R, DePinho RA. Chronic bile duct injury associated with fibrotic matrix microenvironment provokes cholangiocarcinoma in p53-deficient mice. Cancer Res. 2006;66(13):6622–7. https://doi.org/10.1158/0008-5472.CAN-05-4609.

73. Cadamuro M, Stecca T, Brivio S, Mariotti V, Fiorotto R, Spirli C, Strazzabosco M, Fabris L. The deleterious interplay between tumor epithelia and stroma in cholangiocarcinoma. Biochim Biophys Acta Mol basis Dis. 2018;1864(4 Pt B):1435–43. https://doi.org/10.1016/j.bbadis.2017.07.028.
74. Walrath JC, Hawes JJ, Van Dyke T, Reilly KM. Genetically engineered mouse models in cancer 638 research. Adv Cancer Res. 2010;106:113–64.
75. Xu X, Kobayashi S, Qiao W, Li C, Xiao C, Radaeva S, Stiles B, Wang RH, Ohara N, Yoshino T, LeRoith D, Torbenson MS, Gores GJ, Wu H, Gao B, Deng CX. Induction of intrahepatic cholangiocellular carcinoma by liver-specific disruption of Smad4 and Pten in mice. J Clin Invest. 2006;116(7):1843–52. https://doi.org/10.1172/JCI27282.
76. Horie Y, Suzuki A, Kataoka E, Sasaki T, Hamada K, Sasaki J, Mizuno K, Hasegawa G, Kishimoto H, Iizuka M, Naito M, Enomoto K, Watanabe S, Mak TW, Nakano T. Hepatocyte-specific Pten deficiency results in steatohepatitis and hepatocellular carcinomas. J Clin Invest. 2004;113(12):1774–83. https://doi.org/10.1172/JCI20513.
77. O'Dell MR, Huang JL, Whitney-Miller CL, Deshpande V, Rothberg P, Grose V, Rossi RM, Zhu AX, Land H, Bardeesy N, Hezel AF. Kras(G12D) and p53 mutation cause primary intrahepatic cholangiocarcinoma. Cancer Res. 2012;72(6):1557–67. https://doi.org/10.1158/0008-5472.CAN-11-3596.
78. Rizvi S, Gores GJ. Emerging molecular therapeutic targets for cholangiocarcinoma. J Hepatol. 2017;67(3):632–44. https://doi.org/10.1016/j.jhep.2017.03.026.
79. Ikenoue T, Terakado Y, Nakagawa H, Hikiba Y, Fujii T, Matsubara D, Noguchi R, Zhu C, Yamamoto K, Kudo Y, Asaoka Y, Yamaguchi K, Ijichi H, Tateishi K, Fukushima N, Maeda S, Koike K, Furukawa Y. Corrigendum: a novel mouse model of intrahepatic cholangiocarcinoma induced by liver-specific Kras activation and Pten deletion. Sci Rep. 2017;7:39567. https://doi.org/10.1038/srep39567.
80. Borger DR, Tanabe KK, Fan KC, Lopez HU, Fantin VR, Straley KS, Schenkein DP, Hezel AF, Ancukiewicz M, Liebman HM, Kwak EL, Clark JW, Ryan DP, Deshpande V, Dias-Santagata D, Ellisen LW, Zhu AX, Iafrate AJ. Frequent mutation of isocitrate dehydrogenase (IDH)1 and IDH2 in cholangiocarcinoma identified through broad-based tumor genotyping. Oncologist. 2012;17(1):72–9. https://doi.org/10.1634/theoncologist.2011-0386.
81. Saha SK, Parachoniak CA, Ghanta KS, Fitamant J, Ross KN, Najem MS, Gurumurthy S, Akbay EA, Sia D, Cornella H, Miltiadous O, Walesky C, Deshpande V, Zhu AX, Hezel AF, Yen KE, Straley KS, Travins J, Popovici-Muller J, Gliser C, Ferrone CR, Apte U, Llovet JM, Wong KK, Ramaswamy S, Bardeesy N. Corrigendum: mutant IDH inhibits HNF-4alpha to block hepatocyte differentiation and promote biliary cancer. Nature. 2015;528(7580):152. https://doi.org/10.1038/nature16136.
82. Hofmann JJ, Zovein AC, Koh H, Radtke F, Weinmaster G, Iruela-Arispe ML. Jagged1 in the portal vein mesenchyme regulates intrahepatic bile duct development: insights into Alagille syndrome. Development. 2010;137(23):4061–72. https://doi.org/10.1242/dev.052118.
83. Zender S, Nickeleit I, Wuestefeld T, Sorensen I, Dauch D, Bozko P, El-Khatib M, Geffers R, Bektas H, Manns MP, Gossler A, Wilkens L, Plentz R, Zender L, Malek NP. A critical role for notch signaling in the formation of cholangiocellular carcinomas. Cancer Cell. 2016;30(2):353–6. https://doi.org/10.1016/j.ccell.2016.07.005.
84. Yuan D, Huang S, Berger E, Liu L, Gross N, Heinzmann F, Ringelhan M, Connor TO, Stadler M, Meister M, Weber J, Ollinger R, Simonavicius N, Reisinger F, Hartmann D, Meyer R, Reich M, Seehawer M, Leone V, Hochst B, Wohlleber D, Jors S, Prinz M, Spalding D, Protzer U, Luedde T, Terracciano L, Matter M, Longerich T, Knolle P, Ried T, Keitel V, Geisler F, Unger K, Cinnamon E, Pikarsky E, Huser N, Davis RJ, Tschaharganeh DF, Rad R, Weber A, Zender L, Haller D, Heikenwalder M. Kupffer cell-derived Tnf triggers cholangiocellular tumorigenesis through JNK due to chronic mitochondrial dysfunction and ROS. Cancer Cell. 2017;31(6):771–89. e776. https://doi.org/10.1016/j.ccell.2017.05.006.
85. Nakagawa H, Suzuki N, Hirata Y, Hikiba Y, Hayakawa Y, Kinoshita H, Ihara S, Uchino K, Nishikawa Y, Ijichi H, Otsuka M, Arita J, Sakamoto Y, Hasegawa K, Kokudo N, Tateishi K,

Koike K. Biliary epithelial injury-induced regenerative response by IL-33 promotes cholangiocarcinogenesis from peribiliary glands. Proc Natl Acad Sci U S A. 2017;114(19):E3806–15. https://doi.org/10.1073/pnas.1619416114.
86. Tipanee J, VandenDriessche T, Chuah MK. Transposons: moving forward from preclinical studies to clinical trials. Hum Gene Ther. 2017;28(11):1087–104. https://doi.org/10.1089/hum.2017.128.
87. Yamada D, Rizvi S, Razumilava N, Bronk SF, Davila JI, Champion MD, Borad MJ, Bezerra JA, Chen X, Gores GJ. IL-33 facilitates oncogene-induced cholangiocarcinoma in mice by an interleukin-6-sensitive mechanism. Hepatology. 2015;61(5):1627–42. https://doi.org/10.1002/hep.27687.
88. Yant SR, Meuse L, Chiu W, Ivics Z, Izsvak Z, Kay MA. Somatic integration and long-term transgene expression in normal and haemophilic mice using a DNA transposon system. Nat Genet. 2000;25(1):35–41. https://doi.org/10.1038/75568.
89. Suda T, Liu D. Hydrodynamic gene delivery: its principles and applications. Mol Ther. 2007;15(12):2063–9. https://doi.org/10.1038/sj.mt.6300314.
90. Carlson CM, Frandsen JL, Kirchhof N, McIvor RS, Largaespada DA. Somatic integration of an oncogene-harboring sleeping beauty transposon models liver tumor development in the mouse. Proc Natl Acad Sci U S A. 2005;102(47):17059–64. https://doi.org/10.1073/pnas.0502974102.
91. Zhang S, Wang J, Wang H, Fan L, Fan B, Zeng B, Tao J, Li X, Che L, Cigliano A, Ribback S, Dombrowski F, Chen B, Cong W, Wei L, Calvisi DF, Chen X. Hippo cascade controls lineage commitment of liver tumors in mice and humans. Am J Pathol. 2018;188(4):995–1006. https://doi.org/10.1016/j.ajpath.2017.12.017.
92. Fan B, Malato Y, Calvisi DF, Naqvi S, Razumilava N, Ribback S, Gores GJ, Dombrowski F, Evert M, Chen X, Willenbring H. Cholangiocarcinomas can originate from hepatocytes in mice. J Clin Invest. 2012;122(8):2911–5. https://doi.org/10.1172/JCI63212.
93. Che L, Fan B, Pilo MG, Xu Z, Liu Y, Cigliano A, Cossu A, Palmieri G, Pascale RM, Porcu A, Vidili G, Serra M, Dombrowski F, Ribback S, Calvisi DF, Chen X. Jagged 1 is a major notch ligand along cholangiocarcinoma development in mice and humans. Oncogenesis. 2016;5(12):e274. https://doi.org/10.1038/oncsis.2016.73.
94. Tschaharganeh DF, Chen X, Latzko P, Malz M, Gaida MM, Felix K, Ladu S, Singer S, Pinna F, Gretz N, Sticht C, Tomasi ML, Delogu S, Evert M, Fan B, Ribback S, Jiang L, Brozzetti S, Bergmann F, Dombrowski F, Schirmacher P, Calvisi DF, Breuhahn K. Yes-associated protein up-regulates Jagged-1 and activates the notch pathway in human hepatocellular carcinoma. Gastroenterology. 2013;144(7):1530–42. e1512. https://doi.org/10.1053/j.gastro.2013.02.009.
95. Zhang S, Song X, Cao D, Xu Z, Fan B, Che L, Hu J, Chen B, Dong M, Pilo MG, Cigliano A, Evert K, Ribback S, Dombrowski F, Pascale RM, Cossu A, Vidili G, Porcu A, Simile MM, Pes GM, Giannelli G, Gordan J, Wei L, Evert M, Cong W, Calvisi DF, Chen X. Pan-mTOR inhibitor MLN0128 is effective against intrahepatic cholangiocarcinoma in mice. J Hepatol. 2017;67(6):1194–203. https://doi.org/10.1016/j.jhep.2017.07.006.
96. Li X, Tao J, Cigliano A, Sini M, Calderaro J, Azoulay D, Wang C, Liu Y, Jiang L, Evert K, Demartis MI, Ribback S, Utpatel K, Dombrowski F, Evert M, Calvisi DF, Chen X. Co-activation of PIK3CA and yap promotes development of hepatocellular and cholangiocellular tumors in mouse and human liver. Oncotarget. 2015;6(12):10102–15. https://doi.org/10.18632/oncotarget.3546.
97. Dong M, Liu X, Evert K, Utpatel K, Peters M, Zhang S, Xu Z, Che L, Cigliano A, Ribback S, Dombrowski F, Cossu A, Gordan J, Calvisi DF, Evert M, Liu Y, Chen X. Efficacy of MEK inhibition in a K-Ras-driven cholangiocarcinoma preclinical model. Cell Death Dis. 2018;9(2):31. https://doi.org/10.1038/s41419-017-0183-4.
98. Xue W, Chen S, Yin H, Tammela T, Papagiannakopoulos T, Joshi NS, Cai W, Yang G, Bronson R, Crowley DG, Zhang F, Anderson DG, Sharp PA, Jacks T. CRISPR-mediated

direct mutation of cancer genes in the mouse liver. Nature. 2014;514(7522):380–4. https://doi.org/10.1038/nature13589.
99. Doudna JA, Charpentier E. Genome editing. The new frontier of genome engineering with CRISPR-Cas9. Science. 2014;346(6213):1258096. https://doi.org/10.1126/science.1258096.
100. Seehawer M, Heinzmann F, D'Artista L, Harbig J, Roux PF, Hoenicke L, Dang H, Klotz S, Robinson L, Dore G, Rozenblum N, Kang TW, Chawla R, Buch T, Vucur M, Roth M, Zuber J, Luedde T, Sipos B, Longerich T, Heikenwalder M, Wang XW, Bischof O, Zender L. Necroptosis microenvironment directs lineage commitment in liver cancer. Nature. 2018;562(7725):69–75. https://doi.org/10.1038/s41586-018-0519-y.
101. Ko KS, Peng J, Yang H. Animal models of cholangiocarcinoma. Curr Opin Gastroenterol. 2013;29(3):312–8. https://doi.org/10.1097/MOG.0b013e32835d6a3e.
102. Lampis A, Carotenuto P, Vlachogiannis G, Cascione L, Hedayat S, Burke R, Clarke P, Bosma E, Simbolo M, Scarpa A, Yu S, Cole R, Smyth E, Mateos JF, Begum R, Hezelova B, Eltahir Z, Wotherspoon A, Fotiadis N, Bali MA, Nepal C, Khan K, Stubbs M, Hahne JC, Gasparini P, Guzzardo V, Croce CM, Eccles S, Fassan M, Cunningham D, Andersen JB, Workman P, Valeri N, Braconi C. MIR21 drives resistance to heat shock protein 90 inhibition in cholangiocarcinoma. Gastroenterology. 2018;154(4):1066–79. e1065. https://doi.org/10.1053/j.gastro.2017.10.043.
103. Cho SY, Kang W, Han JY, Min S, Kang J, Lee A, Kwon JY, Lee C, Park H. An integrative approach to precision cancer medicine using patient-derived xenografts. Mol Cells. 2016;39(2):77–86. https://doi.org/10.14348/molcells.2016.2350.
104. Jung J, Seol HS, Chang S. The generation and application of patient-derived xenograft model for cancer research. Cancer Res Treat. 2018;50(1):1–10. https://doi.org/10.4143/crt.2017.307.
105. Cavalloni G, Peraldo-Neia C, Sassi F, Chiorino G, Sarotto I, Aglietta M, Leone F. Establishment of a patient-derived intrahepatic cholangiocarcinoma xenograft model with KRAS mutation. BMC Cancer. 2016;16:90. https://doi.org/10.1186/s12885-016-2136-1.
106. Wang Y, Ding X, Wang S, Moser CD, Shaleh HM, Mohamed EA, Chaiteerakij R, Allotey LK, Chen G, Miyabe K, McNulty MS, Ndzengue A, Barr Fritcher EG, Knudson RA, Greipp PT, Clark KJ, Torbenson MS, Kipp BR, Zhou J, Barrett MT, Gustafson MP, Alberts SR, Borad MJ, Roberts LR. Antitumor effect of FGFR inhibitors on a novel cholangiocarcinoma patient derived xenograft mouse model endogenously expressing an FGFR2-CCDC6 fusion protein. Cancer Lett. 2016;380(1):163–73. https://doi.org/10.1016/j.canlet.2016.05.017.
107. Jang SY, Bae HI, Lee IK, Park HK, Cho CM. Successful xenograft of endoscopic ultrasound-guided fine-needle aspiration specimen from human extrahepatic cholangiocarcinoma into an immunodeficient mouse. Gut Liver. 2015;9(6):805–8. https://doi.org/10.5009/gnl14279.
108. Cavalloni G, Peraldo-Neia C, Varamo C, Casorzo L, Dell'Aglio C, Bernabei P, Chiorino G, Aglietta M, Leone F. Establishment and characterization of a human intrahepatic cholangiocarcinoma cell line derived from an Italian patient. Tumor Biol. 2016;37(3):4041–52. https://doi.org/10.1007/s13277-015-4215-3.
109. Hernandez MC, Yang L, Leiting JL, Sugihara T, Bergquist JR, Ivanics T, Graham R, Truty MJ. Successful secondary engraftment of pancreatic ductal adenocarcinoma and cholangiocarcinoma patient-derived Xenografts after previous failed primary engraftment. Transl Oncol. 2019;12(1):69–75. https://doi.org/10.1016/j.tranon.2018.09.008.
110. Wu Z, Boonmars T, Nagano I, Boonjaraspinyo S, Srinontong P, Ratasuwan P, Narong K, Nielsen PS, Maekawa Y. Significance of S100P as a biomarker in diagnosis, prognosis and therapy of opisthorchiasis-associated cholangiocarcinoma. Int J Cancer. 2016;138(2):396–408. https://doi.org/10.1002/ijc.29721.
111. Cardinale V, Renzi A, Carpino G. Profiles of cancer stem cell subpopulations in cholangiocarcinomas. Am J Pathol. 2015;185:1724–39.
112. Huynh H, Choo SP, Toh HC, Tai WM, Chung AY, Chow PK, Ong R, Soo KC. Comparing the efficacy of sunitinib with sorafenib in xenograft models of human hepatocellular carcinoma:

mechanistic explanation. Curr Cancer Drug Targets. 2011;11(8):944–53. https://doi.org/10.2174/156800911797264716.

113. Sirica AE, Zhang Z, Lai GH, Asano T, Shen XN, Ward DJ, Mahatme A, Dewitt JL. A novel "patient-like" model of cholangiocarcinoma progression based on bile duct inoculation of tumorigenic rat cholangiocyte cell lines. Hepatology. 2008;47(4):1178–90. https://doi.org/10.1002/hep.22088.

114. Rizvi S, Fischbach SR, Bronk SF, Hirsova P, Krishnan A, Dhanasekaran R, Smadbeck JB, Smoot RL, Vasmatzis G, Gores GJ. YAP-associated chromosomal instability and cholangiocarcinoma in mice. Oncotarget. 2018;9(5):5892–905. https://doi.org/10.18632/oncotarget.23638.

Chapter 23
Organoid Models of Cholangiocarcinoma

Timothy Gilbert, Marc Quinn, Christopher Goldring, Daniel Palmer, Chiara Braconi, and Hassan Malik

Abbreviations

AFP	Alpha fetoprotein
CCA	Cholangiocarcinoma
CRC	Colorectal cancer
ECM	Extracellular matrix
HCC	Hepatocellular carcinoma
HTS	High-throughput screening
iCCA	Intrahepatic cholangiocarcinoma
pCCA	Perihilar cholangiocarcinoma
PDTX	Patient-derived tumour xenograft
PDO	Patient-derived organoid
TME	Tumour microenvironment
WES	Whole-exome sequencing

T. Gilbert (✉) · H. Malik
Department of Hepato-Biliary Surgery, Aintree University Hospital, Liverpool University Hospitals NHS Foundation Trust, Liverpool, UK
e-mail: timothy.gilbert@liverpoolft.nhs.uk; Hassan.malik@liverpoolft.nhs.uk

M. Quinn · C. Goldring · D. Palmer
Sherrington Building, Institute of Translational Medicine, University of Liverpool, Liverpool, UK
e-mail: l.m.quinn@liverpool.ac.uk; c.e.p.goldring@liverpool.ac.uk; Daniel.palmer@liverpool.ac.uk

C. Braconi
Institute of Cancer Sciences, Beatson West of Scotland Cancer Centre, University of Glasgow, Glasgow, UK
e-mail: Chiara.braconi@glasgow.ac.uk

J. H. Tabibian (ed.), *Diagnosis and Management of Cholangiocarcinoma*,
https://doi.org/10.1007/978-3-030-70936-5_23

The Case for Organoids

One of the major hurdles in furthering our understanding and treatment of cancer is the ability to produce models that faithfully recapture the in vivo cancer phenotype and environment [1]. Historically, animal cancer models have made important contributions, yet they are inherently limited as they do not adequately reflect the histological architecture or genetic heterogeneity of human cancers [2]. Two-dimensional (2D) cell culture using human immortalised cancer cell lines has also contributed tremendously to cancer research; however, cell lines used to generate these models have often undergone significant selection and adaption to enable successful expansion over many generations [3]. As a result, many cell lines have undergone substantial genotypic drift and no longer reflect the underlying heterogeneity of the original tumour [3]. Moreover, 2D culture is inherently limited as it does not enable cell-cell interactions in 3D (as they would be in vivo); such interactions are important for our understanding of tumour biology as they are involved in regulating important cellular activities such as differentiation, proliferation, gene expression, and drug response [4]. In addition, cells within a tumour are often exposed to differing concentration gradients of signalling molecules, nutrients, and waste products, whereas cells in 2D culture are exposed uniformly with direct contact to the culture medium. Patient-derived tumour xenografts (PDTXs) are another commonly used cancer model that involves transplanting fresh human tumour tissue into immunodeficient mice; however, issues with graft uptake for certain tumour types along with the general expense and time-consuming nature of the technique are limitations. Equally, many PDTXs undergo mouse-specific tumour evolution, thus limiting their clinical relevance [5] (Table 23.1).

The requirement for more functionally representative tissue models led to the development of novel culture techniques. One such technique, using patient-derived epithelial stem cells embedded in a 3D cellular matrix, results in the growth of self-renewing, self-organising 3D organotypic structures called ‘organoids’ [6]. This culture technique was pioneered by Sato et al., who first demonstrated that an organoid could be established from a single leucine-rich repeat-containing G protein-coupled receptor 5 (LGR5) intestinal stem cell [7]. Organ-specific adaptations to this technique have enabled organoids to be established from a wide range of healthy human tissues (breast, colon· liver, pancreas, prostate, stomach, lung) [8–15] and more recently from human cancers including colon, pancreas, prostate, liver, and bile duct [14, 16–20]. These patient-derived organoid models (PDOs) are able to more faithfully recapture the genotypic and phenotypic expression of the source tissue and better reflect the natural cellular environment compared to 2D culture systems [17, 21]. Furthermore, as they are established from patient-specific tissue, they provide a useful platform for drug discovery projects [18, 22, 23]. PDOs also hold the potential to drive a more personalised approach to medicine through the molecular characterisation and targeted drug testing of a patient’s own tumour prior to treatment [22, 24, 25]. The ability to grow matched normal and cancerous

Table 23.1 Comparison of 2D cell lines, PDTX, and organoid models for cancer research

Feature	2D cell lines	PDTX	Organoids
Cost	Low	High	Moderate
Ease of maintenance	Low maintenance	High maintenance	Moderate/high maintenance
Resource consumption	Low	High	Moderate
Long-term expansion	Immortalised for long-term expansion	Limited long-term expansion	Can be expanded long term and retains source tumour features
Source tissue	Immortalised cell lines	Tissue-specific cells	Tissue-specific stem cells
Morphology	2D monolayer	Cell clusters within 3D environment	Self-organising 3D structures, mimicking organ structure.
In vivo features	Limited cell-cell interactions Homogeneous cell line derived from a single cell Poor retention of histological and mutational landscape of source tissue	Cell-cell interactions Cell-stromal interaction Cellular heterogeneity Histological and phenotypic features of source tissues	Cell-cell interactions Cellular heterogeneity retains histological and mutational landscape of original tumour
Genetic manipulation for cancer modelling	Amenable	No	Amenable
Incorporation of immune system	None	None	Can be co-cultured
Tumour/stromal interactions	None	Stromal interaction with murine host	Can be co-cultured
Drug testing	Suitable for HTS Highly sensitive due to 2D structure – limited translation to in vivo effects	Not suitable for HTS Better predictor of in vivo response	Patient-specific responses Suitable for personalised therapy. Can predict in vivo drug response Possible to have matched normal controls

Key: *HTS* high-throughput screening, *PDTX* patient-derived tumour xenograft

tissue from the same patient also provides a valuable control in comparative studies. In light of these benefits and the promise PDOs hold in advancing our understanding of cancer biology, they have become a rapidly expanding field and were named by Nature as 'method of the year' in 2017 [26].

In this chapter we review the development of PDOs as a model for cholangiocarcinoma (CCA). We highlight some current applications of PDOs, including their potential role in drug development and personalised medicine, whilst also discussing some present limitations.

Development of Organoid Models in CCA

CCA is amongst the most aggressive GI malignancies, with overall 5-year survival between 5% and 10% [27–29]. Whilst comparatively rare, the incidence of CCA is rising globally [27, 28, 30]. Surgical resection remains the only curative treatment option. However, the majority of patients will present with advanced disease that is not surgically curative and that often displays a stubborn chemo resistance [31, 32]. Given the poor prognosis, there is clearly an unmet clinical need to develop novel treatments that are able to effectively combat CCA. Until now the lack of reproducible in vitro models that mimic the in vivo properties of CCA has frustrated attempts at understanding the underlying tumour biology, rationalising current treatments protocols, and identifying novel therapies.

Establishment of CCA Organoids in Long-Term In Vitro Culture

Based on the work that first established the growth of healthy liver organoids from human tissue [10, 15], Boutier et al. were the first group to successfully establish PDOs from patients with primary liver cancers [20]. Using a novel culture protocol, they successfully established PDOs from eight different patients including specimens of HCC ($n = 3$), intrahepatic/perihilar CCA ($n = 3$), and combined HCC/CCA (CHC; $n = 2$) [20]. Interestingly, the investigators found a strong correlation between the establishment rate of the organoids and the proliferation index of the original tumour [20]. Thus, the efficiency in establishing an organoid culture was higher in samples derived from poorly differentiated tumours as opposed to samples from well-differentiated lesions. Following this work, other groups have also been successful in establishing patient-derived CCA organoids [33–37]. These PDOs are sustainable over the long term, being expanded up to a year in culture [34]. The success rates for establishment of CCA organoids vary between 50% and 100% [33–37]. Where establishments rates are low, this is often due to non-tumoural tissue contaminating the samples and outcompeting the cancer cells [20, 34], essentially leading to the growth of a 'healthy' organoid.

CCA Organoids Maintain the Histopathological Features of the Source Tumour

Microscopic examination of CCA PDOs shows them to retain the architecture of the parental tissue with the atypical histological features of the cancerous cells corresponding to the differentiated adenocarcinomas from which they are derived [34]. Equally, they display a preference for forming cystic glandular domains and grow in cribriform patterns, with the cancerous cells seen to be invading tubular structures, as observed in the original patient samples [20, 33, 34, 37]. Immunohistochemistry for tumour-specific markers show CCA organoids to express known markers for CCA and the biliary tract such as the epithelial marker EpCAM [20]. They are also shown to be highly positive for the expression of cytokeratin 7 (CK7) and 19 (CK19) and the mucin marker mucicarmine (MUC1), consistent with patterns in the originating tumour samples [20, 33–37]. Similarly, CCA PDOs are shown not to express AFP, a well-established marker for HCC [20].

CCA Organoids Maintain Histology and Metastatic Potential in Vivo

Subsequent analyses have sought to establish whether the histopathological features of CCA PDOs can be maintained in vivo. To establish this, several groups orthotopically transplanted their organoids into immunodeficient mice [20, 33, 36]. Histological analysis of the xenograft organoid tissue revealed cancerous growths with a strong desmoplastic stromal reaction, a typical CCA feature and one seen in the original patient samples [38], even though this was not observed in the organoids whilst in vitro (due to an absence of stromal cells). This finding in the xenograft organoid tissue suggests that the ability to induce a desmoplastic reaction and reproduce the tumour microenvironment (TME) in vivo is intrinsically programmed into CCA cells [36]. Similarly, Boutier et al. also saw a strong stromal reaction on histology following implantation of their organoids [20]. The xenograft tissue also showed tumours forming glandular structures with proliferative cells growing in cribriform patterns reminiscent of the corresponding patient's original tumour tissue [20]. In addition, the metastatic potential of organoids in culture is also preserved. This was demonstrated by the formation of lung metastases in NOD-acid gamma (NSG) mice following injection of their kidney capsule with a PDO from a patient with metastatic CCA [33].

CCA Organoids Retain Genetic Alterations Present in the Original Tumour

Whilst important to ensure that organoid cultures are histologically representative of their source tissue, it is equally important that their genetic and mutational landscape is also preserved. A primary failing of immortalised cancer cells is that substantial genetic modifications within these cell lines mean they no longer reflect the underlying heterogeneity of the original tumour. It is important that cancer models maintain the genetic mutations of the parental tumour if they are to be used as clinically relevant models to interrogate the mutational processes underpinning carcinogenesis or as platforms to identify therapeutic targets. Saito et al. compared gene expression profiles by performing whole-exome sequencing (WES) of their CCA

PDOs and corresponding primary tumour tissue [34]. This analysis showed high concordance rates between the two, with an average 88% of genetic variants observed in the patient's tumour being retained in the organoid. Similar genetic comparisons performed by Lampis et al. confirmed that the genetic background of their CCA PDOs closely matched that of the parental biopsy, with a Spearman r correlation score of 0.96. Likewise, the transcriptome of the PDO closely reflected that of the parental tissue (Spearman r score of 0.91 for housekeeping genes and 0.61 for the whole transcriptome [$p < 0.0001$]) [33]. These observations provide confirmation that it is possible for CCA PDOs to retain the genomic landscape of the original tumour from which they are derived.

Applications of Organoids in CCA Research

A Biobank for CCA Research

PDOs can be passaged and cryopreserved, much like 2D immortal cell lines, whilst simultaneously maintaining the genetic and histological features of the source tumour. Currently, PDO biobanks have been established for breast and colorectal cancer [8]. The development of a CCA biobank from a wide range of individuals will provide the ideal material to assess the overall genetic landscape of CCA and identify common genetic mutations. In turn, biobanks will then provide a valuable repository for drug screening programmes. In combination with matched normal tissue, these biobanks could also be used in help to predict drug toxicity, thus providing valuable insight for preclinical studies.

A Model to Understand CCA Carcinogenesis

Identification and in-depth understanding of cancer-driving genetic mutations is critical to understanding the nature of carcinogenesis. PDOs can be used as a platform to study the initiation and progression of this process by driving healthy organoids towards cancer through engineered genetic mutations [39, 40, 42] (Fig. 23.1). This was first demonstrated by two groups who transformed healthy human intestinal organoids into adenomas by using genome editing technology to introduce combinations of common CRC oncogene mutations including APC, SMAD4, TP53, KRAS, and PIK3CA [40, 41]. Via similar mechanisms, murine liver organoids have been used to examine the effects of certain genetic mutations on the initiation and progression of iCCA [43]. In this study, no single genetic alteration was found to induce tumour transformation; however, mutant KRAS, in conjunction with repression of tumour suppressor genes, did induce tumour development. Additionally, two presumed oncogenes (mutant Pik3ca and FGFR2-AHCYL) showed to be only modest drivers of carcinogenesis [43]. More recently Artegiani et al. engineered CCA PDOs from healthy human cholangiocytes by introducing four common CCA

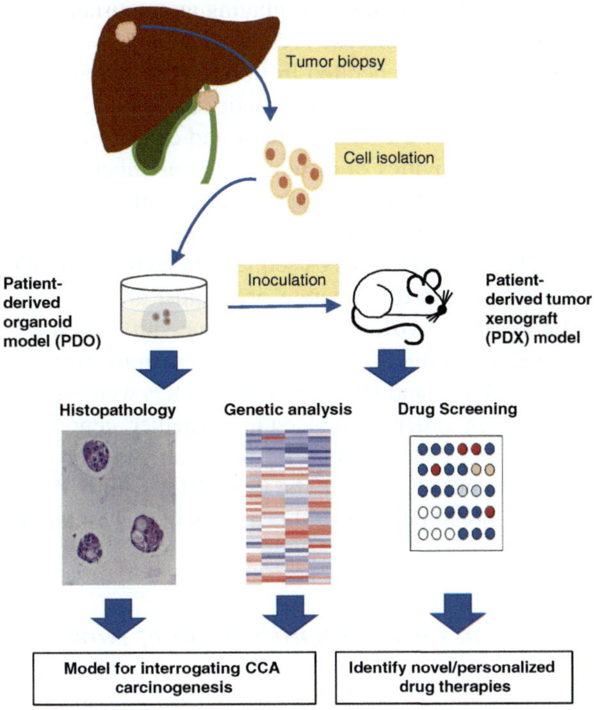

Fig. 23.1 Analysis of cholangiocarcinoma tumour biology using patient-derived tumour models

mutations (TP53, PTEN, SMAD4, and NF1) [83]. These studies highlight the potential of gene-edited organoid systems to identify and validate key driver mutations underpinning carcinogenesis.

Importantly, organoids can also be used to investigate the complex interactions between genetic mutations and niche factors within the extracellular matrix (ECM) that help drive carcinogenesis. For instance, Fujii et al., by using different combinations of growth factors in their culture media, identified the niches that supported or inhibited growth of their mutated CRC organoids. Results from this study showed that organoids carrying mutations in APC, CTNNB1, and TCF7L2 could grow without Wnt activators (Wnt3A/R-spondin1), whilst mutation of the KRAS gene and the PI3K pathway led to EGF-independent growth [84]. This demonstrates that organoids with different carcinogenic mutations have a distinct dependence on different niche factors and thereby serve as an effective tool to help understand the interaction between the genetic mutations and TME during carcinogenesis [24].

A Model of Intra-Tumoural Heterogeneity

Intra-tumoural heterogeneity arises as tumours inherently harbour unstable genomes, and consequently, individual tumour cells in different parts of the same tumour may contain separate sets of genetic mutations [44, 85]. This heterogeneity is increasingly recognised as playing an important role in tumour progression, chemoresistance, and disease recurrence [44, 45]. To reflect this situation, individual organoids can be generated from different regions of the same parent tumour. This then enables the analysis of genetic, epigenetic, and transcriptomic profiles of different regions of the same tumour and can subsequently be used to help determine the drug sensitivities of different tumour subclones. Initially explored in organoid models of CRC [46], this has more recently been replicated in CCA [35]. In said study, investigators generated six PDOs from different regions of the same resected iCCA. WES as well as RNA sequencing of the six PDOs showed a variety of genetic mutations across the separate organoids: all PDOs showed mutations in KMT2C and PTCHD3, two displayed a frame-shift mutation in fibroblast growth factor receptor 1 (FGFR1), and further mutations were also seen in FMN2, USP2, ARID1B, RTK, and HDAC5. These PDOs were then treated with a panel of different drugs in order to understand whether genomic profiles could predict drug response. For example, FGFR1 mutation should correlate with an increased sensitivity to ponatinib. Indeed, the two PDOs with FGFR1 mutations were killed by of 10 μM of ponatinib, whilst those without this mutation survived [35].

A Platform for the Identification of Novel Therapeutics in CCA

As highlighted above, PDOs can act as an important platform for drug discovery projects whilst helping explore the mechanisms underlying drug sensitivity and resistance (Fig. 23.1). Ling et al. recently tested 129 different therapeutic compounds on 27 PDOs derived from 5 patients (3 iCCA and 2 HCC) [35]. Of the 129 drugs tested, only 9 showed effectiveness across all CCA organoid lines. The remainder showed interpatient variability in terms of response. Interestingly, amongst the drugs that showed the most interpatient divergence were gemcitabine and cisplatin, which are traditionally used as a front-line chemotherapy agents in CCA [35, 47].

A similar drug discovery project using high-throughput screening (HTS) techniques on a large library of 484 targeted small molecules assessed impact of these compounds on the viability of iCCA and extrahepatic CCA human cell lines [33]. From this small-molecule library, HSP90 inhibitors were shown to be particularly effective, with the highest activity recorded for the HSP90 inhibitor, AUY922 [33]. To assess the clinical relevance of these findings, the authors then assessed AUY922 activity in PDOs established from liver biopsies of a patient with chemo-resistant iCCA. The PDOs were shown to be sensitive to AUY922 in both in vivo culture and xenograft models, with sensitivity significantly enhanced after inducible inhibition of MIR2I [33], an oncogenic microRNA known to modulate drug sensitivity and drive CCA carcinogenesis [48, 49]. These studies highlight the utility of organoid models in screening for novel therapeutic but also open the possibility of developing a more personalised approach to medicine through identification of patient-specific drug sensitivities. In this regard Saito et al. correlated the gene expression profiles of their CCA PDOs with sensitivity to the anti-epidermal growth factor receptor (EGFR) tyrosine kinase inhibitors, erlotinib [34]. The effect of EGFR inhibitors has previously been shown to be associated with KRAS mutation status [50]. However, in the setting of CCA, erlotinib was shown to function independent of KRAS mutation. In contrast, reduced sensitivity to erlotinib was shown to correlate with increased expression of the CPB2 gene, which was also associated with poorer overall patient survival [34].

Personalised Medicine and 'Live' Drug Screening in CCA

As discussed PDOs are valuable tools for screening multiple novel therapeutic agents and also hold the potential to generate a more personalised approach to anti-cancer therapies. However, their ability to actually predict 'real-world' clinical outcomes in patients has remained unclear. PDOs were recently included in a phase I/II clinical trial that involved 71 patients with advanced CRC or gastro-oesophageal cancer [51]. In this trial, investigators compared the in vitro response of anticancer agents in the PDO with the in vivo clinical response of the corresponding trial patient. On comparing the matched organoid and patient clinical response, they found PDOs to have 100% sensitivity, 93% specificity, 88% positive predictive value, and 100% negative predictive value in forecasting the in vivo patient response to drug treatment [51]. This suggests that PDOs can faithfully recapture clinical patient responses and could be used to develop personalised treatment programmes within the lifetime of the patient. A further use for organoids in personalised medicine is to grow matched cancer organoid and healthy liver and kidney tissue from an individual which can then be used to model drug- and dose-related toxicities on normal patient tissue whilst simultaneously assessing for therapeutic response in the cancer organoid.

Limitations of Organoid Models

Although organoids are widely regarded as a highly promising in vitro model, limitations are still present. The 3D structure helps better recapitulate the cell-to-cell arrangement of the parental tumour; however, as organoids are solely epithelial cell-derived, they lack the stromal tissue, blood vessels, and immune cells that make up the whole extracellular environment [39, 52]. This is important as we know the interaction between the extracellular environment, host immune system, and cancer cells play a key role in disease progression, tumour angiogenesis, and response to drug treatment [53–57]. For example, under healthy circumstances, the rigidity of the ECM provides tumour suppressor functions [58]. However, in the presence of a tumour, an increase in the rigidity of the ECM by cancer-associated fibroblasts and stimulation of the YAP pathway facilitates an increase in malignant behaviour

[59–61]. As a result, almost all CCA patients exhibit a high expression of YAP and its co-activator TAZ [60, 62]. Likewise, modulation of the TME by MMP-7 and MMP-9 and an increased expression of periostin are associated with a worse prognosis and development of lymph node metastases [63–65]. Similarly, lower survival rates, higher recurrence rates, and increased metastasis are all linked to angiogenesis and lymphangiogenesis in CCA [66–69]. A focus on developing in vitro organoid models that more fully incorporate the whole TME would provide better mechanistic insight into its role in disease progression and provide potential targets for therapeutic intervention [70–73]. Combining organoids with a more representative TME has been attempted by several groups who have co-cultured organoids with lymphocytes and stromal cells [74–82]; further studies are required to better address these issues. Notably, the successful co-culture of organoids with immune cells is of particular importance when looking to provide an accurate model for immunotherapy agents.

Summary

PDOs hold much promise in helping advance our understanding of CCA, with clear advantages over traditional 2D cell culture. In addition to being able to be grown at high efficiencies, expanded over many generations, and cryopreserved in biobanks, they maintain the histological and mutational genetic landscape of the source tumour from which they are derived. This makes them ideal platforms to functionally dissect the underlying tumour biology and explore novel drug targets for all solid tumours, including CCA. Future studies with the development of co-culture techniques will undoubtedly refine organoid models to include more aspects of the extracellular environment with the aim of generating a sophisticated organoid with full representation of the TME. In terms of patient treatment, PDOs have the potential to significantly alter the treatment paradigm in CCA, changing the current systemic approach to patient treatment to a more personalised programme, whereby combinations of anticancer drugs can be given based on the mutational profile and sensitivity of the individual patient's tumour.

References

1. Kamb A. What's wrong with our cancer models? Nat Rev Drug Discov. 2005;4(2):161–5.
2. Cheon DJ, Orsulic S. Mouse models of cancer. Annu Rev Pathol. 2011;6:95–119.
3. Drost J, Clevers H. Organoids in cancer research. Nat Rev Cancer. 2018;18(7):407–18.
4. Baker BM, Chen CS. Deconstructing the third dimension: how 3D culture microenvironments alter cellular cues. J Cell Sci. 2012;125(Pt 13):3015–24.
5. Ben-David U, Ha G, Tseng YY, Greenwald NF, Oh C, Shih J, et al. Patient-derived xenografts undergo mouse-specific tumor evolution. Nat Genet. 2017;49(11):1567–75.

6. Lancaster MA, Knoblich JA. Organogenesis in a dish: modeling development and disease using organoid technologies. Science. 2014;345(6194):1247125.
7. Sato T, Vries RG, Snippert HJ, van de Wetering M, Barker N, Stange DE, et al. Single Lgr5 stem cells build crypt-villus structures in vitro without a mesenchymal niche. Nature. 2009;459(7244):262–5.
8. Sachs N, de Ligt J, Kopper O, Gogola E, Bounova G, Weeber F, et al. A living biobank of breast cancer organoids captures disease heterogeneity. Cell. 2018;172(1–2):373–86.e10.
9. Jung P, Sato T, Merlos-Suarez A, Barriga FM, Iglesias M, Rossell D, et al. Isolation and in vitro expansion of human colonic stem cells. Nat Med. 2011;17(10):1225–7.
10. Huch M, Gehart H, van Boxtel R, Hamer K, Blokzijl F, Verstegen MM, et al. Long-term culture of genome-stable bipotent stem cells from adult human liver. Cell. 2015;160(1–2):299–312.
11. Chua CW, Shibata M, Lei M, Toivanen R, Barlow LJ, Bergren SK, et al. Single luminal epithelial progenitors can generate prostate organoids in culture. Nat Cell Biol. 2014;16(10):951–61, 1-4.
12. Bartfeld S, Bayram T, van de Wetering M, Huch M, Begthel H, Kujala P, et al. In vitro expansion of human gastric epithelial stem cells and their responses to bacterial infection. Gastroenterology. 2015;148(1):126–36.e6.
13. Turco MY, Gardner L, Hughes J, Cindrova-Davies T, Gomez MJ, Farrell L, et al. Long-term, hormone-responsive organoid cultures of human endometrium in a chemically defined medium. Nat Cell Biol. 2017;19(5):568–77.
14. Boj SF, Hwang CI, Baker LA, Chio II, Engle DD, Corbo V, et al. Organoid models of human and mouse ductal pancreatic cancer. Cell. 2015;160(1–2):324–38.
15. Broutier L, Andersson-Rolf A, Hindley CJ, Boj SF, Clevers H, Koo BK, et al. Culture and establishment of self-renewing human and mouse adult liver and pancreas 3D organoids and their genetic manipulation. Nat Protoc. 2016;11(9):1724–43.
16. Sato T, Stange DE, Ferrante M, Vries RG, Van Es JH, Van den Brink S, et al. Long-term expansion of epithelial organoids from human colon, adenoma, adenocarcinoma, and Barrett's epithelium. Gastroenterology. 2011;141(5):1762–72.
17. van de Wetering M, Francies HE, Francis JM, Bounova G, Iorio F, Pronk A, et al. Prospective derivation of a living organoid biobank of colorectal cancer patients. Cell. 2015;161(4):933–45.
18. Crespo M, Vilar E, Tsai SY, Chang K, Amin S, Srinivasan T, et al. Colonic organoids derived from human induced pluripotent stem cells for modeling colorectal cancer and drug testing. Nat Med. 2017;23(7):878–84.
19. Gao D, Vela I, Sboner A, Iaquinta PJ, Karthaus WR, Gopalan A, et al. Organoid cultures derived from patients with advanced prostate cancer. Cell. 2014;159(1):176–87.
20. Broutier L, Mastrogiovanni G, Verstegen MM, Francies HE, Gavarro LM, Bradshaw CR, et al. Human primary liver cancer-derived organoid cultures for disease modeling and drug screening. Nat Med. 2017;23(12):1424–35.
21. Birgersdotter A, Sandberg R, Ernberg I. Gene expression perturbation in vitro--a growing case for three-dimensional (3D) culture systems. Semin Cancer Biol. 2005;15(5):405–12.
22. Kondo J, Inoue M. Application of cancer organoid model for drug screening and personalized therapy. Cells. 2019;8(5):470.
23. Lee SH, Hu W, Matulay JT, Silva MV, Owczarek TB, Kim K, et al. Tumor evolution and drug response in patient-derived organoid models of bladder cancer. Cell. 2018;173(2):515–28.e17.
24. Fan H, Demirci U, Chen P. Emerging organoid models: leaping forward in cancer research. J Hematol Oncol. 2019;12(1):142.
25. Jabs J, Zickgraf FM, Park J, Wagner S, Jiang X, Jechow K, et al. Screening drug effects in patient-derived cancer cells links organoid responses to genome alterations. Mol Syst Biol. 2017;13(11):955.
26. Method of the year 2017: organoids. Nature Methods. 2018;15(1):1.
27. Rizvi S, Gores GJ. Pathogenesis, diagnosis, and management of cholangiocarcinoma. Gastroenterology. 2013;145(6):1215–29.
28. Razumilava N, Gores GJ. Cholangiocarcinoma. Lancet. 2014;383(9935):2168–79.

29. Razumilava N, Gores GJ. Classification, diagnosis, and management of cholangiocarcinoma. Clin Gastroenterol Hepatol. 2013;11(1):13–21.e1; quiz e3–4.
30. Patel N, Benipal B. Incidence of cholangiocarcinoma in the USA from 2001 to 2015: a US cancer statistics analysis of 50 states. Cureus. 2019;11(1):e3962.
31. Marin JJG, Lozano E, Herraez E, Asensio M, Di Giacomo S, Romero MR, et al. Chemoresistance and chemosensitization in cholangiocarcinoma. Biochim Biophys Acta Mol Basis Dis. 2018;1864(4 Pt B):1444–53.
32. Mavros MN, Economopoulos KP, Alexiou VG, Pawlik TM. Treatment and prognosis for patients with intrahepatic cholangiocarcinoma: systematic review and meta-analysis. JAMA Surg. 2014;149(6):565–74.
33. Lampis A, Carotenuto P, Vlachogiannis G, Cascione L, Hedayat S, Burke R, et al. MIR21 drives resistance to heat shock protein 90 inhibition in cholangiocarcinoma. Gastroenterology. 2018;154(4):1066–79.e5.
34. Saito Y, Muramatsu T, Kanai Y, Ojima H, Sukeda A, Hiraoka N, et al. Establishment of patient-derived organoids and drug screening for biliary tract carcinoma. Cell Rep. 2019;27(4):1265–76.e4.
35. Li L, Knutsdottir H, Hui K, Weiss MJ, He J, Philosophe B, et al. Human primary liver cancer organoids reveal intratumor and interpatient drug response heterogeneity. JCI Insight. 2019;4(2).
36. Nuciforo S, Fofana I, Matter MS, Blumer T, Calabrese D, Boldanova T, et al. Organoid models of human liver cancers derived from tumor needle biopsies. Cell Rep. 2018;24(5):1363–76.
37. Saito Y, Nakaoka T, Muramatsu T, Ojima H, Sukeda A, Sugiyama Y, et al. Induction of differentiation of intrahepatic cholangiocarcinoma cells to functional hepatocytes using an organoid culture system. Sci Rep. 2018;8(1):2821.
38. Hogdall D, Lewinska M, Andersen JB. Desmoplastic tumor microenvironment and immunotherapy in cholangiocarcinoma. Trends Cancer. 2018;4(3):239–55.
39. van Tienderen GS, Groot Koerkamp B, JNM IJ, van der Laan LJW, Verstegen MMA. Recreating tumour complexity in a dish: organoid models to study liver cancer cells and their extracellular environment. Cancers (Basel). 2019;11(11):1706.
40. Drost J, van Jaarsveld RH, Ponsioen B, Zimberlin C, van Boxtel R, Buijs A, et al. Sequential cancer mutations in cultured human intestinal stem cells. Nature. 2015;521(7550):43–7.
41. Matano M, Date S, Shimokawa M, Takano A, Fujii M, Ohta Y, et al. Modeling colorectal cancer using CRISPR-Cas9-mediated engineering of human intestinal organoids. Nat Med. 2015;21(3):256–62.
42. Li X, Nadauld L, Ootani A, Corney DC, Pai RK, Gevaert O, et al. Oncogenic transformation of diverse gastrointestinal tissues in primary organoid culture. Nat Med. 2014;20(7):769–77.
43. Ochiai M, Yoshihara Y, Maru Y, Tetsuya M, Izumiya M, Imai T, et al. Kras-driven heterotopic tumor development from hepatobiliary organoids. Carcinogenesis. 2019.
44. McGranahan N, Swanton C. Clonal heterogeneity and tumor evolution: past, present, and the future. Cell. 2017;168(4):613–28.
45. Burrell RA, McGranahan N, Bartek J, Swanton C. The causes and consequences of genetic heterogeneity in cancer evolution. Nature. 2013;501(7467):338–45.
46. Roerink SF, Sasaki N, Lee-Six H, Young MD, Alexandrov LB, Behjati S, et al. Intra-tumour diversification in colorectal cancer at the single-cell level. Nature. 2018;556(7702):457–62.
47. Valle J, Wasan H, Palmer DH, Cunningham D, Anthoney A, Maraveyas A, et al. Cisplatin plus gemcitabine versus gemcitabine for biliary tract cancer. N Engl J Med. 2010;362(14):1273–81.
48. Lu L, Byrnes K, Han C, Wang Y, Wu T. miR-21 targets 15-PGDH and promotes cholangiocarcinoma growth. Mol Cancer Res. 2014;12(6):890–900.
49. Wang LJ, He CC, Sui X, Cai MJ, Zhou CY, Ma JL, et al. MiR-21 promotes intrahepatic cholangiocarcinoma proliferation and growth in vitro and in vivo by targeting PTPN14 and PTEN. Oncotarget. 2015;6(8):5932–46.

50. Massarelli E, Varella-Garcia M, Tang X, Xavier AC, Ozburn NC, Liu DD, et al. KRAS mutation is an important predictor of resistance to therapy with epidermal growth factor receptor tyrosine kinase inhibitors in non-small-cell lung cancer. Clin Cancer Res. 2007;13(10):2890–6.
51. Vlachogiannis G, Hedayat S, Vatsiou A, Jamin Y, Fernandez-Mateos J, Khan K, et al. Patient-derived organoids model treatment response of metastatic gastrointestinal cancers. Science. 2018;359(6378):920–6.
52. Fatehullah A, Tan SH, Barker N. Organoids as an in vitro model of human development and disease. Nat Cell Biol. 2016;18(3):246–54.
53. Chen Z, Guo P, Xie X, Yu H, Wang Y, Chen G. The role of tumour microenvironment: a new vision for cholangiocarcinoma. J Cell Mol Med. 2019;23(1):59–69.
54. Fabris L, Perugorria MJ, Mertens J, Bjorkstrom NK, Cramer T, Lleo A, et al. The tumour microenvironment and immune milieu of cholangiocarcinoma. Liver Int. 2019;39(Suppl 1):63–78.
55. Rimassa L, Personeni N, Aghemo A, Lleo A. The immune milieu of cholangiocarcinoma: from molecular pathogenesis to precision medicine. J Autoimmun. 2019;100:17–26.
56. Wang M, Zhao J, Zhang L, Wei F, Lian Y, Wu Y, et al. Role of tumor microenvironment in tumorigenesis. J Cancer. 2017;8(5):761–73.
57. Junttila MR, de Sauvage FJ. Influence of tumour micro-environment heterogeneity on therapeutic response. Nature. 2013;501(7467):346–54.
58. Bissell MJ, Hines WC. Why don't we get more cancer? A proposed role of the microenvironment in restraining cancer progression. Nat Med. 2011;17(3):320–9.
59. Dobrokhotov O, Samsonov M, Sokabe M, Hirata H. Mechanoregulation and pathology of YAP/TAZ via hippo and non-hippo mechanisms. Clin Transl Med. 2018;7(1):23.
60. Sugihara T, Isomoto H, Gores G, Smoot R. YAP and the hippo pathway in cholangiocarcinoma. J Gastroenterol. 2019;54(6):485–91.
61. Calvo F, Ege N, Grande-Garcia A, Hooper S, Jenkins RP, Chaudhry SI, et al. Mechanotransduction and YAP-dependent matrix remodelling is required for the generation and maintenance of cancer-associated fibroblasts. Nat Cell Biol. 2013;15(6):637–46.
62. Van Haele M, Moya IM, Karaman R, Rens G, Snoeck J, Govaere O, et al. YAP and TAZ heterogeneity in primary liver cancer: an analysis of its prognostic and diagnostic role. Int J Mol Sci. 2019;20(3):638.
63. Riener MO, Fritzsche FR, Soll C, Pestalozzi BC, Probst-Hensch N, Clavien PA, et al. Expression of the extracellular matrix protein periostin in liver tumours and bile duct carcinomas. Histopathology. 2010;56(5):600–6.
64. Shirabe K, Shimada M, Kajiyama K, Hasegawa H, Gion T, Ikeda Y, et al. Expression of matrix metalloproteinase-9 in surgically resected intrahepatic cholangiocarcinoma. Surgery. 1999;126(5):842–6.
65. Hirashita T, Iwashita Y, Ohta M, Komori Y, Eguchi H, Yada K, et al. Expression of matrix metalloproteinase-7 is an unfavorable prognostic factor in intrahepatic cholangiocarcinoma. J Gastrointest Surg. 2012;16(4):842–8.
66. Thelen A, Scholz A, Weichert W, Wiedenmann B, Neuhaus P, Gessner R, et al. Tumor-associated angiogenesis and lymphangiogenesis correlate with progression of intrahepatic cholangiocarcinoma. Am J Gastroenterol. 2010;105(5):1123–32.
67. Sha M, Jeong S, Wang X, Tong Y, Cao J, Sun HY, et al. Tumor-associated lymphangiogenesis predicts unfavorable prognosis of intrahepatic cholangiocarcinoma. BMC Cancer. 2019;19(1):208.
68. Thelen A, Scholz A, Benckert C, Weichert W, Dietz E, Wiedenmann B, et al. Tumor-associated lymphangiogenesis correlates with lymph node metastases and prognosis in hilar cholangiocarcinoma. Ann Surg Oncol. 2008;15(3):791–9.
69. Sha M, Jeong S, Chen XS, Tong Y, Cao J, Sun HY, et al. Expression of VEGFR-3 in intrahepatic cholangiocarcinoma correlates with unfavorable prognosis through lymphangiogenesis. Int J Biol Sci. 2018;14(10):1333–42.

70. Heits N, Heinze T, Bernsmeier A, Kerber J, Hauser C, Becker T, et al. Influence of mTOR-inhibitors and mycophenolic acid on human cholangiocellular carcinoma and cancer associated fibroblasts. BMC Cancer. 2016;16:322.
71. Wu CE, Chen MH, Yeh CN. mTOR inhibitors in advanced biliary tract cancers. Int J Mol Sci. 2019;20(3):500.
72. Adeva J, Sangro B, Salati M, Edeline J, La Casta A, Bittoni A, et al. Medical treatment for cholangiocarcinoma. Liver Int. 2019;39(Suppl 1):123–42.
73. Rizvi S, Gores GJ. Emerging molecular therapeutic targets for cholangiocarcinoma. J Hepatol. 2017;67(3):632–44.
74. Cattaneo CM, Dijkstra KK, Fanchi LF, Kelderman S, Kaing S, van Rooij N, et al. Tumor organoid–T-cell coculture systems. Nat Protoc. 2020;15(1):15–39.
75. Dijkstra KK, Cattaneo CM, Weeber F, Chalabi M, van de Haar J, Fanchi LF, et al. Generation of tumor-reactive T cells by co-culture of peripheral blood lymphocytes and tumor organoids. Cell. 2018;174(6):1586–98.e12.
76. Neal JT, Li X, Zhu J, Giangarra V, Grzeskowiak CL, Ju J, et al. Organoid modeling of the tumor immune microenvironment. Cell. 2018;175(7):1972–88.e16.
77. Tsai S, McOlash L, Palen K, Johnson B, Duris C, Yang Q, et al. Development of primary human pancreatic cancer organoids, matched stromal and immune cells and 3D tumor microenvironment models. BMC Cancer. 2018;18(1):335.
78. Lee JH, Kim SK, Khawar IA, Jeong SY, Chung S, Kuh HJ. Microfluidic co-culture of pancreatic tumor spheroids with stellate cells as a novel 3D model for investigation of stroma-mediated cell motility and drug resistance. J Exp Clin Cancer Res. 2018;37(1):4.
79. Neal JT, Kuo CJ. Organoids as models for neoplastic transformation. Annu Rev Pathol. 2016;11:199–220.
80. Li X, Ootani A, Kuo C. An air-liquid Interface culture system for 3D organoid culture of diverse primary gastrointestinal tissues. Methods Mol Biol. 2016;1422:33–40.
81. Finnberg NK, Gokare P, Lev A, Grivennikov SI, MacFarlane AW, Campbell KS, et al. Application of 3D tumoroid systems to define immune and cytotoxic therapeutic responses based on tumoroid and tissue slice culture molecular signatures. Oncotarget. 2017;8(40):66747–57.
82. Ootani A, Li X, Sangiorgi E, Ho QT, Ueno H, Toda S, et al. Sustained in vitro intestinal epithelial culture within a Wnt-dependent stem cell niche. Nat Med. 2009;15(6):701–6.
83. Artegiani B, van Voorthuijsen L, Lindeboom RGH, Seinstra D, Heo I, Tapia P, et al. Probing the tumor suppressor function of BAP1 in CRISPR-engineered human liver organoids. Cell Stem Cell. 2019;24(6):927–43.
84. Fujii M, Shimokawa M, Date S, Takano A, Matano M, Nanki K, et al. A colorectal tumor organoid library demonstrates progressive loss of niche factor requirements during tumorigenesis. Cell Stem Cell. 2016;18(6):827–38.
85. Gerlinger M, Rowan AJ, Horswell S, Math M, Larkin J, et al. Endesfelder DIntratumor heterogeneity and branched evolution revealed by multiregion sequencing. N Engl J Med. 2012;366(10):883–92.

Chapter 24
The Tumor Environment: Cholangiocarcinoma-Associated Fibroblasts and Beyond

Anja Moncsek and Joachim C. Mertens

Abbreviations

Bcl-2 proteins	B-cell lymphoma-2 proteins
CAFs	Cancer-associated fibroblasts
CCA	Cholangiocarcinoma
CCL2	CC-chemokine ligand 2
CXCL	C-X-C motif ligand
ECM	Extracellular matrix
EGFR	Epidermal growth factor receptor
ERK	Extracellular signal-regulated kinase
FAP	Fibroblast activation protein
FGF	Fibroblast growth factor
HB-EGF	Heparin-binding epidermal growth factor
HGF	Hepatocyte growth factor
HSCs	Hepatic stellate cells
MCP1	Monocyte chemoattractant protein 1
MDSCs	Myeloid-derived suppressor cells
PD-L1	Programmed death-ligand 1
PDGF	Platelet-derived growth factor
PI3K	Phosphatidylinositol 3-kinase
TAM	Tumor-associated macrophage
TANs	Tumor-associated neutrophils
TGF	Transforming growth factor
TILs	Tumor-infiltrating lymphocytes
TME	Tumor microenvironment
TNF	Tumor necrosis factor
TRAIL	TNF-related apoptosis-inducing ligand
αSMA	alpha-smooth muscle actin

A. Moncsek · J. C. Mertens (✉)
Gastroenterology and Hepatology, University Hospital Zürich, Zürich, Switzerland
e-mail: joachim.mertens@usz.ch

J. H. Tabibian (ed.), *Diagnosis and Management of Cholangiocarcinoma*,
https://doi.org/10.1007/978-3-030-70936-5_24

Introduction to the Tumor Microenvironment in Cholangiocarcinoma

Malignant cancers are in fact a complex tissue consisting of the cancer cells and nonmalignant stromal cells with their cell-cell interactions and respective extracellular matrix (ECM) [1, 2], forming the so-called tumor microenvironment (TME). Over the last decade, the TME in cholangiocarcinoma (CCA) has gained increasing interest, and we have seen a surge in research into this particular compartment of CCA. Often arising from a chronic inflammatory background, cholangiocarcinoma has long been known as a "stroma-rich" cancer, characterized by an extensive fibrous tissue around the often small clusters of cancer cells (Fig. 24.1) [3]. In most CCA, the tumor stroma makes up the largest part of the tumor tissue. Therefore, the hypothesis has been for some time that the vast stromal compartment plays a more important role in the biology of this devastating malignancy [4].

The TME consists of a variety of cells including cancer-associated fibroblasts (CAFs), inflammatory cells, and endothelial cells. Inside this multicellular compartment, CAFs are able to shape the (premalignant) microenvironment by remodeling the ECM and recruiting and interacting with cells of the innate and adaptive immune response, thereby supporting cancer initiation and progression.

More specific studies into the overall gene expression profile of the stromal compartment have revealed gene signatures that correlate with worse clinical outcome. Among differentially expressed genes are receptors and ligands of the chemokine (CXCR4, CCR7, CCL2, CCL5, CCL19, CCL21) and interleukin (IL) family (IL3RA, IL7R, IL-10RA, IL-18RAP, IL-6, IL-16, IL-33) [7]. Moreover,

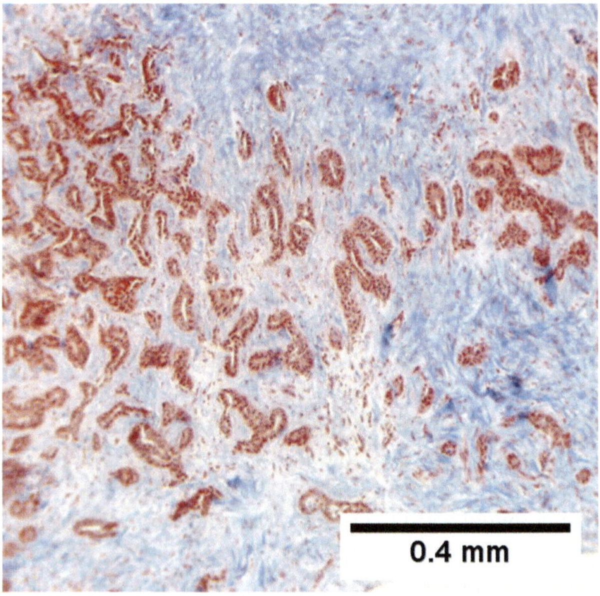

Fig. 24.1 Trichrome stain shows spread of tumor into scar with collagen deposition (Photography by TexasPathologistMSW [5] is licensed under CC BY-SA 4.0 [6])

overexpression of genes such as KIAA0101 (proliferating cell nuclear antigen-associated factor), transforming growth factor (TGF)-β2, laminin subunit γ2, and osteopontin, has been found in the stromal compartment of CCA [8]. An increased stromal expression of CAF marker alpha-smooth muscle actin (αSMA) was reported as an independent prognostic factor for overall and disease-free survival [9, 10].

In this chapter, we review the different components of the CCA microenvironment. We focus on CAFs, their origin, heterogeneity, and activation. We further address different immune cells subpopulations in CCA, their cellular cross talk with CAFs, as well as their potential application for therapeutic intervention.

Cancer-Associated Fibroblasts

The most abundant cell types in CCA are activated stromal fibroblasts, also referred to CAFs [11]. This cell type is of mesenchymal origin and often outnumbers all other cells in the tumor, including the tumor cells themselves [12]. Many studies have highlighted the pivotal role of CAFs in the CCA microenvironment and the importance of cross talk among CAFs and cancer cells with respect to tumor development, progression, and even drug resistance [9, 12–15].

The phenotype of a CAF is that of an activated fibroblast. These cells characteristically express αSMA, vimentin, S100A4 or fibroblast-specific protein 1, fibroblast activation protein alpha (FAP), fibronectin, and collagen type I [16]. They secrete an array of growth factors, especially platelet-derived growth factor (PDGF) in its variant PDGF-BB, TGF-β, CCL2, CXCL12 (also referred to as stromal-derived factor-1), CXCL14, insulin-like growth factor, fibroblast growth factor (FGF), heparin-binding epidermal growth factor (HB-EGF), hepatocyte growth factor (HGF), and granulocyte-macrophage colony-stimulating factor [11] and are proliferative. Interestingly, the activated state of a CAF comes at the cost of increased apoptosis sensitivity induced by altered expression of B-cell lymphoma-2 (*Bcl-2*) family proteins – a state termed "apoptotic priming" [17].

Origin and Heterogeneity

Regarding the origins of CAFs, several sources have been proposed. The most obvious are resident intrahepatic periportal fibroblasts. A second and probably the most important source of CAFs are likely hepatic stellate cells (HSCs) from the perisinusoidal space of Disse. HSCs have been identified as an important source of activated fibroblasts in various models of biliary fibrosis [18, 19]. In addition, circulating mesenchymal stem cells from the bone marrow are a third likely source of CAFs in CCA. The hypothesis of epithelial to mesenchymal transition has been debated controversially but has not been confirmed so far [19–21]. This heterogeneity of origin and phenotype poses a challenge with regard to identifying specific CAF markers and biological functions of CAFs in cancer development.

Activation

In contrast to the tissue resident fibroblasts of the organ affected by the tumor, CAFs are generally in an activated cell state. A large number of markers have been proposed and described to identify and further characterize CAFs in tumor tissue. Many of these markers show different expression depending on the tissue type origin, the subtype of CAF, and possibly the stage of tumor development [22, 23].

One the most well-known markers is αSMA, which is found overexpressed in CAFs of many tumors. In CCA, high expression of αSMA is an indicator of poor prognosis and is correlated with larger, less differentiated tumors that metastasize more readily [24]. It has been proposed that the high αSMA positivity of CAFs from hepato- and pancreatobiliary cancers is due to their origin from stellate cells [25]. Another commonly found marker is PDGFRα, which has been attributed to a fibroblast origin of CAFs [26]. Among the many additional CAF markers, fibulin-2 and desmin as well as glial fibrillary acidic protein have been interpreted as indicators of the heterogeneous sources of CAFs in CCA, namely, HSCs and portal fibroblasts [27].

As we begin to better understand the phenotype and role of CAFs in CCA, the concept that cancer cells "educate" surrounding mesenchymal cells to transform into several CAF subtypes that serve different functions in the TME has been suggested in CCA, similar to pancreatic carcinoma [28, 29]. This could explain the multitude of functions that have been attributed to CAFs such as tumor cell growth, metastasis, ECM remodeling, or angiogenesis. Even more importantly, different populations of CAFs within the tumor could also explain pro- and anti-tumorigenic effects of CAFs. The mechanisms by which CCA cells "educate" mesenchymal cells to become CAFs are still under investigation. Tumor-derived PDGF and TGF-β are probably the most important stimulating factors that trigger CAF development [30]. Besides these, an ever more detailed panel of CAF-promoting stimuli is evolving and includes inflammatory signals such as IL-1, IL-6, and tumor necrosis factor (TNF) but also direct contact signals via Notch or properties of the ECM (Fig. 24.2). In an elegant review by Kalluri et al., these factors are summarized [22].

Pro- and Anti-tumorigenic Functions of CAF

CAFs exhibit a variety of *functions and interactions* within the CCA microenvironment. CAFs directly interact with CCA cells and have been found to modulate CCA cell behavior, resulting in more aggressive growth and invasiveness. Cultivation of

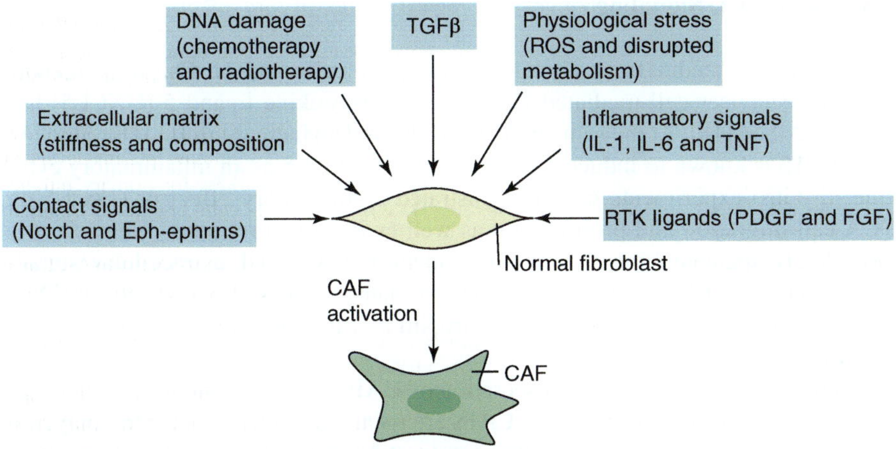

Fig. 24.2 Diverse mechanisms of cancer-associated fibroblast (CAF) activation. This schematic highlights the multiple mechanisms that can contribute to CAF activation. FGF fibroblast growth factor, PDGF platelet-derived growth factor, ROS reactive oxygen species, RTK receptor tyrosine kinase, TGF-β transforming growth factor-β, TNF tumor necrosis factor (Figure reprinted from Sahai et al. [31] is licensed under CC BY-SA 4.0 [6])

CCA cells in conditioned medium from CAFs as well as co-cultivation of these two cell types leads to an increase in proliferation and migration of CCA cells [9, 32]. Moreover, co-cultivation of CAFs and CCA cells from a syngeneic rat model in more sophisticated three-dimensional cultures systems has been reported to lead to a change in growth behavior, with increased duct formation by the CCA cells [33]. Other studies suggest that CAFs could inhibit apoptosis of normal biliary epithelial cells and by this promote the proliferation of these cells in the very early stages of cholangiocarcinogenesis [9].

CAF and PDGF Signaling

Among the various signaling molecules mediating CAF-CCA cell interaction in CCA, PDGF has been of particular interest. CAF-derived PDGF-BB in the TME binds to PDGFRβ, which is highly expressed on the CCA cell surface [34]. In a recent study, PDGF-BB-induced resistance of CCA cells to TNF-related apoptosis-inducing ligand (TRAIL)-mediated apoptosis by activating the Hedgehog signaling pathway [35]. At the same time, PDGF-BB acts in an autocrine fashion, binding to PDGFRβ on HSCs and CAFs and inducing fibroblast migration [36]. The PDGF-PDGFRβ signal and downstream effects in CAFs are further propagated by activation of intracellular Rho GTPases, via induction of Rac1 and Cdc42, as well as activation of the JNK pathway [21]. Upon treatment with PDGF, CAFs have been reported to acquire a more spindle-like shape and increased expression of αSMA in vitro [37].

CAF and CXCL Signaling

In conditioned media from co-cultures of CCA cells and HSCs, a remarkable increase of cancer cell-mediated C-X-C motif chemokine ligand 5 (CXCL5) has been described [14]. At the same time, CAF showed an increase in IL-1β production [33]. IL-1β is known to induce the expression of CXCL5 as an inflammatory cytokine. In vitro experiments have demonstrated a stimulatory effect of CXCL5 on CCA cell migration and proliferation as well as invasive properties. This effect is most likely mediated via CXCR2-dependent PI3/Akt and extracellular signal-regulated kinase (ERK) 1/2 activation [33]. Furthermore, CXCL5 has been described as a chemokine that strongly drives neutrophil recruitment into the tissue in different diseases [38, 39].

In contrast, thrombospondin-1 secretion by CAFs appears to induce immunosuppression via TGF-β activation [40]. CAFs are meanwhile seen as a central player in tumor immune mechanisms and tumor-promoting immunosuppression. Effects of CAFs on tumor immunity are discussed further below.

CXCL12, or stromal cell-derived factor-1, is secreted by CAFs as a ligand of the CXCR4 and CXCR7 chemokine receptors that act in a G protein-coupled manner. Together with molecules from the interleukin family, it regulates the recruitment of endothelial cells and leukocytes in inflammation and malignancy. CAFs have been described as one of the primary sources of CXCL12, and the CXCL12 / CXCR4 axis has been found as important tumor promoter in various malignancies [41, 42], including gallbladder carcinoma [43]. Overexpression of CXLC12 is associated with poor prognosis in CCA [44]. In vitro, CXCL12 promotes cell survival and invasive growth of CCA cells. The mechanism is most likely an upregulation of anti-apoptotic Bcl-2 and activation of phosphatidylinositol 3-kinase (PI3K) and ERK 1/2 pathways [45]. This effect could be further enhanced through the overexpression of CXCR4 in CCA cells, induced by CAF-secreted HGF or tumor-associated macrophage (TAM)-released TNF-α [46, 47]. CXLC12 also seems to act in an autocrine and paracrine fashion, not only acting on CCA cells but also activating quiescent HSC and stromal fibroblasts to a CAF phenotype [45].

CAF and EGF Signaling

The interplay between CAF and CCA cells also relies on the HB-EGF/epidermal growth factor receptor (EGFR) signaling axis. Activating EGFR mutations and overexpression are among the most common alterations in CCA and have been linked to worse prognosis in CCA patients [7, 48, 49], while HB-EGF as an EGFR ligand has been implicated in cancer development [50]. This interaction of CAF-derived HB-EGF and EGFR on CCA cells has also been characterized in vitro [37]. CCA cells were reported to demonstrate enhanced proliferative, migratory, and invasive activity when incubated with HB-EGF-conditioned media from activated fibroblasts. In addition, HB-EGF-treated CCA cells have been found to overexpress TGF-β and thereby further stimulate CAFs to secrete EGF in a paracrine fashion [51].

CAF and Pro-angiogenic Signaling

CAFs have a well-known pro-angiogenic role, as they represent a main source of vascular endothelial growth factor A (VEGFA) in the TME [52]. In a VEGF-independent way, CAFs further support neoangiogenesis by PDGF and FGF2 as well as osteopontin release [53]. The recruitment of endothelial cells and bone marrow-derived monocytes via the CXCL12 pathway is another mechanism of pro-angiogenic CAF effects [54].

Besides their evident pro-tumorigenic effects, CAFs, or at least certain subpopulations thereof, do exert antitumor effects. These are primarily mediated through regulation of antitumor immunity. In genetically engineered mouse models of pancreatic cancer, depletion of αSMA-positive CAFs was (surprisingly) shown to result in more aggressive, enhanced tumor growth [55]. These findings underscore that the role of CAFs in the tumor is more complex and multidimensional than merely forming the soil for cancer growth.

Druggable Targets in CAFs

As previously mentioned, CAFs exhibit an increased sensitivity to apoptotic stimuli. This is due to changes in the expression of apoptosis-regulating Bcl-2 proteins. In vitro as well as in a rat model of CCA, the pro-apoptotic BH3 mimetic navitoclax was effective in depleting CAFs by inducing apoptosis and subsequently improved survival in the animal model [17].

Inhibiting PDGF, its receptor PDGFR or downstream activation of the Hedgehog pathway, for example, by imatinib mesylate or cyclopamine, has been shown to promote cancer cell apoptosis in vitro and in a murine CCA model [34, 35]. Of importance, reduction of tumor growth and vascularization was seen in models of co-implanted xenografts only, supporting the concept that HSCs or CAFs are pivotal for activation of the Hedgehog pathway [56]. PDGFRβ-directed therapy with sorafenib has been explored in a clinical trial for advanced ICC, with some beneficial effect [57].

In another study, inhibition of TGF-β signaling was similarly found to result in reduced CCA growth in a rat model [58].

Targeting the EGFR signaling axis is currently being explored in clinical trials [59, 60], as are other approaches.

Reprogramming of Cellular Immunity

CAFs can be activated by tumor cells but also interact with other cells types by secreting a multitude of factors to modulate the TME, thereby influencing innate and adaptive immune responses. Thus, CAFs have a crucial influence on the recruitment of immune cells such as macrophages, monocytes, and neutrophils into the tumor [61]. In other tumor entities such as lymphoma or breast cancer, CAF-mediated recruitment of macrophages has been shown to promote tumor growth and metastasis [62, 63]. More detailed knowledge regarding CAF subpopulations suggests that a distinct phenotype of inflammatory CAFs are primarily responsible for contributing to an inflammatory milieu [64].

Extracellular Matrix

The ECM is a noncellular mixture of macromolecules, including fibrous proteins such as collagen, fibronectin, laminin, and tenascin, and proteoglycans [65]. By providing structural signals for tumor growth and migration, the ECM can favor tumor progression.

Besides cancer cells, CAFs are able to produce ECM macromolecules but also ECM remodeling enzymes such as lysyl oxidases (LOXs) and matrix metalloproteinase (MMPs). LOX enzymes increase the crosslinking of collagen and elastin, thereby contributing to increased stiffness of the TME [66]. It has been demonstrated for many cancers that LOX levels are elevated in and correlate with tumor progression [67]. In CCA, increased LOXL2 expression correlates with αSMA expression and poor overall survival [68]. LOX inhibitors have been tested in combination with anticancer drugs to improve drug delivery. LOX inhibition was found to improve the diffusion of doxorubicin in a 3D spheroid model using four different mouse tumor cell lines [69] and demonstrated potent antitumor activities in vitro and in vivo in breast and pancreatic cancers [70, 71]. However, recent clinical trials failed to show enhancement of anticancer benefits in breast and colorectal cancer [63, 72].

Tissue stiffness can lead to increased malignancy through activation of the intracellular mechanosensor yes-associated protein (YAP), the effector protein of the Hippo pathway [73]. CCA patients show an upregulated expression of YAP and its transcriptional coactivator with PDZ-binding motif (TAZ). Moreover, increased nuclear localization of YAP correlates with metastasis and poor prognosis [74, 75]. *Lentivirus*-mediated silencing of YAP has been shown to increase tumor sensitivity to chemotherapy and inhibit CCA tumorigenesis both in vivo and in vitro [75].

To migrate through the stiff matrix, cancer cells produce matrix-degrading MMPs. MMP2 and MMP9 are increased in many cancer types [76]. CAFs have been shown to be the major producer of MMP2 in mouse lung tumors [77]. In CCA, CAF-mediated expression of MMP1, MMP2, MMP3, and MMP9 is associated with tumor aggressiveness [78, 79]. In addition, MMP9 expression correlates with CCA progression and metastasis [80]. Thus, MMP inhibition might be a new target for future cancer therapy. To date, however, although more than 50 MMP inhibitors have been investigated in clinical trials, none of them showed antitumor effects. Thus, more research is needed to unravel the, to some extent controversial, impact of MMPs on cancer.

Immune Cells

In order to escape immune surveillance and killing by cytotoxic lymphocytes, cancer cells manipulate their environment toward a tolerant and immunosuppressive setting. In addition to the cancer cells themselves, CAFs are central players in shaping the TME (Fig. 24.3). Both CAF and cancer cells communicate extensively with tumor-infiltrating immune cells from the innate and adaptive immune system, thereby stimulating immune suppression, angiogenesis, and tumor progression. The impact of immune cells on CCA is summarized in Table 24.1.

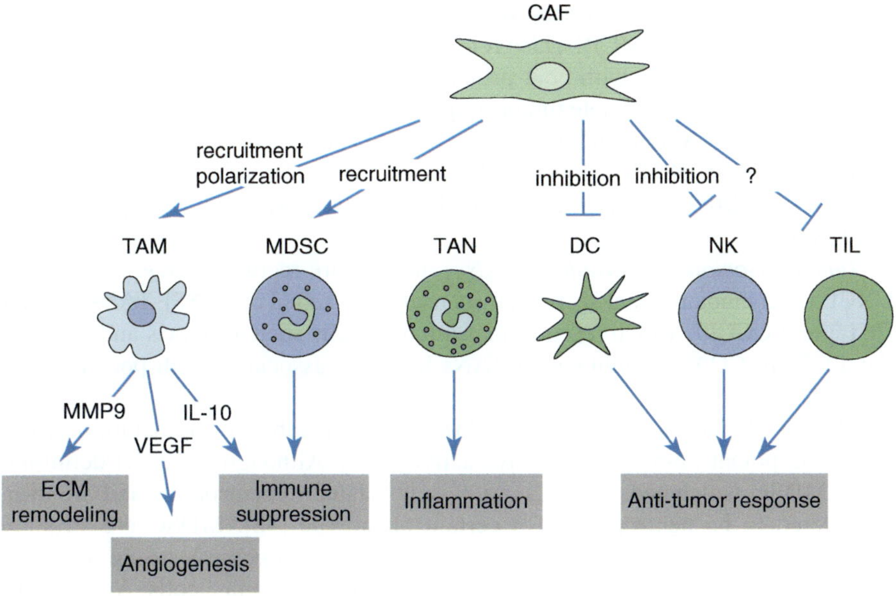

Fig. 24.3 Influence of cancer-associated fibroblasts (CAFs) on regulation and function of immune cells in cholangiocarcinoma. By mediating soluble factors, CAFs support the recruitment and activity of immune cells in the tumor microenvironment. CAFs favor M2 polarization of tumor-associated macrophages (TAMs) that support tumor progression via remodeling of the extracellular matrix (ECM), stimulation of angiogenesis and enhancing immune suppression. In addition, CAFs are able to recruit immunosuppressive myeloid-derived suppressor cells (MDSCs). On the other hand, CAFs inhibit the activity of dendritic cells (DCs) and natural killer cells (NKs). Whether CCA-derived CAFs can affect tumor-infiltrating lymphocytes (TILs), as demonstrated for other cancers, is not yet fully understood

Table 24.1 Impact of immune cell components on cholangiocarcinoma

Immune cell component	Impact on cholangiocarcinoma
TAMs	Immunosuppressive via IL-10 secretion and T-cell suppression ECM remodeling via MPP9 secretion Angiogenesis via VAGF secretion
TANs	Recruitment of other immunosuppressive immune cells
MDSCs	Immunosuppressive regulation other immune cells (inhibition of T and NK cells)
DCs	Tumor inhibition via recruitment and activation of lymphocytes
NKs	Tumor inhibition via cancer cell cytotoxicity
TILs	Tumor inhibition

Components of the Innate Immune Response

Tumor-associated macrophages (TAMs) are alternatively activated, pro-tumorigenic M2-like macrophages that mediate their immunosuppressive properties via ECM remodeling, angiogenesis, and suppression of T-cell activity/proliferation. CAFs have been demonstrated to recruit M2 macrophages via secretion of monocyte chemoattractant protein 1 (MCP1), also referred to as CCL2 [81]. In CCA, the M2-like phenotype is associated with poor prognosis and metastasis [82]. TAMs secrete a variety of factors that promote tumor progression on many levels such as angiogenesis (VEGFA), ECM remodeling (TGF-β, MMP9), antigen presentation, and immunosuppression (IL-10) [83]. In CCA, TAMs are the main source of MMP9, and the number of MMP9-secreting TAMs is significantly correlated with patient survival [84].

Tumor-associated neutrophils (TANs) in CCA are recruited predominantly by CXCL5, a chemoattractant secreted by cancer and stromal cells [85]. TANs express CCL2 and CCL17, which recruit other immune cells such as TAMs and Tregs to the TME. In CCA, the number of TANs has been associated with poor prognosis [86].

Myeloid-derived suppressor cells (MDSCs) are a subset of immature myeloid cells with potent immunosuppressive activity [87]. Although the exact definition of an MDSC is debated, MDSCs are closely related to neutrophils and are even considered to be neutrophils of a certain phenotype [88]. MDSC are strongly increased in pathological conditions such as cancer and possess strong immunosuppressive activities, regulating the function of other immune cells. Among others, MDSC inhibit cytotoxic T cells and NK cells via antigen-dependent and antigen-independent mechanisms. In CCA, a specific FAP-positive CAF subset enhances MDSC recruitment via CCL2/MCP1 secretion, thereby mediating tumor-promoting inflammation and immunosuppression [89]. Nevertheless, the contribution of MDSC to CCA progression is relatively unexplored, and further studies are needed.

Dendritic cells (DCs) are a heterogeneous group of functionally specialized antigen-presenting cells, uniquely able to initiate the adaptive immune response by presenting immunogenetic peptides via antigen-presenting major histocompatibility complex (MHC) class I and II molecules to naïve T cells [90]. Hence, DCs induce a cellular immune response that involves both CD4+ T helper and cytolytic CD8+ T cells.

CAFs are able to mediate immunosuppression on DCs via downregulation of MHC class II molecules in a TGF-β-dependent manner, thus reducing the capability to activate cytotoxic T cells [91]. In CCA patients, mature DCs might be able to enhance CD8- and CD4-positive cell infiltration into cancers, since increased numbers of mature DCs at the invasive margin correlate significantly with the number of CD8-positive or CD4-positive T cells in the cancerous region [92]. In addition, CCA patients with increased numbers of mature DCs have a significantly lower incidence of lymph node metastasis and a better outcome [92]. Immunotherapy using mature DCs loaded with aspartate-β-hydroxylase, a highly expressed tumor-associated cell surface protein, has been reported to induce antigen-specific immunity, cytotoxicity against tumor cells, and inhibition of tumor growth in a syngeneic rat model of CCA [93].

In addition to the abovementioned immune cells, the liver hosts an abundance of *natural killer* (NK) cells, which are important mediators of immunological tolerance in the liver [94]. NK cells are able to recognize and eliminate abnormal cells such as cancer cells. In CCA, genetic variants of the NK cell receptor NKG2D are associated with development of CCA in PSC patients [95]. Furthermore, treatment of CCA cells with cytokine-activated killer cells (including acNK and T cells) and cetuximab has been shown to enhance cytotoxic efficiency on cancer cells in vitro [96]. In vivo, infusion of ex vivo-expanded human NK cells in HuCCT-1 tumor-bearing nude mice has similarly been found to result in significant inhibition of CCA [97].

Components of the Adaptive Immune Response

Tumor-infiltrating lymphocytes (TILs) are a heterogeneous group of immune cells that are recruited from the blood into the tumor to eliminate cancer cells. TILs include CD8+ cytotoxic T cells, CD4 + T helper cells, Foxp3+ regulatory T cells, and B lymphocytes.

Biliary tract cancer patients with increased numbers of tumor-infiltrating CD4+, CD8+, and FoxP3+ T lymphocytes showed a significantly longer overall survival [98]. Analysis of the adaptive immune system in CCA is based primarily on immunohistochemical studies. Although adaptive immune response components decrease with CCA progression, more than half of CCAs are positive for CD4+ and CD8+ TILs [98], and an increased number of TILs are associated with improved overall patient survival [99, 100]. Interestingly, CD8+ TILs are predominantly located within the tumor tissue and CD4+ TILs in the peritumoral area [101].

Regulatory T cells, which express FoxP3, play a role in promoting antigen tolerance and immunosuppression in different malignancies. In CCA, FoxP3 expression is associated with a worse prognosis in CCA [102].

In cancer therapy, adoptive T-cell therapy is an approach to increase the number of endogenous/autologous activated cytotoxic T lymphocytes in the TME. Ongoing clinical trials evaluate the benefit of adoptive immunotherapy in biliary tract cancers in combination with additional therapeutic approaches [103].

Among TILs, B cells represent only a minor proportion in CCA. However, it has been observed that their presence is associated with a favorable prognosis [98].

Exosomes: Biological Role and Clinical Implications

Exosomes are small, lipid bilayer extracellular vesicles of endosomal origin with an average size of 100 nm in diameter. Depending on their origin, exosomes can contain a variety of cellular components including proteins, mRNAs, miRNAs, lipids, and metabolites. Although exosomes have been described already in the early 1980s [104, 105], the physiological role remains largely unknown, but over the last decade, the general interest of the scientific community has evolved exponentially [106]. Recent studies suggest a role in near and long-distance intracellular communication, thereby affecting various physiological and pathological conditions such as immune response, mammalian reproduction, viral infection, cardiovascular disease, and cancer. Most cell types, including cancer cells, can release exosomes. Interestingly, tumor cells exhibit an enhanced production of these extracellular vesicles and have been shown to promote tumor growth, ECM remodeling, angiogenesis, metastasis, and resistance to therapy in various cancer types [22]. Cancer cell-derived exosomes are enriched in immunosuppressive and pro-tumorigenic molecules including death receptor ligands such as Fas-ligand (FasL) or TRAIL, check point receptor ligands such as programmed death-ligand 1 (PD-L1), and inhibitory cytokines such as IL-10 and TGF-β1 [107]. Most studies suggest that cancer-derived exosomes are able to reprogram their microenvironment to favour tumor progression. Well-studied stromal recipient cells are CAFs and immune cells.

Recent studies in liver cancer suggest that CCA-derived extracellular vesicles (in most cases exosomes) carry oncogenic proteins that promote CCA growth and progression [108]. Although there appear to be no differences in serum concentrations of extracellular vesicle in patients with PSC, CCA, and healthy controls [108], intravesicular differences do exist; indeed, well-characterized cancer-associated miRNAs are significantly up- and downregulated in CCA-derived exosomes compared with normal cholangiocyte-derived exosomes and controls [109]. Given that exosomes are released into body fluids such as blood and urine, they have potential as noninvasive biomarkers. CCA-derived exosomes contain molecules with relvant diagnostic potential. Arbelaiz et al. identified several proteins differentially expressed between the serum extracellular vesicles of PSC, CCA, and healthy patients. In particular, fibrinogen gamma chain, alpha-1-acid glycoprotein 1, and S100A8 showed the best differential diagnostic capacity whereas ficolin-2 and inter-alpha-trypsin inhibitor heavy chain H4, among others, showing higher diagnostic value than the traditional serum tumor marker carbohydrate antigen 19–9 [108]. Of note, although serum concentrations of extracellular vesicles are not elevated in CCA patients, biliary concentrations of extracellular vesicles are significantly increased in CCA patients [110]. Furthermore, a panel of miRNAs (miR-191, miR-486-3p, miR-1274b) are upregulated in bile extracellular vesicles of CCA patients [110].

Due to their membrane structure, exosomes could serve as natural carriers of therapeutic agents for cancer therapy as well. An interesting candidate for extracellular vesicle-based CCA therapy is miR-195, a fibroblast-derived extracellular vesicle cargo that is downregulated in human CCA cells and was demonstrated to inhibit CCA growth in vitro and in vivo [111]. Therapeutic delivery of miR-195 might therefore be a future therapeutic approach.

Conclusions

Cholangiocarcinoma epitomizes the concept of a stroma-driven malignancy. The stromal part of the cancer not only forms the largest part of the tumor but contains several nonmalignant cell populations that together with their respective signals must be considered crucial for tumor development and progression. First and foremost, CAFs are the most abundant cell type in CCA and contribute essential growth factors and ECM components that promote CCA growth. Cancer-associated immune cells of the stromal compartment further contribute to the highly complex and heterogenous tumor microenvironment. Deciphering, understanding, and specifically targeting the CCA stroma hold the promise to contribute effective therapies for this still dismal disease.

References

1. Quail DF, Joyce JA. Microenvironmental regulation of tumor progression and metastasis. Nat Med. 2013;19(11):1423–37.
2. Greaves M, Maley CC. Clonal evolution in cancer. Nature. 2012;481(7381):306–13.
3. Razumilava N, Gores GJ. Cholangiocarcinoma. Lancet. 2014;383(9935):2168–79.
4. Sirica AE, Gores GJ. Desmoplastic stroma and cholangiocarcinoma: clinical implications and therapeutic targeting. Hepatology. 2014;59(6):2397–402.
5. TexasPathologistMSW. 2016. Available from: https://commons.wikimedia.org/wiki/File:4_CCA_1_680x512px.tif.
6. https://creativecommons.org/licenses/by-sa/4.0/deed.en.
7. Andersen JB, Spee B, Blechacz BR, Avital I, Komuta M, Barbour A, et al. Genomic and genetic characterization of cholangiocarcinoma identifies therapeutic targets for tyrosine kinase inhibitors. Gastroenterology. 2012;142(4):1021–31. e15.
8. Sulpice L, Rayar M, Desille M, Turlin B, Fautrel A, Boucher E, et al. Molecular profiling of stroma identifies osteopontin as an independent predictor of poor prognosis in intrahepatic cholangiocarcinoma. Hepatology. 2013;58(6):1992–2000.
9. Chuaysri C, Thuwajit P, Paupairoj A, Chau-In S, Suthiphongchai T, Thuwajit C. Alpha-smooth muscle actin-positive fibroblasts promote biliary cell proliferation and correlate with poor survival in cholangiocarcinoma. Oncol Rep. 2009;21(4):957–69.
10. Okabe H, Beppu T, Hayashi H, Ishiko T, Masuda T, Otao R, et al. Hepatic stellate cells accelerate the malignant behavior of cholangiocarcinoma cells. Ann Surg Oncol. 2011;18(4):1175–84.
11. Cadamuro M, Stecca T, Brivio S, Mariotti V, Fiorotto R, Spirli C, et al. The deleterious interplay between tumor epithelia and stroma in cholangiocarcinoma. Biochim Biophys Acta Mol basis Dis. 2018;1864(4 Pt B):1435–43.
12. Sirica AE. The role of cancer-associated myofibroblasts in intrahepatic cholangiocarcinoma. Nat Rev Gastroenterol Hepatol. 2011;9(1):44–54.
13. Mertens J, Stuber K, Wunderlich P, Ladewig J, Kesavan JC, Vandenberghe R, et al. APP processing in human pluripotent stem cell-derived neurons is resistant to NSAID-based gamma-secretase modulation. Stem Cell Reports. 2013;1(6):491–8.
14. Brivio S, Cadamuro M, Strazzabosco M, Fabris L. Tumor reactive stroma in cholangiocarcinoma: the fuel behind cancer aggressiveness. World J Hepatol. 2017;9(9):455–68.
15. Gentilini A, Pastore M, Marra F, Raggi C. The role of stroma in cholangiocarcinoma: the intriguing interplay between fibroblastic component, immune cell subsets and tumor epithelium. Int J Mol Sci. 2018;19(10):2885.

16. Cadamuro M, Morton SD, Strazzabosco M, Fabris L. Unveiling the role of tumor reactive stroma in cholangiocarcinoma: an opportunity for new therapeutic strategies. Transl Gastrointest Cancer. 2013;2(3):130–44.
17. Mertens JC, Fingas CD, Christensen JD, Smoot RL, Bronk SF, Werneburg NW, et al. Therapeutic effects of deleting cancer-associated fibroblasts in cholangiocarcinoma. Cancer Res. 2013;73(2):897–907.
18. Mederacke I, Hsu CC, Troeger JS, Huebener P, Mu X, Dapito DH, et al. Fate tracing reveals hepatic stellate cells as dominant contributors to liver fibrosis independent of its aetiology. Nat Commun. 2013;4:2823.
19. Leyva-Illades D, McMillin M, Quinn M, Demorrow S. Cholangiocarcinoma pathogenesis: role of the tumor microenvironment. Transl Gastrointest Cancer. 2012;1(1):71–80.
20. Brivio S, Cadamuro M, Fabris L, Strazzabosco M. Epithelial-to-mesenchymal transition and cancer invasiveness: what can we learn from cholangiocarcinoma? J Clin Med. 2015;4(12):2028–41.
21. Cadamuro M, Nardo G, Indraccolo S, Dall'olmo L, Sambado L, Moserle L, et al. Platelet-derived growth factor-D and Rho GTPases regulate recruitment of cancer-associated fibroblasts in cholangiocarcinoma. Hepatology. 2013;58(3):1042–53.
22. Kalluri R. The biology and function of fibroblasts in cancer. Nat Rev Cancer. 2016;16(9):582–98.
23. Liao Z, Tan ZW, Zhu P, Tan NS. Cancer-associated fibroblasts in tumor microenvironment - accomplices in tumor malignancy. Cell Immunol. 2019;343:103729.
24. Sha M, Jeong S, Qiu BJ, Tong Y, Xia L, Xu N, et al. Isolation of cancer-associated fibroblasts and its promotion to the progression of intrahepatic cholangiocarcinoma. Cancer Med. 2018;7(9):4665–77.
25. Ferdek PE, Jakubowska MA. Biology of pancreatic stellate cells-more than just pancreatic cancer. Pflugers Arch. 2017;469(9):1039–50.
26. Lynch MD, Watt FM. Fibroblast heterogeneity: implications for human disease. J Clin Invest. 2018;128(1):26–35.
27. Vaquero J, Aoudjehane L, Fouassier L. Cancer-associated fibroblasts in cholangiocarcinoma. Curr Opin Gastroenterol. 2020;36(2):63–9.
28. Ohlund D, Handly-Santana A, Biffi G, Elyada E, Almeida AS, Ponz-Sarvise M, et al. Distinct populations of inflammatory fibroblasts and myofibroblasts in pancreatic cancer. J Exp Med. 2017;214(3):579–96.
29. Neuzillet C, Tijeras-Raballand A, Ragulan C, Cros J, Patil Y, Martinet M, et al. Inter- and intra-tumoural heterogeneity in cancer-associated fibroblasts of human pancreatic ductal adenocarcinoma. J Pathol. 2019;248(1):51–65.
30. Ostman A, Augsten M. Cancer-associated fibroblasts and tumor growth--bystanders turning into key players. Curr Opin Genet Dev. 2009;19(1):67–73.
31. Sahai E, Astsaturov I, Cukierman E, DeNardo DG, Egeblad M, Evans RM, et al. A framework for advancing our understanding of cancer-associated fibroblasts. Nat Rev Cancer. 2020;20(3):174–86.
32. Heits N, Heinze T, Bernsmeier A, Kerber J, Hauser C, Becker T, et al. Influence of mTOR-inhibitors and mycophenolic acid on human cholangiocellular carcinoma and cancer associated fibroblasts. BMC Cancer. 2016;16:322.
33. Okabe H, Beppu T, Hayashi H, Horino K, Masuda T, Komori H, et al. Hepatic stellate cells may relate to progression of intrahepatic cholangiocarcinoma. Ann Surg Oncol. 2009;16(9):2555–64.
34. Fingas CD, Mertens JC, Razumilava N, Bronk SF, Sirica AE, Gores GJ. Targeting PDGFR-beta in cholangiocarcinoma. Liver Int. 2012;32(3):400–9.
35. Fingas CD, Bronk SF, Werneburg NW, Mott JL, Guicciardi ME, Cazanave SC, et al. Myofibroblast-derived PDGF-BB promotes Hedgehog survival signaling in cholangiocarcinoma cells. Hepatology. 2011;54(6):2076–88.

36. Porsch H, Mehic M, Olofsson B, Heldin P, Heldin CH. Platelet-derived growth factor beta-receptor, transforming growth factor beta type I receptor, and CD44 protein modulate each other's signaling and stability. J Biol Chem. 2014;289(28):19747–57.
37. Claperon A, Mergey M, Aoudjehane L, Ho-Bouldoires TH, Wendum D, Prignon A, et al. Hepatic myofibroblasts promote the progression of human cholangiocarcinoma through activation of epidermal growth factor receptor. Hepatology. 2013;58(6):2001–11.
38. Disteldorf EM, Krebs CF, Paust HJ, Turner JE, Nouailles G, Tittel A, et al. CXCL5 drives neutrophil recruitment in TH17-mediated GN. J Am Soc Nephrol. 2015;26(1):55–66.
39. Zhou SL, Zhou ZJ, Hu ZQ, Li X, Huang XW, Wang Z, et al. CXCR2/CXCL5 axis contributes to epithelial-mesenchymal transition of HCC cells through activating PI3K/Akt/GSK-3beta/Snail signaling. Cancer Lett. 2015;358(2):124–35.
40. Silzle T, Randolph GJ, Kreutz M, Kunz-Schughart LA. The fibroblast: sentinel cell and local immune modulator in tumor tissue. Int J Cancer. 2004;108(2):173–80.
41. Sugihara H, Ishimoto T, Yasuda T, Izumi D, Eto K, Sawayama H, et al. Cancer-associated fibroblast-derived CXCL12 causes tumor progression in adenocarcinoma of the esophagogastric junction. Med Oncol. 2015;32(6):618.
42. Domanska UM, Kruizinga RC, Nagengast WB, Timmer-Bosscha H, Huls G, de Vries EG, et al. A review on CXCR4/CXCL12 axis in oncology: no place to hide. Eur J Cancer. 2013;49(1):219–30.
43. Lee HJ, Lee K, Lee DG, Bae KH, Kim JS, Liang ZL, et al. Chemokine (C-X-C motif) ligand 12 is associated with gallbladder carcinoma progression and is a novel independent poor prognostic factor. Clin Cancer Res. 2012;18(12):3270–80.
44. Okamoto K, Tajima H, Nakanuma S, Sakai S, Makino I, Kinoshita J, et al. Angiotensin II enhances epithelial-to-mesenchymal transition through the interaction between activated hepatic stellate cells and the stromal cell-derived factor-1/CXCR4 axis in intrahepatic cholangiocarcinoma. Int J Oncol. 2012;41(2):573–82.
45. Gentilini A, Rombouts K, Galastri S, Caligiuri A, Mingarelli E, Mello T, et al. Role of the stromal-derived factor-1 (SDF-1)-CXCR4 axis in the interaction between hepatic stellate cells and cholangiocarcinoma. J Hepatol. 2012;57(4):813–20.
46. Campbell DJ, Dumur CI, Lamour NF, Dewitt JL, Sirica AE. Novel organotypic culture model of cholangiocarcinoma progression. Hepatol Res. 2012;42(11):1119–30.
47. Ohira S, Sasaki M, Harada K, Sato Y, Zen Y, Isse K, et al. Possible regulation of migration of intrahepatic cholangiocarcinoma cells by interaction of CXCR4 expressed in carcinoma cells with tumor necrosis factor-alpha and stromal-derived factor-1 released in stroma. Am J Pathol. 2006;168(4):1155–68.
48. Gwak GY, Yoon JH, Shin CM, Ahn YJ, Chung JK, Kim YA, et al. Detection of response-predicting mutations in the kinase domain of the epidermal growth factor receptor gene in cholangiocarcinomas. J Cancer Res Clin Oncol. 2005;131(10):649–52.
49. Chong DQ, Zhu AX. The landscape of targeted therapies for cholangiocarcinoma: current status and emerging targets. Oncotarget. 2016;7(29):46750–67.
50. Sagmeister S, Drucker C, Losert A, Grusch M, Daryabeigi A, Parzefall W, et al. HB-EGF is a paracrine growth stimulator for early tumor prestages in inflammation-associated hepatocarcinogenesis. J Hepatol. 2008;49(6):955–64.
51. Vaquero J, Lobe C, Fouassier L. Unveiling resistance mechanisms to EGFR inhibitors in cholangiocarcinoma. Oncotarget. 2018;9(99):37274–5.
52. De Palma M, Biziato D, Petrova TV. Microenvironmental regulation of tumour angiogenesis. Nat Rev Cancer. 2017;17(8):457–74.
53. Hou X, Kumar A, Lee C, Wang B, Arjunan P, Dong L, et al. PDGF-CC blockade inhibits pathological angiogenesis by acting on multiple cellular and molecular targets. Proc Natl Acad Sci U S A. 2010;107(27):12216–21.
54. Orimo A, Gupta PB, Sgroi DC, Arenzana-Seisdedos F, Delaunay T, Naeem R, et al. Stromal fibroblasts present in invasive human breast carcinomas promote tumor growth and angiogenesis through elevated SDF-1/CXCL12 secretion. Cell. 2005;121(3):335–48.

55. Ozdemir BC, Pentcheva-Hoang T, Carstens JL, Zheng X, Wu CC, Simpson TR, et al. Depletion of carcinoma-associated fibroblasts and fibrosis induces immunosuppression and accelerates pancreas cancer with reduced survival. Cancer Cell. 2014;25(6):719–34.
56. Kim Y, Kim MO, Shin JS, Park SH, Kim SB, Kim J, et al. Hedgehog signaling between cancer cells and hepatic stellate cells in promoting cholangiocarcinoma. Ann Surg Oncol. 2014;21(8):2684–98.
57. Pan TT, Wang W, Jia WD, Xu GL. A single-center experience of sorafenib monotherapy in patients with advanced intrahepatic cholangiocarcinoma. Oncol Lett. 2017;13(5):2957–64.
58. Ling H, Roux E, Hempel D, Tao J, Smith M, Lonning S, et al. Transforming growth factor beta neutralization ameliorates pre-existing hepatic fibrosis and reduces cholangiocarcinoma in thioacetamide-treated rats. PLoS One. 2013;8(1):e54499.
59. Rizvi S, Khan SA, Hallemeier CL, Kelley RK, Gores GJ. Cholangiocarcinoma - evolving concepts and therapeutic strategies. Nat Rev Clin Oncol. 2018;15(2):95–111.
60. Mahipal A, Kommalapati A, Tella SH, Lim A, Kim R. Novel targeted treatment options for advanced cholangiocarcinoma. Expert Opin Investig Drugs. 2018;27(9):709–20.
61. Monteran L, Erez N. The dark side of fibroblasts: cancer-associated fibroblasts as mediators of immunosuppression in the tumor microenvironment. Front Immunol. 2019;10:1835.
62. Pollard JW. Tumour-educated macrophages promote tumour progression and metastasis. Nat Rev Cancer. 2004;4(1):71–8.
63. Hecht JR, Benson AB 3rd, Vyushkov D, Yang Y, Bendell J, Verma U. A phase II, randomized, double-blind, placebo-controlled study of simtuzumab in combination with FOLFIRI for the second-line treatment of metastatic KRAS mutant colorectal adenocarcinoma. Oncologist. 2017;22(3):243–e23.
64. Biffi G, Oni TE, Spielman B, Hao Y, Elyada E, Park Y, et al. IL1-induced JAK/STAT signaling is antagonized by TGFbeta to shape CAF heterogeneity in pancreatic ductal adenocarcinoma. Cancer Discov. 2019;9(2):282–301.
65. Frantz C, Stewart KM, Weaver VM. The extracellular matrix at a glance. J Cell Sci. 2010;123(Pt 24):4195–200.
66. Tenti P, Vannucci L. Lysyl oxidases: linking structures and immunity in the tumor microenvironment. Cancer Immunol Immunother. 2020;69(2):223–35.
67. Trackman PC. Lysyl oxidase isoforms and potential therapeutic opportunities for fibrosis and cancer. Expert Opin Ther Targets. 2016;20(8):935–45.
68. Bergeat D, Fautrel A, Turlin B, Merdrignac A, Rayar M, Boudjema K, et al. Impact of stroma LOXL2 overexpression on the prognosis of intrahepatic cholangiocarcinoma. J Surg Res. 2016;203(2):441–50.
69. Schutze F, Rohrig F, Vorlova S, Gatzner S, Kuhn A, Ergun S, et al. Inhibition of lysyl oxidases improves drug diffusion and increases efficacy of cytotoxic treatment in 3D tumor models. Sci Rep. 2015;5:17576.
70. Park JS, Lee JH, Lee YS, Kim JK, Dong SM, Yoon DS. Emerging role of LOXL2 in the promotion of pancreas cancer metastasis. Oncotarget. 2016;7(27):42539–52.
71. Chang J, Lucas MC, Leonte LE, Garcia-Montolio M, Singh LB, Findlay AD, et al. Preclinical evaluation of small molecule LOXL2 inhibitors in breast cancer. Oncotarget. 2017;8(16):26066–78.
72. Benson AB 3rd, Wainberg ZA, Hecht JR, Vyushkov D, Dong H, Bendell J, et al. A phase II randomized, double-blind, placebo-controlled study of simtuzumab or placebo in combination with gemcitabine for the first-line treatment of pancreatic adenocarcinoma. Oncologist. 2017;22(3):241–e15.
73. Liu AM, Xu MZ, Chen J, Poon RT, Luk JM. Targeting YAP and Hippo signaling pathway in liver cancer. Expert Opin Ther Targets. 2010;14(8):855–68.
74. Van Haele M, Moya IM, Karaman R, Rens G, Snoeck J, Govaere O, et al. YAP and TAZ heterogeneity in primary liver cancer: an analysis of its prognostic and diagnostic role. Int J Mol Sci. 2019;20(3):638.
75. Pei T, Li Y, Wang J, Wang H, Liang Y, Shi H, et al. YAP is a critical oncogene in human cholangiocarcinoma. Oncotarget. 2015;6(19):17206–20.

76. Liu T, Zhou L, Li D, Andl T, Zhang Y. Cancer-associated fibroblasts build and secure the tumor microenvironment. Front Cell Dev Biol. 2019;7:60.
77. Bates AL, Pickup MW, Hallett MA, Dozier EA, Thomas S, Fingleton B. Stromal matrix metalloproteinase 2 regulates collagen expression and promotes the outgrowth of experimental metastases. J Pathol. 2015;235(5):773–83.
78. Terada T, Okada Y, Nakanuma Y. Expression of immunoreactive matrix metalloproteinases and tissue inhibitors of matrix metalloproteinases in human normal livers and primary liver tumors. Hepatology. 1996;23(6):1341–4.
79. Prakobwong S, Yongvanit P, Hiraku Y, Pairojkul C, Sithithaworn P, Pinlaor P, et al. Involvement of MMP-9 in peribiliary fibrosis and cholangiocarcinogenesis via Rac1-dependent DNA damage in a hamster model. Int J Cancer. 2010;127(11):2576–87.
80. Sun Q, Zhao C, Xia L, He Z, Lu Z, Liu C, et al. High expression of matrix metalloproteinase-9 indicates poor prognosis in human hilar cholangiocarcinoma. Int J Clin Exp Pathol. 2014;7(9):6157–64.
81. Zhang J, Chen L, Xiao M, Wang C, Qin Z. FSP1+ fibroblasts promote skin carcinogenesis by maintaining MCP-1-mediated macrophage infiltration and chronic inflammation. Am J Pathol. 2011;178(1):382–90.
82. Thanee M, Loilome W, Techasen A, Namwat N, Boonmars T, Pairojkul C, et al. Quantitative changes in tumor-associated M2 macrophages characterize cholangiocarcinoma and their association with metastasis. Asian Pac J Cancer Prev. 2015;16(7):3043–50.
83. Hasita H, Komohara Y, Okabe H, Masuda T, Ohnishi K, Lei XF, et al. Significance of alternatively activated macrophages in patients with intrahepatic cholangiocarcinoma. Cancer Sci. 2010;101(8):1913–9.
84. Subimerb C, Pinlaor S, Khuntikeo N, Leelayuwat C, Morris A, McGrath MS, et al. Tissue invasive macrophage density is correlated with prognosis in cholangiocarcinoma. Mol Med Rep. 2010;3(4):597–605.
85. Zhou SL, Dai Z, Zhou ZJ, Chen Q, Wang Z, Xiao YS, et al. CXCL5 contributes to tumor metastasis and recurrence of intrahepatic cholangiocarcinoma by recruiting infiltrative intratumoral neutrophils. Carcinogenesis. 2014;35(3):597–605.
86. Shen M, Hu P, Donskov F, Wang G, Liu Q, Du J. Tumor-associated neutrophils as a new prognostic factor in cancer: a systematic review and meta-analysis. PLoS One. 2014;9(6):e98259.
87. Gabrilovich DI. Myeloid-derived suppressor cells. Cancer Immunol Res. 2017;5(1):3–8.
88. Shaul ME, Fridlender ZG. Tumour-associated neutrophils in patients with cancer. Nat Rev Clin Oncol. 2019;16(10):601–20.
89. Yang X, Lin Y, Shi Y, Li B, Liu W, Yin W, et al. FAP Promotes Immunosuppression by Cancer-Associated Fibroblasts in the Tumor Microenvironment via STAT3-CCL2 Signaling. Cancer Res. 2016;76(14):4124–35.
90. Patente TA, Pinho MP, Oliveira AA, Evangelista GCM, Bergami-Santos PC, Barbuto JAM. Human dendritic cells: their heterogeneity and clinical application potential in cancer immunotherapy. Front Immunol. 2018;9:3176.
91. Flavell RA, Sanjabi S, Wrzesinski SH, Licona-Limon P. The polarization of immune cells in the tumour environment by TGFbeta. Nat Rev Immunol. 2010;10(8):554–67.
92. Takagi S, Miyagawa S, Ichikawa E, Soeda J, Miwa S, Miyagawa Y, et al. Dendritic cells, T-cell infiltration, and Grp94 expression in cholangiocellular carcinoma. Hum Pathol. 2004;35(7):881–6.
93. Noda T, Shimoda M, Ortiz V, Sirica AE, Wands JR. Immunization with aspartate-beta-hydroxylase-loaded dendritic cells produces antitumor effects in a rat model of intrahepatic cholangiocarcinoma. Hepatology. 2012;55(1):86–97.
94. Mikulak J, Bruni E, Oriolo F, Di Vito C, Mavilio D. Hepatic natural killer cells: organ-specific sentinels of liver immune homeostasis and physiopathology. Front Immunol. 2019;10:946.
95. Melum E, Karlsen TH, Schrumpf E, Bergquist A, Thorsby E, Boberg KM, et al. Cholangiocarcinoma in primary sclerosing cholangitis is associated with NKG2D polymorphisms. Hepatology. 2008;47(1):90–6.

96. Morisaki T, Umebayashi M, Kiyota A, Koya N, Tanaka H, Onishi H, et al. Combining cetuximab with killer lymphocytes synergistically inhibits human cholangiocarcinoma cells in vitro. Anticancer Res. 2012;32(6):2249–56.
97. Jung IH, Kim DH, Yoo DK, Baek SY, Jeong SH, Jung DE, et al. In vivo study of natural killer (NK) cell cytotoxicity against cholangiocarcinoma in a nude mouse model. In Vivo. 2018;32(4):771–81.
98. Goeppert B, Frauenschuh L, Zucknick M, Stenzinger A, Andrulis M, Klauschen F, et al. Prognostic impact of tumour-infiltrating immune cells on biliary tract cancer. Br J Cancer. 2013;109(10):2665–74.
99. Oshikiri T, Miyamoto M, Shichinohe T, Suzuoki M, Hiraoka K, Nakakubo Y, et al. Prognostic value of intratumoral CD8+ T lymphocyte in extrahepatic bile duct carcinoma as essential immune response. J Surg Oncol. 2003;84(4):224–8.
100. Lim YJ, Koh J, Kim K, Chie EK, Kim B, Lee KB, et al. High ratio of programmed cell death protein 1 (PD-1)(+)/CD8(+) tumor-infiltrating lymphocytes identifies a poor prognostic subset of extrahepatic bile duct cancer undergoing surgery plus adjuvant chemoradiotherapy. Radiother Oncol. 2015;117(1):165–70.
101. Kasper HU, Drebber U, Stippel DL, Dienes HP, Gillessen A. Liver tumor infiltrating lymphocytes: comparison of hepatocellular and cholangiolar carcinoma. World J Gastroenterol. 2009;15(40):5053–7.
102. Dunne RF, Findeis-Hosey J, Bratton L, Figueroa N, Belt B, McMahon L, et al. Association of FoxP3 expression with worse outcomes in cholangiocarcinoma: Evidence to support the use of immunotherapy. J Clin Oncol. 2016;34(15_suppl):e15631.
103. Blair AB, Murphy A. Immunotherapy as a treatment for biliary tract cancers: a review of approaches with an eye to the future. Curr Probl Cancer. 2018;42(1):49–58.
104. Harding C, Stahl P. Transferrin recycling in reticulocytes: pH and iron are important determinants of ligand binding and processing. Biochem Biophys Res Commun. 1983;113(2):650–8.
105. Pan BT, Johnstone RM. Fate of the transferrin receptor during maturation of sheep reticulocytes in vitro: selective externalization of the receptor. Cell. 1983;33(3):967–78.
106. Olaizola P, Lee-Law PY, Arbelaiz A, Lapitz A, Perugorria MJ, Bujanda L, et al. MicroRNAs and extracellular vesicles in cholangiopathies. Biochim Biophys Acta Mol basis Dis. 2018;1864(4 Pt B):1293–307.
107. Whiteside TL. Exosomes and tumor-mediated immune suppression. J Clin Invest. 2016;126(4):1216–23.
108. Arbelaiz A, Azkargorta M, Krawczyk M, Santos-Laso A, Lapitz A, Perugorria MJ, et al. Serum extracellular vesicles contain protein biomarkers for primary sclerosing cholangitis and cholangiocarcinoma. Hepatology. 2017;66(4):1125–43.
109. Kitdumrongthum S, Metheetrairut C, Charoensawan V, Ounjai P, Janpipatkul K, Panvongsa W, et al. Dysregulated microRNA expression profiles in cholangiocarcinoma cell-derived exosomes. Life Sci. 2018;210:65–75.
110. Li L, Masica D, Ishida M, Tomuleasa C, Umegaki S, Kalloo AN, et al. Human bile contains microRNA-laden extracellular vesicles that can be used for cholangiocarcinoma diagnosis. Hepatology. 2014;60(3):896–907.
111. Li L, Piontek K, Ishida M, Fausther M, Dranoff JA, Fu R, et al. Extracellular vesicles carry microRNA-195 to intrahepatic cholangiocarcinoma and improve survival in a rat model. Hepatology. 2017;65(2):501–14.

Chapter 25
Glycosylation in Cholangiocarcinoma Development and Metastasis: Diagnostic and Therapeutic Considerations

Atit Silsirivanit, Chatchai Phoomak, and Sopit Wongkham

Abbreviations

5-FU	5-fluorouracil
DON	6-Diazo-5-oxo-L-norleucine
MAN1A1	α1-mannosidase 1A
AFP	Alpha-fetoprotein
AFU	Alpha-L-fucosidase
Asn	Asparagine
BB	Benign bile tract disease
CA19–9	Carbohydrate antigen 19–9
CA-S27	Carbohydrate antigen-S27
Cer	Ceramide
CERS	Ceramide synthase
CCA	Cholangiocarcinoma
Dol-P	Dolichol phosphate
EMT	Epithelial to mesenchymal transition
ECCA	Extrahepatic CCA
FA2H	Fatty acid-2-hydroxylase
FOXO3	Forkhead box O3
Fuc	Fucose
FUT	Fucosyltransferase
Gal	Galactose

A. Silsirivanit (✉) · S. Wongkham
Department of Biochemistry, and Center for Translational Medicine, Faculty of Medicine, Khon Kaen University, Khon Kaen, Thailand
e-mail: atitsil@kku.ac.th; sopit@kku.ac.th

C. Phoomak
Department of Therapeutic Radiology, Yale University School of Medicine, New Haven, CT, USA
e-mail: chatchai.phoomak@yale.edu

J. H. Tabibian (ed.), *Diagnosis and Management of Cholangiocarcinoma*,
https://doi.org/10.1007/978-3-030-70936-5_25

GalCer	Galactosylceramide
GalT	Galactosyltransferase
GalNAcT5	GalNAc-transferase 5
Glc	Glucose
GlcCer	Glucosylceramide
GFAT	Glutamine-fructose amidotransferase
GSL	Glycosphingolipid
HC	Healthy controls
hnRNP-K	Heterogeneous nuclear ribonucleoprotein-K
HE4	Human epididymis protein 4
LacCer	Lactosylceramide
MAL	*Maackia amurensis* lectin
MAL-SG	MAL-II-binding glycan
Man	Mannose
MMP	Matrix metalloproteinase
mAb	Monoclonal antibody
MUC	Mucin
GalNAc	*N*-acetylgalactosamine
GlcNAc	*N*-acetylglucosamine
GlcNAc-T	*N*-acetylglucosaminyltransferase
NEU	Neuraminidase
POFUT1	O-fucosyltransferase 1
OGP	O-GlcNAcylated protein
OGT	O-linked β-N-acetylglucosaminyltransferase
OST	Oligosaccharyltransferase
PSA	*Pisum sativum* agglutinin
PSC	Primary sclerosing cholangitis
PSA	Prostate-specific antigen
SNA	*Sambucus nigra* agglutinin
Ser	Serine
sLe^a	Sialyl-Lewis A
sLe^x	Sialyl-Lewis X
sTn	Sialyl-Tn
ST	Sialyltransferase
SNAG	SJA-binding *N*-acetylgalactosamine-associated glycan
SNA-SG	SNA-binding glycan
SJA	*Sophora japonica* agglutinin
SBA	Soybean agglutinin
TFG	Terminal α1,2-fucose glycan
Thr	Threonine
GalNAc-T	UDP-GalNAc-polypeptide GalNAc-transferase
UEA-I	*Ulex europaeus* agglutinin-I
UDP-GlcNAc	Uridine diphospho-N-acetylglucosamine

VVL	*Vicia villosa* lectin
VBG	VVL-binding GalNAc glycan
WFA	*Wisteria floribunda* agglutinin
XIAP	X-linked inhibitor of apoptosis protein
Xyl	Xylose
OGA	β-*N*-acetylglucosaminidase

Introduction

Glycosylation is an enzymatic process that modifies glycans, lipids, or proteins with sugar molecules. The biosynthesis of glycan branches is effectuated through a specific set of glycosylation machinery, e.g., glycosyltransferases and glycosidases, sugar transporters, and activated sugar donors. The resulting glycan microheterogeneity and complexity is intricately involved with many physiological processes, e.g., cell identity, cell-cell cross talk, and cell-environment interactions. The specific terminal glycan modification can confer unique function and properties to oligosaccharides and is often regulated during ontogeny and cellular differentiation [1].

Changes in glycan patterns have been observed as early events in several pathological conditions and used as biomarkers of many diseases, including cancer. Alteration of glycan structure of cell surface glycoproteins was first reported in SV-40-transformed murine fibroblasts [2]. Since then, the significance of glycan patterns in tumor development and progression has been extensively studied [3]. At present, it is well accepted that aberrant glycosylation is a universal feature of cancer cells and plays a crucial role in cancer biology [4]. Aberrant glycans that modify the cell surface or the secreted glycoproteins of cancer cells can be potential cancer biomarkers [5] and therapeutically targeted and manipulated to provide a new avenue to improving cancer treatment [6]. Advancements in high-throughput approaches for glycome analysis have accelerated the glycoproteomics-based discovery of glyco-biomarkers and drawn much attention from researchers to investigate glycomics for medical applications. Lectin-based approaches [7–10] and mass spectrometry [11, 12] have been applied to determine the aberrant glycosylation in clinical samples from cholangiocarcinoma (CCA) patients.

In this chapter, we present a broad overview of cellular glycosylation processes and the dysregulation of glycosylation in cancer. We then describe the aberrant glycosylation, in core (N- and O-glycosylation) and peripheral glycosylation (fucosylation, sialylation) as well as O-GlcNAcylation and glycosphingolipid synthesis, in the development and progression of CCA. Lastly, we explore the potential of using these glycosylated products to improve diagnosis and treatment of CCA.

Glycans and Glycosylation in Biology

Biochemistry of Glycans

Glycans reported in eukaryotic cells can be classified according to the linkage to proteins or lipids and include glycoproteins, proteoglycans, sulfated glycosaminoglycans, hyaluronan, and glycosphingolipids (GSLs) [13, 14]. A glycoprotein is a glycoconjugate in which a protein carries one or more glycans attached to a polypeptide chain, mostly via N- or O-linkages [15]. An *N*-linked glycosylation refers to the co- or posttranslational modification of a polypeptide with an oligosaccharide that is covalently linked to the amide nitrogen of an asparagine (Asn) residue and can be classified into three main types: high-mannose, complex, and hybrid types [16]. N-glycosylation is the most common glycosylation observed in a large number of proteins synthesized in humans. O-linked glycosylation refers to the post-translational linkage of an oligosaccharide to the OH group of a serine (Ser) or threonine (Thr) residue of a polypeptide. The first sugar that attaches to Ser or Thr can be mannose (Man), fucose (Fuc), galactose (Gal), glucose (Glc), *N*-acetylgalactosamine (GalNAc), *N*-acetylglucosamine (GlcNAc), or xylose (Xyl). An attachment of GalNAc to Ser/Thr is the most common O-glycosylation of membrane-bound and secreted glycoproteins such as mucin (MUC) glycoproteins; therefore, O-linked GalNAc modifications are generally called mucin-type glycosylation. One of the polypeptide N-acetylgalactosaminyltransferases (GalNAc-Ts) transfers a GalNAc to Ser or Thr of the specific proteins in different cell types and organs [17]. The oligosaccharide is further extended with Gal and GlcNAc, forming eight types of core mucin O-glycan [18, 19]. In addition, the linkage of Ser/Thr with a single molecule of GlcNAc, called O-GlcNAcylation, is another O-glycosylation that has been aggressively studied in the past decade. Several nucleocytoplasmic proteins, especially transcription factors, have been identified as O-GlcNAcylated proteins [20].

Proteoglycans are a polymeric glycoconjugate that contains one or more glycosaminoglycan chains, linear polysaccharides, and uronic acid or galactose, attached to a core protein [21, 22]. Hyaluronan is one of the glycosaminoglycans; it is unique from other classes of glycosaminoglycans in that it is not further modified by sulfation or by epimerization of the glucuronic acid moiety to iduronic acid [22]. A GSL consists of a glycan usually attached via glucose or galactose to the terminal primary hydroxyl group of the lipid moiety ceramide, which is composed of a long chain base (sphingosine) and a fatty acid; therefore, they can be neutral or acidic [21, 22]. A ganglioside is an acidic glycolipid containing one or more residues of sialic acid [23]. All forms of glycosylation are synthesized in the endoplasmic reticulum (ER) and Golgi apparatus, except O-GlcNAcylation.

Glycosylation Process

Unlike DNA, RNA, and protein, glycan structure is not directly encoded from the genome; rather, it is tightly regulated by a cellular process called "glycosylation" [13]. Particular glycan structures are generated and sequentially modified by a variety of glycosyltransferases and glycosidases as well as the presence of sugar donors inside the cells [19]. The sub-compartmentalization of glycan biosynthesis in the Golgi apparatus can also modulate the order of glycosylation [19]. A variety of glycan structures mediate the diversity and complexity of cellular biology. Furthermore, glycan structures and production can reflect small changes in intra- or extracellular environment.

Protein N-linked glycosylation is compartmentalized in the ER. The biosynthesis of N-glycan precursors begins on the outer leaflet of the ER and is completed in the ER lumen, with proficiently glycosylated proteins then being exported to the Golgi apparatus for further elongation and addition of peripheral glycans moieties (Fig. 24.1) [16, 24, 25]. The biosynthesis of the core oligosaccharide (14-sugar glycan) for N-glycan requires several known enzymes. Firstly, the sugar moieties are sequentially added to the dolichol phosphate (Dol-P) on the outer part of the ER membrane by the asparagine-linked glycosylation family of glycosyltransferases [16, 24]. The mature oligosaccharide is then transferred to the acceptor protein in the sequence of asparagine-X-serine/threonine (X can be any amino acid except proline) by the oligosaccharyltransferase (OST) complex [24, 25]. The glucoses of the core oligosaccharide are then removed by glycosidase I–II. Generally, glycoproteins exiting ER to Golgi contain either eight or nine mannose residues of N-glycans. In the *cis*-Golgi, the oligomannoses are trimmed by α-mannosidases to form Man5, an important intermediate glycoform for synthesizing hybrid and complex N-glycans [16, 19]. In the last step of N-glycan processing, the biosynthesis of hybrid and complex N-glycans is started in the *medial* Golgi by adding and branching of GlcNAc to mannose residues via the action of N-acetylglucosaminyltransferases (GlcNAc-Ts) [16]. There are several glycosyltransferases, including galactosyltransferases (GalTs), fucosyltransferases (FUTs), and sialyltransferases (STs) involved in the extension of N-glycans to form mature N-glycans which ordinarily occur in the *trans* Golgi [16, 19].

Different from N-glycosylation, the synthesis of O-linked glycan is initiated by the addition of a monosaccharide to a Ser or Thr residue followed by the stepwise-elongation into an oligosaccharide chain. Biosynthesis of mucin-type O-linked glycosylation is initiated in the Golgi apparatus by the transfer of a GalNAc to a Ser or Thr residue on the peptide chain by one of the UDP-GalNAc enzymes (Fig. 25.1) [18]. The Tn antigen is further elongated to form complex O-glycan by several glycosyltransferases [18, 19].

GSL biosynthesis starts with an addition of the first sugar to ceramide (Cer) and then transfer of subsequent sugars by glycosyltransferases. Cer is synthesized at the

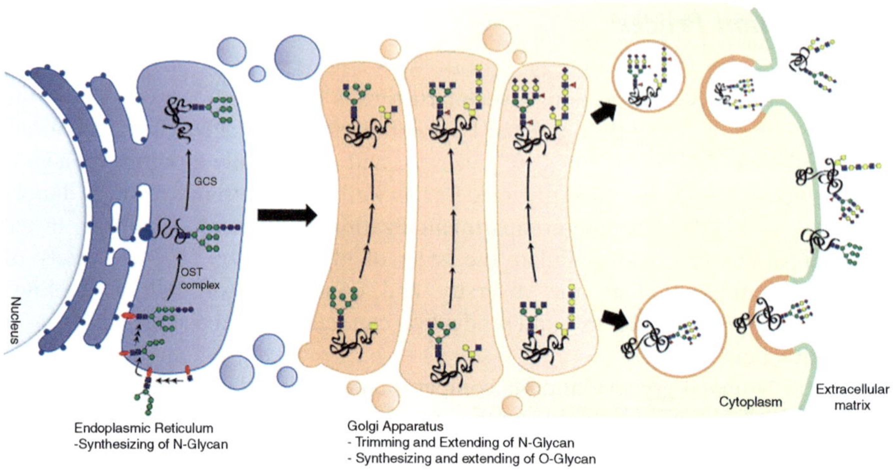

Fig. 25.1 Biosynthesis of protein glycosylation in mammalian cells. N-glycosylation is started in the ER by the synthesis of core *N*-glycan on a dolichol phosphate and then transferred to the peptide and elongated to a more complex oligosaccharide in the Golgi apparatus. Mucin-type O-glycosylation is started and sequentially modified in the Golgi apparatus by several glycosyltransferases to form the complex oligosaccharides

outer part of the ER and consequently equilibrates to the luminal part and transfers to the Golgi apparatus (Fig. 25.2) [26, 27]. Glucosylceramide (GlcCer) is synthesized at the cytoplasmic face of the ER and *cis*-Golgi apparatus and then flipped into the Golgi lumen, where it is further elongated by a series of glycosyltransferases. In contrast, galactosylceramide (GalCer) is synthesized inside of the ER lumen and consequentially traffics through the Golgi, where it can be sulfated to form sulfatide [26, 27].

The Significance of Glycans and Glycosylation in Medicine

Glycosylation is one of the important co- and/or posttranslational modifications required for modulating the normal biological function of cells and is necessary to control protein folding, conformation, localization, stability, and activity [14, 28]. Glycans have various structures and biophysical roles, including surface antigens, adhesion molecules, signaling receptors, cell-cell recognition, and cell-matrix interactions [29–31]. In addition, glycan elements in the matrix, such as proteoglycans, are important for maintaining tissue structure, porosity, and integrity [31]. Therefore, aberration of glycosylation has been shown to be involved in many human diseases, including cancer [28–30].

Several glycan/glycoprotein antigens have been used for detecting and monitoring the growth status of tumors. For CCA, these include carbohydrate antigen 19–9 (CA19–9), i.e., sialyl-Lewis A (sLe^{a}), attached to mucin glycoproteins and

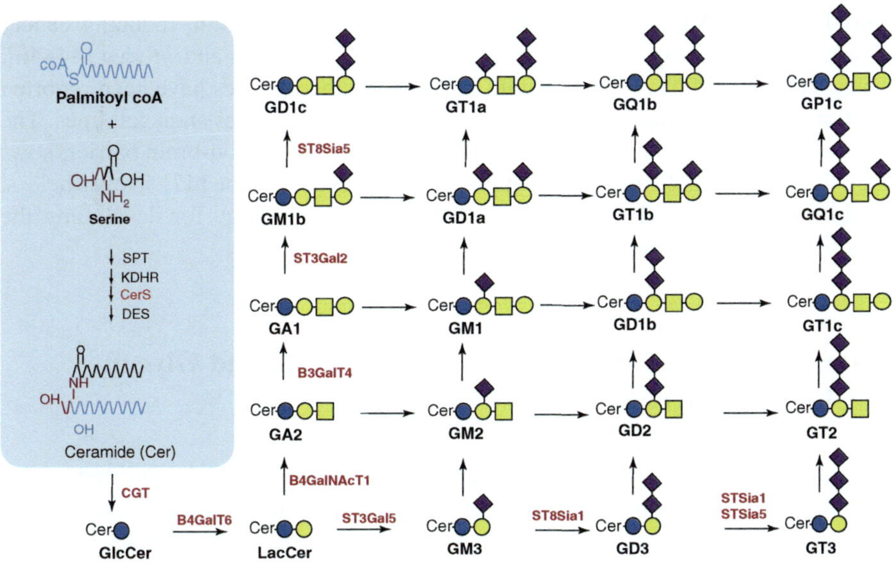

Fig. 25.2 Synthesis of GSLs. The synthesis of GSL starts with CER synthesis by ceramide synthase (CERS) and related enzymes, followed by sequential glycosylation processes with different glycosyltransferases

gangliosides and MUC5AC for screening, surveillance, and prognosis [34–36]. Examples in other tumors include CA15–3 (a sialylated O-glycan on MUC1), CA27–29 (recognizes MUC1), and HER2 for breast cancer; CEA for colon cancer; CA125 (i.e., MUC16) and human epididymis protein 4 (HE4) for ovarian cancer; alpha-fetoprotein (AFP) and its fucosylated form (i.e., AFP-L3) for hepatocellular carcinoma (HCC); sialyl-Lewis X (sLe^x)-related glycans for lung and breast cancers; prostate-specific antigen (PSA) for prostate cancer; and thyroglobulin for thyroid cancer [32, 33]. Although many candidate glycan/glycoprotein markers have been suggested, most of them yield only limited accuracy for cancer screening, diagnosis, prognosis, and/or monitoring. Therefore, the discovery of new biomarkers focused on carbohydrate antigens may improve the quality of diagnostic and prognostic predictions of particular cancers.

From a therapeutic perspective, inhibition of protein glycosylation using the antibiotic tunicamycin (*in vitro*) can induce cancer cell apoptosis and reduce metastasis of cancer cells via several mechanisms, e.g., ER-stress activation, reduction of stemness ability, inhibition of signaling pathways (TNF-related apoptosis-inducing ligand, MAPK/Erk, EGFR, IGF-1R, and several RTKs), induction of drug sensitivity, etc. [37–40]. Tunicamycin, however, has not been used in humans due to its severe side effects [41, 42]. Several plant lectins have been shown to inhibit progression of cancer [43]; however, lectins again might cause side effects in human patients such as aggregation of red blood cells. Recently, 5-[(Dimethylamino)sulfonyl]-N-(5-methyl-2-thiazolyl)-2-(1-pyrrolidinyl)-benzamide (NGI-1, ML414), a new inhibitor of protein glycosylation, was established [44].

NGI-1 targets OST subunit and blocks N-linked glycosylation, reducing cancer growth and increasing cancer sensitivity to radiation *in vitro* and *in vivo* [44–46]. The synergistic effects of NGI-1 with other chemotherapeutics have been reported in glioma and non-small cell lung cancer, especially in drug-resistant cell lines. The low solubility of NGI-1 and its ability to pass through the blood-brain barrier, however, limit the benefit of this compound in cancer treatment [47]. Nevertheless, inhibition of protein glycosylation is still a potential strategy for developing the effective therapy for cancer.

Clinical Relevance of Aberrant Glycosylation and Glycans in Cholangiocarcinoma

Alteration of glycosylation and elevation of cancer-associated glycans and glycoproteins in CCA have been increasingly reported. The aberrantly expressed glycoconjugates play important roles in CCA progression and are potentially useful as markers for detection of the disease. Direct evidence to demonstrate the alteration of glycosylation in CCA has been discovered by glycomics using lectin-based approaches [7–10] and mass spectrometry [11, 12]. The collective evidence suggests that glycosylation is globally altered in CCA. The alterations can be observed either in N-linked and O-linked glycosylations [12, 48–50]. Peripheral glycosylating processes, including fucosylation and sialylation, and synthesis of glycosphingolipids have also been found to be altered in CCA [51–53], as described below.

N-Glycans

Alteration in specific N-glycans can serve as a distinct molecular signature for cancer progression. Circulating N-glycoprotein/N-glycoform markers are suggested to be useful for diagnosis, disease monitoring, and assessment of clinical outcomes. Most serum/plasma N-glycoproteins are synthesized by the hepatobiliary system and reflect the status of the liver. In-depth analysis of the glycans in the serum/plasma of CCA patients may facilitate the discovery of novel diagnostic/therapeutic markers of CCA.

The plasma glycoproteome of patients with CCA ($n = 60$) and control group who were negative for hepatobiliary diseases ($n = 95$) was determined by Chang et al. using liquid chromatography-tandem mass spectrometry [11]. The analyses revealed four proteins closely related to tumor progression and prognosis of hepatobiliary malignancies. Of these, galectin-3-binding protein, also named MAC-2-binding protein, was found to be highly correlated with tumor stage, tumor grade, recurrence-free survival, and overall survival of CCA patients. Talabnin et al. used positive nanospray ionization-linear ion trap mass spectrometry (NSI-MS^n) to determine the serum glycoproteomes and aberrant N-glycans in eight CCA patients compared to four healthy controls [12]. Similar glycan patterns with different relative quantities were obtained. The levels of high-mannose type N-glycan, M6N2, and the complex tri-antennary N-glycan containing a core fucose and terminal tri-sialic acid, NeuAc3H3N3M3N2F, were significantly increased, while levels of M9N2 were decreased, in CCA patients compared to healthy controls. The association of these glycans with clinicopathological features of patients, however, was not observed in this cohort.

For extrahepatic CCA (ECCA), the N-glycome profiling patterns in serum were determined using DNA sequencer-assisted fluorophore-assisted capillary electrophoresis (DSA-FACE) in 106 ECCA patients compared to 60 benign bile tract disease (BBD) and 89 healthy controls [54]. Different N-glycan patterns were observed in CCA vs. BBD and CCA vs. healthy controls, suggesting the N-glycan pattern specific to the disease condition and the potential use of these N-glycans as diagnostic markers. In addition, high levels of branching fucosylated tri-antennary and tetra-antennary N-glycans but not CA19–9 were correlated with positive lymph node metastasis. Using logistic regression coefficients, the authors constructed a mathematical formula for specific N-glycans to separate ECCA patients from normal controls with a higher diagnostic power than CA19–9. The combination of an N-glycan peak and CA19–9 improved the diagnostic accuracy of CA19–9 from 90.8% to 94.4% [54]. Moreover, N-glycan profiles but not CA19–9 levels in pre- and postoperative sera were significantly different. These data suggest circular N-glycan markers as novel and noninvasive markers in the diagnosis and progression monitoring of CCA.

O-Glycans

Alterations of O-glycosylation and an increase in O-glycans can be applied to the diagnosis and prognostic prediction of many types of cancer [5, 55]. In addition, these glycans have also been found to play significant roles in cancer progression and therapeutic resistances [17, 56, 57].

Increases in cancer-associated O-glycans in patient tissues and sera are possibly triggered by the overexpression of carrier glycoproteins. In CCA, elevation of mucin glycoproteins, such as MUC5AC and MUC1, was reported in tissues and sera [34, 36, 58, 59]. MUC5AC was elevated in CCA comparing with normal bile ducts [58, 59] and was demonstrated to be a good candidate for a diagnostic and prognostic marker for CCA. A high level of serum MUC5AC was associated with high tumor stage and short survival of CCA patients [59]. MUC1 and its glycoforms were found to be elevated in CCA [58, 60, 61], and high levels of MUC1 in CCA was associated with vascular invasion and shorter survival of patients [58]. These mucins also play significant roles in CCA progression and metastasis [62, 63].

Not only the elevation of carrier proteins but also the variation of glycan pattern may have clinical significance in CCA. Truncated mucin-type O-glycans such as Tn antigen (GalNAc-Ser/Thr), sialyl-Tn (sTn, Sia-GalNAc-Ser/Thr), Thomsen-Friedenreich antigen (T antigen, Gal-GalNAc-Ser/Thr), and sialyl-T antigen (Sia-Gal-GalNAc-Ser/Thr) are elevated and appear to play important roles in progression and metastasis of cancers; therefore, studies on the potential of using these antigens as targets for immunotherapy have been recently performed [64]. In CCA, Tn-, STn, and T-antigens were found to be elevated in CCA cells [48, 65]; the methods for detection these antigens in patients' sera are being continuously developed [66, 67].

There are many lines of evidence pointing to the elevation of O-GalNAc modification or mucin-type glycosylation in CCA [8, 48, 61, 68]. Matsuda et al. analyzed the glycan profiles in CCA and normal bile ducts using lectin microarray and showed that a GalNAc-binding lectin, *Wisteria floribunda* agglutinin (WFA), provided the highest power in differentiating CCA from normal bile duct epithelia [61]. In addition, lectin histochemistry studies revealed that Gal/GalNAc-binding lectins, *Sophora japonica* agglutinin (SJA) and *Vicia villosa* lectins (VVL), provided strong reactivity with hyperplastic/dysplastic bile ducts and CCA compared with normal bile ducts and hepatocytes (Fig. 25.3) [8, 48, 68]. SJA-binding *N*-acetylgalactosamine-associated glycan (SNAG) appeared to be applicable as a diagnostic and prognostic marker for CCA; it was highly detected in sera from CCA patients compared to non-CCA controls and associated with short survival of CCA patients [68]. In addition, VVL-binding GalNAc glycan (VBG) has been found to play important roles in CCA metastasis in vitro [48]. Synthesis of VBG and its metastatic potential were recently shown to be related with the activity of polypeptide GalNAc-transferase 5 (GalNAcT5) in CCA cell lines [48]. Suppression of GalNAcT5 expression significantly reduced the migration and invasion abilities of CCA cell lines, while the overexpression of GalNAcT5 reversed these features. The molecular basis underlying this event involved AKT/ERK signaling pathways. In addition, an immunohistochemistry-based study showed that diffusely positive staining of GalNAcT3 in cancer cells was associated with lymph node metastasis of CCA, suggesting the usefulness of preoperative GalNAcT3 investigation in clinical management [69].

Experiments in animal models are useful to better understand the association of glycan modification and CCA tumor biology. Using a hamster model of liver fluke-associated CCA [70, 71], O-GalNAc modifications, VBG and SNAG, were detected in hyperplastic/dysplastic bile ducts of hamster liver tissues as early as 1 month after liver fluke infection and CCA induction [48, 68]. No signal of VBG and SNAG was detected in normal bile ducts and hepatocytes. This finding suggested the association of VBG and SNAG in the development of carcinogenesis.

Collectively, these observations point to the importance of O-GalNAc modified glycans in CCA development and metastasis, suggesting the possibility of using the enzymes involved in O-GalNAc modification, e.g., GalNAcT5, as a target for CCA treatment in the future.

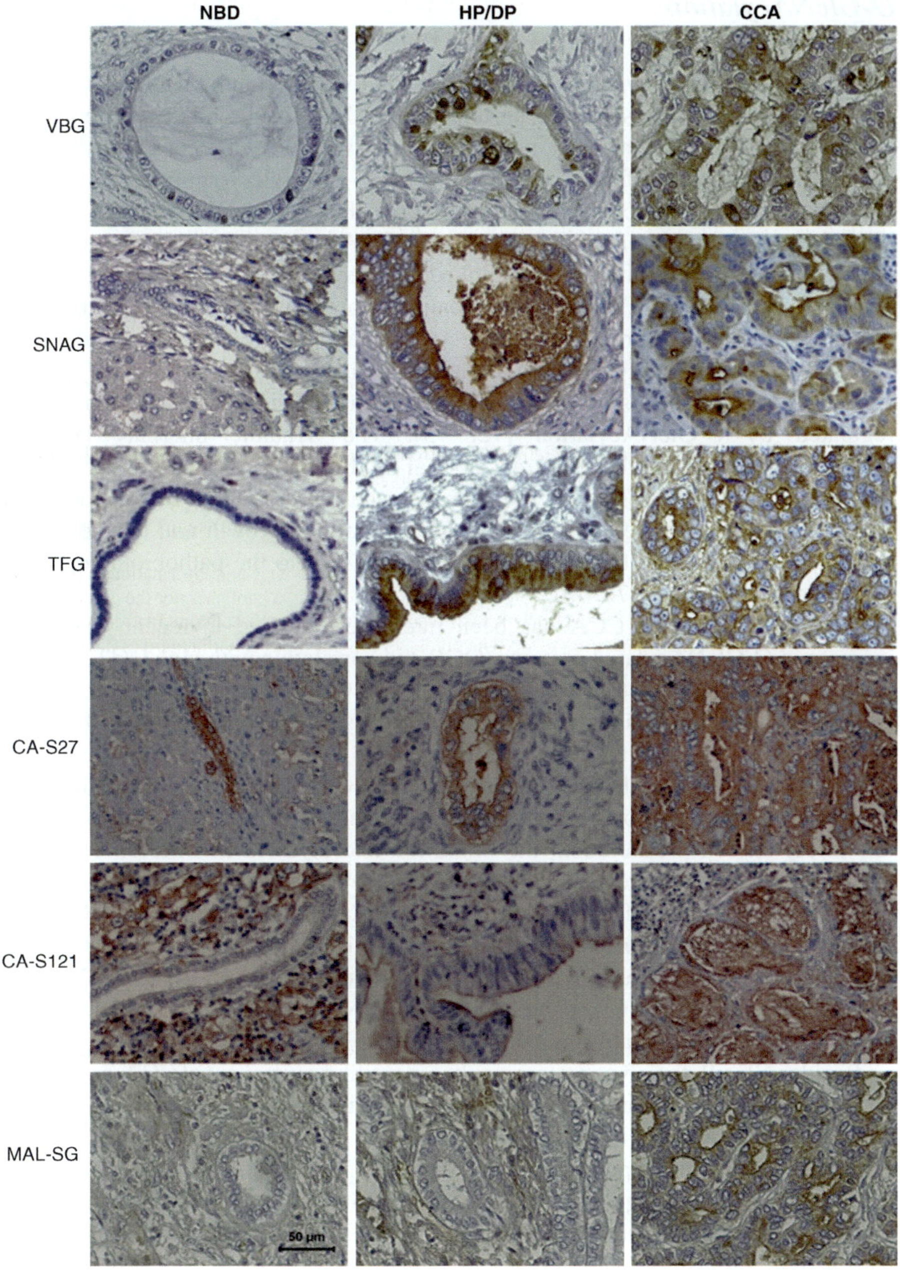

Fig. 25.3 Expression of CCA-associated glycans in patient tissues. Lectin immunohistochemistry staining was used to detect VVL-binding glycan (VBG), SJA-binding GalNAc-associated glycan (SNAG), terminal fucose glycan (TFG), carbohydrate antigen (CA)-S27, CA-S121, and MAL-II-binding glycan (MAL-SG) in CCA tissues. Normal bile ducts (NBD) were for all CCA-associated glycans, except CA-S27. Hyperplastic/dysplastic (HP/DP) bile ducts were positive for all the glycans except MAL-SG, while CCA was positive for all examined glycans. Bar = 50 μm

O-GlcNAcylation

O-GlcNAcylation is a dynamic posttranslational modification by adding a GlcNAc moiety on Ser or Thr residues of proteins via O-β-glycosidic linkage without any elongation. The process is regulated by two enzymes; O-linked β-N-acetylglucosaminyltransferase (OGT) and β-N-acetylglucosaminidase (OGA). OGT transfers GlcNAc from uridine diphospho-N-acetylglucosamine (UDP-GlcNAc) to -OH group of Ser or Thr, whereas OGA catalyzes the reversed reaction. Unlike the general N-linked or O-linked glycosylation, O-GlcNAcylation is a reversible process [20]. The rapid modification of proteins by O-GlcNAcylation can dynamically modulate protein function, stability, and activity. Several cellular processes including transcription regulation, translation control, inhibition of proteasomal degradation, stress response, and modulation of signal transduction can be regulated by O-GlcNAcylation [72, 73]. The dynamic interplay between O-GlcNAcylation and other posttranslational modifications, e.g., phosphorylation, has also been reported [20, 72, 74]. The balance between O-GlcNAcylation and phosphorylation of proteins is required for normal cell growth and development; hence, the alteration of these modifications may lead to the pathobiological processes and then disease [72, 75].

O-GlcNAcylation in CCA has been intensively studied in recent years. An increase in O-GlcNAcylated proteins (OGPs) in correlation with high OGT and low OGA levels was demonstrated in tumor tissues of CCA patients [50]. High expression of OGT (similar to high levels of SNAG, as discussed above [68]) was found to be associated with poor prognosis and shorter survival of CCA patients, suggesting the involvement of O-GlcNAcylation in CCA development and progression. The roles of O-GlcNAcylation on *metastasis* were studied in CCA cell lines; without any effect on cell proliferation, the migration and invasion abilities of CCA cell lines were dramatically reduced when O-GlcNAcylation was suppressed using specific siRNA against OGT. In contrast, enhancing O-GlcNAcylation by siOGA significantly increased migration and invasion abilities of CCA cell lines [76]. This effect was shown to be via O-GlcNAcylation of a transcription factor, NF-κB. Nuclear translocation of NF-κB was regulated by O-GlcNAc modification, which in turn induced expression of matrix metalloprotease enzymes [76].

Besides NF-κB, the glycoproteomics has identified several novel CCA-associated OGPs [77]. Among these, heterogeneous nuclear ribonucleoprotein-K (hnRNP-K) was abundantly detected in highly metastatic CCA cell lines [77]. O-GlcNAcylation was found to be an important modification to mediate nuclear translocation of hnRNP-K, which subsequently activated expression of several downstream genes, including cyclin D1, X-linked inhibitor of apoptosis protein 1 (XIAP1), epithelial to mesenchymal transition (EMT) markers, matrix metalloproteinase 2 (MMP2), and MMP7. Suppression of hnRNP-K negatively affected proliferation, migration, and invasion of CCA cell lines. In addition, immunohistochemistry of tumor tissues from CCA patients revealed that the nuclear localization of hnRNP-K could predict metastatic status and poor patient survival [77].

A recent study in CCA cell lines revealed that O-GlcNAcylation could indirectly mediate the N-glycan pattern of the membrane-bound glycoproteins via α1-mannosidase 1A (MAN1A1), an enzyme that reduces the high-mannose type N-glycan [49]. Suppression of O-GlcNAcylation using si-OGT could reduce the level of high-mannose type N-glycan and consequently repressed metastatic ability of CCA cells. Decreased O-GlcNAcylation was concomitant with the repression of PI3K/Akt and MAPK/Erk signaling pathways, which enhanced the stability of fork-head box O3 (FOXO3), the transcriptional factor regulating MAN1A1 expression [49]. Masking the high-mannose type N-glycan on the CCA cell surface using *Pisum sativum* agglutinin (PSA), a mannose specific lectin, reduced the metastatic ability of CCA cells. The correlation between O-GlcNAcylation, high-mannose type N-glycan, and CCA metastasis was also demonstrated in tumor tissues from CCA patients [49].

Aside from the enzymes OGT and OGA, the concentration of nutrient-sensing UDP-GlcNAc can also modulate intracellular O-GlcNAcylation. UDP-GlcNAc is synthesized via the hexosamine biosynthesis pathway in which glutamine-fructose amidotransferase (GFAT) is a rate-limiting enzyme. Recent studies have indicated an association between diabetes mellitus and poor prognosis of CCA patients. In vitro experiments have demonstrated that high-glucose media can promote the aggressiveness of CCA cells via mediating O-GlcNAcylation [78, 79]. Cultured cells in high-glucose conditions could enhance the expression of OGT and GFAT, resulting in an increase of O-GlcNAcylation and metastatic abilities of CCA cell lines. Vimentin was found to be highly stabilized under high-glucose conditions. The GFAT inhibitor, 6-Diazo-5-oxo-L-norleucine (DON), significantly suppressed O-GlcNAcylation, migration, and vimentin stability of CCA cells [79]. The association between O-GlcNAcylation and the expression level of GFAT in human CCA tissues were also confirmed using immunohistochemistry [79].

These findings strongly suggest that a high level of O-GlcNAcylation supports progressive phenotypes of CCA cells in several ways (Fig. 25.4). CCA-associated OGPs may be of clinical use, either as a prognostic marker or a potential target for CCA treatment. Before use in a clinical setting, however, further preclinical and clinical studies are needed to confirm the true indicators and utility of these CCA-associated OGPs for prognosis and treatment of CCA.

Fucosylation

Fucosylation is a glycosylation step catalyzed by 1 of 13 fucosyltransferases (FUTs) that use GDP-fucose as a donor substrate [81]. FUT adds a fucose to oligosaccharides with through various linkages, providing products with various glycan structures (Fig. 25.5). FUTs can be classified into four subfamilies based on the glycosidic linkage formed. The first group, FUT1 and FUT2, transfers a fucose residue to the terminal galactose to form α1,2-linkage, yielding H blood group antigen and related structures. The second group, α1,3/4-FUTs, FUT3, FUT4, FUT5, FUT6, FUT7, and

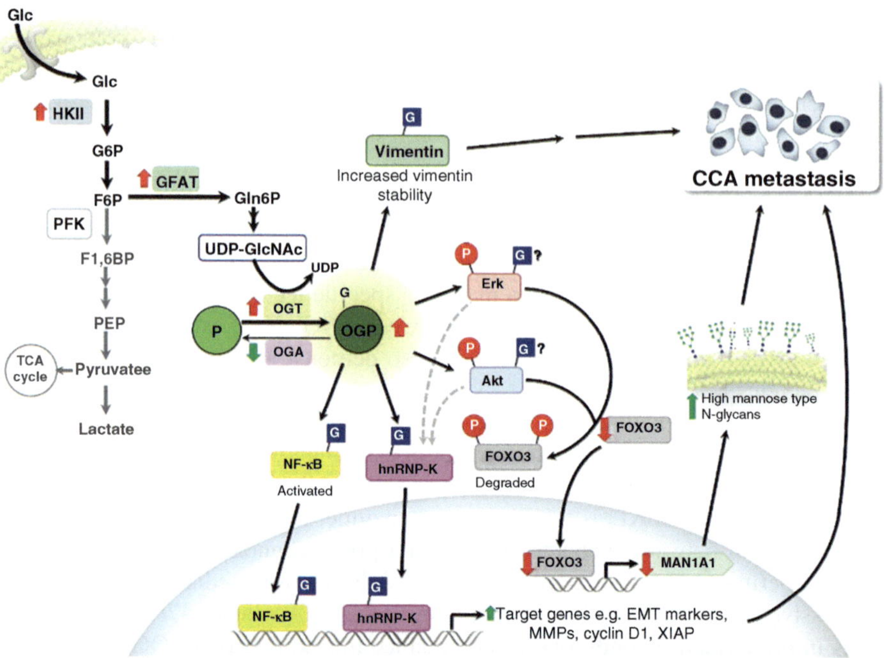

Fig. 25.4 Molecular mechanisms of O-GlcNAcylation promote the progression of CCA cells. In high-glucose conditions, CCA cells might increase glucose uptake and the hexosamine biosynthesis pathway (HBP) via upregulating glutamine-fructose amidotransferase (GFAT), resulting in an increase of UDP-GlcNAc. Together with increased UDP-GlcNAc, OGT is increased while OGA is decreased, leading to the elevation of OGP in CCA cells. Increasing O-GlcNAcylation in CCA cells promotes CCA metastasis via many mechanisms, including (i) induction of nuclear translocation of NF-κB and hnRNP-K, (ii) activation of Akt and Erk signaling pathways, (iii) modulation of vimentin and FOXO3 stability, and (iv) induction of high-mannose type N-glycan at the cell surface

FUT9, is involved in the synthesis of Lewis blood group antigens. The third group is comprised of FUT8, an α1,6-FUT which directly adds a fucose to the innermost GlcNAc of the N-linked oligosaccharides on glycoproteins to produce core fucosylation. Finally, protein O-fucosyltransferase 1 (POFUT1) and POFUT2 transfer a fucose residue via an α-linkage to Ser or Thr to produce O-fucosylation.

Fucose is added to an oligosaccharide chain in the final step in the late cisternae of the Golgi apparatus to increase the complexity of glycan structures. This specific glycan modification can confer unique function and properties to oligosaccharides and is often regulated during ontogeny and cellular differentiation [1]. Abnormal fucosylation has been observed in various disease states including cancer. Monitoring fucosylation changes across the spectrum of carcinogenesis can be useful for early cancer detection and management [57]. Exploring fucosylation in CCA development and progression, therefore, may offer an opportunity for early diagnosis and targeted treatment.

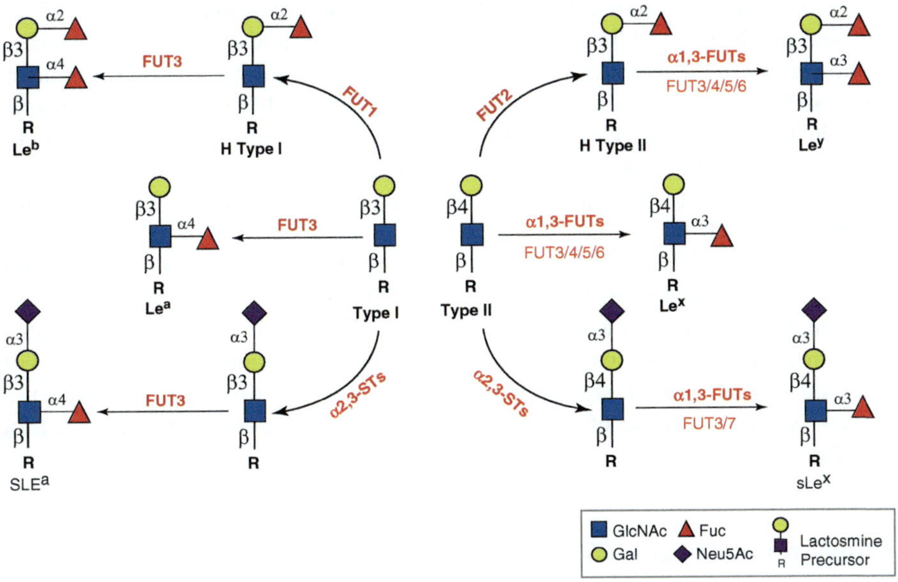

Fig. 25.5 Biosynthesis of carbohydrate terminal Lewis antigens. There are two major groups of Lewis antigens, including Lewis type 1 (left) and Lewis type 2 (right), depending on the type of precursor. Only FUT3 and FUT7 can add fucose to sialic acid-containing glycans (i.e., sialoglycans)

Blood Group Antigens

Fucosylation is involved in the biosynthesis of blood group-related antigens, such as A, B, H, Le^a, Le^b, Le^x, Le^y, sLe^a, and sLe^x. Several fucosylated products are potential biomarkers for CCA. Immunohistochemistry of these blood group-related antigens has been reported in 75 cases of CCA tissues (31 peripheral type and 44 hilar type CCA) [80]. Expression of A, B, and H were detected in the large bile ducts, whereas Le^a, Le^b, and Le^y were variably observed in small and large bile ducts of nonneoplastic tissues. In CCA, expression of the blood group A, Le^a, Le^b, Le^y, and sLe^a antigens were differentially expressed according to the histological type of cancer, suggesting that the distribution of blood group-related antigens may relate to the differentiation of CCA.

Terminal α1, 2-Fucose Glycans

Clinical relevance of terminal α1,2-fucose glycan (TFG) in CCA was reported by Indramanee et al. (2019) [82]. Lectin histochemistry of human CCA tissues using *Ulex europaeus* agglutinin-I (UEA-I) that recognizes TFG was performed in 79 paraffin-embedded tumors from CCA patients [8]. Neither hepatocytes nor normal bile duct epithelia expressed TFG; in contrast, 47% of CCA specimens showed high expression of TFG (Fig. 25.3), which was correlated with shorter patient survival, suggesting aberrant terminal fucosylation in CCA and a possible prognostic indicator. The involvement of TFG in carcinogenesis and progression of CCA has been demonstrated in the liver fluke-associated CCA hamster model. UEA-I lectin histochemistry of hamster liver sections demonstrated that TFG was absent in normal bile duct epithelia but elevated in hyperproliferative bile ducts and gradually increased during CCA development. TFG was expressed in CCA but was negative in all HCC tissues tested, suggesting TFG as a potential biomarker for differentiating CCA from HCC.

Significance of TFG on the efficiency of EGF-EGFR binding and/or activation has also been examined [82]. Suppression of TFG expression using siFUT1 or neutralizing the surface TFG with UEA-I in CCA cell lines effectively inhibited migration, invasion, and adhesion abilities in vitro. The observation was concurrent with the reduction of Akt/Erk signaling and EMT. The effect was further shown to be driven by the decreasing of EGF-EGFR activation that consequently reduced the Akt/Erk cascades.

Carbohydrate Antigen-S27

A novel carbohydrate antigen, CA-S27, recognized by the S27 monoclonal antibody (mAb) [83, 84], was proven to be a Le^a-associated glycan using glycoconjugate microarray [84]. The clinical relevance of CA-S27 was reported by Silsirivanit et al. (2013) [84]. Immunohistochemistry of 45 human CCA tissues revealed a high reactivity of CA-S27 in almost all CCA tissues but not hepatocytes (Fig. 25.3). Additionally, a quantitative determination of serum CA-S27 by sandwich ELISA was developed using the CA-S27 monoclonal antibody and soybean agglutinin. Using this method, serum CA-S27 of CCA patients (n = 96) was found to be significantly higher than those of the control groups (patients with gastrointestinal cancers, HCC, benign hepatobiliary diseases, and healthy subjects [n = 190]) and distinguished CCA patients from controls with 87% sensitivity and 59% specificity. Serum CA-S27 was secreted from CCA tissues, and serum CA-S27 level declined dramatically after tumor removal. Moreover, a high serum CA-S27 level was associated with shorter survival of CCA patients. MUC5AC mucin, a secretory mucin-related to poor prognosis in CCA [36], was shown to be the major glycoprotein possessed by CA-S27 in serum [84].

The significance of CA-S27 in promoting CCA progression was demonstrated in CCA cell lines [84]. FUT3, a key enzyme for Le synthesis was highly expressed in CCA cells with high CA-S27expression. Silencing of FUT3 expression by siFUT3 or neutralizing surface CA-S27 by CA-S27 mAb effectively decreased invasion, migration, adhesion, and proliferation abilities of CCA cells.

Collectively, these data suggest important roles and significance of CA-S27 in CCA. In particular, serum CA-S27 might be a serum marker for diagnosis and progression of CCA, a prognostic factor for clinical outcomes of CCA, and a potential therapeutic target for metastatic CCA.

Carbohydrate Antigen-S121

Carbohydrate antigen-S121 (CA-S121 or CCA-CA) is an unidentified sugar structure recognized by a monoclonal antibody S121 [83]. The glycan epitope was found on MUC5AC mucin and strongly detected in hyperplastic/dysplastic and neoplastic bile duct epithelia but not in normal bile ducts or hepatocytes (Fig. 25.3). Serum CA-S121 assessment by lectin sandwich ELISA was able to distinguish CCA patients from several controls, e.g., healthy individuals, *Opisthorchis viverrini*-infected individuals, patients with benign hepatobiliary diseases, and patients with various gastrointestinal cancers or HCC with 87.63% sensitivity and 89.58% specificity. CCA patients with high serum CA-S121 had a shorter survival than those with low serum CA-S121. Moreover, the combination of serum CA-S121 with serum alkaline phosphatase resulted in sensitivity, specificity, positive predictive value, and negative predictive value all >95% [85]. Using the combination of these two markers may be useful for screening people who are risk of CCA.

sLe^a or CA19–9

sLe^a or CA19–9 has been used clinically since 1997 for diagnosis and surveillance of patients with gastrointestinal cancers, especially CCA, pancreatic adenocarcinoma, and gallbladder adenocarcinoma [86, 87]. Although CA19–9 is not a specific biomarker for CCA, it is the most frequent and best studied marker for identifying CCA in clinical practice. Recently, use of CA19–9 has also been recommended as part of CCA surveillance in primary sclerosing cholangitis (PSC), as discussed in greater detail elsewhere in this book (Chap. 20, Ali et al.) [88–92].

The biosynthesis of CA19–9 is based on the enzymatic activity of FUT3 irrespective of FUT2 activity [93, 94]. In contrast, inactivity of FUT2 increases levels of serum CA19–9 [95]. Based on these observations, Wannhoff A et al. (2013) suggested to use a new optimal cutoff value for CA19–9 based on individual FUT2/3 genotype [96]. The approach could improve the power of CA19–9 in differentiating PSC from CCA with 90% sensitivity and a 43% reduction of false-positive results. Serum CA19–9 and FUT genotyping is clinically beneficial and may enhance the early detection of CCA in clinical practice.

The clinical relevance of sLe^a in CCA has been demonstrated in various studies. For example, Juntavee et al. (2005) found that sLe^a was highly expressed in tissue of the mass-forming type of CCA and correlated well with vascular invasion and unfavorable patient outcomes [51]. The significance of sLe^a in vascular invasion was signified by the fact that CCA cells that possessed high sLe^a expression adhered and transmigrated to IL-1β-activated endothelial cells of the human umbilical vein more than CCA cells without sLe^a expression. Moreover, these abilities were significantly diminished in the presence of neutralizing antibodies specific to either sLe^a or E-selectin.

Fucosylated Fetuin-A and Kininogen

The aberrant N-linked glycans observed in serum can be used as a diagnostic or prognostic marker for specific cancers, including CCA. Betesh et al. used a glycomic approach to analyze and compare N-linked glycans in sera from CCA patients and controls. Increased levels of serum alpha-1,6 linked core and alpha 1,3 linked outer arm fucosylation in CCA patients were noted [97]. Furthermore, the fucosylated proteome of sera from CCA patients identified numerous fucosylated glycoproteins, e.g., alpha-2-macroglobulin, kininogen, hemopexin, fetuin-A, and ceruloplasmin. The relative proportion of fucosylation of these proteins was further determined using lectin fluorophore-linked immunosorbent assay (lectin-FLISA). The technique detects the amount of fucosylation present on an equal number of captured molecules independently of the total amount of protein tested. Of these, fucosylated fetuin-A and kininogen were significantly elevated in sera from CCA patients compared with those from PSC. Fucosylated fetuin-A could differentiate PSC from CCA with 62% sensitivity and 90% specificity, while fucosylated kininogen could differentiate CCA from the control group with similar diagnostic performance. In addition, these markers, either used alone or in combination, provide better detection of CCA than CA-19-9, indicating the potential of these two glycoproteins as diagnostic markers for CCA [97].

Alpha-L-Fucosidase

Alpha-L-fucosidase (AFU), a lysosomal enzyme, hydrolyzes the cleavage of fucose α-1,2, α-1,3, α-1,4, and α-1,6 linkages in the glycosylation chains to maintain homeostasis of fucose metabolism. It has been used as a tumor marker for various cancers, e.g., HCC and colorectal cancer [98, 99]. A high level of serum AFU has been shown to be associated with poor outcomes in HCC [100], though the reversed outcome was observed in breast cancer [101]. For CCA, AFU activity in serum was determined in 148 intrahepatic CCA cases by an automated analyzer. Based on ROC analysis and a cutoff of AFU <20.85 U/L, it was found that AFU level was an independent prognostic factor in patients with intrahepatic CCA [102]; patients with a high serum AFU level exhibited better outcomes. Treating CCA cells with AFU diminished the invasion capacity of CCA cells by suppression of MMP-2 and MMP-9 expression. Hence, serum AFU has been proposed to be a prognostic indicator for CCA.

Sialylation

Sialylation, the addition of sialic acid to subterminal sugar residues on oligosaccharides, is an important peripheral glycosylation process for maturation of glycoproteins and glycolipids (Fig. 25.6). The patterns of sialylation in cells are regulated

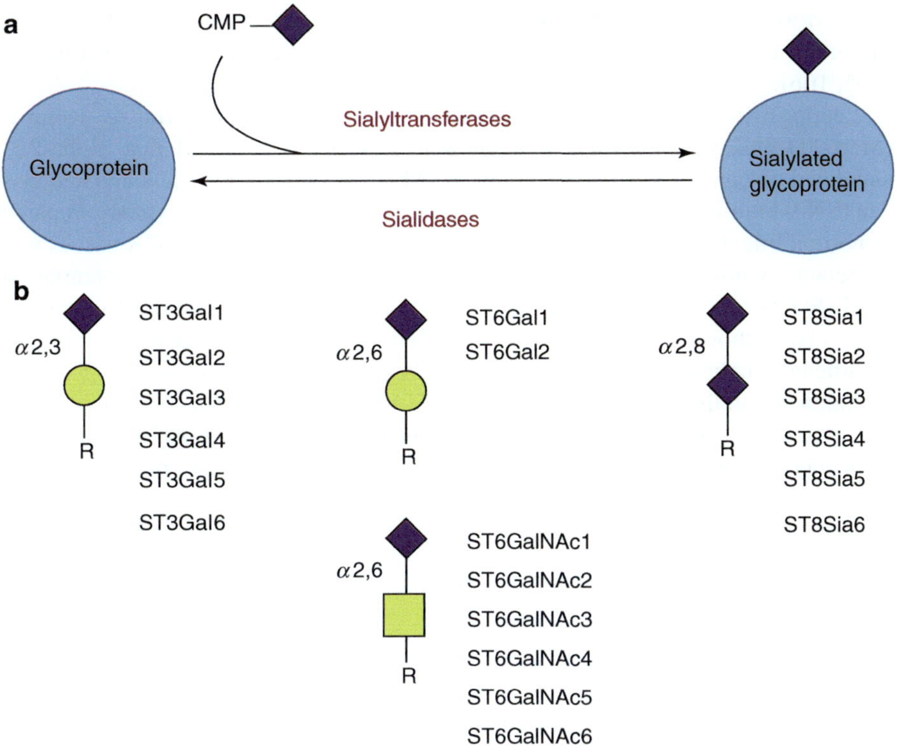

Fig. 25.6 Sialylation in human cells. (**a**) The addition of sialic acid to glycoprotein is catalyzed by sialytransferases (STs) and the removal reaction by sialidases. (**b**) The linkage of sialic acids to subterminal sugar residues is performed by four groups of STs: (1) ST3GalTs for Sia-α2,3-Gal linkage; (2) ST6GalT for Sia-α2,6-Gal linkage; (3) ST6GalNAcT for Sia-α2,6-GalNAc linkage, and (4) ST8Sia for Sia-α2,8-Sia linkage

by levels of nucleotide sugar donor, CMP-sialic acid, and the expressions of sialyltransferases (STs) and sialidases. STs are a family of enzymes responsible for transferring a sialic acid from a nucleotide sugar donor (CMP-sialic acid) to a glycoconjugate acceptor. Desialylation, the process of removing terminal sialic acid from glycoconjugates, is driven by sialidases or neuraminidases (NEUs). Altered expression of STs and/or NEUs, resulting in increases in uncommon sialylated glycans, has been reported in many cancer types [103]. These sialylated glycans were found to promote tumor progression and therapeutic resistance in several cancers.

Accumulating data over the past few decades have demonstrated alterations of sialylation in CCA. Serum sialic acid was found to be increased in CCA patients and capable of differentiating CCA patients from those with benign biliary diseases and healthy controls [104]. The elevation of serum sialic acid in CCA patients may be due to increases in core glycans/glycoproteins such as MU5AC and sLe^a

[34]. Moreover, sialic acid residues on sLe^a or sLe^x (section Fucosylation) are important for the binding of these molecules with E-selectin during extravasation [105, 106].

Lectin histochemistry of CCA tissues using *Maackia amurensis* lectin-II (MAL-II) and *Sambucus nigra* agglutinin (SNA) has revealed that alpha-2,3-sialylated glycan (MAL-II-binding glycan, MAL-SG) and alpha-2,6-sialylated glycan (SNA-binding glycan, SNA-SG) were overexpressed in CCA tissues compared to normal bile ducts (Fig. 25.3) [52]. A high level of MAL-SG in CCA tissues was associated with shorter survival of CCA patients, suggesting the potential of MAL-SG as a prognostic indicator for CCA. In addition, *in vitro* drug sensitivity assays have shown that suppression of sialylation by a sialyltransferase inhibitor significantly enhanced the sensitivity of CCA cell lines to 5-fluorouracil (5-FU), a common chemotherapeutic drug used for CCA treatment [52]. In addition to 5-FU, the involvement of sialylation in drug resistance to cisplatin and paclitaxel has also been reported (in other cancers) [107, 108]; a similar effect may be expected for CCA, in which cisplatin and paclitaxel are also drugs of choice.

Glycosphingolipids

GSLs are an important membrane component which play important roles in forming functional membranous microdomains. Synthesis of GSLs is separated into two phases: (1) CER synthesis and (2) glycosylation (Fig. 25.2). Hydrophobic interactions between the ceramide part of GSLs and other membrane components, such as cholesterol, proteins, and sphingomyelin, are important for determining the functions of microdomains [109–113]. The heterogeneity of GSLs is attributable to either glycan or ceramide compositions [114, 115]. The glycan part of a GSL can be monosaccharide, such as glucose and galactose, or oligosaccharide such as lactose, forming glucosyl-ceramide (GlcCer), galactosylceramide (GalCer), and lactosylceramide (LacCer), respectively. The ceramide part of a GSL can be composed of either hydroxylated or non-hydroxylated forms of fatty acids with C16 to C24. Aberrant expression of GSLs has been reported in many cancers, including breast, endometrial, and lung, and may be due to dysregulated expression of ceramide synthases (CERSs), GTs, and fatty acid-2-hydroxylases (FA2H) [116–122]. Indeed, altered expression of these enzymes has been associated with tumor growth and metastasis [116, 117, 120, 121, 123].

There is limited information regarding GSL expression in CCA. A recent study using LC-MS/MS analysis revealed that GSLs were elevated in CCA tissues compared with the adjacent normal liver [53]. High level of hydroxylated fatty-containing GSL was associated with shorter survival of CCA patients, suggesting the role of fatty acid hydroxylation in tumor progression of CCA [53]. These findings suggest increased activity of GSL-associated enzymes, e.g., ceramide synthase and fatty acid hydroxylase, in CCA as well as potential prognostic implications. Further study, however, is needed in this regard.

Conclusions and Perspectives

Glycoconjugates are one of the major components in cells that modulate key biological and physiological processes to maintain cellular homeostasis. Aberrant glycosylation of cell surface molecules alters cellular functions which can contribute to human diseases, including cancer. With the advanced technology in glycobiology research, several glycan structures and functions related to diseases have been revealed. The association of abnormal glycosylation patterns and aggressive phenotypes, e.g., tumor growth and metastasis, have been reported in CCA. Moreover, several CCA-associated glycans have been validated and are applicable for diagnosis and prognostic prediction. Directly targeting the synthesis of these glycans for cancer treatment, however, remains to be validated and is an area of ongoing investigation. A number of glycosylation inhibitors have been developed and studied for their antitumor activities, many of which appear to effectively suppress tumor growth and metastasis and enhance chemosensitivity of cancer cells. A combination of glycosylation inhibitors with other therapeutic agents or therapy may be a promising strategy to improve the treatment of CCA.

Further research into the molecular basis of glycosylation in CCA is expected to enhance understanding of cell-cell interactions, extracellular communications, and cancer immunology and which may reveal new targets for CCA treatment. Furthermore, the integration of large data analysis of glycomics/glycoproteomics and several other "-omics," e.g., genomics, transcriptomics, proteomics as well as metabolomics, in CCA cell lines/tissues from patients will provide an avenue for greater impact on developing novel approaches for the screening, diagnosis, prognosis, and targeted treatment for this highly lethal malignancy.

Acknowledgments We are grateful for the support from the Integration and Innovation Research grant (I62-01-02); the Center for Translational Medicine, Faculty of Medicine; and Mekong Health Science Research Institute (12/2561), Khon Kaen University, Thailand.

References

1. Becker DJ, Lowe JB. Fucose: biosynthesis and biological function in mammals. Glycobiology. 2003;13(7):41R–53R.
2. Meezan E, Wu HC, Black PH, Robbins PW. Comparative studies on the carbohydrate-containing membrane components of normal and virus-transformed mouse fibroblasts. II. Separation of glycoproteins and glycopeptides by sephadex chromatography. Biochemistry. 1969;8(6):2518–24.
3. Pinho SS, Reis CA. Glycosylation in cancer: mechanisms and clinical implications. Nat Rev Cancer. 2015;15(9):540–55.
4. Munkley J, Elliott DJ. Hallmarks of glycosylation in cancer. Oncotarget. 2016;7(23):35478–89.
5. Kailemia MJ, Park D, Lebrilla CB. Glycans and glycoproteins as specific biomarkers for cancer. Anal Bioanal Chem. 2017;409(2):395–410.
6. Munkley J, Mills IG, Elliott DJ. The role of glycans in the development and progression of prostate cancer. Nat Rev Urol. 2016;13(6):324–33.

7. Hirabayashi J, Yamada M, Kuno A, Tateno H. Lectin microarrays: concept, principle and applications. Chem Soc Rev. 2013;42(10):4443–58.
8. Indramanee S, Silsirivanit A, Pairojkul C, Wongkham C, Wongkham S. Aberrant glycosylation in cholangiocarcinoma demonstrated by lectin-histochemistry. Asian Pac J Cancer Prev. 2012;13 Suppl:119–24.
9. Kuno A, Matsuda A, Unno S, Tan B, Hirabayashi J, Narimatsu H. Differential glycan analysis of an endogenous glycoprotein: toward clinical implementation--from sample pretreatment to data standardization. Methods Mol Biol. 2014;1200:265–85.
10. Matsuda A, Kuno A, Matsuzaki H, Kawamoto T, Shikanai T, Nakanuma Y, et al. Glycoproteomics-based cancer marker discovery adopting dual enrichment with Wisteria floribunda agglutinin for high specific glyco-diagnosis of cholangiocarcinoma. J Proteome. 2013;85:1–11.
11. Chang TT, Cheng JH, Tsai HW, Young KC, Hsieh SY, Ho CH. Plasma proteome plus site-specific N-glycoprofiling for hepatobiliary carcinomas. J Pathol Clin Res. 2019;5(3):199–212.
12. Talabnin K, Talabnin C, Ishihara M, Azadi P. Increased expression of the high-mannose M6N2 and NeuAc3H3N3M3N2F tri-antennary N-glycans in cholangiocarcinoma. Oncol Lett. 2018;15(1):1030–6.
13. Varki A, Kornfeld S. Historical background and overview. In: Varki A, Cummings RD, Esko JD, Stanley P, Hart GW, et al., editors. Essentials of glycobiology. New York: Cold Spring Harbor; 2015. p. 1–18.
14. Varki A. Biological roles of glycans. Glycobiology. 2017;27(1):3–49.
15. Spiro RG. Protein glycosylation: nature, distribution, enzymatic formation, and disease implications of glycopeptide bonds. Glycobiology. 2002;12(4):43R–56R.
16. Stanley P, Taniguchi N, Aebi M. N-Glycans. In: Varki A, Cummings RD, Esko JD, Stanley P, Hart GW, et al., editors. Essentials of glycobiology. New York: Cold Spring Harbor; 2015. p. 99–111.
17. Bennett EP, Mandel U, Clausen H, Gerken TA, Fritz TA, Tabak LA. Control of mucin-type O-glycosylation: a classification of the polypeptide GalNAc-transferase gene family. Glycobiology. 2012;22(6):736–56.
18. Brockhausen I, Stanley P. O-GalNAc glycans. In: Varki A, Cummings RD, Esko JD, Stanley P, Hart GW, et al., editors. Essentials of glycobiology. New York: Cold Spring Harbor; 2015. p. 113–23.
19. Stanley P. Golgi glycosylation. Cold Spring Harb Perspect Biol. 2011;3(4)
20. Hart GW, Housley MP, Slawson C. Cycling of O-linked beta-N-acetylglucosamine on nucleocytoplasmic proteins. Nature. 2007;446(7139):1017–22.
21. Mouw JK, Ou G, Weaver VM. Extracellular matrix assembly: a multiscale deconstruction. Nat Rev Mol Cell Biol. 2014;15(12):771–85.
22. Schaefer L, Schaefer RM. Proteoglycans: from structural compounds to signaling molecules. Cell Tissue Res. 2010;339(1):237–46.
23. Yu RK, Tsai YT, Ariga T, Yanagisawa M. Structures, biosynthesis, and functions of gangliosides–an overview. J Oleo Sci. 2011;60(10):537–44.
24. Aebi M. N-linked protein glycosylation in the ER. Biochim Biophys Acta. 2013;1833(11):2430–7.
25. Kelleher DJ, Gilmore R. An evolving view of the eukaryotic oligosaccharyltransferase. Glycobiology. 2006;16(4):47R–62R.
26. D'Angelo G, Capasso S, Sticco L, Russo D. Glycosphingolipids: synthesis and functions. FEBS J. 2013;280(24):6338–53.
27. Schnaar RL, Kinoshita T. Glycosphingolipids. In: Varki A, Cummings RD, Esko JD, Stanley P, Hart GW, et al., editors. Essentials of glycobiology. New York: Cold Spring Harbor; 2015. p. 125–35.
28. Li X, Wang X, Tan Z, Chen S, Guan F. Role of glycans in cancer cells undergoing epithelial-mesenchymal transition. Front Oncol. 2016;6:33.
29. Ghazarian H, Idoni B, Oppenheimer SB. A glycobiology review: carbohydrates, lectins and implications in cancer therapeutics. Acta Histochem. 2011;113(3):236–47.

30. Freeze HH, Kinoshita T, Varki A. Glycans in acquired human diseases. In: Varki A, Cummings RD, Esko JD, Stanley P, Hart GW, et al., editors. Essentials of glycobiology. New York: Cold Spring Harbor; 2015. p. 583–95.
31. Varki A, Gagneux P. Biological functions of glycans. In: Varki A, Cummings RD, Esko JD, Stanley P, Hart GW, et al., editors. Essentials of glycobiology. New York: Cold Spring Harbor; 2015. p. 77–88.
32. Kirwan A, Utratna M, O'Dwyer ME, Joshi L, Kilcoyne M. Glycosylation-based serum biomarkers for cancer diagnostics and prognostics. Biomed Res Int. 2015;2015:490531.
33. Stowell SR, Ju T, Cummings RD. Protein glycosylation in cancer. Annu Rev Pathol. 2015;10:473–510.
34. Wongkham S, Sheehan JK, Boonla C, Patrakitkomjorn S, Howard M, Kirkham S, et al. Serum MUC5AC mucin as a potential marker for cholangiocarcinoma. Cancer Lett. 2003;195(1):93–9.
35. Xuan J, Li J, Zhou Z, Zhou R, Xu H, Wen W. The diagnostic performance of serum MUC5AC for cholangiocarcinoma: a systematic review and meta-analysis. Medicine (Baltimore). 2016;95(24):e3513.
36. Boonla C, Wongkham S, Sheehan JK, Wongkham C, Bhudhisawasdi V, Tepsiri N, et al. Prognostic value of serum MUC5AC mucin in patients with cholangiocarcinoma. Cancer. 2003;98(7):1438–43.
37. Barkeer S, Chugh S, Karmakar S, Kaushik G, Rauth S, Rachagani S, et al. Novel role of O-glycosyltransferases GALNT3 and B3GNT3 in the self-renewal of pancreatic cancer stem cells. BMC Cancer. 2018;18(1):1157.
38. Wu J, Chen S, Liu H, Zhang Z, Ni Z, Chen J, et al. Tunicamycin specifically aggravates ER stress and overcomes chemoresistance in multidrug-resistant gastric cancer cells by inhibiting N-glycosylation. J Exp Clin Cancer Res. 2018;37(1):272.
39. Abhari BA, McCarthy N, Le Berre M, Kilcoyne M, Joshi L, Agostinis P, et al. Smac mimetic suppresses tunicamycin-induced apoptosis via resolution of ER stress. Cell Death Dis. 2019;10(3):155.
40. Hou H, Ge C, Sun H, Li H, Li J, Tian H. Tunicamycin inhibits cell proliferation and migration in hepatocellular carcinoma through suppression of CD44s and the ERK1/2 pathway. Cancer Sci. 2018;109(4):1088–100.
41. Foufelle F, Fromenty B. Role of endoplasmic reticulum stress in drug-induced toxicity. Pharmacol Res Perspect. 2016;4(1):e00211.
42. Chang JY, Korolev VV. Specific toxicity of tunicamycin in induction of programmed cell death of sympathetic neurons. Exp Neurol. 1996;137(2):201–11.
43. Yau T, Dan X, Ng CC, Ng TB. Lectins with potential for anti-cancer therapy. Molecules. 2015;20(3):3791–810.
44. Lopez-Sambrooks C, Shrimal S, Khodier C, Flaherty DP, Rinis N, Charest JC, et al. Oligosaccharyltransferase inhibition induces senescence in RTK-driven tumor cells. Nat Chem Biol. 2016;12(12):1023–30.
45. Baro M, Lopez Sambrooks C, Quijano A, Saltzman WM, Contessa J. Oligosaccharyltransferase inhibition reduces receptor tyrosine kinase activation and enhances glioma radiosensitivity. Clin Cancer Res. 2019;25(2):784–95.
46. Lopez Sambrooks C, Baro M, Quijano A, Narayan A, Cui W, Greninger P, et al. Oligosaccharyltransferase inhibition overcomes therapeutic resistance to EGFR tyrosine kinase inhibitors. Cancer Res. 2018;78(17):5094–106.
47. Wahl DR, Lawrence TS. No sugar added: a new strategy to inhibit glioblastoma receptor tyrosine kinases. Clin Cancer Res. 2019;25(2):455–6.
48. Detarya M, Sawanyawisuth K, Aphivatanasiri C, Chuangchaiya S, Saranaruk P, Sukprasert L, et al. The O-GalNAcylating enzyme GALNT5 mediates carcinogenesis and progression of cholangiocarcinoma via activation of AKT/ERK signaling. Glycobiology. 2020;30(5):312–24.
49. Phoomak C, Silsirivanit A, Park D, Sawanyawisuth K, Vaeteewoottacharn K, Wongkham C, et al. O-GlcNAcylation mediates metastasis of cholangiocarcinoma through FOXO3 and MAN1A1. Oncogene. 2018;37(42):5648–65.

50. Phoomak C, Silsirivanit A, Wongkham C, Sripa B, Puapairoj A, Wongkham S. Overexpression of O-GlcNAc-transferase associates with aggressiveness of mass-forming cholangiocarcinoma. Asian Pac J Cancer Prev. 2012;13 Suppl:101–5.
51. Juntavee A, Sripa B, Pugkhem A, Khuntikeo N, Wongkham S. Expression of sialyl Lewis(a) relates to poor prognosis in cholangiocarcinoma. World J Gastroenterol. 2005;11(2):249–54.
52. Wattanavises S, Silsirivanit A, Sawanyawisuth K, Cha'on U, Waraasawapati S, Saentaweesuk W, et al. Increase of MAL-II binding alpha2,3-sialylated glycan is associated with 5-FU resistance and short survival of cholangiocarcinoma patients. Medicina (Kaunas). 2019;55(12)
53. Silsirivanit A, Phoomak C, Teeravirote K, Wattanavises S, Seubwai W, Saengboonmee C, et al. Overexpression of HexCer and LacCer containing 2-hydroxylated fatty acids in cholangiocarcinoma and the association of the increase of LacCer (d18:1-h23:0) with shorter survival of the patients. Glycoconj J. 2019;36(2):103–11.
54. Wang M, Fang M, Zhu J, Feng H, Warner E, Yi C, et al. Serum N-glycans outperform CA19-9 in diagnosis of extrahepatic cholangiocarcinoma. Electrophoresis. 2017;38(21):2749–56.
55. Silsirivanit A. Glycosylation markers in cancer. Adv Clin Chem. 2019;89:189–213.
56. Tarp MA, Clausen H. Mucin-type O-glycosylation and its potential use in drug and vaccine development. Biochim Biophys Acta. 2008;1780(3):546–63.
57. Vajaria BN, Patel PS. Glycosylation: a hallmark of cancer? Glycoconj J. 2017;34(2):147–56.
58. Boonla C, Sripa B, Thuwajit P, Cha-On U, Puapairoj A, Miwa M, et al. MUC1 and MUC5AC mucin expression in liver fluke-associated intrahepatic cholangiocarcinoma. World J Gastroenterol. 2005;11(32):4939–46.
59. Bamrungphon W, Prempracha N, Bunchu N, Rangdaeng S, Sandhu T, Srisukho S, et al. A new mucin antibody/enzyme-linked lectin-sandwich assay of serum MUC5AC mucin for the diagnosis of cholangiocarcinoma. Cancer Lett. 2007;247(2):301–8.
60. Xu H, Inagaki Y, Tang W, Guo Q, Wang F, Seyama Y, et al. Elevation of serum KL-6 mucin levels in patients with cholangiocarcinoma. Hepato-Gastroenterology. 2008;55(88):2000–4.
61. Matsuda A, Kuno A, Kawamoto T, Matsuzaki H, Irimura T, Ikehara Y, et al. Wisteria floribunda agglutinin-positive mucin 1 is a sensitive biliary marker for human cholangiocarcinoma. Hepatology. 2010;52(1):174–82.
62. Danese E, Ruzzenente A, Montagnana M, Lievens PM. Current and future roles of mucins in cholangiocarcinoma-recent evidences for a possible interplay with bile acids. Ann Transl Med. 2018;6(17):333.
63. Kasprzak A, Adamek A. Mucins: the old, the new and the promising factors in hepatobiliary carcinogenesis. Int J Mol Sci. 2019;20(6)
64. Fu C, Zhao H, Wang Y, Cai H, Xiao Y, Zeng Y, et al. Tumor-associated antigens: Tn antigen, sTn antigen, and T antigen. HLA. 2016;88(6):275–86.
65. Sasaki M, Yamato T, Nakanuma Y. Expression of sialyl-Tn, Tn and T antigens in primary liver cancer. Pathol Int. 1999;49(4):325–31.
66. Rangel MGH, Silva MLS. Detection of the cancer-associated T antigen using an Arachis hypogaea agglutinin biosensor. Biosens Bioelectron. 2019;141:111401.
67. Tanaka-Okamoto M, Hanzawa K, Mukai M, Takahashi H, Ohue M, Miyamoto Y. Correlation of serum sialyl Tn antigen values determined by immunoassay and SRM based method. Anal Biochem. 2018;544:42–8.
68. Saentaweesuk W, Silsirivanit A, Vaeteewoottacharn K, Sawanyawisuth K, Pairojkul C, Cha'on U, et al. Clinical significance of GalNAcylated glycans in cholangiocarcinoma: values for diagnosis and prognosis. Clin Chim Acta. 2018;477:66–71.
69. Inoue T, Eguchi T, Oda Y, Nishiyama K, Fujii K, Izumi H, et al. Expression of GalNAc-T3 and its relationships with clinicopathological factors in 61 extrahepatic bile duct carcinomas analyzed using stepwise sections - special reference to its association with lymph node metastases. Mod Pathol. 2007;20(2):267–76.
70. Thamavit W, Bhamarapravati N, Sahaphong S, Vajrasthira S, Angsubhakorn S. Effects of dimethylnitrosamine on induction of cholangiocarcinoma in Opisthorchis viverrini-infected Syrian golden hamsters. Cancer Res. 1978;38(12):4634–9.

71. Thamavit W, Kongkanuntn R, Tiwawech D, Moore MA. Level of Opisthorchis infestation and carcinogen dose-dependence of cholangiocarcinoma induction in Syrian golden hamsters. Virchows Arch B Cell Pathol Incl Mol Pathol. 1987;54(1):52–8.
72. Hart GW, Slawson C, Ramirez-Correa G, Lagerlof O. Cross talk between O-GlcNAcylation and phosphorylation: roles in signaling, transcription, and chronic disease. Annu Rev Biochem. 2011;80:825–58.
73. Yang X, Qian K. Protein O-GlcNAcylation: emerging mechanisms and functions. Nat Rev Mol Cell Biol. 2017;18(7):452–65.
74. Hu P, Shimoji S, Hart GW. Site-specific interplay between O-GlcNAcylation and phosphorylation in cellular regulation. FEBS Lett. 2010;584(12):2526–38.
75. Caldwell SA, Jackson SR, Shahriari KS, Lynch TP, Sethi G, Walker S, et al. Nutrient sensor O-GlcNAc transferase regulates breast cancer tumorigenesis through targeting of the oncogenic transcription factor FoxM1. Oncogene. 2010;29(19):2831–42.
76. Phoomak C, Vaeteewoottacharn K, Sawanyawisuth K, Seubwai W, Wongkham C, Silsirivanit A, et al. Mechanistic insights of O-GlcNAcylation that promote progression of cholangiocarcinoma cells via nuclear translocation of NF-kappaB. Sci Rep. 2016;6:27853.
77. Phoomak C, Park D, Silsirivanit A, Sawanyawisuth K, Vaeteewoottacharn K, Detarya M, et al. O-GlcNAc-induced nuclear translocation of hnRNP-K is associated with progression and metastasis of cholangiocarcinoma. Mol Oncol. 2019;13(2):338–57.
78. Saengboonmee C, Seubwai W, Pairojkul C, Wongkham S. High glucose enhances progression of cholangiocarcinoma cells via STAT3 activation. Sci Rep. 2016;6:18995.
79. Phoomak C, Vaeteewoottacharn K, Silsirivanit A, Saengboonmee C, Seubwai W, Sawanyawisuth K, et al. High glucose levels boost the aggressiveness of highly metastatic cholangiocarcinoma cells via O-GlcNAcylation. Sci Rep. 2017;7:43842.
80. Minato H, Nakanuma Y, Terada T. Expression of blood group-related antigens in cholangiocarcinoma in relation to non-neoplastic bile ducts. Histopathology. 1996;28(5):411–9.
81. Ma B, Simala-Grant JL, Taylor DE. Fucosylation in prokaryotes and eukaryotes. Glycobiology. 2006;16(12):158R–84R.
82. Indramanee S, Sawanyawisuth K, Silsirivanit A, Dana P, Phoomak C, Kariya R, et al. Terminal fucose mediates progression of human cholangiocarcinoma through EGF/EGFR activation and the Akt/Erk signaling pathway. Sci Rep. 2019;9(1):17266.
83. Silsirivanit A, Araki N, Wongkham C, Pairojkul C, Narimatsu Y, Kuwahara K, et al. A novel serum carbohydrate marker on mucin 5AC: values for diagnostic and prognostic indicators for cholangiocarcinoma. Cancer. 2011;117(15):3393–403.
84. Silsirivanit A, Araki N, Wongkham C, Vaeteewoottacharn K, Pairojkul C, Kuwahara K, et al. CA-S27: a novel Lewis a associated carbohydrate epitope is diagnostic and prognostic for cholangiocarcinoma. Cancer Sci. 2013;104(10):1278–84.
85. Pattanapairoj S, Silsirivanit A, Muisuk K, Seubwai W, Cha'on U, Vaeteewoottacharn K, et al. Improve discrimination power of serum markers for diagnosis of cholangiocarcinoma using data mining-based approach. Clin Biochem. 2015;48(10–11):668–73.
86. Safi F, Schlosser W, Kolb G, Beger HG. Diagnostic value of CA 19-9 in patients with pancreatic cancer and nonspecific gastrointestinal symptoms. J Gastrointest Surg. 1997;1(2):106–12.
87. Wozniak MA, Modzelewska K, Kwong L, Keely PJ. Focal adhesion regulation of cell behavior. Biochim Biophys Acta. 2004;1692(2–3):103–19.
88. Ali AH, et al. Surveillance for hepatobiliary cancers in patients with primary sclerosing cholangitis. Hepatology. 2018;67(6):2338–51.
89. Charatcharoenwitthaya P, et al. Utility of serum tumor markers, imaging, and biliary cytology for detecting cholangiocarcinoma in primary sclerosing cholangitis. Hepatology. 2008;48(4):1106–17.
90. Fung BM, Lindor KD, Tabibian JH. Cancer risk in primary sclerosing cholangitis: epidemiology, prevention, and surveillance strategies. World J Gastroenterol. 2019;25(6):659–71.
91. Lindor KD, et al. ACG clinical guideline: primary sclerosing cholangitis. Am J Gastroenterol. 2015;110(5):646–59. quiz 660

92. Tabibian JH, Ali AH, Lindor KD. Primary Sclerosing cholangitis, part 2: cancer risk, prevention, and surveillance. Gastroenterol Hepatol (N Y). 2018;14(7):427–32.
93. Mollicone R, Reguigne I, Kelly RJ, Fletcher A, Watt J, Chatfield S, et al. Molecular basis for Lewis alpha(1,3/1,4)-fucosyltransferase gene deficiency (FUT3) found in Lewis-negative Indonesian pedigrees. J Biol Chem. 1994;269(33):20987–94.
94. Nishihara S, Narimatsu H, Iwasaki H, Yazawa S, Akamatsu S, Ando T, et al. Molecular genetic analysis of the human Lewis histo-blood group system. J Biol Chem. 1994;269(46):29271–8.
95. Narimatsu H, Iwasaki H, Nakayama F, Ikehara Y, Kudo T, Nishihara S, et al. Lewis and secretor gene dosages affect CA19-9 and DU-PAN-2 serum levels in normal individuals and colorectal cancer patients. Cancer Res. 1998;58(3):512–8.
96. Wannhoff A, Hov JR, Folseraas T, Rupp C, Friedrich K, Anmarkrud JA, et al. FUT2 and FUT3 genotype determines CA19-9 cut-off values for detection of cholangiocarcinoma in patients with primary sclerosing cholangitis. J Hepatol. 2013;59(6):1278–84.
97. Betesh L, Comunale MA, Wang M, Liang H, Hafner J, Karabudak A, et al. Identification of fucosylated Fetuin-A as a potential biomarker for cholangiocarcinoma. Proteomics Clin Appl. 2017;11(9–10)
98. Delacadena M, Fernandez J, Decarlos A, Martinezzorzano V, Gilmartin E, Rodriguezberrocal F. Low levels of alpha-L-fucosidase activity in colorectal cancer are due to decreased amounts of the enzymatic protein and are related with Dukes' stage. Int J Oncol. 1996;9(4):747–54.
99. Deugnier Y, David V, Brissot P, Mabo P, Delamaire D, Messner M, et al. Serum alpha-L-fucosidase: a new marker for the diagnosis of primary hepatic carcinoma? Hepatology. 1984;4(5):889–92.
100. Wang K, Guo W, Li N, Shi J, Zhang C, Lau WY, et al. Alpha-1-fucosidase as a prognostic indicator for hepatocellular carcinoma following hepatectomy: a large-scale, long-term study. Br J Cancer. 2014;110(7):1811–9.
101. Yuan K, Listinsky CM, Singh RK, Listinsky JJ, Siegal GP. Cell surface associated alpha-L-fucose moieties modulate human breast cancer neoplastic progression. Pathol Oncol Res. 2008;14(2):145–56.
102. Shuang Z, Mao Y, Lin G, Wang J, Huang X, Chen J, et al. Alpha-L-fucosidase serves as a prognostic Indicator for intrahepatic cholangiocarcinoma and inhibits its invasion capacity. Biomed Res Int. 2018;2018:8182575.
103. Munkley J, Scott E. Targeting aberrant sialylation to treat cancer. Medicines (Basel). 2019;6(4)
104. Wongkham S, Boonla C, Kongkham S, Wongkham C, Bhudhisawasdi V, Sripa B. Serum total sialic acid in cholangiocarcinoma patients: an ROC curve analysis. Clin Biochem. 2001;34(7):537–41.
105. Ben-David T, Sagi-Assif O, Meshel T, Lifshitz V, Yron I, Witz IP. The involvement of the sLe-a selectin ligand in the extravasation of human colorectal carcinoma cells. Immunol Lett. 2008;116(2):218–24.
106. Trinchera M, Aronica A, Dall'Olio F. Selectin ligands sialyl-lewis a and sialyl-lewis x in gastrointestinal cancers. Biology (Basel). 2017;6(1)
107. Rillahan CD, Antonopoulos A, Lefort CT, Sonon R, Azadi P, Ley K, et al. Global metabolic inhibitors of sialyl- and fucosyltransferases remodel the glycome. Nat Chem Biol. 2012;8(7):661–8.
108. Schultz MJ, Swindall AF, Wright JW, Sztul ES, Landen CN, Bellis SL. ST6Gal-I sialyltransferase confers cisplatin resistance in ovarian tumor cells. J Ovarian Res. 2013;6(1):25.
109. Chiricozzi E, Ciampa MG, Brasile G, Compostella F, Prinetti A, Nakayama H, et al. Direct interaction, instrumental for signaling processes, between LacCer and Lyn in the lipid rafts of neutrophil-like cells. J Lipid Res. 2015;56(1):129–41.
110. Diaz-Rohrer BB, Levental KR, Simons K, Levental I. Membrane raft association is a determinant of plasma membrane localization. Proc Natl Acad Sci U S A. 2014;111(23):8500–5.
111. Iwabuchi K, Prinetti A, Sonnino S, Mauri L, Kobayashi T, Ishii K, et al. Involvement of very long fatty acid-containing lactosylceramide in lactosylceramide-mediated superoxide generation and migration in neutrophils. Glycoconj J. 2008;25(4):357–74.

112. Ohno Y, Suto S, Yamanaka M, Mizutani Y, Mitsutake S, Igarashi Y, et al. ELOVL1 production of C24 acyl-CoAs is linked to C24 sphingolipid synthesis. Proc Natl Acad Sci U S A. 2010;107(43):18439–44.
113. Prinetti A, Loberto N, Chigorno V, Sonnino S. Glycosphingolipid behaviour in complex membranes. Biochim Biophys Acta. 2009;1788(1):184–93.
114. Hakomori S. Glycosphingolipids in cellular interaction, differentiation, and oncogenesis. Annu Rev Biochem. 1981;50:733–64.
115. Hakomori SI, Handa K. GM3 and cancer. Glycoconj J. 2015;32(1–2):1–8.
116. Alderson NL, Hama H. Fatty acid 2-hydroxylase regulates cAMP-induced cell cycle exit in D6P2T schwannoma cells. J Lipid Res. 2009;50(6):1203–8.
117. Chen J, Li X, Ma D, Liu T, Tian P, Wu C. Ceramide synthase-4 orchestrates the cell proliferation and tumor growth of liver cancer in vitro and in vivo through the nuclear factor-kappaB signaling pathway. Oncol Lett. 2017;14(2):1477–83.
118. Patt LM, Grimes WJ. Cell surface glycolipid and glycoprotein glycosyltransferases of normal and transformed cells. J Biol Chem. 1974;249(13):4157–65.
119. Schiffmann S, Sandner J, Birod K, Wobst I, Angioni C, Ruckhaberle E, et al. Ceramide synthases and ceramide levels are increased in breast cancer tissue. Carcinogenesis. 2009;30(5):745–52.
120. Suzuki M, Cao K, Kato S, Komizu Y, Mizutani N, Tanaka K, et al. Targeting ceramide synthase 6-dependent metastasis-prone phenotype in lung cancer cells. J Clin Invest. 2016;126(1):254–65.
121. Wang S, Beeghly-Fadiel A, Cai Q, Cai H, Guo X, Shi L, et al. Gene expression in triple-negative breast cancer in relation to survival. Breast Cancer Res Treat. 2018;171(1):199–207.
122. Wegner M, Neddermann D, Piorunska-Stolzmann M, Jagodzinski PP. Role of epigenetic mechanisms in the development of chronic complications of diabetes. Diabetes Res Clin Pract. 2014;105(2):164–75.
123. Nagano M, Takahara K, Fujimoto M, Tsutsumi N, Uchimiya H, Kawai-Yamada M. Arabidopsis sphingolipid fatty acid 2-hydroxylases (AtFAH1 and AtFAH2) are functionally differentiated in fatty acid 2-hydroxylation and stress responses. Plant Physiol. 2012;159(3):1138–48.

Chapter 26
The Investigative Therapeutic Pipeline for Cholangiocarcinoma: Insights from Model Systems

Luca Maroni and Marco Marzioni

Abbreviations

S100A8	S100 calcium-binding protein A8
AUC	area under the curve
BilIN	biliary intraepithelial neoplasia
CAF	cancer-associated fibroblast
CCA	cholangiocarcinoma
DNMT	DNA methyltransferase
EGFR	endothelial growth factor receptor
ERCP	endoscopic retrograde cholangiopancreatography
FGFR2	fibroblast growth factor receptor 2
HATs	histone acetyltransferases
HDACs	histone deacetylases
HIF	hypoxia-inducible factor
HMGB1	high-mobility group box 1
HRH3	H3 histamine receptor
IDH	isocitrate dehydrogenase
IPNLs	intraductal papillary neoplasms of the liver
LOXL2	lysyl oxidase-like 2
MSCs	derived mesenchymal stem cells
ncRNAs	noncoding RNAs
NGF-β	nerve growth factor-β
OS	overall survival
PCR	polymerase chain reaction
PDGF	platelet-derived growth factor
PFS	progression-free survival
PR	partial response

L. Maroni (✉) · M. Marzioni
Department of Gastroenterology and Hepatology, Università Politecnica delle Marche, Ancona, Italy
e-mail: l.maroni@univpm.it; m.marzioni@univpm.it

J. H. Tabibian (ed.), *Diagnosis and Management of Cholangiocarcinoma*,
https://doi.org/10.1007/978-3-030-70936-5_26

PSC	primary sclerosing cholangitis
RIPK1	receptor-interacting protein kinase 1
TGF-β	transforming growth factor
TLR4	Toll-like receptor 4
VEGF	vascular endothelial growth factor

Introduction

Preclinical and clinical research on cholangiocarcinoma (CCA) has traditionally lagged behind relative to a variety of other tumors. This may be explained in part by the fact that CCA has been regarded as a rare tumor, especially in Western countries, and until recently has attracted only marginal attention from researchers and industry. In the last 20 years, however, the incidence of CCA has steadily risen worldwide, and it represents the second most common hepatic tumor after hepatocellular carcinoma. Moreover, a recent series of basic science studies, supported by advances in technology, have begun to shed light in the pathophysiology of CCA, which is characterized by extensive heterogeneity of the tumor, intricate genomic and epigenetic alterations, and a complex microenvironment and immunologic landscape.

The application of next-generation sequencing in CCA has unveiled a number of genetic alterations that are consistently found in intrahepatic and extrahepatic CCA. In particular, mutations in the isocitrate dehydrogenase (IDH1/IDH2), fibroblast growth factor receptor 2 (FGFR2) fusion, and mutations in cell proliferation genes (KRAS, BRAF, and HER family) offer the possibility to explore the use of different small molecules to selectively block intracellular pathways involved in CCA. Current use of such targeted therapies and their possible development in future years has been extensively discussed in Chap. 21.

Here, we specifically address the recent advances in angiogenesis, epigenetic modifications, and alterations of the Wnt/β-catenin pathway in the pathogenesis of CCA, as informed in large part by model systems, with a special attention to molecular pathways that may be amenable of clinical implementation in the diagnosis, prognostic stratification, or treatment of patients.

Angiogenesis and Lymphangiogenesis

The ability to form new blood and lymphatic vessels from preexisting vasculature is a fundamental feature of many solid tumors. Neovascularization is indeed paramount to provide proper oxygenation and nutrient supply for tumor growth and undoubtedly influence the development of distant metastases. CCA is a highly desmoplastic tumor and displays a limited number of newly developed blood vessels, while tumor-associated lymphangiogenesis is pronounced. Early lymph node metastases are indeed frequent at presentation (though in some cases may be difficult to accurate detect) and deeply influence the prognosis of the disease, whereas distant metastases occur in later phases [1]. Nonetheless, CCA tissues have been shown to express a number to growth factors that are involved in sustaining de novo formation of blood and lymphatic vessels and in orchestrating complex interactions with the tumor microenvironment.

Angiogenesis in CCA

The expression of vascular endothelial growth factor (VEGF), the main molecule involved in neoangiogenesis, has been consistently shown in CCA. The VEGF family comprises different isoforms (VEGF-A, VEGF-B, VEGF-C, VEGF-D, VEGF-E, and placenta growth factor) which are secreted by a number of cells and interact with corresponding receptors (VEGF-R). Among the members of the family, VEGF-A binds to VEGF-R1 and VEGF-R2 and mainly mediates the formation and permeability of new blood vessels. VEGF-C and VEGF-D, in turn, bind to VEGF-R3 and are involved in lymphangiogenesis (Fig. 26.1) [2].

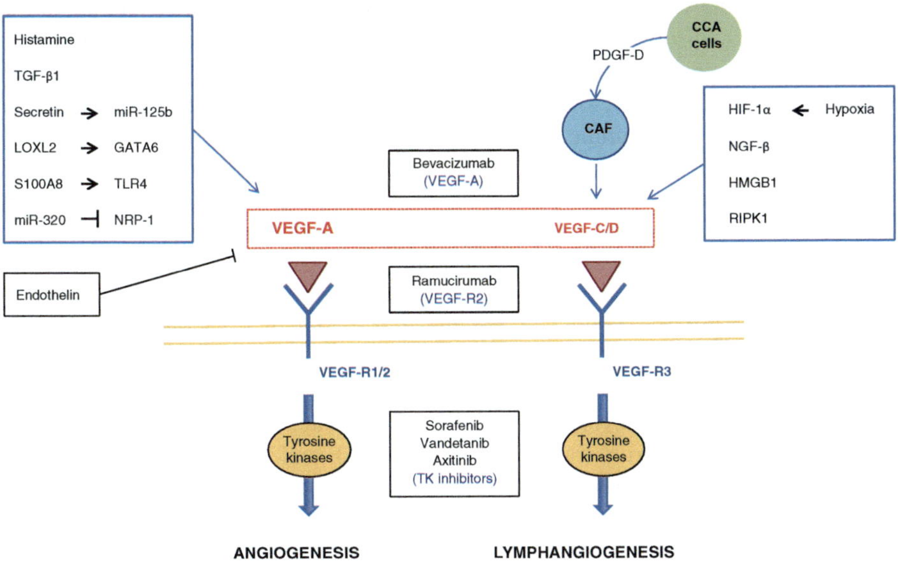

Fig. 26.1 Activation of the VEGF/VEGF-R signaling pathways in the pathogenesis of CCA. Molecular pathways preferentially implicated in the activation or repression of VEGF-A are depicted in the left side of the panel. Pathways preferentially involved in the regulation of VEGF-C/D are represented in the right side of the panel. Small molecules that have been evaluated in the treatment of CCA are depicted in the middle of the panel (pathways blocked by each molecule in brackets)

Previous immunohistochemical studies showed that VEGF expression is present in both intra- and extrahepatic CCA (53.8% and 59.2%, respectively), with a positive correlation with intrahepatic metastases [3]. In extrahepatic CCA, increased immunoreactivity against VEGF was correlated with a significantly higher overall mortality and a trend toward lymph node metastasis and peritoneal recurrence [4]. Expression of VEGF and its receptors (VEGF-R1 and VEGF-R2) has been confirmed in resected specimens of CCA, in which a coexpression of TGF-β1 and its receptors were demonstrated [5]. A more recent systematic review demonstrated that, based on data available, expression of VEGF-A was significantly higher in intrahepatic CCA compared to extrahepatic CCA [6]. These data are partially in contrast with a previous study showing that VEGF-A expression was more frequent in distal CCA compared to perihilar CCA and correlated with increased vascular density [7].

The secretion of VEGF is triggered in many cells by hypoxia, which stimulates the induction of a series of hypoxia-inducible factors. In addition to stimulating new vessel formation, the role of VEGF secretion as a paracrine factor modulating cholangiocytes pathophysiology, especially in terms of proliferation, has been evaluated. In vitro studies have demonstrated that proliferating cholangiocytes express VEGF-A, VEGF-C, VEGF-R2, and VEGF-R3 and that blocking this pathway decreases biliary cell proliferation [8]. In CCA cell lines, transcription of VEGF is induced by transforming growth factor-β1 (TGF-β1), which has also been found overexpressed in CCA tissue [5]. Multiple studies have evaluated a number of pathways that regulate VEGF secretion. Such studies offer a deeper understanding of the molecular mechanisms behind VEGF secretion in cholangiocytes and represent the basis to devise possible therapeutic strategies to be tested in clinical trials. The effect of VEGF on cholangiocyte proliferation is modulated, at least in part, by the activation of the H3 histamine receptor (HRH3). Both in vitro and in vivo, the activation of HRH3 in biliary cells decreases the expression of VEGF-A and VEGF-C and inhibits CCA growth in a protein kinase C-dependent manner [9]. Long-term administration of histamine, however, has been showed to increase CCA proliferation and VEGF secretion; such effects could be reversed by blocking histidine decarboxylase, the enzyme responsible for histamine synthesis [10].

Additional regulation of the VEGF pathway is mediated by secretin. After biliary damage, cholangiocytes produce secretin that, in a paracrine fashion, results in upregulation of VEGF via modulation of microRNA 125b and let7a levels [11]. Endothelin-1, which is overexpressed in CCA tissue, has also been showed to reduce cholangiocyte proliferation as well as VEGF and VEGF-R expression both in vitro and in vivo [12]. The list of pathways modulating the VEGF axis has grown even more in recent years. Peng et al. demonstrated in vitro that the scavenger receptor cysteine-rich domain of lysyl oxidase-like 2 (LOXL2) physically interacts with GATA-binding protein 6 (GATA6), which in turn stimulates VEGF synthesis and secretion. In human CCA samples, expression of LOXL2 and GATA6 was associated with poor overall survival and disease-free survival [13]. S100 calcium-binding protein A8 (S100A8) regulates in vitro the expression of VEGF via activation of the Toll-like receptor 4 (TLR4)/NF-κB pathway [14]. Finally, microRNA 320 has been recently shown to downregulate the expression of neuropilin-1

(NRP-1), a multifunctional receptor involved in tumor development, growth, and metastasis, which in turn stimulates the expression of VEGF [15].

Collectively, these data strongly indicate that modulation of angiogenesis may be of therapeutic interest in the treatment of CCA. It seems plausible that, in the clinical context, the regulation of VEGF expression may be under the control of many different pathways and that mutual interactions between such pathways need to be taken into account when devising possible new treatments.

Lymphangiogenesis in CCA

The development of a rich intra- and peri-tumoral lymphatic vasculature with subsequent early lymph node metastases is a characteristic feature of CCA. In intrahepatic CCA patients, the degree of tumor-associated lymphangiogenesis evaluated by immunohistochemistry for podoplanin (a specific lymphatic vessel marker) correlated with increased lymphatic metastases, recurrence of the tumor after surgery, and reduced overall survival (OS) [16]. Lymphatic vessel density in tumor specimens has been shown to correlate to lymph node metastasis and to be an independent negative prognostic factor also in perihilar CCA [17]. In fact, tumor spread to regional lymph nodes has been consistently demonstrated to strongly impact the prognosis of CCA patients, with median survival as low as 15 months for lymph node-positive compared to 37 months in lymph node-negative patients [18, 19]. Aishima et al. showed that in intrahepatic CCA patients, the lymphatic vessel density is lower in the tumor center and much more pronounced at the periphery of the tumor, especially in poorly differentiated CCA. Interestingly, while no correlation was found between proliferation of lymphatic vessels and development of metastasis, the expression of VEGF-C by tumor cells was associated with lymph node metastasis [20]. High expression of VEGF-C in CCA has been confirmed by various other studies, with positive percentages comprised between 40% and 75% of the patients [21–23].

The generation of a prominent lymphatic vasculature may be stimulated in CCA by the overexpression of hypoxia-inducible factor (HIF)-1α, in a similar fashion to a mechanism described for multiple others tumors. HIF-1α is induced in response to cancer-related intratumoral hypoxia and regulates the transcription of many genes involved in cell survival and invasion, including the expression of VEGFs [24]. HIF-1α expression has been shown to be prominent in a majority of CCA tissues (66%), again with a positive correlation with lymph node metastasis [25]. Moreover, in an in vitro model, hypoxia induces the expression of a number of genes involved in tumor progression and chemoresistance in CCA cells [26]. The regulation of lymphangiogenesis in CCA may also involve a complex interplay between CCA cells and the tumor microenvironment (see Chap. 24 for greater detail). In fact, CCA cells secrete platelet-derived growth factor (PDGF)-D, which is functional to recruit cancer-associated fibroblast (CAF) in the tumor stroma [27]. The binding of PDGF-D to its cognate receptor on CAF induces the release of VEGF-A and VEGF-C, which in turn mediates lymphatic vasculature expansion and permeability with invasion of CCA cells [28]. VEGF-C expression in CCA seems also under the control of different growth and transcription factors. In vitro, nerve growth factor-β (NGF-β) overexpression induced the upregulation of VEGF-C, which stimulated the proliferation and migration of lymphatic endothelial cells [29]. In addition, the high-mobility group box 1 (HMGB1), a proinflammatory cytokine, has been shown to be involved in VEGF-C secretion in intrahepatic CCA cells [30]. More recently, Li et al. demonstrated that receptor-interacting protein kinase 1 (RIPK1), a newly described mediator in proinflammatory and apoptotic pathways, is upregulated in CCA tissue compared to nonneoplastic control. In vitro, silencing of RIPK1 reduced protein expression of VEGF-C, while, in vivo, it inhibited lymphangiogenesis in a orthotopic CCA model in null mice [31].

Given the strong negative impact on prognosis, the molecular mechanisms regulating tumor-associated lymphangiogenesis appear therefore as possible candidates for therapeutic targeting in CCA. It remains of paramount importance to clearly identify the interactions between CCA cells and the tumor microenvironment, which are responsible for vasculature changes, in order to devise specific and effective treatments.

Angiogenesis Inhibition in Preclinical and Clinical Trials

A possible role of anti-antiangiogenic agents in the treatment of CCA has been investigated in a number of preclinical and clinical trials. Bevacizumab, a recombinant monoclonal antibody that inhibits VEGF-A and is already available for clinical use, was shown to reduce the growth of CCA in an in vivo xenograft mouse model. Treatment with bevacizumab, however, also induced the expression of HIF-1α and its responsive genes such as VEGF and carbonic anhydrases, creating the bases for a possible drug resistance. Intriguingly, the addition of acetazolamide, a carbonic anhydrase inhibitor, improved the antiproliferative effect of the treatment [32]. Bevacizumab has also been tested in multiple phase 2 clinical trials. Zhu et al. reported favorable tolerability of the administration of bevacizumab in combination with gemcitabine and oxaliplatin (GEMOX) in 35 patients with advanced biliary tract cancers, including 25 patients with CCA. In the CCA subgroup, partial response (PR) was achieved in 41% of patients, with a median progression-free survival (PFS) and OS of 7.6 and 14.2 months, respectively [33]. The combination of bevacizumab and erlotinib, an inhibitor of endothelial growth factor receptor (EGFR), has also shown promising results in a phase 2 trial of 53 patients with advanced biliary tract cancer, including 43 patients with intra- or extrahepatic CCA. In this study, 12% of patients achieved PR, and 51% had stable disease without severe adverse events [34]. After failure of first-line treatment (gemcitabine plus oxaliplatin-based), the administration of folinic acid, fluorouracil, and irinotecan (FOLFIRI) plus bevacizumab in metastatic intrahepatic CCA patients showed a response rate of 38.4% and a disease control rate of 84.5% [35]. More recently, Iyer et al. reported the results of the combination of bevacizumab and gemcitabine plus capecitabine in 50 patients with gallbladder cancer (22%), intrahepatic CCA (58%), and extrahepatic CCA (20%). Median PFS of 8.1 months (95% confidence interval, 5.3–9.9) and a median OS of 10.2 months (95% confidence interval, 7.5–13.7) were reported for the combination therapy [36].

Preliminary results have also been reported for ramucirumab, a fully human monoclonal antibody blocking VEGF-R2. Patients with advanced biliary tract cancer and a prior treatment with gemcitabine-based regimens were treated with ramucirumab (8 mg/kg every 2 weeks) until progression. Median PFS and OS of 2.73 months and 6.31 months, respectively, were reported with six patients presenting a prolonged PFS of more than 24 months [37]. Ramucirumab has also been investigated in combination with pembrolizumab, an immune checkpoint inhibitor blocking the PD-1 receptor, in patients with metastatic CCA with progression after first-line treatment. However, the results of the study were suboptimal, with a median PFS and OS of 1.6 months and 6.4 months, respectively [38].

Much research has also been conducted evaluating the efficacy of drugs inhibiting tyrosine kinases, which are involved in the activation of a number of intracellular pathways controlled by growth factor receptors. Sorafenib is an orally available tyrosine kinase inhibitor acting on VEGF-R, PDGF receptor, and RAF kinases, currently employed in the treatment of hepatocellular carcinoma. A preclinical study demonstrated a favorable effect of sorafenib on CCA. In vivo, oral administration of sorafenib significantly reduced the growth of a subcutaneous xenograft CCA model and prolonged the survival of mice subjected to an intraperitoneal CCA dissemination model [39]. However, results of clinical trials were inferior to expectations. One phase 2 study was terminated because of failure to meet the meet the requirement of a minimum of one confirmed PR [40]. Another study showed a very low PFS (2.3 months) and median OS (4.4 months) in patients with advanced biliary tract tumors treated with sorafenib as a single agent [41]. Also combination trials have been disappointing and showed no significant improvement with the addition of sorafenib compared to standard chemotherapy alone [42, 43].

An alternative possibility has been offered by vandetanib, a tyrosine kinase inhibitor of VEGF-R and EGFR. In a preclinical study, vandetanib incubations had an antiproliferative effect on TKKK cells, a human CCA cell line derived from Japanese patients, and reduced the growth of a TKKK subcutaneous xenograft model. Interestingly, the effect of vandetanib was present only in cells with high VEGF and EGFR expression and lack of KRAS mutations, suggesting that CCA patients with similar molecular characteristics may benefit the most from the treatment [44]. Vandetanib has been investigated also in a phase 2 randomized, multicenter trial comparing its efficacy as monotherapy or in combination with gemcitabine in patients with advanced biliary tract cancers. Unfortunately, despite no major side effects being reported, PFS did not differ significantly between groups (105 days for vandetanib alone vs. 114 days for vandetanib plus gemcitabine vs. 148 days for gemcitabine plus placebo) [45].

Axitinib, an inhibitor of VEGF-R1/2/3, also showed promising results in vivo. Takahashi et al. showed that oral administration of axitinib inhibited the subcutaneous growth of two xenograft models based on the injection of NCC-BD1 and TKKK cells lines [46]. Axitinib has been investigated in only five patients with advanced biliary tract cancer and with progressive disease under a gemcitabine-based regimen. Partial response was achieved in one patient; OS and PFS ranged from 2.0 to 19.9 months and 1.5 to 7.4 months, respectively [47].

Despite encouraging in the preclinical setting, the results of clinical trials of selective inhibitors of lymphangiogenesis or more broad tyrosine kinase inhibitors do not currently justify their widespread use in clinical practice. The very limited efficacy of such molecules in the human setting may be due to the extreme heterogeneity of CCA patients and tumors, combined with enhanced chemoresistance profiles. Undoubtedly, given the increasing incidence of CCA worldwide, future studies will have to include large populations in multicenter clinical trials. A careful selection of the patients, based on specific molecular features of the tumor, will also be paramount for unveiling effective treatments in the era of precision medicine.

Epigenetic Modifications

Epigenetic modifications are a series of heritable and nonheritable changes in gene expression that do not require modification of the DNA sequence. The main epigenetic mechanisms described so far are DNA methylation, histone modification, and noncoding RNAs. A number of studies have demonstrated that tumor tissues display early and profound epigenetic changes that are believed to contribute to tumor development and progression. In particular, epigenetic modifications are involved in silencing of tumor suppressor genes and overexpression of oncogenes. Moreover, the study of epigenetic changes may offer interesting possibilities in terms of early detection of CCA and therapeutic implications [48].

DNA Methylation

DNA methylation involves the transfer of a methyl group to cytosine residues of DNA, which is catalyzed by various DNA methyltransferase (DNMT) enzymes. This process occurs specifically in CpG sites of the genome and results in failure of transcription and gene silencing. Lee et al. initially reported that, using a methylation-specific polymerase chain reaction (PCR), a selected panel of 18 genes and loci was frequently mutated in a cohort of 79 resected intrahepatic CCA patients, while normal bile ducts showed no methylation at the same sites. Interestingly, OS was shorter in patients with CpG island methylation of APC, p16, and TIMP3 than in the patients without methylation [49]. Using methylation-specific PCR of limited target loci, a number of reports have subsequently showed that methylation occurs in the promoter region of various oncosuppressor genes, including p16, p14, DAPK1,

E-cadherin, and MLH1, among others (Table 26.1) [50–55]. More recently, Goeppert et al. performed a global methylation analysis by methyl-CpG immunoprecipitation combined with whole-genome CpG island array in 18 patients with CCA (intrahepatic and extrahepatic combined). Hypomethylation was more frequent than hypermethylation, and a differential methylation was present in the promoter regions of a number of cancer-related pathways including Wnt, TGF-β, and PI3K signaling pathways [56].

DNA methylation appears to be an early event in CCA carcinogenesis, with possible important implications for early diagnosis. A significant proportion of

Table 26.1 List of the most frequently differentially methylated gene in CCA and in premalignant biliary lesions

Gene	Sample	Methylation status	% positive	Reference
APC	iCCA eCCA	Hypermethylated	26.6–47.2% 44.4%	[49, 52] [52]
p16	iCCA eCCA CCA IPNL	Hypermethylated	17.7–48.6% 54.3–80% 26.1–76% 54.6%	[49, 52] [52, 54] [53, 55] [57]
p14	iCCA eCCA CCA	Hypermethylated	8.9–30% 46% 25%	[49, 52] [52] [53]
TIMP3	iCCA	Hypermethylated	8.9%	[49]
E-cadherin	iCCA eCCA CCA	Hypermethylated	21.5–48.6% 40% 34.8%	[49, 52] [52, 53] [55]
RASSF-1	iCCA eCCA CCA	Hypermethylated	48.6% 83.3% 30.4%	[52] [52] [55]
DAPK1	iCCA eCCA CCA	Hypermethylated	0–7.6% 5.7–40% 17.4%	[49, 52] [52, 53] [55]
MLH1	iCCA eCCA CCA	Hypermethylated	18.5% 32–46.6% 13%	[52] [52, 54] [55]
CHFR	CCA	Hypermethylated	17.4%	[55]
RUNX3	CCA BilIN	Hypermethylated	78.3% >30%	[55] [58]
MGMT	iCCA eCCA	Hypermethylated	27% 40–49%	[52] [52, 55]
TMEFF2	BilIN	Hypermethylated	>80%	[58]
HOXA1	BilIN	Hypermethylated	>50%	[58]
NEUROG1	BilIN	Hypermethylated	>30%	[58]
LINE-1	BilIN	Hypomethylated		[58]
SAT2	BilIN	Hypomethylated		[58]

Data on methylation frequency are reported for intrahepatic CCA (iCCA) or extrahepatic CCA (eCCA) when available. *IPNL* intraductal papillary neoplasm of the liver, *BilIN* biliary intraepithelial neoplasia intraductal papillary neoplasms of the liver (IPNLs), a precursor lesion of CCA, showed hypermethylation at the p16^{INK4a} promoter region, which correlated with decreased protein expression [57]. In parallel, biliary intraepithelial neoplasia (BilIN), the premalignant lesion of extrahepatic CCA, has been shown to harbor increased methylation levels of TMEFF2, HOXA1, NEUROG1, and RUNX3 compared to normal bile duct tissue. The methylation levels of the same genes increased even further in extrahepatic CCA samples, suggesting that cancer-specific CpG island hypermethylation occurs early in CCA development [58]. Klump et al. evaluated the promoter methylation of p16 ^{INK4a} and p14^{ARF} in bile samples obtained during endoscopic retrograde cholangiopancreatography (ERCP) of extrahepatic CCA patients, PSC patients, and control subjects. p16 ^{INK4a} was found to be methylated in 53% of patients with CCA and only in 6% of controls, suggesting its possible role in the diagnostic workup, especially in cases of diagnostic uncertainty [59]. In a small cohort of patients with extrahepatic CCA, the evaluation of the methylation index of HOXA1 and NEUROG1 in samples obtained from brush cytology was shown to be superior to standard cytology alone [60]. Andresen et al. tested by methylation-specific PCR a total of 13 candidate genes in a 39 CCA and 54 nonmalignant tissue samples and, subsequently, in biliary brush samples of 15 CCA and 20 nonmalignant PSC controls. The four best performing genes (CDO1, CNRIP1, SEPT9, and VIM) were subsequently evaluated in a validation cohort of 34 CCA and 34 PSC controls, obtaining a sensitivity of 85%, a specificity of 98%, and an area under the ROC curve (AUC) of 0.944 [61]. The evaluation of the methylation of a five-gene panel comprising CCND2, CDH13, GRIN2B, RUNX3, and TWIST1 also showed very promising results (sensitivity of 83%, superior to standard cytology) when employed directly in bile samples collected during ERCP [62]. More recently, the evaluation of the methylation status of candidate genes has been attempted also in serum cell-free DNA (cfDNA), which consists of DNA fragments released into the blood mainly by apoptotic and necrotic tumor cells. The assessment of methylation of OPCML and HOXD9, quantified by methylation-sensitive high-resolution melting, showed a AUC of 0.850 and 0.789, respectively. The combination of both genes reached values of sensitivity and specificity of 62.50% and 100% and a positive predictive values and negative predictive value of 100% and 72.72%, respectively [63].

Taken together, these data show that the study of DNA methylation pattern in CCA may not only deepen our understanding on the complex epigenetic regulation of the disease but also offer concrete new option for earlier and more sensitive detection of biliary cancers in the clinical practice.

Histone Modifications

In the nucleus of eukaryotic cells, genomic DNA is normally associated with a number of proteins in the form of chromatin. The nucleosome, which is the functional unit of chromatin, is composed of 147 base pairs of DNA wrapped around a histone protein octamer that is formed of two subunits of histone H2A, H2B, H3, and H4. Posttranslational modifications of histones, which include acetylation, methylation, and phosphorylation, are essential in regulating all aspects of DNA-directed process such as replication, transcription, and repair [64]. In particular, histone acetylation mediated by histone acetyltransferases (HATs) and histone deacetylation mediated by histone deacetylases (HDACs) have been known to result in activation and repression of transcription, respectively.

In vitro, treatment of CCA cell lines (QBC939, KMBC and OZ) with trichostatin A, a known HDAC inhibitor, significantly reduced cell proliferation. In a xenograft model using gallbladder cancer cell, trichostatin A also reduced the subcutaneous growth of the tumor in vivo [65]. In the preclinical setting, a similar effect on CCA cell growth has been confirmed by a number of studies investigating the role of different HDAC inhibitors (valproic acid, NVP-LAQ824, NVP-LBH589) [66]. The effect of the HDAC inhibitor MS-275 on CCA cells lines is mediated by induction of apoptosis, as suggested by the activation of caspase-3, upregulation of Bax, and downregulation of Bcl-2 in treated cells [67]. Moreover, treatment of CCA cell lines with trichostatin A or valproic acid induced the expression of E-cadherin and zonulin-1, both epithelial markers, and reduced migration and invasion as compared to cells treated only with gemcitabine, suggesting a possible role of HDAC inhibitor in suppressing the epithelial-mesenchymal transition of CCA cells [68].

In the clinical setting, in intrahepatic CCA, expression of HDAC correlated with higher tumor stage; moreover, the expression of HDAC was associated with a poorer prognosis and worse disease-free survival rate [69]. The expression of HDAC2 and HDAC3, measured by PCR, Western blot, and immunohistochemistry, was also found to be induced in about half of 26 cases of CCA; HDAC2 and HDAC3 correlated with a shorter OS and were identified as independent prognostic factors on multivariate Cox regression analysis [70]. Conversely, the expression of HDAC8 has been shown to be downregulated in intrahepatic CCA tissues compared with nonmalignant corresponding bile ducts; lower HDAC8 expression also correlated with lymph node metastases and poor prognosis [71].

Despite promising preclinical studies and encouraging results in the management of other solid tumors, data regarding the use of HDAC inhibitors clinically in the treatment of CCA are currently lacking [72]. The use of valproic acid in combination with S-1, an oral fluoropyrimidine derivative, was preliminarily tested in a phase 1/2 study enrolling a total of 12 patients with advanced pancreatobiliary cancers (7 pancreatic cancer, 4 CCA, and 1 gallbladder cancer). A PR was reported only in one patient, while a stable disease was obtained in 91.7% of patients, with grade 3–4 adverse events in about 20% of cases [73]. A clinical trial testing the effect of entinostat, an oral class I HDAC inhibitor, in combination with nivolumab is currently recruiting patients (NCT03250273) [74]. Moreover, a clinical trial evaluating HDAC6 inhibition with KA2507 in advanced biliary tract cancer is expected to start recruiting patients in the near future (NCT04186156) [75].

Noncoding RNAs

Noncoding RNAs (ncRNAs) comprise a group of single-stranded RNA sequences that are not translated into proteins but regulate gene expression with complex post-transcriptional modulation. Based on the their length, ncRNAs are divided into long ncRNAs (>200 nucleotides long) and small ncRNAs (<200 nucleotides long); the latter includes microRNA (miR), small interfering RNA, piwi-RNA, and small nucleolar RNA [76].

A number of ncRNAs have been investigated in CCA. Among them, miRs are so far the most studied, with selective miRs having been found to be upregulated or downregulated in CCA [77]. miR-21, miR-141, and miR-200b have been shown to be highly upregulated in malignant cholangiocytes in vitro. Interestingly, miR-21 regulated the PTEN-mediated activation of PI 3-kinase signaling, and its inhibition increased the sensitivity to gemcitabine [78]. Using a miR array in five primary CCAs and five control bile duct specimens, Selaru et al. confirmed that miR-21 is overexpressed in human CCA. In vitro, miR-21 regulated the expression of programmed cell death 4 and tissue inhibitor of metalloproteinases 3 [79]. Contrasting results regarding the possible use of miR-21 as a serum marker for CCA have been reported in the literature. For instance, Correa-Gallego et al. reported a significant overexpression in the serum levels of miR-21 and miR-221 in a cohort of patients formed by 25 intrahepatic CCA patients and 7 healthy controls, with an AUC of 0.94 when using miR-21 levels to discriminate between cases and controls [80]. In contrast, in a cohort of 50 CCA patients, 15 hepatolithiasis patients, and 15 healthy volunteers, serum miR-21 levels were suboptimal in discriminating between cases and controls (AUC of 0.871, which was inferior to the performance of CA 19-9 in this study), though they were significantly correlated with clinical stage, invasion, lymphatic vessel infiltration, metastasis, and poor survival [81].

In recent years, the list of upregulated or downregulated miRs in CCA has grown exponentially, and this aspect has been reviewed in detail elsewhere [77, 82]. Many studies have focused on single miRs, while others have provided a more thorough expression profile of cancer tissue compared to control samples. In the latter case, among the many miRs identified, only a small proportion of miRs was consistently found to be differently expressed in tumoral tissues by different studies. For example, miR-21 was found to be upregulated in human CCA cell lines and in two in human CCA tissue profiling studies [78, 83, 84], while miR-200c was downregulated in two distinct studies [83, 84]. The small sample size of the majority of the studies, given the intrinsic rarity of CCA and the lack of large international collaborative studies, may have influenced the results of the investigations (e.g., inadequate study power). Altogether, apart from the important role of miRs in the pathophysiological alterations of CCA on a molecular level, the available literature seems to show a significant potential for miRs as biomarkers. Along with the results previously reported for miR-21, a number of different miRs have shown promising results in different studies. For example, serum levels of miR-29 were found to be significantly increased in a cohort of 66 CCA patients compared to 66 controls, with an AUC of 0.899 and sensitivity and specificity of 84.8% and 81.8%, respectively, in distinguishing CCA from controls [85]. Moreover, serum levels of miR-122 were significantly more elevated in CCA patients than in PSC patients, despite the latter showing increased levels compared to healthy individuals; the AUC of miR-122 (0.818) was slightly better than the AUC of CA 19.9 (0.778) for discriminating between CCA and PSC patients, but this difference did not reach statistical significance [86].

An important aid in the diagnosis of CCA may also come from the evaluation of miRs directly in bile samples collected during ERCP procedures. Voigtländer et al. reported that miR-412, miR-640, miR-1537, and miR-3189 bile levels were significantly higher in patients with PSC or PSC-related CCA than in patients with sporadic CCA. More importantly, the same miRs were significantly different also in PSC or PSC-related CCA patients, suggesting their possible role in detecting the neoplastic transformation of cholangiocytes during the course of PSC [87]. Along the same lines, by using a microarray platform screening 1209 miRs, miR-30d-5p and miR-92a-3p were found to be upregulated in bile of CCA patients compared to patients with benign biliary obstruction. In a validation cohort of 37 CCA patients and 48 controls, bile miR-30d-5p demonstrated an AUC of 0.730, with a sensitivity of 81.1% and a specificity of 60.5%, and outperformed serum levels of CA 19.9 and CEA [88]. Since RNA samples may degrade relatively fast in bile samples, the validity of measuring miRs in whole bile samples has been questioned by some investigators. Moreover, the different protocols used in terms of storing and processing samples and analyzing the data (with special reference to internal controls for miR evaluation) make the interpretation of the available studies difficult. A promising solution may come from the evaluation of miRs in biliary extracellular vesicles, which contain abundant and stable RNA material. In this context, one study found that a panel of miRs in extracellular vesicles could correctly identify CCA patients with a sensitivity of 67% and specificity of 96% [89].

Alterations in the Wnt/β-catenin Signaling Pathway

The Wnt/β-catenin signaling is an evolutionarily conserved pathway that is fundamental for cell fate determination during embryogenesis, cell proliferation, and migration [90]. In recent years, after the initial report that the APC gene driving the development of familial adenomatous polyposis interacts with β-catenin, a number of studies have confirmed the involvement of the Wnt/β-catenin signaling in many cancers [91]. High nuclear expression of β-catenin, evaluated by immunohistochemistry, has been reported in a small proportion (about 16%) of intrahepatic CCA [92]. In perihilar CCA, substantial expression (between 10 and 49% of cells) of Wnt2 and β-catenin has been shown in about 80% and 50%, respectively, of tumors [93]. Interestingly, mutations of the β-catenin gene at exon 3 (containing the element responsible for Wnt signaling) was not detected in any of 55 intrahepatic CCA samples, suggesting an alternative mechanism of deregulation in CCA [94].

Tokumoto et al. also reported a low frequency of β-catenin mutations (8.3%) in a cohort of 24 surgically resected samples of intrahepatic CCA patients; however, expression levels of downstream target genes of the Wnt/β-catenin signaling were significantly upregulated [95]. Boulter et al. clearly demonstrated that the Wnt/β-catenin pathway plays a crucial role in CCA; in CCA tissue samples, the expression of Wnt target genes and of Wnt ligands WNT7B and WNT10A were significantly increased in comparison with matched noncancerous tissues [96].

Wnt ligands seem to be produced by macrophages derived from the bone marrow and infiltrating the tumor stroma. After transplantation of GFP-expressing bone marrow into irradiated rats subjected to a chemically induced model of CCA, the majority of tumor-associated macrophages were GFP-positive. Moreover, depletion of macrophages with different strategies resulted in reduced Wnt7b expression in xenograft CCA models and reduced tumor burden. The effect of two small molecules ICG-001 and C-59, inhibitors of CTNNB1 and PORCN, respectively, was also tested in xenograft CCA models and a chemically induced CCA model and found that both reduced the occurrence and volume of tumors [96]. The Wnt/β-catenin pathway may also be activated by cancer stem cells, a subpopulation of cancer cells that are present in the tumor microenvironment [97]. Wang et al. demonstrated that the presence of human umbilical cord-derived mesenchymal stem cells (MSCs) in a xenograft model of CCA significantly increases tumor volume, metastatic potential, and chemoresistance. In vitro, incubation of CCA cells with MSC-conditioned media resulted in nuclear translocation of β-catenin and upregulation of Wnt target genes [98]. Additional details of the molecular regulation of the Wnt/β-catenin pathway in CCA have also emerged lately. For example, osteopontin, a chemokine-like phosphorylated glycoprotein, was found to be upregulated in both serum and CCA tissue and to promote phosphorylation and nucleus accumulation of β-catenin, thereby activating the pathway and sustaining CCA growth and metastasis [99]. Moreover, the SRC-like adaptor protein (SLAP), an adaptor protein that regulates signal transduction of various cell surface receptors, seems to be downregulated in CCA, thus enabling the activation of the Wnt/β-catenin pathway [100]. Preliminary results from a phase 1 clinical trial with DKN-01, an antibody directed against the inhibitor of the canonical Wnt/β-catenin DKK1, demonstrated a reasonable safety profile when administered with gemcitabine in advanced biliary tract cancers [101]. A phase 2 clinical trial investigating the response rate of DKN-01 and nivolumab in previously treated patients with CCA is currently recruiting patients (NCT04057365) [102].

Conclusions

CCA is an extremely heterogeneous malignancy, and intensive basic and translational studies have only recently started to shed light on the complex molecular landscape of the disease. The application of next-generation sequencing to the CCA genome has enabled a deeper understanding of the genetic alterations sustaining tumor progression and identified a number of possible targets for early diagnosis and treatment. In parallel, epigenetic modifications are actively studied as possible pivotal factors in CCA development, and a number of alterations have been identified.

Despite multiple encouraging results that have come from basic studies in in vitro and in vivo models, the outcome of the majority of clinical trials has been below the expectations of researchers, clinicians, and patients. Looking ahead, international collaborative studies will undoubtedly be useful in order to reach large enough patient cohorts, with specific clinical and molecular CCA characteristics. Current results of clinical trials are in fact hampered by small sample size and nonuniform patient characteristic. The heterogeneity of CCA in terms of anatomical, genetic, epigenetic, and molecular differences needs to be taken into account when testing new treatments in the human setting, especially in the era of precision medicine.

References

1. Blechacz B. Cholangiocarcinoma: current knowledge and new developments. Gut Liver. 2017;11:13–26. https://doi.org/10.5009/gnl15568.
2. Shibuya M. Vascular Endothelial Growth Factor (VEGF) and its receptor (VEGFR) signaling in angiogenesis: a crucial target for anti- and pro-angiogenic therapies. Genes Cancer. 2011;2:1097–105. https://doi.org/10.1177/1947601911423031.
3. Yoshikawa D, Ojima H, Iwasaki M, Hiraoka N, Kosuge T, Kasai S, Hirohashi S, Shibata T. Clinicopathological and prognostic significance of EGFR, VEGF, and HER2 expression in cholangiocarcinoma. Br J Cancer. 2008;98:418–25. https://doi.org/10.1038/sj.bjc.6604129.
4. Hida Y, Morita T, Fujita M, Miyasaka Y, Horita S, Fujioka Y, Nagashima K, Katoh H. Vascular endothelial growth factor expression is an independent negative predictor in extrahepatic biliary tract carcinomas. Anticancer Res. 1999;19:2257–60.
5. Benckert C, Jonas S, Cramer T, Von Marschall Z, Schafer G, Peters M, Wagner K, Radke C, Wiedenmann B, Neuhaus P, et al. Transforming growth factor beta 1 stimulates vascular endothelial growth factor gene transcription in human cholangiocellular carcinoma cells. Cancer Res. 2003;63:1083–92.
6. Wiggers JK, Ruys AT, Groot Koerkamp B, Beuers U, ten Kate FJ, van Gulik TM. Differences in immunohistochemical biomarkers between intra- and extrahepatic cholangiocarcinoma: a systematic review and meta-analysis. J Gastroenterol Hepatol. 2014;29:1582–94. https://doi.org/10.1111/jgh.12620.
7. Guedj N, Zhan Q, Perigny M, Rautou PE, Degos F, Belghiti J, Farges O, Bedossa P, Paradis V. Comparative protein expression profiles of hilar and peripheral hepatic cholangiocarcinomas. J Hepatol. 2009;51:93–101. https://doi.org/10.1016/j.jhep.2009.03.017.
8. Gaudio E, Barbaro B, Alvaro D, Glaser S, Francis H, Ueno Y, Meininger CJ, Franchitto A, Onori P, Marzioni M, et al. Vascular endothelial growth factor stimulates rat cholangiocyte proliferation via an autocrine mechanism. Gastroenterology. 2006;130:1270–82. https://doi.org/10.1053/j.gastro.2005.12.034.
9. Francis H, Onori P, Gaudio E, Franchitto A, DeMorrow S, Venter J, Kopriva S, Carpino G, Mancinelli R, White M, et al. H3 histamine receptor-mediated activation of protein kinase Calpha inhibits the growth of cholangiocarcinoma in vitro and in vivo. Mol Cancer Res. 2009;7:1704–13. https://doi.org/10.1158/1541-7786.MCR-09-0261.
10. Francis H, DeMorrow S, Venter J, Onori P, White M, Gaudio E, Francis T, Greene JF Jr, Tran S, Meininger CJ, et al. Inhibition of histidine decarboxylase ablates the autocrine tumorigenic effects of histamine in human cholangiocarcinoma. Gut. 2012;61:753–64. https://doi.org/10.1136/gutjnl-2011-300007.

11. Glaser S, Meng F, Han Y, Onori P, Chow BK, Francis H, Venter J, McDaniel K, Marzioni M, Invernizzi P, et al. Secretin stimulates biliary cell proliferation by regulating expression of microRNA 125b and microRNA let7a in mice. Gastroenterology. 2014;146:1795–1808 e1712. https://doi.org/10.1053/j.gastro.2014.02.030.
12. Fava G, Demorrow S, Gaudio E, Franchitto A, Onori P, Carpino G, Glaser S, Francis H, Coufal M, Marucci L, et al. Endothelin inhibits cholangiocarcinoma growth by a decrease in the vascular endothelial growth factor expression. Liver Int. 2009;29:1031–42. https://doi.org/10.1111/j.1478-3231.2009.01997.x.
13. Peng T, Deng X, Tian F, Li Z, Jiang P, Zhao X, Chen G, Chen Y, Zheng P, Li D, et al. The interaction of LOXL2 with GATA6 induces VEGFA expression and angiogenesis in cholangiocarcinoma. Int J Oncol. 2019;55:657–70. https://doi.org/10.3892/ijo.2019.4837.
14. Pan S, Hu Y, Hu M, Xu Y, Chen M, Du C, Cui J, Zheng P, Lai J, Zhang Y, et al. S100A8 facilitates cholangiocarcinoma metastasis via upregulation of VEGF through TLR4/NFkappaB pathway activation. Int J Oncol. 2020;56:101–12. https://doi.org/10.3892/ijo.2019.4907.
15. Zhu H, Jiang X, Zhou X, Dong X, Xie K, Yang C, Jiang H, Sun X, Lu J. Neuropilin-1 regulated by miR-320 contributes to the growth and metastasis of cholangiocarcinoma cells. Liver Int. 2018;38:125–35. https://doi.org/10.1111/liv.13495.
16. Sha M, Jeong S, Wang X, Tong Y, Cao J, Sun HY, Xia L, Xu N, Xi ZF, Zhang JJ, et al. Tumor-associated lymphangiogenesis predicts unfavorable prognosis of intrahepatic cholangiocarcinoma. BMC Cancer. 2019;19:208. https://doi.org/10.1186/s12885-019-5420-z.
17. Thelen A, Scholz A, Benckert C, Weichert W, Dietz E, Wiedenmann B, Neuhaus P, Jonas S. Tumor-associated lymphangiogenesis correlates with lymph node metastases and prognosis in hilar cholangiocarcinoma. Ann Surg Oncol. 2008;15:791–9. https://doi.org/10.1245/s10434-007-9774-0.
18. Jutric Z, Johnston WC, Hoen HM, Newell PH, Cassera MA, Hammill CW, Wolf RF, Hansen PD. Impact of lymph node status in patients with intrahepatic cholangiocarcinoma treated by major hepatectomy: a review of the National Cancer Database. HPB (Oxford). 2016;18:79–87. https://doi.org/10.1016/j.hpb.2015.07.006.
19. Choi SB, Kim KS, Choi JY, Park SW, Choi JS, Lee WJ, Chung JB. The prognosis and survival outcome of intrahepatic cholangiocarcinoma following surgical resection: association of lymph node metastasis and lymph node dissection with survival. Ann Surg Oncol. 2009;16:3048–56. https://doi.org/10.1245/s10434-009-0631-1.
20. Aishima S, Nishihara Y, Iguchi T, Taguchi K, Taketomi A, Maehara Y, Tsuneyoshi M. Lymphatic spread is related to VEGF-C expression and D2-40-positive myofibroblasts in intrahepatic cholangiocarcinoma. Mod Pathol. 2008;21:256–64. https://doi.org/10.1038/modpathol.3800985.
21. Park BK, Paik YH, Park JY, Park KH, Bang S, Park SW, Chung JB, Park YN, Song SY. The clinicopathologic significance of the expression of vascular endothelial growth factor-C in intrahepatic cholangiocarcinoma. Am J Clin Oncol. 2006;29:138–42. https://doi.org/10.1097/01.coc.0000204402.29830.08.
22. Zhao R, Chang Y, Liu Z, Liu Y, Guo S, Yu J, Wang J. Effect of vascular endothelial growth factor-C expression on lymph node metastasis in human cholangiocarcinoma. Oncol Lett. 2015;10:1011–5. https://doi.org/10.3892/ol.2015.3309.
23. Sha M, Jeong S, Chen XS, Tong Y, Cao J, Sun HY, Xia L, Xu N, Wang X, Han LZ, et al. Expression of VEGFR-3 in intrahepatic cholangiocarcinoma correlates with unfavorable prognosis through lymphangiogenesis. Int J Biol Sci. 2018;14:1333–42. https://doi.org/10.7150/ijbs.26045.
24. Semenza GL. Targeting HIF-1 for cancer therapy. Nat Rev Cancer. 2003;3:721–32. https://doi.org/10.1038/nrc1187.
25. Thongchot S, Yongvanit P, Loilome W, Seubwai W, Phunicom K, Tassaneeyakul W, Pairojkul C, Promkotra W, Techasen A, Namwat N. High expression of HIF-1alpha, BNIP3 and PI3KC3: hypoxia-induced autophagy predicts cholangiocarcinoma survival and metastasis. Asian Pac J Cancer Prev. 2014;15:5873–8. https://doi.org/10.7314/apjcp.2014.15.14.5873.

26. Seubwai W, Kraiklang R, Wongkham C, Wongkham S. Hypoxia enhances aggressiveness of cholangiocarcinoma cells. Asian Pac J Cancer Prev. 2012;13(Suppl):53–8.
27. Cadamuro M, Nardo G, Indraccolo S, Dall'olmo L, Sambado L, Moserle L, Franceschet I, Colledan M, Massani M, Stecca T, et al. Platelet-derived growth factor-D and Rho GTPases regulate recruitment of cancer-associated fibroblasts in cholangiocarcinoma. Hepatology. 2013;58:1042–53. https://doi.org/10.1002/hep.26384.
28. Cadamuro M, Brivio S, Mertens J, Vismara M, Moncsek A, Milani C, Fingas C, Cristina Malerba M, Nardo G, Dall'Olmo L, et al. Platelet-derived growth factor-D enables liver myofibroblasts to promote tumor lymphangiogenesis in cholangiocarcinoma. J Hepatol. 2019;70:700–9. https://doi.org/10.1016/j.jhep.2018.12.004.
29. Yue XJ, Xu LB, Zhu MS, Zhang R, Liu C. Over-expression of nerve growth factor-beta in human cholangiocarcinoma QBC939 cells promote tumor progression. PLoS One. 2013;8:e62024. https://doi.org/10.1371/journal.pone.0062024.
30. Xu YF, Ge FJ, Han B, Yang XQ, Su H, Zhao AC, Zhao MH, Yang YB, Yang J. High-mobility group box 1 expression and lymph node metastasis in intrahepatic cholangiocarcinoma. World J Gastroenterol. 2015;21:3256–65. https://doi.org/10.3748/wjg.v21.i11.3256.
31. Li CZ, Lin YX, Huang TC, Pan JY, Wang GX. Receptor-interacting protein kinase 1 promotes Cholangiocarcinoma proliferation and Lymphangiogenesis through the activation protein 1 pathway. Onco Targets Ther. 2019;12:9029–40. https://doi.org/10.2147/OTT.S215276.
32. Vaeteewoottacharn K, Kariya R, Dana P, Fujikawa S, Matsuda K, Ohkuma K, Kudo E, Kraiklang R, Wongkham C, Wongkham S, et al. Inhibition of carbonic anhydrase potentiates bevacizumab treatment in cholangiocarcinoma. Tumour Biol. 2016;37:9023–35. https://doi.org/10.1007/s13277-016-4785-8.
33. Zhu AX, Meyerhardt JA, Blaszkowsky LS, Kambadakone AR, Muzikansky A, Zheng H, Clark JW, Abrams TA, Chan JA, Enzinger PC, et al. Efficacy and safety of gemcitabine, oxaliplatin, and bevacizumab in advanced biliary-tract cancers and correlation of changes in 18-fluorodeoxyglucose PET with clinical outcome: a phase 2 study. Lancet Oncol. 2010;11:48–54. https://doi.org/10.1016/S1470-2045(09)70333-X.
34. Lubner SJ, Mahoney MR, Kolesar JL, Loconte NK, Kim GP, Pitot HC, Philip PA, Picus J, Yong WP, Horvath L, et al. Report of a multicenter phase II trial testing a combination of biweekly bevacizumab and daily erlotinib in patients with unresectable biliary cancer: a phase II consortium study. J Clin Oncol. 2010;28:3491–7. https://doi.org/10.1200/JCO.2010.28.4075.
35. Guion-Dusserre JF, Lorgis V, Vincent J, Bengrine L, Ghiringhelli F. FOLFIRI plus bevacizumab as a second-line therapy for metastatic intrahepatic cholangiocarcinoma. World J Gastroenterol. 2015;21:2096–101. https://doi.org/10.3748/wjg.v21.i7.2096.
36. Iyer RV, Pokuri VK, Groman A, Ma WW, Malhotra U, Iancu DM, Grande C, Saab TB. A multicenter phase II study of gemcitabine, Capecitabine, and Bevacizumab for locally advanced or metastatic biliary tract cancer. Am J Clin Oncol. 2018;41:649–55. https://doi.org/10.1097/COC.0000000000000347.
37. Mizrahi J, Javle MM, Xiao L, Varadhachary GR, Raghav KPS, Wolff RA, Shroff RT. A phase II study of ramucirumab for advanced, pre-treated biliary cancers. J Clin Oncol. 2018;36:4081. https://doi.org/10.1200/JCO.2018.36.15_suppl.4081.
38. Arkenau HT, Martin-Liberal J, Calvo E, Penel N, Krebs MG, Herbst RS, Walgren RA, Widau RC, Mi G, Jin J, et al. Ramucirumab plus Pembrolizumab in patients with previously treated advanced or metastatic biliary tract cancer: nonrandomized, open-label, phase I trial (JVDF). Oncologist. 2018;23:1407–e1136. https://doi.org/10.1634/theoncologist.2018-0044.
39. Sugiyama H, Onuki K, Ishige K, Baba N, Ueda T, Matsuda S, Takeuchi K, Onodera M, Nakanuma Y, Yamato M, et al. Potent in vitro and in vivo antitumor activity of sorafenib against human intrahepatic cholangiocarcinoma cells. J Gastroenterol. 2011;46:779–89. https://doi.org/10.1007/s00535-011-0380-3.
40. El-Khoueiry AB, Rankin CJ, Ben-Josef E, Lenz HJ, Gold PJ, Hamilton RD, Govindarajan R, Eng C, Blanke CD. SWOG 0514: a phase II study of sorafenib in patients with unre-

sectable or metastatic gallbladder carcinoma and cholangiocarcinoma. Investig New Drugs. 2012;30:1646–51. https://doi.org/10.1007/s10637-011-9719-0.
41. Bengala C, Bertolini F, Malavasi N, Boni C, Aitini E, Dealis C, Zironi S, Depenni R, Fontana A, Del Giovane C, et al. Sorafenib in patients with advanced biliary tract carcinoma: a phase II trial. Br J Cancer. 2010;102:68–72. https://doi.org/10.1038/sj.bjc.6605458.
42. Moehler M, Maderer A, Schimanski C, Kanzler S, Denzer U, Kolligs FT, Ebert MP, Distelrath A, Geissler M, Trojan J, et al. Gemcitabine plus sorafenib versus gemcitabine alone in advanced biliary tract cancer: a double-blind placebo-controlled multicentre phase II AIO study with biomarker and serum programme. Eur J Cancer. 2014;50:3125–35. https://doi.org/10.1016/j.ejca.2014.09.013.
43. Lee JK, Capanu M, O'Reilly EM, Ma J, Chou JF, Shia J, Katz SS, Gansukh B, Reidy-Lagunes D, Segal NH, et al. A phase II study of gemcitabine and cisplatin plus sorafenib in patients with advanced biliary adenocarcinomas. Br J Cancer. 2013;109:915–9. https://doi.org/10.1038/bjc.2013.432.
44. Yoshikawa D, Ojima H, Kokubu A, Ochiya T, Kasai S, Hirohashi S, Shibata T. Vandetanib (ZD6474), an inhibitor of VEGFR and EGFR signalling, as a novel molecular-targeted therapy against cholangiocarcinoma. Br J Cancer. 2009;100:1257–66. https://doi.org/10.1038/sj.bjc.6604988.
45. Santoro A, Gebbia V, Pressiani T, Testa A, Personeni N, Arrivas Bajardi E, Foa P, Buonadonna A, Bencardino K, Barone C, et al. A randomized, multicenter, phase II study of vandetanib monotherapy versus vandetanib in combination with gemcitabine versus gemcitabine plus placebo in subjects with advanced biliary tract cancer: the VanGogh study. Ann Oncol. 2015;26:542–7. https://doi.org/10.1093/annonc/mdu576.
46. Takahashi H, Ojima H, Shimizu H, Furuse J, Furukawa H, Shibata T. Axitinib (AG-013736), an oral specific VEGFR TKI, shows potential therapeutic utility against cholangiocarcinoma. Jpn J Clin Oncol. 2014;44:570–8. https://doi.org/10.1093/jjco/hyu045.
47. Okano N, Kasuga A, Kawai K, Kobayashi T, Naruge D, Nagashima F, Furuse J. Axitinib for Gemcitabine-refractory advanced biliary tract cancer: report of 5 cases. Anticancer Res. 2017;37:3711–5. https://doi.org/10.21873/anticanres.11743.
48. Sharma S, Kelly TK, Jones PA. Epigenetics in cancer. Carcinogenesis. 2010;31:27–36. https://doi.org/10.1093/carcin/bgp220.
49. Lee S, Kim WH, Jung HY, Yang MH, Kang GH. Aberrant CpG island methylation of multiple genes in intrahepatic cholangiocarcinoma. Am J Pathol. 2002;161:1015–22. https://doi.org/10.1016/S0002-9440(10)64262-9.
50. Nakaoka T, Saito Y, Saito H. Aberrant DNA methylation as a biomarker and a therapeutic target of Cholangiocarcinoma. Int J Mol Sci. 2017;18 https://doi.org/10.3390/ijms18061111.
51. Sandhu DS, Shire AM, Roberts LR. Epigenetic DNA hypermethylation in cholangiocarcinoma: potential roles in pathogenesis, diagnosis and identification of treatment targets. Liver Int. 2008;28:12–27. https://doi.org/10.1111/j.1478-3231.2007.01624.x.
52. Yang B, House MG, Guo M, Herman JG, Clark DP. Promoter methylation profiles of tumor suppressor genes in intrahepatic and extrahepatic cholangiocarcinoma. Mod Pathol. 2005;18:412–20. https://doi.org/10.1038/modpathol.3800287.
53. Tannapfel A, Sommerer F, Benicke M, Weinans L, Katalinic A, Geissler F, Uhlmann D, Hauss J, Wittekind C. Genetic and epigenetic alterations of the INK4a-ARF pathway in cholangiocarcinoma. J Pathol. 2002;197:624–31. https://doi.org/10.1002/path.1139.
54. Koga Y, Kitajima Y, Miyoshi A, Sato K, Kitahara K, Soejima H, Miyazaki K. Tumor progression through epigenetic gene silencing of O(6)-methylguanine-DNA methyltransferase in human biliary tract cancers. Ann Surg Oncol. 2005;12:354–63. https://doi.org/10.1245/ASO.2005.07.020.
55. Tozawa T, Tamura G, Honda T, Nawata S, Kimura W, Makino N, Kawata S, Sugai T, Suto T, Motoyama T. Promoter hypermethylation of DAP-kinase is associated with poor survival in primary biliary tract carcinoma patients. Cancer Sci. 2004;95:736–40. https://doi.org/10.1111/j.1349-7006.2004.tb03254.x.

56. Goeppert B, Konermann C, Schmidt CR, Bogatyrova O, Geiselhart L, Ernst C, Gu L, Becker N, Zucknick M, Mehrabi A, et al. Global alterations of DNA methylation in cholangiocarcinoma target the Wnt signaling pathway. Hepatology. 2014;59:544–54. https://doi.org/10.1002/hep.26721.
57. Ishikawa A, Sasaki M, Sato Y, Ohira S, Chen MF, Huang SF, Oda K, Nimura Y, Nakanuma Y. Frequent p16ink4a inactivation is an early and frequent event of intraductal papillary neoplasm of the liver arising in hepatolithiasis. Hum Pathol. 2004;35:1505–14. https://doi.org/10.1016/j.humpath.2004.08.014.
58. Kim BH, Cho NY, Shin SH, Kwon HJ, Jang JJ, Kang GH. CpG island hypermethylation and repetitive DNA hypomethylation in premalignant lesion of extrahepatic cholangiocarcinoma. Virchows Arch. 2009;455:343–51. https://doi.org/10.1007/s00428-009-0829-4.
59. Klump B, Hsieh CJ, Dette S, Holzmann K, Kiebetalich R, Jung M, Sinn U, Ortner M, Porschen R, Gregor M. Promoter methylation of INK4a/ARF as detected in bile-significance for the differential diagnosis in biliary disease. Clin Cancer Res. 2003;9:1773–8.
60. Prachayakul V, Kanchanapermpoon J, Thuwajit C, Boonyaarunnate T, Pongpaibul A, Chobson P, Thuwajit P. DNA methylation markers improve the sensitivity of endoscopic retrograde Cholangiopancreatography-based brushing cytology in Extrahepatic Cholangiocarcinoma. Technol Cancer Res Treat. 2017;16:1252–8. https://doi.org/10.1177/1533034617748090.
61. Andresen K, Boberg KM, Vedeld HM, Honne H, Jebsen P, Hektoen M, Wadsworth CA, Clausen OP, Lundin KE, Paulsen V, et al. Four DNA methylation biomarkers in biliary brush samples accurately identify the presence of cholangiocarcinoma. Hepatology. 2015;61:1651–9. https://doi.org/10.1002/hep.27707.
62. Shin SH, Lee K, Kim BH, Cho NY, Jang JY, Kim YT, Kim D, Jang JJ, Kang GH. Bile-based detection of extrahepatic cholangiocarcinoma with quantitative DNA methylation markers and its high sensitivity. J Mol Diagn. 2012;14:256–63. https://doi.org/10.1016/j.jmoldx.2012.01.014.
63. Wasenang W, Chaiyarit P, Proungvitaya S, Limpaiboon T. Serum cell-free DNA methylation of OPCML and HOXD9 as a biomarker that may aid in differential diagnosis between cholangiocarcinoma and other biliary diseases. Clin Epigenetics. 2019;11:39. https://doi.org/10.1186/s13148-019-0634-0.
64. Tessarz P, Kouzarides T. Histone core modifications regulating nucleosome structure and dynamics. Nat Rev Mol Cell Biol. 2014;15:703–8. https://doi.org/10.1038/nrm3890.
65. Xu LN, Wang X, Zou SQ. Effect of histone deacetylase inhibitor on proliferation of biliary tract cancer cell lines. World J Gastroenterol. 2008;14:2578–81. https://doi.org/10.3748/wjg.14.2578.
66. Mastoraki A, Schizas D, Charalampakis N, Naar L, Ioannidi M, Tsilimigras D, Sotiropoulou M, Moris D, Vassiliu P, Felekouras E. Contribution of histone deacetylases in prognosis and therapeutic management of Cholangiocarcinoma. Mol Diagn Ther. 2020; https://doi.org/10.1007/s40291-020-00454-x.
67. Baradari V, Hopfner M, Huether A, Schuppan D, Scherubl H. Histone deacetylase inhibitor MS-275 alone or combined with bortezomib or sorafenib exhibits strong antiproliferative action in human cholangiocarcinoma cells. World J Gastroenterol. 2007;13:4458–66. https://doi.org/10.3748/wjg.v13.i33.4458.
68. Wang JH, Lee EJ, Ji M, Park SM. HDAC inhibitors, trichostatin A and valproic acid, increase Ecadherin and vimentin expression but inhibit migration and invasion of cholangiocarcinoma cells. Oncol Rep. 2018;40:346–54. https://doi.org/10.3892/or.2018.6441.
69. Morine Y, Shimada M, Iwahashi S, Utsunomiya T, Imura S, Ikemoto T, Mori H, Hanaoka J, Miyake H. Role of histone deacetylase expression in intrahepatic cholangiocarcinoma. Surgery. 2012;151:412–9. https://doi.org/10.1016/j.surg.2011.07.038.
70. He JC, Yao W, Wang JM, Schemmer P, Yang Y, Liu Y, Qian YW, Qi WP, Zhang J, Shen Q, et al. TACC3 overexpression in cholangiocarcinoma correlates with poor prognosis and is a potential anti-cancer molecular drug target for HDAC inhibitors. Oncotarget. 2016;7:75441–56. https://doi.org/10.18632/oncotarget.12254.

71. Zhu YJ, Xu Q, Shao MY, Cao XY, Wu ZR, Chen YW, Bu H, Shi YJ. Decreased expression of HDAC8 indicates poor prognosis in patients with intrahepatic cholangiocarcinoma. Hepatobiliary Pancreat Dis Int. 2019;18:464–70. https://doi.org/10.1016/j.hbpd.2019.07.006.
72. Suraweera A, O'Byrne KJ, Richard DJ. Combination therapy with histone deacetylase inhibitors (HDACi) for the treatment of cancer: achieving the full therapeutic potential of HDACi. Front Oncol. 2018;8:92. https://doi.org/10.3389/fonc.2018.00092.
73. Iwahashi S, Utsunomiya T, Imura S, Morine Y, Ikemoto T, Arakawa Y, Saito Y, Ishikawa D, Shimada M. Effects of valproic acid in combination with S-1 on advanced pancreatobiliary tract cancers: clinical study phases I/II. Anticancer Res. 2014;34:5187–91.
74. A clinical trial of Entinostat in combination with Nivolumab for patients with previously treated unresectable or metastatic Cholangiocarcinoma and pancreatic Adenocarcinoma. https://ClinicalTrials.gov/show/NCT03250273.
75. A study of selective HDAC6 inhibition with KA2507 in advanced Biliary tract cancer. https://ClinicalTrials.gov/show/NCT04186156.
76. Esteller M. Non-coding RNAs in human disease. Nat Rev Genet. 2011;12:861–74. https://doi.org/10.1038/nrg3074.
77. Zheng B, Jeong S, Zhu Y, Chen L, Xia Q. miRNA and lncRNA as biomarkers in cholangiocarcinoma(CCA). Oncotarget. 2017;8:100819–30. https://doi.org/10.18632/oncotarget.19044.
78. Meng F, Henson R, Lang M, Wehbe H, Maheshwari S, Mendell JT, Jiang J, Schmittgen TD, Patel T. Involvement of human micro-RNA in growth and response to chemotherapy in human cholangiocarcinoma cell lines. Gastroenterology. 2006;130:2113–29. https://doi.org/10.1053/j.gastro.2006.02.057.
79. Selaru FM, Olaru AV, Kan T, David S, Cheng Y, Mori Y, Yang J, Paun B, Jin Z, Agarwal R, et al. MicroRNA-21 is overexpressed in human cholangiocarcinoma and regulates programmed cell death 4 and tissue inhibitor of metalloproteinase 3. Hepatology. 2009;49:1595–601. https://doi.org/10.1002/hep.22838.
80. Correa-Gallego C, Maddalo D, Doussot A, Kemeny N, Kingham TP, Allen PJ, D'Angelica MI, DeMatteo RP, Betel D, Klimstra D, et al. Circulating plasma levels of MicroRNA-21 and MicroRNA-221 are potential diagnostic markers for primary intrahepatic Cholangiocarcinoma. PLoS One. 2016;11:e0163699. https://doi.org/10.1371/journal.pone.0163699.
81. Liu CH, Huang Q, Jin ZY, Xie F, Zhu CL, Liu Z, Wang C. Circulating microRNA-21 as a prognostic, biological marker in cholangiocarcinoma. J Cancer Res Ther. 2018;14:220–5. https://doi.org/10.4103/0973-1482.193125.
82. Howell JA, Khan SA. The role of miRNAs in cholangiocarcinoma. Hepatol Oncol. 2016;3:167–80. https://doi.org/10.2217/hep-2015-0003.
83. Karakatsanis A, Papaconstantinou I, Gazouli M, Lyberopoulou A, Polymeneas G, Voros D. Expression of microRNAs, miR-21, miR-31, miR-122, miR-145, miR-146a, miR-200c, miR-221, miR-222, and miR-223 in patients with hepatocellular carcinoma or intrahepatic cholangiocarcinoma and its prognostic significance. Mol Carcinog. 2013;52:297–303. https://doi.org/10.1002/mc.21864.
84. Chen L, Yan HX, Yang W, Hu L, Yu LX, Liu Q, Li L, Huang DD, Ding J, Shen F, et al. The role of microRNA expression pattern in human intrahepatic cholangiocarcinoma. J Hepatol. 2009;50:358–69. https://doi.org/10.1016/j.jhep.2008.09.015.
85. Wang LJ, Zhang KL, Zhang N, Ma XW, Yan SW, Cao DH, Shi SJ. Serum miR-26a as a diagnostic and prognostic biomarker in cholangiocarcinoma. Oncotarget. 2015;6:18631–40. https://doi.org/10.18632/oncotarget.4072.
86. Loosen SH, Lurje G, Wiltberger G, Vucur M, Koch A, Kather JN, Paffenholz P, Tacke F, Ulmer FT, Trautwein C, et al. Serum levels of miR-29, miR-122, miR-155 and miR-192 are elevated in patients with cholangiocarcinoma. PLoS One. 2019;14:e0210944. https://doi.org/10.1371/journal.pone.0210944.

87. Voigtlander T, Gupta SK, Thum S, Fendrich J, Manns MP, Lankisch TO, Thum T. MicroRNAs in serum and bile of patients with primary Sclerosing cholangitis and/or Cholangiocarcinoma. PLoS One. 2015;10:e0139305. https://doi.org/10.1371/journal.pone.0139305.
88. Han HS, Kim MJ, Han JH, Yun J, Kim HK, Yang Y, Kim KB, Park SM. Bile-derived circulating extracellular miR-30d-5p and miR-92a-3p as potential biomarkers for cholangiocarcinoma. Hepatobiliary Pancreat Dis Int. 2020;19:41–50. https://doi.org/10.1016/j.hbpd.2019.10.009.
89. Li L, Masica D, Ishida M, Tomuleasa C, Umegaki S, Kalloo AN, Georgiades C, Singh VK, Khashab M, Amateau S, et al. Human bile contains microRNA-laden extracellular vesicles that can be used for cholangiocarcinoma diagnosis. Hepatology. 2014;60:896–907. https://doi.org/10.1002/hep.27050.
90. MacDonald BT, Tamai K, He X. Wnt/beta-catenin signaling: components, mechanisms, and diseases. Dev Cell. 2009;17:9–26. https://doi.org/10.1016/j.devcel.2009.06.016.
91. Zhan T, Rindtorff N, Boutros M. Wnt signaling in cancer. Oncogene. 2017;36:1461–73. https://doi.org/10.1038/onc.2016.304.
92. Settakorn J, Kaewpila N, Burns GF, Leong AS. FAT, E-cadherin, beta catenin, HER 2/neu, Ki67 immuno-expression, and histological grade in intrahepatic cholangiocarcinoma. J Clin Pathol. 2005;58:1249–54. https://doi.org/10.1136/jcp.2005.026575.
93. Chen W, Liang J, Huang L, Cai J, Lei Y, Lai J, Liang L, Zhang K. Characterizing the activation of the Wnt signaling pathway in hilar cholangiocarcinoma using a tissue microarray approach. Eur J Histochem. 2016;60:2536. https://doi.org/10.4081/ejh.2016.2536.
94. Sugimachi K, Taguchi K, Aishima S, Tanaka S, Shimada M, Kajiyama K, Sugimachi K, Tsuneyoshi M. Altered expression of beta-catenin without genetic mutation in intrahepatic cholangiocarcinoma. Mod Pathol. 2001;14:900–5. https://doi.org/10.1038/modpathol.3880409.
95. Tokumoto N, Ikeda S, Ishizaki Y, Kurihara T, Ozaki S, Iseki M, Shimizu Y, Itamoto T, Arihiro K, Okajima M, et al. Immunohistochemical and mutational analyses of Wnt signaling components and target genes in intrahepatic cholangiocarcinomas. Int J Oncol. 2005;27:973–80.
96. Boulter L, Guest RV, Kendall TJ, Wilson DH, Wojtacha D, Robson AJ, Ridgway RA, Samuel K, Van Rooijen N, Barry ST, et al. WNT signaling drives cholangiocarcinoma growth and can be pharmacologically inhibited. J Clin Invest. 2015;125:1269–85. https://doi.org/10.1172/JCI76452.
97. Wu HJ, Chu PY. Role of cancer stem cells in Cholangiocarcinoma and therapeutic implications. Int J Mol Sci. 2019;20 https://doi.org/10.3390/ijms20174154.
98. Wang W, Zhong W, Yuan J, Yan C, Hu S, Tong Y, Mao Y, Hu T, Zhang B, Song G. Involvement of Wnt/beta-catenin signaling in the mesenchymal stem cells promote metastatic growth and chemoresistance of cholangiocarcinoma. Oncotarget. 2015;6:42276–89. https://doi.org/10.18632/oncotarget.5514.
99. Zheng Y, Zhou C, Yu XX, Wu C, Jia HL, Gao XM, Yang JM, Wang CQ, Luo Q, Zhu Y, et al. Osteopontin promotes metastasis of intrahepatic cholangiocarcinoma through recruiting MAPK1 and mediating Ser675 phosphorylation of beta-Catenin. Cell Death Dis. 2018;9:179. https://doi.org/10.1038/s41419-017-0226-x.
100. Wang Y, He X, Wei Y, Liu L, Wang W, Li N. SRC-like adaptor protein negatively regulates Wnt signaling in intrahepatic cholangiocarcinoma. Oncol Lett. 2019;17:2745–53. https://doi.org/10.3892/ol.2019.9901.
101. Eads JR, Goyal L, Stein S, El-Khoueiry AB, Manji GA, Abrams TA, Landau SB, Sirard CA. Phase I study of DKN-01, an anti-DKK1 antibody, in combination with gemcitabine (G) and cisplatin (C) in patients (pts) with advanced biliary cancer. J Clin Oncol. 2016;34:e15603. https://doi.org/10.1200/JCO.2016.34.15_suppl.e15603.
102. Study of the combination of DKN-01 and Nivolumab in previously treated patients with advanced Biliary Tract Cancer (BTC). https://ClinicalTrials.gov/show/NCT04057365.

Index

J. H. Tabibian (ed.), *Diagnosis and Management of Cholangiocarcinoma*,
https://doi.org/10.1007/978-3-030-70936-5

N

O

R

GPSR Compliance

The European Union's (EU) General Product Safety Regulation (GPSR) is a set of rules that requires consumer products to be safe and our obligations to ensure this.

If you have any concerns about our products, you can contact us on ProductSafety@springernature.com

In case Publisher is established outside the EU, the EU authorized representative is:

Springer Nature Customer Service Center GmbH
Europaplatz 3
69115 Heidelberg, Germany

Batch number: 10726133

Printed by Printforce, the Netherlands